Multiple Imputation and its Application

Statistics in Practice

Founding Editor

Vic Barnett
Nottingham Trent University, UK

Statistics in Practice is an important international series of texts which provide detailed coverage of statistical concepts, methods and worked case studies in specific fields of investigation and study.

With sound motivation and many worked practical examples, the books show in down-to-earth terms how to select and use an appropriate range of statistical techniques in a particular practical field within each title's special topic area.

The books provide statistical support for professionals and research workers across a range of employment fields and research environments. Subject areas covered include medicine and pharmaceutics; industry, finance and commerce; public services; the earth and environmental sciences, and so on.

The books also provide support to students studying statistical courses applied to the above areas. The demand for graduates to be equipped for the work environment has led to such courses becoming increasingly prevalent at universities and colleges.

It is our aim to present judiciously chosen and well-written workbooks to meet everyday practical needs. Feedback of views from readers will be most valuable to monitor the success of this aim.

Multiple Imputation and its Application

Second Edition

James R. Carpenter
London School of Hygiene & Tropical Medicine, London, UK
MRC Clinical Trials Unit, University College London, UK

Jonathan W. Bartlett
London School of Hygiene & Tropical Medicine, London, UK

Tim P. Morris
MRC Clinical Trials Unit, University College London, UK

Angela M. Wood
University of Cambridge, Cambridge, UK

Matteo Quartagno
MRC Clinical Trials Unit at University College London, UK

Michael G. Kenward
Ashkirk, UK

WILEY

This edition first published 2023

Edition History: John Wiley & Sons Ltd (1e, 2013)

Registered Offices
John Wiley & Sons, Inc., 111 River Street, Hoboken, NJ 07030, USA
John Wiley & Sons Ltd, The Atrium, Southern Gate, Chichester, West Sussex, PO19 8SQ, UK

For details of our global editorial offices, customer services, and more information about Wiley products visit us at www.wiley.com.

Wiley also publishes its books in a variety of electronic formats and by print-on-demand. Some content that appears in standard print versions of this book may not be available in other formats.

Library of Congress Cataloging-in-Publication Data applied for

ISBN: 9781119756088 (Hardback); 9781119756095 (Adobe PDF); 9781119756101 (ePub)

Cover design: Wiley
Cover image: Courtesy of Harvey Goldstein

Set in 10/12pt TimesLTStd by Straive, Chennai, India

Contents

Preface to the second edition

No study of any complexity manages to collect all the intended data. Analysis of the resulting partially collected data must therefore address the issues raised by the missing data. Beyond simply estimating the proportion of missing values, the interplay between the substantive questions and the reasons for the missing data is crucial. There is no simple, universal, solution.

Suppose, for a substantive question at hand, the consequences of missing data in terms of bias and loss of precision are non-trivial. Then the analyst must make a set of assumptions about the reasons, or mechanisms, causing data to be missing, and perform an inferentially valid analysis under these assumptions. In this regard, analysis of a partially observed dataset is the same as any statistical analysis; the difference is that when data are missing we cannot assess the validity of these assumptions in the way we might do in a regression analysis, for example. Hence, sensitivity analysis, where we explore the robustness of inference to different assumptions about the reasons for missing data, is important.

Given a set of assumptions about the reasons data are missing, there are a number of statistical methods for carrying out the analysis. These include the expectation-maximization (EM) algorithm, inverse probability (of non-missingness) weighting, a full Bayesian analysis and, depending on the setting, a direct application of maximum likelihood. These methods, and those derived from them, each have their own advantages in particular settings. We focus on multiple imputation for its practical utility, broad applicability, and relatively straightforward application. Since the first edition was published ten years ago, new applications of multiple imputation have continued to emerge and we have had to be selective in what we cover. The topics included are those we have found most relevant for our research and teaching.

Like the first edition, the book is divided into three parts. Part I lays the foundations, with an introductory chapter outlining the issues raised by missing data, followed by a chapter describing the theoretical foundations of multiple imputation. Part II describes the application of multiple imputation for standard regression analyses, explaining how MI can be used for continuous, categorical, and ordinal data. Part III describes how to apply MI in a range of practical settings, specifically analysis with non-linear relationships, analysis of survival data, development and validation of prognostic models, analysis with multilevel data structures, sensitivity analysis, handling measurement error, analysis involving weights, and causal inference. We conclude with a chapter outlining some broad practical points on the application of multiple imputation. While readers may wish to read only specific relevant chapters in Part III, Chapter 14 is intended to be relevant to all readers. We illustrate ideas with a range of examples from the medical and social sciences, reflecting the wide application that MI has seen in recent years.

Each chapter concludes with a range of exercises, designed to consolidate and deepen understanding of the material. The computer-based exercises have been designed with `R` and `Stata` users in mind. The book's home page at https://missingdata.lshtm.ac.uk contains both (i) hints for the exercises (including suggestions for `R` and `Stata` code) and (ii) full solutions where applicable.

We welcome feedback from readers. Please email `james.carpenter@lshtm.ac.uk` in the first instance.

James R. Carpenter, Jonathan W. Bartlett, Tim P. Morris,
Angela M. Wood, Matteo Quartagno and Mike G. Kenward
September 2022

Data acknowledgements

We are grateful to the following:

1. AstraZeneca for permission to use data from the 5-arm asthma study in examples in Chapters 1, 3, 6, and 10;
2. GlaxoSmithKline for permission to use data from the dental pain study in Chapter 4;
3. Mike English (Director, Child and Newborn Health Group, Nairobi, Kenya) for permission to data from a multi-faceted intervention to implement guidelines and improve admission paediatric care in Kenyan district hospitals in Chapter 9;
4. Peter Blatchford for permission to use data from the Class Size Study (Blatchford *et al.*, 2002) in Chapter 9;
5. Sara Schroter for permission to use data from the study to improve the quality of peer review in Chapter 10.

In Chapter 12, we used data from the Millennium Cohort Study available through the UK Data Service (ukdataservice.ac.uk), study number 2000031.

In Chapters 1, 5, 9, and 10, we have analysed data from the Youth Cohort Time Series for England, Wales, and Scotland, 1984–2002 First Edition, Colchester, Essex, published by and freely available from the UK Data Archive, Study Number SN 5765. Thanks to Vernon Gayle for introducing us to these data.

In Chapter 6, we have analysed data from theAlzheimer's Disease Neuro-imaging Initiative (ADNI) database (adni.loni.ucla.edu). As such, the investigators within the ADNI contributed to the design and implementation of ADNI and/or provided data but did not participate in analysis or writing of this book. A complete listing of ADNI investigators can be found at http://adni.loni.usc.edu/wp-content/uploads/how_to_apply/ADNI_Acknowledgement_List.pdf.

The ADNI was launched in 2003 as a public–private partnership, led by Principal Investigator Michael W. Weiner, MD. The primary goal of ADNI has been to test whether serial magnetic resonance imaging (MRI), positron emission tomography (PET), other biological markers, and clinical and neuropsychological assessment can be combined to measure the progression of mild cognitive impairment (MCI) and early Alzheimer's disease (AD). For up-to-date information, see www.adni-info.org.

Data collection and sharing for this project was funded by the ADNI (National Institutes of Health Grant U01 AG024904) and DOD ADNI (Department of Defense award number W81XWH-12-2-0012). ADNI is funded by the National Institute on Aging, the National Institute of Biomedical Imaging and Bioengineering, and through generous contributions from the following: AbbVie, Alzheimer's Association; Alzheimer's Drug Discovery Foundation; Araclon Biotech; BioClinica, Inc.; Biogen; Bristol-Myers Squibb Company; CereSpir, Inc.; Cogstate; Eisai Inc.; Elan Pharmaceuticals, Inc.; Eli Lilly and Company; EuroImmun; F. Hoffmann-La Roche Ltd and its affiliated company Genentech, Inc.; Fujirebio; GE Healthcare; IXICO Ltd.; Janssen Alzheimer Immunotherapy Research & Development, LLC.; Johnson & Johnson Pharmaceutical Research & Development LLC.; Lumosity; Lundbeck; Merck & Co., Inc.; Meso Scale Diagnostics, LLC.; NeuroRx Research; Neurotrack Technologies; Novartis Pharmaceuticals Corporation; Pfizer Inc.; Piramal Imaging; Servier; Takeda Pharmaceutical Company; and Transition Therapeutics. The Canadian Institutes of Health Research is providing funds to support ADNI clinical sites in Canada. Private sector contributions are facilitated by the Foundation for the National Institutes of Health (www.fnih.org). The grantee organisation is the Northern California Institute for Research and Education, and the study is coordinated by the Alzheimer's Therapeutic Research Institute at the University of Southern California. ADNI data are disseminated by the Laboratory for Neuro Imaging at the University of Southern California.

In Chapter 11, we have analysed data from the US National Health and Nutrition Examination Survey (NHANES), which is freely available from the US Centers for Disease Control and Prevention. We thank the participants and survey organisers of NHANES.

Acknowledgements

No book of this kind is written in a vacuum, and we are grateful to many friends and colleagues.

In particular, we would like to thank the following for discussions and/or inputs that have contributed to this book or shaped our thinking through the years: John Carlin, Orlagh Carroll, Stephen Cole, Suzie Cro, Rhian Daniel, Dan Jackson, Ruth Keogh, Katherine Lee, Clemence Leyrat, Geert Molenberghs, Tra My Pham, Freya Roberts, James Roger, Jeremy Saxe, Shaun Seaman, Jonathan Sterne, Kate Tilling, and Ian White.

Specific thanks to Tetiana Gorbach for checking the exercises in Chapter 2.

James would like to acknowledge many years' collaboration with Harvey Goldstein, who died in 2020.

James would like to thank Mike Elliott, Rod Little, Trivellore Raghunathan, and Jeremy Taylor for facilitating a visit to the Institute for Social Research and Department of Biostatistics at the University of Michigan, Ann Arbor, in Summer 2011, when the first draft of the first edition was written.

Thanks to Tim Collier for the anecdote in Section 1.3.

We also gratefully acknowledge funding support from the ESRC (three-year fellowship for James Carpenter, RES-063-27-0257, and follow-on funding RES-189-25-0103) and MRC (grants G0900724, G0900701 and G0600599, MC_UU_12023/21, MC_UU_12023/29, MC_UU_00004/07, MC_UU_00004/09 and MC_UU_00004/06, MR/T023953/1).

We would also like to thank Richard Davies and Kathryn Sharples at Wiley for their encouragement and support with the first edition, and Kimberly Monroe-Hill and Alison Oliver for their support and patient encouragement with the second edition.

Lastly, thanks to our families for their forbearance and understanding over the course of this project.

Despite the encouragement and support of those listed above, the text inevitably contains errors and shortcomings, for which we take full responsibility.

James R. Carpenter, Jonathan W. Bartlett, Tim P. Morris,
Angela M. Wood, Matteo Quartagno, and Mike G. Kenward
September 2022

Glossary

Indices and symbols

i	indexes units, often individuals
j	indexes variables in the dataset
n	total number of units in the dataset
p	depending on context, number of variables in the dataset or number of parameters in a statistical model
W, X, Y, Z	random variables
$Y_{i,j}$	ith observation on jth variable, $i = 1, \ldots, n; j = 1, \ldots, p$
R	response indicator, where $R_i = 1$ denotes observed data for unit i and $R_i = 0$ indicates missing data
θ	generic parameter
$\boldsymbol{\theta}$	generic parameter column vector, typically p by 1
$\alpha, \beta, \gamma, \delta$	regression coefficients
$\boldsymbol{\beta}$	column vector of regression coefficients, typically p by 1.
$*$	a random draw, typically from a probability distribution but sometimes data/a datum
$U(.)$	a generic score statistic

Matrices

$\boldsymbol{\Omega}$	Matrix, typically of dimension $p \times p$
$\boldsymbol{\Omega}_{i,j}$	i, jth element of $\boldsymbol{\Omega}$
$\boldsymbol{\Omega}^T$	Transpose of $\boldsymbol{\Omega}$, so that $\boldsymbol{\Omega}^T_{i,j} = \boldsymbol{\Omega}_{i,j}$
$\mathbf{Y}_j = (Y_{1,j}, \ldots, Y_{n,j})^T$	n by 1 column vector of observations on variable j
$\text{tr}(\boldsymbol{\Omega})$	Sum of diagonal elements of $\boldsymbol{\Omega}$, i.e. $\sum \boldsymbol{\Omega}_{i,i}$ known as the trace of the matrix

Abbreviations

CAR	censoring at random
CNAR	censoring not at random
EM	expectation maximisation
FCS	full conditional specification

FEV_1	forced expiratory volume in one second (measured in litres)
FMI	fraction of missing information
IPW	inverse probability weighting
IV	instrumental variable
MAR	missing at random
MCAR	missing completely at random
MI	multiple imputation
MNAR	missing not at random
PMM	predictive mean matching

Probability distributions

$f(\,.\,)$	Probability distribution function
$F(\,.\,)$	Cumulative distribution function
$\|$	to be verbalised 'given' or 'conditional on', as in $f(Y\|X)$ 'the probability distribution function of Y given [conditional on] X'

Miscellaneous

We use the terms *complete records* and *incomplete records* rather than *complete cases* and *incomplete cases*, respectively.
For generic regression of Y on $\mathbf{X}$, we use the terms *outcome* or *dependent variable* for Y and *covariates* or *independent variables* for X.

PART I

FOUNDATIONS

1

Introduction

Collecting, analysing, and drawing inferences from data are central to research in the medical and social sciences. Unfortunately, for any number of reasons, it is rarely possible to collect all the intended data. The ubiquity of missing data, and the problems this poses for both analysis and inference, has spawned a substantial statistical literature dating from 1950s. At that time, when statistical computing was in its infancy, many analyses were only feasible because of the carefully planned balance in the dataset (for example the same number of observations on each unit). Missing data meant the available data for analysis were unbalanced, thus complicating the planned analysis and in some instances rendering it infeasible. Early work on the problem was therefore largely computational (e.g. Healy and Westmacott, 1956, Afifi and Elashoff, 1966, Orchard and Woodbury, 1972, Dempster *et al.*, 1977).

The wider question of the consequences of non-trivial proportions of missing data for inference was neglected until the seminal paper by Rubin (1976). This set out a typology for assumptions about the reasons for missing data and sketched their implications for analysis and inference. It marked the beginning of a broad stream of research about the analysis of partially observed data. The literature is now huge and continues to grow, both as methods are developed for large and complex data structures, and as increasing computer power and suitable software enables researchers to apply these methods.

For a broad overview of the literature, a good place to start for applied statisticians is Little and Rubin (2019). They give a good overview of likelihood methods and an introduction to multiple imputation. Allison (2002) presents a less technical overview. Schafer (1997) is more algorithmic, focusing on the expectation maximisation (EM) algorithm and imputation using the multivariate normal and general location model. Molenberghs and Kenward (2007) focus on clinical studies, while Daniels and Hogan (2008) focus on longitudinal studies with a Bayesian emphasis.

Multiple Imputation and its Application, Second Edition.
James R. Carpenter, Jonathan W. Bartlett, Tim P. Morris, Angela M. Wood, Matteo Quartagno and Michael G. Kenward.

The above books concentrate on the parametric approaches. However, there is also a growing literature based around using inverse probability weighting, in the spirit of Horvitz and Thompson (1952), and associated doubly robust methods. In particular, we refer to the work of Robins and colleagues (e.g. Robins and Rotnitzky, 1995, Scharfstein *et al.*, 1999). Vansteelandt *et al.* (2009) give an accessible introduction to these developments. A comparison with multiple imputation in a simple setting is given by Carpenter *et al.* (2006). The pros and cons are debated in Kang and Schafer (2007) and the theory is brought together by Tsiatis (2006).

This book is concerned with a particular statistical method for analysing and drawing inferences from incomplete data called *multiple imputation* (MI). Initially proposed by Rubin (1987) in the context of surveys, increasing awareness among researchers about the possible effects of missing data (e.g. Klebanoff and Cole, 2008) has led to an upsurge of interest (e.g. Sterne *et al.* (2009), Kenward and Carpenter (2007), Schafer (1999a), Rubin (1996)), fuelled by the increasing availability of software and computing power.

MI is attractive because it is both practical and widely applicable. Well-developed statistical software (see, for example, issue 45 of the Journal of Statistical Software) has placed MI within the reach of most researchers in the medical and social sciences, whether or not they have undertaken advanced training in statistics. However, the increasing use of MI in a range of settings beyond that originally envisaged has led to a bewildering proliferation of algorithms and software. Further, the implications of the underlying assumptions in the context of the data at hand are often unclear.

We are writing for researchers in the medical and social sciences with the aim of clarifying the issues raised by missing data, outlining the rationale for MI, explaining the motivation and relationship between the various imputation algorithms and describing and illustrating its application in various settings and to some complex data structures.

Throughout most of the book (with the partial exception of Chapter 8), we will assume that a key aim of analysis with incomplete data is to recover the information lost due to missing data. More specifically, we will take the 'substantive model' as the model that would be used with complete data. We can then define certain desirable properties of our estimator with incomplete data. First, it should be unbiased for the value of the parameter we would see with complete data. Second, it should have low variance. Third, we should have a reliable variance formula and a means of constructing confidence intervals with the advertised coverage.

In the context of multiple imputation, it is worth noting that these remain our aims; the aim of multiple imputation is not to accurately predict the missing values. Rubin (1996) describes it as follows:

> 'Judging the quality of missing data procedures by their ability to recreate the individual missing values [...] does not lead to choosing procedures that result in valid inference, which is our objective'.

An objection may be that the ability to perfectly predict missing values *would* result in valid inference; however, in our view, this hypothetical scenario would be one in which data are not really 'missing'.

Central to the analysis of partially observed data is an understanding of why the data are missing and the implications of this for the analysis. This is the focus of the remainder of this chapter. Introducing some of the examples that run through the book, we show how Rubin's typology (Rubin, 1976) provides the foundational framework for understanding the implications of missing data.

1.1 Reasons for missing data

In this section, we consider possible reasons for missing data, illustrate these with examples, and note some preliminary implications for inference. We use the word 'possible' advisedly, since we can rarely be sure of the mechanism giving rise to missing data. Instead, a range of possible mechanisms are consistent with the observed data. In practice, we therefore wish to analyse the data under different mechanisms to establish the robustness of our inference in the face of uncertainty about the missingness mechanism.

All datasets consist of a series of *units* each of which provides information on a series of *items*. For example, in a cross-sectional questionnaire survey, the units would be individuals, and the items their answers to the questions. In a household survey, the units would be households, and the items information about the household and members of the household. In longitudinal studies, units would typically be individuals, while items would be longitudinal data from those individuals. In this book, units

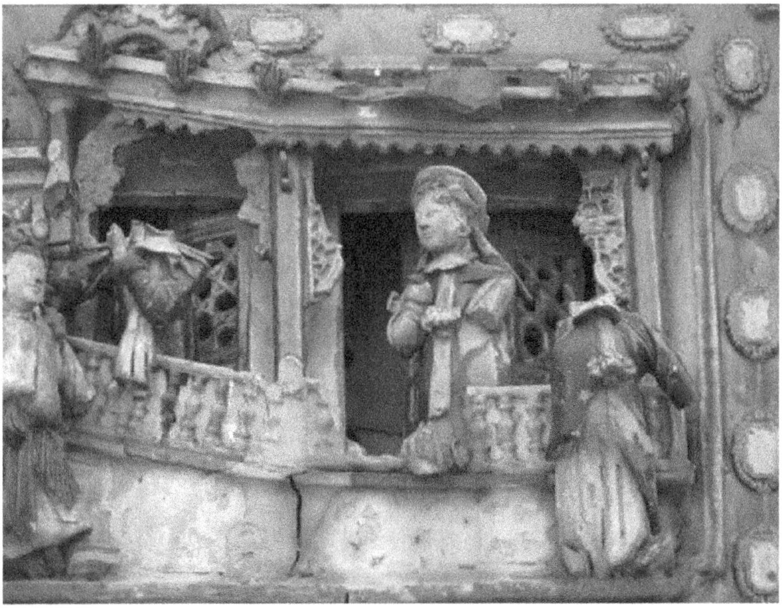

Figure 1.1 Detail from a senior mandarin's house front in New Territories, Hong Kong.

therefore correspond to the highest level in multi-level (i.e. hierarchical) data, and unless stated otherwise, data from different units are statistically independent.

Within this framework, it is useful to distinguish between units where all the information is missing, termed *unit non-response* and units who contribute partial information, termed *item non-response*. The statistical issues are the same in both cases and both can in principle be handled by MI. However, the main focus of this book is the latter.

Example 1.1 Mandarin tableau

Figure 1.1, which is also shown on the book's cover, shows part of the frontage of a senior mandarin's house in the New Territories, Hong Kong. We suppose interest focuses on characteristics of the figurines, for example their number, height, facial characteristics, and dress. Unit non-response then corresponds to missing figurines, and item non-response to damaged – hence, partially observed – figurines. □

1.2 Examples

We now introduce two key examples, which we return to throughout the book.

Example 1.2 Youth Cohort Study (YCS)

The Youth Cohort Study of England and Wales (YCS) is an ongoing UK government-funded representative survey of pupils in England and Wales at school-leaving age (School year 11, age 16–17) (UK Data Archive, 2007). Each year that a new cohort is surveyed, detailed information is collected on each young person's experience of education, and their qualifications, as well as information on employment and training. A limited amount of information is collected on their personal characteristics, family, home circumstances, and aspirations.

Over the life cycle of the YCS, different organisations have had responsibility for the structure and timings of data collection. Unfortunately, the documentation of older cohorts is poor. Croxford *et al.* (2007) have deposited a harmonised dataset that comprises YCS cohorts from 1984 to 2002 (UK Data Archive Study Number 5765 dataset). We consider data from pupils attending comprehensive schools from five YCS cohorts; these pupils reached the end of Year 11 in 1990, 1993, 1995, 1997, and 1999.

We explore relationships between Year 11 educational attainment (the General Certificate of Secondary Education) and key measures of social stratification. The units are pupils, and the items are measurements on these pupils, and a non-trivial number of items are partially observed. □

Example 1.3 Randomised controlled trial of patients with chronic asthma

We consider data from a five-arm asthma clinical trial to assess the efficacy and safety of budesonide, a second-generation glucocorticosteroid, on patients with chronic asthma. Four hundred and seventy-three patients with chronic asthma were enrolled in the 12-week randomised, double-blind, multi-centre parallel-group trial, which compared the effect of a daily dose of 200, 400, 800, or 1600 mcg of budesonide with placebo.

Key outcomes of clinical interest include patients' peak expiratory flow rate (their maximum speed of expiration in litres/minute) and their forced expiratory volume, FEV_1 (the volume of air, in litres, the patient with fully inflated lungs can breathe out in one second). In summary, the trial found a statistically significant dose–response effect for the mean change from baseline over the study for both morning peak expiratory flow, evening peak expiratory flow, and FEV_1 at the 5% level.

Budesonide-treated patients also showed reduced asthma symptoms and bronchodilator use compared with placebo, while there were no clinically significant differences in treatment-related adverse experiences between the treatment groups. Further details about the conduct of the trial, its conclusions, and the variables collected can be found elsewhere (Busse *et al.*, 1998). Here, we focus on FEV_1 and confine our attention to the placebo and lowest active dose arms. FEV_1 was collected at baseline, then 2, 4, 8, and 12 weeks after randomisation. The intention was to compare FEV_1 across treatment arms at 12 weeks. However (excluding three patients whose participation in the study was intermittent), only 37 out of 90 patients in the placebo arm, and 71 out of 90 patients in the lowest active dose arm, still remained in the trial at 12 weeks. □

1.3 Patterns of missing data

It is very important to investigate the patterns of missing data before embarking on a formal analysis. This can throw up vital information that might otherwise be overlooked and may even allow the missing data to be traced. For example, when analysing the new wave of a longitudinal survey, a colleague's careful examination of missing data patterns established that many of the missing questionnaires could be traced to a set of cardboard boxes. These turned out to have been left behind in a move. They were recovered, and the data entered.

Most statistical software now has tools for describing the pattern of missing data. Key questions concern the extent and patterns of missing values, and whether the pattern is *monotone* (as described in the next paragraph), as if it is, this can considerably speed up and simplify the analysis.

Missing data in a set of p variables are said to follow a *monotone missingness pattern* if the variables can be re-ordered such that, for every unit i and variable j,

1. if unit i is observed on variable j, where $j = 2, \dots, p$ it is observed on all variables $j' < j$, and
2. if unit i is missing on variable j, where $j = 2, \dots, p$ it is missing on all variables $j' > j$.

A natural setting for the occurrence of monotone missing data is a longitudinal study, where units are observed either until they are lost to follow up, or the study concludes. A monotone pattern is thus inconsistent with patterns of interim missing data, where some units are observed for a period, missing for the subsequent period, but then observed. Questionnaires may also give rise to monotone missing data patterns when individuals systematically answer each question in turn from the beginning till they either stop or complete the questionnaire. In other settings, it may be possible to re-order items to achieve a monotone pattern.

Example 1.2 Youth Cohort Study *(ctd)*

Table 1.1 shows the covariates we consider from the YCS. There are no missing data in the variables *cohort* and *boy*. The missingness pattern for General Certificate of Secondary Education (GCSE) score and the remaining two variables is shown in Table 1.2. In this example, it is not possible to re-order the variables (items) to obtain a monotone pattern due, for example to pattern 3 ($N = 697$). □

Example 1.3 Asthma study *(ctd)*

Table 1.3 shows the withdrawal pattern for the placebo and lowest active dose arms (all the patients are receiving their randomised medication). We have removed three patients with unusual interim missing data from Table 1.3 and all our analyses. The remaining missingness pattern is monotone in both treatment arms. □

Table 1.1 YCS variables for exploring the relationship between Year 11 attainment and social stratification.

Variable name	Description
Cohort	Year of data collection: 1990, ’93, ’95, ’97, ’99
Boy	Indicator variable for boys
Occupation	Parental occupation, categorised as managerial, intermediate, or working
Ethnicity	Categorised as Bangladeshi, Black, Indian, other Asian, Other, Pakistani, or White

Table 1.2 Pattern of missing values in the YCS data.

Pattern	GCSE score	Occupation	Ethnicity	No.	% of total
1	✓	✓	✓	55145	87%
2	✓	·	✓	6821	11%
3	·	✓	✓	697	1%
4	✓	·	·	592	1%

Table 1.3 Asthma study: withdrawal pattern by treatment arm.

Dropout pattern	Mean FEV_1 (litres) measured at week					Number	Percent
	0	2	4	8	12		
			Placebo arm				
1	✓	✓	✓	✓	✓	37	40
2	✓	✓	✓	✓	·	15	16
3	✓	✓	✓	·	·	22	24
4	✓	✓	·	·	·	16	17
			Lowest active arm				
1	✓	✓	✓	✓	✓	71	78
2	✓	✓	✓	✓	·	8	9
3	✓	✓	✓	·	·	8	9
4	✓	✓	·	·	·	3	3

1.3.1 Consequences of missing data

Our focus is on the practical implications of missing data for both parameter estimation and inference. Unfortunately, the two are often conflated so that a computational method for parameter estimation when data are missing is said to have 'solved' or 'handled' the missing data issue. Since, with missing data, computational methods only lead to valid inference under specific assumptions, this attitude is likely to lead to misleading inferences.

In this context, it may be helpful to draw an analogy with the sampling process used to collect the data. If an analyst is presented with a spreadsheet containing columns of numerical data, they can analyse the data (calculate means of variables, regress variables on each other, and so forth). However, they cannot draw any inferences unless they are told how and from whom the data were collected. This information is external to the numerical values of the variables.

We may think of the missing data mechanism as a second stage in the sampling process, but one that is not under our control. It acts on the data we intended to collect and leaves us with a partially observed dataset. Once again, the missing data mechanism cannot usually be definitively identified from the observed data, although the observed data may indicate plausible mechanisms (e.g. response may be negatively correlated with age). Thus, we will need to make an assumption about the missingness mechanism in order to draw inference. The process of making this assumption is quite separate from the statistical methods we use for parameter estimation, etc. Further, to the extent that the missing data mechanism cannot be definitively identified from the data, we will often wish to check the sensitivity of our inferences to a range of missingness mechanisms that are consistent with the observed data. The reason this book focuses on the statistical method of MI is that it provides a computationally feasible approach to the analysis for a wide range of problems under a range of missingness mechanisms.

We therefore begin with a typology for the mechanisms causing, or generating, the missing data. Later in this chapter, we will see that consideration of these mechanisms in the context of the analysis at hand clarifies the assumptions under which a simple analysis, such as restriction to complete records, will be valid. It also clarifies when more sophisticated computational approaches such as MI will be valid and informs the way they are conducted. We stress again that the mechanism causing the missing data can rarely be definitively established. Thus, we will often wish to explore the sensitivity of our inferences to a range of plausible missingness mechanisms; a process we call *sensitivity analysis*.

From a general standpoint, missing data may cause two problems: loss of efficiency and bias.

First, loss of efficiency or information is an inevitable consequence of missing data. Unfortunately, the extent of information loss is not directly linked to the proportion of incomplete records. Instead, it is intrinsically linked to the analysis question. When crossing the road, the rear of the oncoming traffic is hidden from view – the data are missing. However, these missing data do not bear on the question at hand – will I make it across the road safely. While the proportion of missing data about each oncoming vehicle is substantial, information loss is negligible. Conversely, when estimating the prevalence of a rare disease, a small proportion of missing observations could have a disproportionate impact on the resulting estimate.

Faced with an incomplete dataset, most software automatically restricts analysis to complete records. As we illustrate below, the consequence of this for loss of information is not always easy to predict. Nevertheless, in many settings, it will be important to include the information from partially complete records. Not least of the reasons for this is the time and money it has taken to collect even the partially complete records. Under certain assumptions about the missingness mechanism, we shall see that MI provides a natural way to do this.

Second, and perhaps more fundamentally, the subset of complete records may not be representative of the population under study. Restricting analysis to complete records may then lead to biased inference. The extent of such bias depends on the statistical behaviour of the missing data. A formal framework to describe this behaviour is thus fundamental. Such a framework was first elucidated in a seminal paper by Rubin (1976). To describe this, we need some definitions.

In this book, we follow Rubin's definitions, which characterizes observation-level independences. A second definition, which characterizes missingness mechanisms in terms of variable-level independences, has been recently introduced by Mohan and Pearl (2020).

1.4 Inferential framework and notation

For clarity, we take a frequentist approach to inference. This is not essential nor necessarily desirable; indeed, we will see that MI is essentially a Bayesian method with good frequentist properties. Often, as Chapter 2 shows, formally showing these frequentist properties is most difficult theoretically.

We suppose we have a sample of n units, which will often be individuals, from a population that for practical inferential purposes can be considered infinite. Let $\mathbf{Y}_i = (Y_{i,1}, Y_{i,2}, \ldots, Y_{i,p})^T$ denote the p variables we intended to collect from the ith unit, $i = 1, \ldots, n$. We wish to use these data to make inferences about a set of p population parameters $\boldsymbol{\theta} = (\theta_1, \ldots, \theta_p)^T$.

For each unit $i = 1, \ldots, n$ let $\mathbf{Y}_{i,O}$ denote the subset of p variables that are observed, and $\mathbf{Y}_{i,M}$ denote the subset that are missing. Thus, for different individuals, $\mathbf{Y}_{i,O}$ and $\mathbf{Y}_{i,M}$ may well be different subsets of the p variables. If no data are missing, $\mathbf{Y}_{i,M}$ will be empty.

Next, again for each individual $i = 1, \ldots, n$ and variable $j = 1, \ldots, p$, let $R_{i,j} = 1$ if $Y_{i,j}$ is observed and $R_{i,j} = 0$ if $Y_{i,j}$ is missing. Let $\mathbf{R}_i = (R_{i,1}, \ldots, R_{i,p})^T$. Consistent with the definition of monotone missingness patterns on p. 8, the pattern is monotone if the p variables can be re-ordered so that for each unit i,

$$R_{i,j} = 0 \implies R_{i,j'} = 0 \quad \text{for } j' = j + 1, \ldots, p. \tag{1.1}$$

The missing value mechanism is then formally defined as

$$\Pr(\mathbf{R}_i | \mathbf{Y}_i), \tag{1.2}$$

that is to say the probability of observing unit i's data given their potentially unseen values $\mathbf{Y}_i$. It is important to note that in what follows we assume that unit i's data exist (or at least existed). In other words, if it were possible for us to have been in the right place at the right time, we would have been able to observe the complete data. What (1.2) describes, therefore, is the probability that the data collection we were able to undertake on unit i yielded values of $Y_{i,1}, \ldots, Y_{i,S}$. Thus (at least until we consider sensitivity analysis for clinical trials in Chapter 12), the missing data are not counter-factual, in the sense of what might have happened if a patient had taken a different drug from the one they actually took, or a child had gone to a different school from the one they actually attended.

Example 1.1 Mandarin tableau *(ctd)*

Here, $\mathbf{Y}_i$ takes the form of observations on the $n = 4$ figurines, describing for example their size and dress. $R_{i,j}$ indicates those observations that are missing on figurine i because its head is missing. Originally, of course, all the heads were present so we can refer to the underlying values of the unobserved variables. □

Example 1.2 Youth Cohort Study (YCS) *(ctd)*

Here, underlying values of missing GCSE score, parental occupation, and ethnicity exist, and given sufficient time and money, we would be able to discover many of them. □

Example 1.3 Asthma study *(ctd)*

Were resources not limited, researchers could have visited each patient in their home at each of the scheduled follow-up times to record their data. □

We now come to the three classes of missing data mechanism. These describe how the probability of seeing the data depends on the observed and unobserved (but potentially observable or underlying) values. In general, depending on the context, we will think of the same mechanism applying either to all $i = 1, \ldots, n$ units in the dataset, or to an independent subset of them.

1.4.1 Missing completely at random (MCAR)

We say data are *missing completely at random* (MCAR) if the probability of a value being missing is unrelated to the observed and unobserved data on that unit. Algebraically,

$$\Pr(\mathbf{R}_i|\mathbf{Y}_i) = \Pr(\mathbf{R}_i). \tag{1.3}$$

Since, when data are MCAR, the chance of the data being missing is unrelated to the values, the observed data are therefore representative of the population. However, relative to the data we intended to collect, information has been lost.

Example 1.1 Mandarin tableau *(ctd)*

Suppose we wish to summarise facial characteristics of the figurines, e.g. average head circumference. If the missing heads are MCAR, a valid estimate is obtained from the observed heads. Although valid, it is imprecise relative to an estimate based on all the heads.

Before moving on, note that the MCAR assumption is made for a specific analysis, it is not a property of the tableau. It may be plausible to assume that headgear is MCAR, while heads may systematically be missing because of racial characteristics. Or, if we step back from the tableau, we may see that missing heads correspond to missing, or recently replaced, roof tiles. If so, the mechanism causing the missing data is clear; however, the assumption of MCAR is still likely to be appropriate, because the mechanism causing the missing data is unlikely to bear on (i.e. is likely statistically independent of) the analysis question.

Similarly, in certain settings, we may find that the variables predictive of missing data are independent of the substantive analysis at hand. This is consistent with the MCAR assumption: analysis of the complete records will be unbiased, but some precision is lost. □

Example 1.2 Youth Cohort Study *(ctd)*

If data are MCAR in the YCS study, valid inference would be obtained from the 55,145 complete records (Table 1.2). However, omitting the 8934 individuals with partial information means inferences are less precise than they could be. □

Example 1.3 Asthma study *(ctd)*

Assuming data are MCAR, a valid estimate of the overall mean in each group at 12 weeks is obtained by simply averaging the 37 available observations in the placebo group and the 71 available observations in the active group. This gives, respectively, 2.05 l (s.e. 0.09) and 2.23 l (s.e. 0.10). □

1.4.2 Missing at random (MAR)

We say data are *missing at random (MAR)* if *given, or conditional on, the observed data* the probability distribution of $\mathbf{R}_i$ is independent of the unobserved data. Recalling that for individual i we can partition $\mathbf{Y}_i$ as $(\mathbf{Y}_{i,O}, \mathbf{Y}_{i,M})$ we can express this mathematically as

$$\Pr(\mathbf{R}_i|\mathbf{Y}_i) = \Pr(\mathbf{R}_i|\mathbf{Y}_{i,O}). \tag{1.4}$$

This does not mean – as is sometimes supposed – that the probability of observing a variable on an individual is independent of the value of that variable. Quite the contrary, under MAR the chance of observing a variable may depend on its value. Crucially though, given the observed data, this dependence is broken. Consider the following example:

Example 1.4 Income and job type

Suppose we survey 100 employees of job types A and B for their income. Only 157 reveal their income, as shown in Figure 1.2. The figure shows that employees with higher incomes are less likely to divulge them: the probability of observing a variable depends on its value. However, if within job type A, the probability of observing income does not depend on income, and within job type B, the probability of observing income does not depend on income, then income is missing at random given job type.

The immediate consequence of this is that the mean of the observed incomes, marginal to (or aggregating over) job type, is biased downwards. The data were generated with a mean income of £60,000 in job type A and £30,000 in job type B, so that the true mean income is £45,000. Contrast the observed mean income of

$$(68 \times 60{,}927 + 89 \times 29{,}566)/157 = £43{,}149.$$

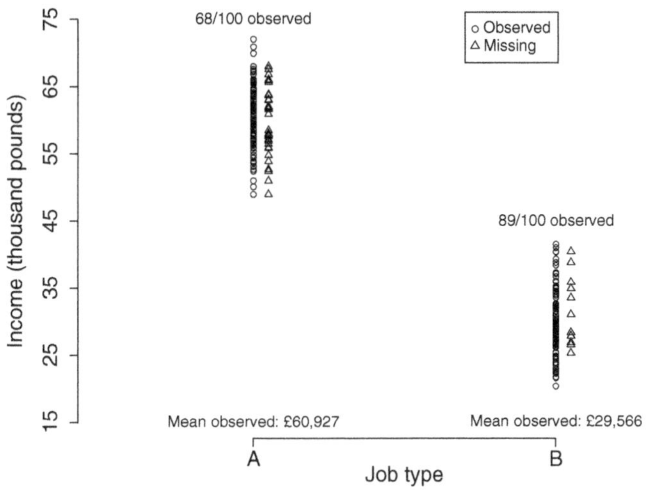

Figure 1.2 Plot of 200 hypothetical incomes against job type.

We note three further points. First, if within job type, the probability of observing income does not depend on income, it follows that:

1. To say 'income is MAR' is incomplete; we need instead to specify the variable which we assume makes income conditionally independent of job type. We could say

   'income is MAR, dependent on job type'

   or, perhaps more explicitly,

   'within categories of job type, income is MCAR'.

2. If income is MAR dependent on job type,

   - in job type A, the distribution of unobserved and observed incomes is the same, and
   - in job type B, the distribution of unobserved and observed incomes is the same.

   Formally, let variable $Y_{i,1}$ be income and $Y_{i,2}$ be job type. Job type is always observed so $R_{i,2} = 1$ for all individuals i. The statement 'income is MAR dependent on job type' is expressed

   $$\Pr(R_{i,1} = 1 | Y_{i,1}, Y_{i,2}) = \Pr(R_{i,1} = 1 | Y_{i,2}). \tag{1.5}$$

   Now consider what this implies for the distribution of income given job type. By repeatedly using the definition of conditional probability

   $$\begin{aligned}\Pr(Y_{i,1} | Y_{i,2}, R_{i,1} = 1) &= \frac{\Pr(Y_{i,1}, Y_{i,2}, R_{i,1} = 1)}{\Pr(Y_{i,2}, R_{i,1} = 1)} \\ &= \frac{\Pr(R_{i,1} = 1 | Y_{i,1}, Y_{i,2}) \Pr(Y_{i,1}, Y_{i,2})}{\Pr(R_{i,1} = 1 | Y_{i,2}) \Pr(Y_{i,2})} \\ &= \Pr(Y_{i,1} | Y_{i,2}),\end{aligned} \tag{1.6}$$

   where the last step follows from MAR, i.e. (1.5). The argument (1.6) holds if income is not observed, $R_{i,1} = 0$. Thus, under MAR, the distribution of income within job type is the same in the observed data, the unobserved data, and the population.
   In this case, to estimate the marginal income we average the observed income in each job type and then scale up:

   $$(100 \times 60{,}927 + 100 \times 29{,}566)/200 = £45{,}247. \tag{1.7}$$

   Notice that to obtain this estimate, we did not need to explicitly specify how the probability of observing income depends on job type; merely that given job type, it does not depend on income.

3. The statement 'income is MAR dependent on job type' is an untestable assumption. The data we would need to test it (represented by the triangles in Figure 1.2) are missing!

Of course, were it observed, we could 'test the MAR assumption' in two ways: first a logistic regression, for example:

$$\text{logit } \Pr(R_{i,1} = 1) = \alpha_0 + \alpha_1 Y_{i,1} + \alpha_2 Y_{i,2} + \alpha_3 Y_{i,1} Y_{i,2};$$

if MAR is true, then the hypothesis $\alpha_1 = \alpha_3 = 0$ is true. Or we could fit a corresponding regression:

$$\mathrm{E}(Y_{i,1}) = \beta_0 + \beta_1 Y_{i,2} + \beta_2 R_{i,1} + \beta_3 Y_{i,2} R_{i,1};$$

if MAR is true, then the hypothesis $\beta_2 = \beta_3 = 0$ is true. □

This simple example draws out the following general points:

1. Statements relating the probability of observing data to the values of data have direct consequences for conditional distributions of the data.
2. Under the MAR assumption, the precise missing data mechanism need not be specified; indeed, the precise form can be different for different individuals.

These two points together mean that the MAR mechanism is much more subtle than might at first appear; these subtleties can manifest themselves unexpectedly.

Example 1.4 Income and job type *(ctd)*

Suppose the mechanism causing the missing income differed for each of the 200 individuals, that is

$$\text{logit } \Pr(R_{i,1} = 1) = \alpha_{0,i} + \alpha_{1,i} Y_{i,2}.$$

Then missing data are still MAR, and (1.7) is still a valid estimate. □

Of course, it may be as contrived to think each individual has their own MAR mechanism as to think that the same mechanism holds for all. In a simple example, this is not important, but in real applications, a blanket assumption of MAR may be very contrived:

Example 1.5 Subtlety of MAR assumption

Suppose we have three variables, $Y_{i,1}, Y_{i,2}, Y_{i,3}$, and we are unfortunate so our dataset contains non-trivial numbers of all possible missingness patterns, as shown in Table 1.4

If the same missingness mechanism applies to all the units, and it is either MAR or MCAR, then it must be MCAR. If we wish to assume data are MAR, we are forced to split the data into groups among which different MAR mechanisms are operating. These groups need not necessarily be defined by the missing data patterns; they could

Table 1.4 Three variables: all possible missing value patterns.

Pattern	Y_1	Y_2	Y_3
1	✓	✓	✓
2	✓	✓	·
3	✓	·	✓
4	·	✓	✓
5	✓	·	·
6	·	✓	·
7	·	·	✓

be defined by characteristics of the units. Settings like this are considered by Harel and Schafer (2009). To illustrate, though, we define groups by the missing data patterns.

For a MAR mechanism, we might assume the following:

- in patterns (1,2) $Y_{i,3}$ is MAR given $Y_{i,1}, Y_{i,2}$;
- in patterns (3,4,7) $Y_{i,1}$ and/or $Y_{i,2}$ is MAR given $Y_{i,3}$; and
- in patterns (5,6) data are MCAR.

In practice, often a relatively small number of the possible missingness patterns predominate, and it is assumptions about these that are important for any analysis. The remaining – relatively infrequent – patterns can often be assumed MCAR, with little risk to the final inference if this assumption is in fact wrong. □

Faced with complex data, there is a temptation to invoke the MAR assumption too readily, especially as this simplifies any analysis using MI. To guard against this, analysts need to be satisfied that any associations assumed to justify the MAR assumption are at least consistent with the observed data. Since consideration of selection mechanisms may not be as straightforward as might first appear, it can also be worth considering the plausibility of MAR from the point of view of the joint and conditional distribution of the data. As (1.6) illustrates, for MAR, we need to be satisfied

1. that conditional distributions of partially observed given fully observed variables do not differ depending on whether the data are observed, and
2. in consequence, the joint distribution of the data can be validly estimated by piecing together the marginal distributions of the observed patterns.

The above discussion explains why we do not regard the MAR assumption as a panacea, but nevertheless often both a plausible and practical starting point for the analysis of partially observed data. In particular, the points drawn out of Example 1.4 are not specific to either the number or type of variables (categorical or quantitative).

Example 1.1 Mandarin tableau *(ctd)*

Here the MAR assumption says that the distribution of head characteristics given body characteristics (i.e. dress, height, etc.,) does not depend on whether the head is present. Thus, under MAR we can estimate the distribution of characteristics of figurines with missing heads from figurines with similar body characteristics.

Notice the two rightmost figurines in Figure 1.1 share the same necktie. Assuming headdress is MAR given necktie, the missing headdress on the rightmost figurine is similar to that on the second rightmost figurine.

Clearly, this assumption cannot be checked from the tableau (data) at hand. However, it might be possible to explore it using other tableaux (i.e. other datasets). If MAR is plausible for headdress given necktie, it does not mean it is plausible for skin colour given necktie. In other words, MAR is an assumption we make for the analysis, not a characteristic of the dataset. For some analyses of partially observed data, it may be plausible; for others not. □

1.4.3 Missing not at random (MNAR)

If the mechanism causing missing data is neither MCAR nor MAR, we say it is missing not at random (MNAR). Under a MNAR mechanism, the probability of an observation being missing depends on the underlying value, and this dependence remains even given the observed data. Mathematically,

$$\Pr(\mathbf{R}_i|\mathbf{Y}_{i,}) \neq \Pr(\mathbf{R}_i|\mathbf{Y}_{i,O}). \tag{1.8}$$

While in some settings MNAR may be more plausible than MAR, analysis under MNAR is considerably harder. This is because under MAR, equation (1.6) showed that conditional distributions of partially observed variables given fully observed variables are the same in units who do, and do not, have the data observed. However, (1.6) does not hold if (1.8) holds.

It follows that inference under MNAR involves an explicit specification of either the selection mechanism or how conditional distributions of partially observed variables given fully observed variables differ between units who do, and do not, have the data observed.

Formally, we can write the joint distribution of unit i's variables, $\mathbf{Y}_i$, and the indicator for observing those variables, $\mathbf{R}_i$ as

$$\Pr(\mathbf{R}_i|\mathbf{Y}_i)\Pr(\mathbf{Y}_i) = \Pr(\mathbf{R}_i, \mathbf{Y}_i) = \Pr(\mathbf{Y}_i|\mathbf{R}_i)\Pr(\mathbf{R}_i). \tag{1.9}$$

In the centre is the joint distribution, and this can be written either as

1. **A selection model**: the LHS of (1.9), i.e. a product of (i) the conditional probability of observing the variables, given their values; and (ii) the marginal distribution of the data, or

2. **A pattern mixture model**: the RHS of (1.9), i.e. a product of (i) the probability distribution of the data within each missingness pattern; and (ii) the marginal probability of the missingness pattern.

Thus, we can specify a MNAR mechanism either by specifying the selection model (which implies the pattern mixture model) or by specifying a pattern mixture model (which implies a selection model). Depending on the context, both approaches may be helpful. Unfortunately, even in apparently simple settings, explicitly calculating the selection implication of a pattern mixture model, or vice versa, can be awkward. We shall see in Chapter 10 that an advantage of multiple imputation is that given a pattern mixture model we can estimate the selection model implications quite easily.

Once again, as the example below shows, MNAR is an assumption for the analysis, not a characteristic of the data.

Example 1.1 Mandarin tableau *(ctd)*

It may be that the figurines with missing heads were wearing a headdress that identified them as a member of a class, or group, that subsequently became very unpopular – causing the heads to be smashed. This MNAR selection mechanism means that we cannot say anything about the typical characteristics of headdress without making untestable assumptions about the characteristics of the missing headdresses. Further, the MNAR assumption implies that the distribution of headdress given body dress is different for figurines with missing and observed heads.

We reiterate, under MNAR any summary statistics, or analyses, require *either* explicit assumptions about the form of the distribution of the missing data given the observed *or* explicit specification of the selection mechanism and the marginal distribution of the full (including unobserved) data. Contrast this with analyses assuming MAR, where these assumptions are made implicitly.

We reiterate a point from the tableau: if head dress was the trigger for missing heads, but the type of head dress worn is not related to physical characteristics of the heads, analyses concerning their physical characteristics could be validly performed under MAR. Just because the heads are MNAR does not mean all analyses require the MNAR assumption. This underlines that, in applications, it is crucial to think carefully about the selection mechanism, and how it affects the analysis question. □

Example 1.6 Income MNAR

To illustrate (1.9), consider a simplified version of the income example above. Suppose that of the 100 people surveyed, 50 have the same income θ_L, and 50 have the same higher income, θ_U. Suppose further that all those with income θ_L disclose it, but only a fraction π of those with income θ_U disclose it.

This is an example of pattern mixture model, i.e. the RHS of (1.9). Let 1[.] be 1 if the statement in brackets is true and 0 otherwise. Then, in this simple example, it is clear what the selection counterpart is

$$\text{Pr(income observed)} = 1 - 0.5 \times 1[\text{income} > \theta_L], \quad \text{and}$$
$$\text{mean income} = (\theta_L + \theta_U)/2.$$

The pattern mixture model implies a selection model.

We now illustrate the same point with a bivariate normal model. Let Y denote income; to keep the algebra simple suppose $Y \sim N(0,1)$, and we drop the index i. Let $R = 1$ if Y is observed, but now let $X \sim N(\mu_x, 1)$ be a normally distributed variable, correlated with Y, which is positive if Y is observed, that is when $R = 1$. We specify the selection model and derive the pattern mixture model.

Let $\Phi(\,.\,)$ be the cumulative distribution of the standard normal, and suppose we choose the selection model as

$$\Pr(R = 1|Y) = \Pr(X > 0|Y) = \Phi(\alpha_0 + \alpha_1 Y). \tag{1.10}$$

Equation (1.10) thus assumes a specific MNAR mechanism, for α_0 and α_1 cannot be estimated from the observed values of Y.

Given (1.10) and the marginal standard normal distribution of Y, the joint distribution of (Y, X) is bivariate normal:

$$\begin{pmatrix} Y \\ X \end{pmatrix} \sim N\left[\begin{pmatrix} 0 \\ \mu_x \end{pmatrix}, \begin{pmatrix} 1 & \rho \\ \rho & 1 \end{pmatrix}\right], \tag{1.11}$$

where $\rho = \text{corr}(Y, X)$. Thus, we have the central term in (1.9). It follows that

$$\Pr(X_i|y_i) \sim N(\mu_x + \rho Y_i, (1 - \rho^2)).$$

Thus,

$$\Pr(X > 0|Y) = \Phi\left(\frac{\mu_x + \rho Y}{\sqrt{1 - \rho^2}}\right) = \Phi\left(\frac{\mu_x}{\sqrt{1 - \rho^2}} + \frac{\rho}{\sqrt{1 - \rho^2}} Y\right). \tag{1.12}$$

Comparing with (1.10) we see $\rho = f(\alpha_1)$ and $\mu_x = g(\alpha_0, \alpha_1)$. Hence, (α_0, α_1) define μ_x, which in turn defines the marginal probability, $\Pr(X > 0)$, of observing Y.

From the bivariate normal (1.11), the distribution of observed income, Y given $R = 1$, is $Y|x > 0$ which is

$$\frac{\phi(y)}{\Phi(\mu_x)} \Phi\left(\frac{\mu_x + \rho y}{\sqrt{1 - \rho^2}}\right) = \frac{\phi(y)}{\Phi\{g(\alpha_0, \alpha_1)\}} \Phi(\alpha_0 + \alpha_1 y). \tag{1.13}$$

A similar result follows for the distribution of unobserved income. Putting this together, we have arrived at the pattern mixture model, the RHS of (1.9). Specification of the selection mechanism, through α_0, α_1, together with the marginal distribution of income, fixes both the marginal probability of observing income and the distribution of the two 'patterns' of data: the seen and unseen incomes.

This is a simple example of the Heckman selection model, which is further discussed in Little and Rubin (2019), Chapter 15. It has also been used as a model for publication bias in meta-analysis (Copas and Shi, 2000). □

The example above illustrates that when data are MNAR, instead of thinking about the selection mechanism, it is equally appropriate to consider differences between conditional distributions of partially observed given fully observed variables. Under MAR, such distributions do not differ depending on whether data are missing or not; under MNAR, they do. Considering the conditional distribution of the observed data, and then exploring the robustness of inference as it is allowed to differ in the unobserved data is therefore a natural way to explore the robustness of inference to an assumption of MAR. Our perspective has two further advantages: (i) the differences can be expressed simply and pictorially, and (ii) MI provides a natural route for inference. Unfortunately, the selection counterparts, or implications, of pattern mixture models are rarely easy to calculate directly, but again MI can help: after imputing missing data under a pattern mixture model, it is straightforward to explore implications for the implied selection model.

Example 1.3 Asthma study *(ctd)*

We illustrate the above using the 12 week data from the asthma study. Suppose first that 12-week response is MAR given treatment group. Then, in each treatment group, the means of unobserved and observed data are the same, so the treatment effect is $2.23 - 2.05 = 0.18$ litres. Suppose we have a MNAR mechanism, and we express this as a pattern mixture model. Let μ_P, μ_A be the mean response under placebo and active treatment. Then

$$\mu_P = 37 \times 2.05 + (90 - 37) \times (2.05 + \Delta_P), \text{ and}$$

$$\mu_A = 71 \times 2.23 + (90 - 71) \times (2.23 + \Delta_A),$$

where Δ_P, Δ_A are the mean differences between observed and unobserved response in the placebo and active groups, respectively.

Figure 1.3 shows how the estimated treatment effect varies as we move away from the assumption of MAR, i.e. that $\Delta_P = \Delta_A = 0$. Since many more patients are missing in the placebo group, the treatment estimate is much more sensitive to departures from MAR in this group.

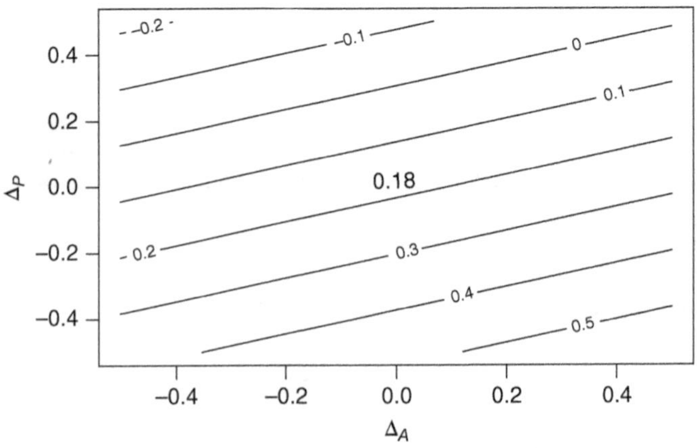

Figure 1.3 Contour-plot of the difference in average FEV_1 (litres) between active and placebo groups, as Δ_P, Δ_A, vary. Under MAR, $\Delta_P = \Delta_A = 0$, and the difference is 0.18 litres.

Notice the inherently arbitrary nature of MNAR: because we cannot estimate Δ_A, Δ_P from the data at hand, all possible values are – in general – equally plausible. This issue is the motivation for our proposed approach to sensitivity analysis in clinical trials of this type in Section 10.4. □

1.4.4 Ignorability

If, under a specific assumption about the missingness mechanism, we can construct a valid analysis that does not require us to explicitly include the model for that missing value mechanism, we term the mechanism, in the context of this analysis, *ignorable*.

A common example of this is a likelihood-based analysis assuming MAR.

However, as we see below there are other settings, where we do not assume MAR, that do not require us to explicitly include the model for the missingness mechanism yet still result in valid inference. For example, as discussed in Section 1.6.2, a complete records regression analysis is valid if data are MNAR-dependent only on the covariates.

1.5 Using observed data to inform assumptions about the missingness mechanism

We have already noted that, given the observed data, we cannot definitively identify the missingness mechanism. Nevertheless, the observed data can help frame plausible assumptions about this – in other words assumptions which are consistent with the observed data. Exploratory analyses of this nature are important for (i) assessing whether a complete case analysis is likely to be biased, and (ii) framing appropriate imputation models. Two key tools for this are summaries (tabular or graphical) of fully observed, or near-fully observed variables, by missingness pattern and logistic regression of missingness indicators on observed or near-fully observed variables.

Example 1.3 Asthma study *(ctd)*

Table 1.5 shows the mean FEV_1 by dropout pattern. In the placebo arm (see Figure 1.4), patterns 3 and 4 have lower FEV_1 at baseline, and for patterns 2–4 FEV_1 declines from baseline to last visit. In the active arm, patterns 1 and 2 show a similar increase of about 0.20 ml, while pattern 3 starts higher and shows little change, while pattern 4 shows marked decline. Notice also the increase in variance in the active arm over time which is different from the placebo arm. This is a common feature of such data and should be reflected in the analysis.

MAR mechanisms which are dependent on treatment and response are consistent with these data. However, there is a suspicion that further decline between the last observed and first missing visit triggered withdrawal, probably followed in the placebo arm by switching to an active treatment. Thus, it would be useful to explore sensitivity of treatment inferences to MNAR, which we do in Chapter 10. □

Table 1.5 Asthma study: mean FEV_1 (litres) at each visit, by dropout pattern and intervention arm.

Dropout pattern	Placebo arm						
	Mean FEV_1 (litres) measured at week					No.	%
	0	2	4	8	12		
1	2.11	2.14	2.07	2.01	2.06	37	40
2	2.31	2.18	1.95	2.13	—	15	16
3	1.96	1.73	1.84	—	—	22	24
4	1.84	1.72	—	—	—	16	17
All patients (mean)	2.06	1.97	1.98	2.04	2.06	90	100
All patients (std.)	0.57	0.67	0.56	0.58	0.55		
	Lowest active arm						
1	2.03	2.22	2.23	2.24	2.23	71	78
2	1.93	1.91	2.01	2.14	—	8	9
3	2.28	2.10	2.29	—	—	8	9
4	2.24	1.84	—	—	—	3	3
All patients (mean)	2.03	2.17	2.22	2.23	2.23	90	100
All patients (std.)	0.65	0.75	0.80	0.85	0.81		

Example 1.2 Youth Cohort Study *(ctd)*

In Table 1.2, we saw that the principal missing data pattern has missing parental occupation. Let $R_i = 1$ if parental occupation is observed, and zero otherwise. Table 1.6 shows the results of various logistic regressions of R on the remaining fully, or near fully observed, variables: GCSE score, ethnicity, gender, and cohort. The receiver operating characteristic (ROC) is an assessment of how well a model discriminates between the missing and observed parental occupation, with a minimum value of 0.5 (no discrimination) and a maximum of 1. Of course, even if the model discriminated perfectly, this would say nothing about differences between observed and unobserved data, i.e. whether the data are MNAR.

We see that GCSE score is the strongest predictor of missing parental occupation (ROC of 0.68), followed by ethnic group (here simplified to white/non-white) and cohort. Gender is a relatively weak predictor. Nevertheless, due to the size of the cohort, all are significant at the 5% level in model 5, which has reasonable discrimination (ROC = 0.74).

Figure 1.5 confirms that GCSE score is substantially higher among those whose parental occupation is observed (mean of 39 versus 28 points, respectively). Further, 10% of children with missing parental occupation have no GCSEs (score 0) compared with 3% who have parental occupation observed.

We conclude the data are consistent with parental occupation missing at random, dependent strongly on GCSE score and ethnic group, but also associated with cohort

Table 1.6 Coefficients (standard errors), and receiver operating characteristic (ROC), from logistic models for the probability of observing parental occupation.

Variable	Models				
	1	2	3	4	5
Cohort '93	−0.085				−0.168
	(0.036)				(0.039)
Cohort '95	0.044				−0.212
	(0.038)				(0.042)
Cohort '97	0.178				−0.032
	(0.040)				(0.043)
Cohort '99	0.135				−0.165
	(0.040)				(0.046)
Boy		−0.053			0.079
		(0.024)			(0.026)
GCSE score			0.037		0.038
			(0.001)		(0.001)
Non-white				−1.723	−1.698
				(0.0288)	(0.031)
ROC	0.53	0.51	0.68	0.62	0.74

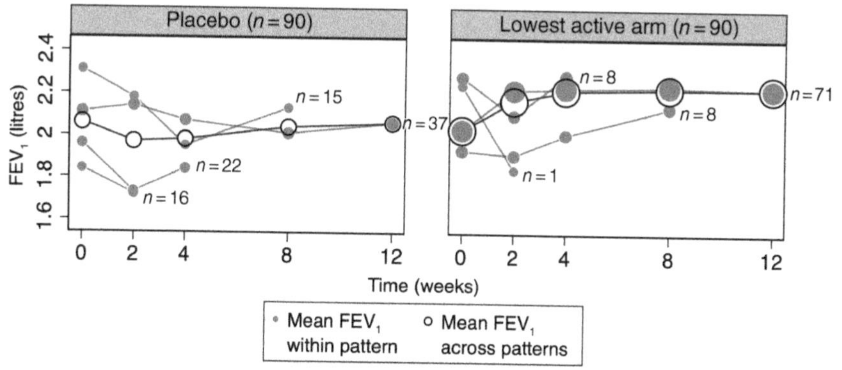

Figure 1.4 Asthma study: mean FEV_1 (litres) at each visit, by randomised arm for each dropout pattern and across dropout patterns, with points weighted according to number of participants contributing to the mean.

and weakly with gender. A relatively small number of values are missing for the other variables. It is plausible to assume these are either MCAR or perhaps MAR given observations on other variables; unless they are strongly MNAR, this will have a negligible impact on subsequent inferences. □

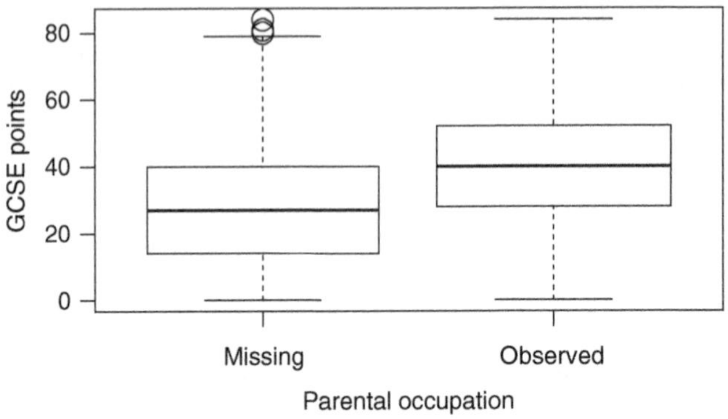

Figure 1.5 Boxplot of GCSE points by whether parental occupation is observed.

1.6 Implications of missing data mechanisms for regression analyses

Usually, we will want to fit some form of regression model to address our substantive questions. Here, we look at the implications in terms of bias and loss of information, of missing data in the response and/or covariates under different missingness mechanisms. We first focus on linear regression; our findings there hold for most other regression models, including relative risk regression and survival analysis. Logistic regression is more subtle; we discuss this in Section 1.6.4.

1.6.1 Partially observed response

Suppose we wish to fit the model

$$Y_i = \beta_0 + \beta_1 X_i + e_i, \quad e_i \overset{i.i.d.}{\sim} N(0, \sigma^2), \quad i = 1, \dots, n, \tag{1.14}$$

but Y is partially observed. Let R_i indicate whether Y_i is observed. For now assume that the X_i is known without error; for example it may be a design variable. Then the contribution to the likelihood for $\boldsymbol{\beta} = (\beta_0, \beta_1)$ from unit i, conditional on X_i, is

$$L_i = \Pr(R_i, Y_i | X_i) = \Pr(R_i | Y_i, X_i) \Pr(Y_i | X_i). \tag{1.15}$$

Assume, as will typically be the case, that the parameters of $\Pr(Y_i|X_i)$, $\boldsymbol{\beta}$, are distinct from the parameters of $\Pr(R_i|Y_i, X_i)$.

Figure 1.2 suggests that provided Y is MAR given the covariates in the model, units with missing response have no information about $\boldsymbol{\beta}$. To see this formally, first observe that as Y_i is MAR given X_i, only the second term on the RHS of (1.15) involves Y; as the first term involves neither Y nor the parameters of $\Pr(Y|X)$ we can ignore it.

Then the contribution to the likelihood for an individual with missing response is obtained by integrating (for discrete variables summing) over all possible values of the missing response variable Y_i, given x_i. This is

$$\int \Pr(Y_i|X_i)dY_i = 1,$$

because we are integrating (summing) over all possible values of Y_i given (β, x_i), so the total probability is 1. Conditional on X, all units with missing Y thus contribute 1 to likelihood for $\boldsymbol{\beta}$, and so have no effect on, or information about, the maximum likelihood estimate of $\boldsymbol{\beta}$.

This may feel counter-intuitive, especially if we have a large number of units with Y missing but X observed. Do they really have no information on the regression?

For linear regression, the answer is yes (there is no information), because the parameter space of the conditional distribution of Y given X is separate from that of the marginal distribution for X. In other words, the mean and variance of X have no information on, and place no restriction on, the parameters of the distribution of $Y|X$. Equivalently, the conditional distribution of $f(Y|X)$ has no information on, and places no restriction on, the marginal distribution of X.

Example 1.3 Asthma study *(ctd)*

To illustrate the above, consider estimating the effect of treatment on 12-week response, adjusting for baseline, setting aside the measurements at 2, 4, and 8 weeks. If we assume that 12-week response is MAR given treatment, then from the above argument, it follows that fitting the regression model,

$$Y_i = \beta_0 + \beta_1 1[\text{treatment} = \text{active}_i] + e_i, \quad e_i \overset{i.i.d.}{\sim} N(0, \sigma^2), \tag{1.16}$$

using the complete records gives a valid estimate of the treatment effect (Table 1.7).

Now suppose, as Table 1.5 suggests that baseline is also predictive of missing 12-week FEV_1; it is also strongly predictive of the actual 12-week FEV_1. Assuming 12-week FEV_1 is MAR given baseline and treatment, we can include baseline in the

Table 1.7 Asthma study: estimated treatment effect fitting treatment, and treatment and baseline. Inference is valid and fully efficient if assumption that data are MAR, dependent on the covariates in the model, is correct.

Covariates	n	Treatment estimate (s.e.)	p-Value
Treat	108	0.172 L (0.149)	0.251
Treat and baseline	108	0.247 L (0.100)	0.016

regression model (1.16). Again, the argument above shows that fitting this model to the observed data is valid and efficient; the results are in Table 1.7. Note that

(a) if baseline were predictive of underlying 12-week response, but given treatment not predictive of observing that response, we would still wish to include it, and

(b) in the unlikely case that baseline were predictive of missing 12-week response, but not related to the actual 12-week response value, there would be no benefit of including it. We explore this study further, taking into account the longitudinal observations, in Chapter 3. □

The above argument extends naturally to partially observed multivariate responses. Suppose we have up to J observations on individual i, denoted $\mathbf{Y}_i = (Y_{i,1}, \dots, Y_{i,J})$. Suppose they are MAR given X_i, and – whatever the pattern of missing data – we partition $\mathbf{Y}_i$ into $\mathbf{Y}_{i,O}$ and $\mathbf{Y}_{i,M}$. Then the contribution of individual i to the likelihood for the regression of $\mathbf{Y}$ on X is

$$\int \Pr(\mathbf{Y}_i|\boldsymbol{\beta}, X_i)\, d\mathbf{Y}_{i,M},$$

in other words the marginal likelihood of the observed data. For the multivariate normal distribution, this is readily calculated; in fact most software fits the model to the observed pattern of response data by default. Once again, in this setting there is no advantage to, or gain from, using multiple imputation.

The last setting we consider in this section is when we have missing response data, but these data are MNAR, given the variables we wish to include in the model of interest. For a direct exposition, we return to univariate Y_i; the extension to multivariate $\mathbf{Y}_i$ is immediate.

Consider (1.15) and let the parameters of $\Pr(R_i|Y_i, X_i)$ be $\boldsymbol{\eta}$ and distinct from those of $\Pr(Y_i|X_i)$, i.e. $\boldsymbol{\beta}$. The contribution to the likelihood from individual i is

$$\int \Pr(R_i, Y_i, X_i)\, dY_i = \Pr(X_i) \int \{\Pr(R_i|\boldsymbol{\eta}, Y_i, X_i) \Pr(Y_i|\boldsymbol{\beta}, X_i)\, dY_i\}. \tag{1.17}$$

We see the likelihood contribution for $\boldsymbol{\beta}$ is now caught up with the selection mechanism; we have to evaluate the integral on the RHS of (1.17) to obtain the contribution of individual i to the likelihood. Failure to do this leads to biased inference for $\boldsymbol{\beta}$.

Example 1.7 Linear regression

To illustrate this, we simulate a sample of 200 observations from the linear regression model

$$\begin{aligned} Y_i &= \beta_0 + \beta_1 X_i + e_i, \quad e_i \overset{i.i.d.}{\sim} N(0, \sigma^2), \quad i = 1, \dots, 200 \\ \text{with } X_i &\overset{i.i.d.}{\sim} N(0, 3.5) \quad i = 1, \dots, 200 \end{aligned} \tag{1.18}$$

and $(\alpha, \beta, \sigma^2) = (5, 1, 4^2)$. These data, together with the fitted regression, are shown in Figure 1.6(a), together with the the least squares fitted line, which has estimated parameters $(\hat{\alpha}, \hat{\beta}) = (4.47, 1.00)$.

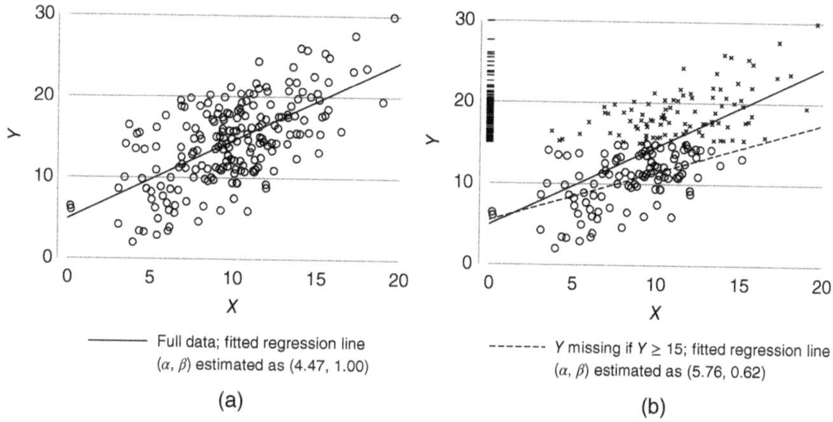

Figure 1.6 Regression lines for simulated data. (a) Fitted regression line to the full data, $n = 200$. (b) Original and fitted line when Y is MNAR, with observed data denoted with a circle, missing data with × and a 'tassle' at the margin showing the values of Y for which X is missing.

Now suppose that some of the Y values are MNAR. Suppose

$$\Pr(Y \text{ is missing}) = \begin{cases} 1 & \text{if } Y_i < 15 \text{ and} \\ 0 & \text{otherwise} \end{cases} \tag{1.19}$$

Starting from the 200 observations shown in the left panel of Figure 1.6, the right panel plots the complete cases that remain under this mechanism. Fitting a regression line to the observed data gives $(\hat{\beta}_0, \hat{\beta}_1) = (5.76, 0.62)$. Because high values of Y, which correspond to high values of X, are likely missing, the intercept is biased slightly up and the slope down. □

Next, suppose that in addition to X, Y we have the fully observed variable Z. We suppose that Y is partially observed, we are interested in the regression of Y on X, that

$$\text{logit } \Pr(R_i = 1) = \alpha_0 + \alpha_1 X_i + \alpha_2 Z_i, \tag{1.20}$$

and that Z is correlated with Y. Then, following from the discussion above, the regression of complete records Y_i on X_i will be biased, because setting Z aside Y_i is MNAR. However, the regression of complete records Y_i on X_i, Z_i will be unbiased and efficient, because given (X, Z), Y is MAR.

1.6.2 Missing covariates

We now consider the regression of Y on X, when Y is fully observed and X is partially observed.

Let $R_1 = 1$ if X_i is observed, and $R_i = 0$ otherwise. Consider the regression of Y on X estimated from the complete records, i.e. given $R_i = 1$. Following (1.6), for each individual pair,

$$\begin{aligned}\Pr(Y_i|X_i, R_i = 1) &= \frac{\Pr(Y_i, X_i, R_i = 1)}{\Pr(X_i, R_i = 1)} \\ &\frac{\Pr(R_i = 1|Y_i, X_i)\Pr(Y_i, X_i)}{\Pr(R_i = 1|X_i)\Pr(X_i)} \\ &\left\{\frac{\Pr(R_i = 1|Y_i, X_i)}{\Pr(R_i = 1|X_i)}\right\}\Pr(Y_i|X_i).\end{aligned} \tag{1.21}$$

Thus, when the missingness mechanism for X, $\Pr(R_i = 1|Y_i, X_i)$, involves the response Y, then restricting the analysis to the complete records gives biased point estimates and invalid inference. This holds whether the missingness mechanism only depends on Y, i.e. MAR, or whether it includes X as well, i.e. MNAR.

Example 1.6 Income *(ctd)*

Consider again the income example, but now suppose we wish to estimate the probability of job type given income, i.e. $\Pr(Z_{2i}|Z_{1i})$. As this is artificial data, we know the data generating mechanism:

$$Z_1 \sim N(60, 5) \text{ for job type 'A'}, \quad \text{and } Z_1 \sim N(30, 5) \text{ for job type 'B'},$$

with $\Pr(\text{job type A}) = \Pr(Z_2 = A) = 0.5$.

Thus,

$$\Pr(Z_2 = A|z_1) = \frac{\Pr(Z_1 = z_1|Z_2 = A)}{\Pr(Z_1 = z_1|Z_2 = A) + \Pr(Z_1 = z_1|Z_2 = B)}.$$

Thus, if $Z_1 = 45$, the probability $Z_2 = A$ is 0.5. In the original data (Figure 1.2), there is no overlap between the groups so again $\Pr(Z_2 = A|Z_1 = 45) = 0.5$. However, from the observed data, we estimate this as $68/(68 + 89) = 0.43$. This illustrates the general point above: in regression when covariates are MAR and the mechanism includes the response, complete records analysis is biased. □

From (1.21), we see that when the missingness mechanism for the covariate does not depend on the response Y_i, the probability of $Y|X$ among the complete records is the same as that in the population. In other words, although the covariate is MNAR, estimating the regression using complete records is unbiased and gives valid inference, although a full likelihood analysis with the correctly specified selection mechanism would be more efficient. Again, we note that the precise form of selection mechanism can vary between units or individuals; its precise form is not relevant to the argument.

Example 1.7 Linear regression *(ctd)*

Continuing with the simulated example, suppose we take the original 200 pairs and set all X values greater than or equal to 12 to missing. This is a strong MNAR mechanism but, given the (possibly unobserved) X value, the probability of X being missing does not depend on Y. Figure 1.7(a) shows the regression of Y on X fitted to the remaining points and the fitted line to the original data. They are very similar. Using the observed points, $(\hat{\beta}_0, \hat{\beta}_1) = (5.73, 0.86)$.

Thus, as (1.21) implies, there is no bias, but some information is lost. In particular, by reducing the range of X, we lose information particularly about β: for an intuition, as to why, imagine that X is only observed if it is equal to 0; then we would be able to estimate α from the observed data but not β.

It is also important to note that (i) in this situation, an analysis under MAR would be biased, but (ii) given the observed data, we cannot conclude that X is MNAR dependent only on X; indeed, it would be plausible to have X MAR, or MNAR dependent on Y and X.

Now consider the setting where the covariate X is MAR depending on outcome Y such that X_i is observed if $Y_i < 15$ and otherwise missing. Here, regression of Y on X among the complete cases is exactly as in Figure 1.6(b). It is of no consequence that there Y was incomplete and here X is incomplete; the analysis of the observed pairs is identical.

Next consider the setting where the covariate, X, is MNAR depending on both X and Y. In this setting, (1.21) implies that regression using the observed pairs only will be biased. Suppose that

$$\Pr(X \text{ is missing}) = \begin{cases} 0 & \text{if } Y < 15 \;\&\; X < 12 \\ 1 & \text{otherwise} \end{cases}$$

Figure 1.7(b) shows the results; the bias is clear. □

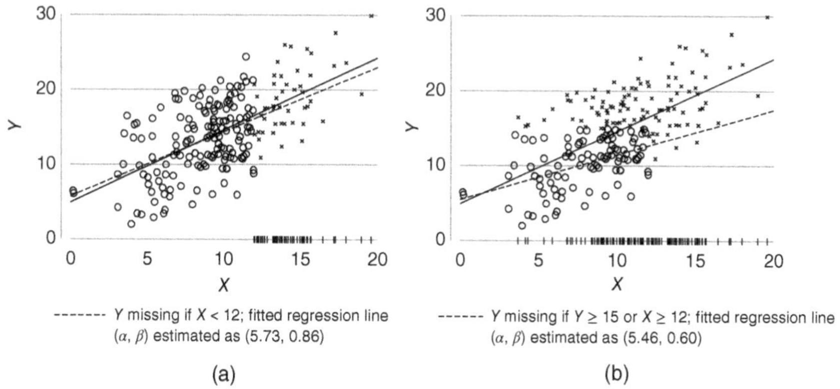

Figure 1.7 Missing covariates: effect of different mechanisms. (a) Effect of missingness dependent on X; (b) effect of missingness dependent on X and Y. Observed data are denoted with a circle; missing data are denoted with × and also a 'tassle' at the margin showing the value of X for which X is missing.

Lastly, consider the case where we have three variables (or sets of variables) X, Y, Z and we are interested in the regression of Y on X. Suppose X is MNAR given X, Z but that if we omit Z there is residual dependence of the missing mechanism on Y so that X is MNAR given X, Y.

In this setting, (1.21) shows us that using the complete records to regress Y on X will be biased; however, using the complete records to regress Y on X, Z will be unbiased for the latter, adjusted relationship. Unfortunately, unless Z is independent of X, so that including Z in the regression does not change the coefficient for X, it is not possible to use this to obtain a valid estimate of the regression of Y on X alone without making additional assumptions. Indeed, even if X is truly independent of Z, under a MNAR mechanism in the observed data, they will typically be correlated.

1.6.3 Missing covariates and response

In our final setting, first suppose we have three variables, X, Y, Z, and that Y and X are MAR given Z. Consider the linear regression of Y on X, Z. Units with X, Y missing contribute

$$\int \Pr(Y|\boldsymbol{\beta}; X, Z)\, dY = 1$$

to the likelihood $\Pr(Y|\boldsymbol{\beta}; X, Z)$. Thus, (1.21) implies the complete records analysis will be unbiased.

When we have additional variables predictive of Y and/or X, then these may be used to recover information on the missing values and, hence, $\boldsymbol{\beta}$.

1.6.4 Subtle issues I: the odds ratio

This and the next two sections consider some more subtle implications of the missingness mechanism for complete records analysis; some readers may prefer to skip to the summary on p. 34.

Bartlett *et al.* (2015a) consider the further complication which arises because some estimators possess a symmetry, which means they can be validly estimated from the complete records under a greater range of missing value mechanisms. The principal example is the odds ratio. Consider Table 1.8. We can either model A, C as binomial random variables with denominator $a+b$, $c+d$, or we can model A, B as binomial random variables with denominator $a+c$, $b+d$. In both cases, estimates and inference for the odds ratio are identical. The first case corresponds to a case-control study, and the latter to a cohort study. Now suppose that the probability of outcome is MNAR dependent on only outcome. Consider the model

$$\text{logit } \Pr(\text{good outcome}) = \beta_0 + \beta_1 \times 1[\text{exposed}].$$

The preceding discussion would lead us to suppose that both β_0 and β_1 will be biased. In fact, β_1 will be unbiased. Symmetry of the odds ratio means inference for this is the same as if we performed a logistic regression of exposure on outcome where

Table 1.8 Typical two-by-two table of counts relating outcome to exposure.

	Unexposed	Exposed
Good outcome	a	b
Poor outcome	c	d

outcome was MNAR dependent only on outcome. However, this is an example of a covariate MNAR, and (1.21) shows that inference using the complete records is valid in this case. The same argument applies if exposure is MAR given outcome. Bias will only occur when estimating β_1 if data are MNAR dependent on both the outcome and covariate.

More generally, we will wish to estimate the log-odds ratio relating outcome, Y, to X for various possible confounders, say Z. Applying the above argument, Y may be MNAR dependent on itself and Z, yet the OR relating X to Y will still be validly estimated from the complete records. Or Y may be MNAR dependent on itself and X, and then the OR relating Z to Y estimated using the complete records is still valid. However, if the MNAR mechanism depends on Y, X, Z, inference from the complete records is generally biased. This argument extends naturally to log-linear models for multi-category, rather than just binary, classifications.

Example 1.8 Odds ratio

Consider synthetic data relating binary outcome, Y, to binary X and a continuous Z. We generate $1 = 1, \dots, 20{,}000$ observations as follows:

$$x_i = \begin{cases} 1 & \text{for } i = 1, \dots, 10000 \\ 0 & \text{for } i = 10{,}001, \dots, 20{,}000 \end{cases},$$

$Z \sim N(0.5 \times (x_i - 0.5), 1)$ and

$$\text{logit } \Pr(Y_i = 1) = \beta_0 + \beta_1 X_i + \beta_2 Z_i. \tag{1.22}$$

where $(\beta_0, \beta_1, \beta_2) = (0,1,1)$.

We may consider either Z or X as the exposure. The relationship is confounded, so the unadjusted odds ratios are both biased.

Table 1.9 shows the mechanisms we consider, the bias we expect from a complete records analysis in a typical regression setting, and what we expect when using logistic regression (i.e. when we estimate log-odds ratios).

Notice that the bias does not depend on which variable has missing data, but instead on the mechanism which differentiates, or selects, the complete records from the rest of the sample. However, the appropriate approach for handling the bias (e.g. multiple imputation) will depend on the variable that is actually missing. For example, if the mechanism depends on Y and X is partially observed, data are MAR.

Table 1.9 Missing data mechanisms and bias on coefficient estimates with typical regression and logistic regression.

Mechanism depends on	Biased estimation of parameters using complete records					
	Typical regression			Logistic regression		
	Constant	Coef. of X	Coef. of Z	Constant	Coef. of X	Coef. of Z
Y	Yes	Yes	Yes	Yes	No	No
X	No	No	No	No	No	No
Z	No	No	No	No	No	No
X,Z	No	No	No	No	No	No
Y,X	Yes	Yes	Yes	Yes	Yes	No
Y,Z	Yes	Yes	Yes	Yes	No	Yes
Y,X,Z	Yes	Yes	Yes	Yes	Yes	Yes

Table 1.10 Empirical illustration of Table 1.9 using logistic regression.

Mechanism depends on	Probability of complete record	Estimated coefficients of		
		constant	X	Z
—	1	−0.03	1.03	1.03
Y	$[1 + \exp(-y)]^{-1}$	0.34	0.99	1.01
X	$[1 + \exp(-x)]^{-1}$	−0.04	1.02	1.00
Z	$[1 + \exp(-z)]^{-1}$	−0.03	0.96	1.03
X,Z	$[1 + \exp\{-(0.5(x - 0.5) + z)\}]^{-1}$	−0.04	0.98	1.03
Y,X	$[1 + \exp\{-(y + 2(x - 0.5))\}]^{-1}$	0.58	0.58	0.99
Y,Z	$[1 + \exp\{-(y + z)\}]^{-1}$	0.38	0.96	0.82
Y,X,Z	$[1 + \exp\{-(y + 2(x - 0.5) + z)\}]^{-1}$	0.63	0.58	0.81

The results of fitting the logistic regression (1.22) for the seven scenarios in Table 1.9 are shown in Table 1.10. We see that when missing data depends on Y, odds ratios for coefficients are only biased if in addition the missingness mechanism depends on the covariates associated with those coefficients. This is a consequence of the symmetry of the logistic link. □

1.6.5 Implication for linear regression

In fact, to first order approximation, the results for the odds ratio hold for linear and probit regression. In the case of linear regression of Y on X, Z, if missingness depends on Y and Z, and the correlation between Y and X is moderate ($|\rho| < 0.75$), then when we estimate the regression using the complete records (i) the largest bias occurs for the coefficient for Z, but (ii) the coefficient for X is markedly less (but not completely) unbiased. As above, this applies even if the actual missing values occur in the variable Z.

This gives an informal guide to the difference between the coefficient estimates we might expect from a complete records analysis and those from an MAR analysis (typically obtained using MI). Because analysis under MAR, whether by MI or another route, is relatively complex – and thus relatively more prone to error – this provides a useful check on the plausibility of the results.

Related to this, Daniel *et al.* (2011) and Lee *et al* (2023) explore how causal diagrams can be used to explore where bias due to missing data may arise. This can be a useful practical guide, both to whether it is worth using MI and to whether the results are consistent with the assumed missingness mechanisms.

Example 1.2 Youth Cohort Study *(ctd)*

Table 1.6 suggests that missing parental occupation depends on GCSE score and ethnicity. The above argument suggests that it is the coefficient for ethnicity that is most likely to be biased in the complete records analysis. After we have described MI for a range of data types, we return to this example at the end of Chapter 5. □

1.6.6 Subtle issues II: sub-sample ignorability

Little and Zhang (2011) describe the related idea of sub-sample ignorable likelihood. Suppose we have four (sets of) variables, and the pattern of missing data shown in Table 1.11. We now make the *sub-sample ignorability* assumption, that is:

1. within pattern 2, missing values of X and Y are MAR, and
2. within pattern 3, W is MNAR, with a mechanism that does not depend on Y.

Consider regression of Y on X, W, Z. Using the arguments developed earlier in this chapter, we see a complete records analysis will be invalid because for observations in pattern 2 the missingness mechanism includes the response. Also, an analysis assuming MAR using observations from all three patterns will also be invalid because data are MNAR in pattern 3. However, using only data from patterns 1 and 2, the

Table 1.11 Missing data patterns for sub-sample ignorable likelihood. As before, '✓' denotes observed, '·' missing, and now '✓·' denotes some observed and some missing.

Pattern	Variables				Number of observations
	Z	W	X	Y	
1	✓	✓	✓	✓	n_1
2	✓	✓	✓·	✓·	n_2
3	✓	·	✓·	✓·	n_3

missingness mechanism is MAR; therefore, an appropriate analysis (e.g. using multiple imputation) in this setting gives valid inference. In essence, this is a partial likelihood analysis, where the MNAR component is set aside.

Thus, by careful consideration of the reasons for missing data, we may be able to get valid inference via MI without recourse to a full MNAR analysis, even if a portion of the data are MNAR. A more formal justification of this approach is given by Little and Zhang (2011), who also present some simulations confirming the validity of inference when the sub-sample ignorability assumption holds, together with an example.

1.6.7 Summary: when restricting to complete records is valid

We have considered above the impact of various missing data mechanisms on regression analyses restricted to complete records. We note that restricting the regression analyses to complete records is generally invalid when the missingness mechanism includes the response. In establishing this, notice that what is important is the variables in the missingness mechanism, rather than variables with the missing data.

Consideration of the variables with missing data is important when deciding how to proceed beyond a complete records analysis. For instance, suppose the missingness mechanism depends on a covariate X and response Y but not on a third covariate, Z. Two possibilities are

1. Y partially observed, and
2. Z partially observed

In case (1) data are MNAR, so an analysis under the MAR assumption (e.g. using multiple imputation) will not be strictly valid. In case (2), we have a covariate MAR, so an analysis under MAR (e.g. using multiple imputation) will be valid.

In case (1), analysis under MAR may nevertheless be less biased, and the sensitivity to MNAR can be readily explored using multiple imputation, as we discuss in Chapter 10.

1.7 Summary

This chapter has introduced the central concepts involved in the analysis of partially observed data. These revolve around the 'reason for the data being missing' – more formally the missingness mechanism, and how this relates to the inferential question at hand. We have described Rubin's typology of missing data mechanisms (Rubin, 1976) and discussed these in the context of regression analysis.

We have stressed the importance of preliminary analysis of the data to identify the principal missingness patterns and elucidate plausible missingness mechanisms. Under particular missingness mechanisms, we have further explored when a regression restricted to complete records analysis is likely to give valid (if inefficient) inference.

The remainder of this book is concerned with using MI to obtain valid inference from partially observed data, predominantly not only under the assumption of MAR but also under the assumption of MNAR. However, there are a number of other methods that could be used to do this: for instance the EM algorithm or a full Bayesian analysis (Clayton *et al.*, 1998). Why MI? The answer is because it is practical for applied researchers in a wide range of settings. The EM algorithm for parameter estimates is not computationally straightforward in general. Further it does not yield standard errors; a further step is required for this. A full Bayesian analysis usually requires specialist programming and will often be computationally demanding, particularly if a range of models have to be fitted.

By contrast, using multiple imputation, the researcher has to specify an appropriate imputation model. Robust software exists in many packages to fit (or approximately fit) this model, from which a series of say K imputed datasets are created. Assuming this has been done properly, the researcher can then fit their model of interest to each of the K imputed datasets in turn, obtaining K point estimates and standard errors. These are combined for final inference using Rubin's rules (Rubin, 1987). These rules are relatively straightforward and perform remarkably well in a wide range of settings.

Thus, once the imputations have been created, inference proceeds using the usual software for fitting the model of interest to the complete records. It is therefore rapid. Further, analysis is not restricted to a single model: a range of models compatible with the imputation model can be explored. In addition, variables that the researcher does not wish to include in the model of interest (e.g. because they are on the causal path) can be included in the imputation model, improving both the plausibility of the MAR assumption and the imputation of the missing values.

Chapter 2 therefore introduces MI and sketches out its theoretical basis, illustrating this using linear regression. Subsequent chapters describe both algorithms for and application of MI to a broad range of social and medical data.

Exercises

1. This exercise is designed to check your understanding of the terms 'marginal' and 'conditional' inference, and the concepts of data being 'MCAR', 'MAR', and 'MNAR'. It can be done without a computer, but it is preferable to use the Excel spreadsheet `chapter1.xls` available from the companion website.

Suppose we have data from previous research on 100 patients' angina grade. We now wish to know these patients' systolic blood pressure. Suppose we write to them and ask them if their blood pressure is low, average, raised, or high.

Assume that the mean systolic blood pressure for the low, average, raised, and high groups is 115, 125, 135, and 145 mmHg, respectively, ignoring for now that such categorisation for a statistical analysis would be a bad idea. Beneath, in Table 1.12, is the truth; i.e. what we would see if each of the 100 patients replied to our letter, telling us whether their blood pressure was low, average, raised, or high.

These data are set up in the `Excel` data sheet `chapter1.xls`.

Table 1.12 Results of fictional blood pressure survey. Each cell is the tally of the number of people in that angina/blood pressure group.

	Blood pressure group (high is 4)				
Angina grade (3 is high)	Low 115 mmHg	Average 125 mmHg	Raised 135 mmHg	High 145 mmHg	Angina grade margin
1	15	5	3	2	25 people
2	10	15	15	10	50 people
3	2	5	6	12	25 people
Blood pressure margin	27	25	24	24	100

Average blood pressure: 129.5 mmHg

Open the file. You should see three tables. The top one shows the true data, as in Table 1.12. The second shows the probability of observing the data in each cell (initially set at 1, or 100%), and the third what we would *expect* to see, given the probabilities in the second table, together with some associated statistics.

Take a moment to familiarise yourself with the spreadsheet and, without changing anything, answer the following questions. These are designed to check your understanding of *marginal* and *conditional* distributions:

(a) What is the true overall average blood pressure?

(b) The true marginal angina grade distribution is 25% in band 1, 50% in band 2, and 25% in the third band. What is the true marginal blood pressure distribution?

(c) What is the *conditional* blood pressure distribution given angina grade 1? What is the conditional blood pressure distribution given angina grade 2? Are they different? Does this make sense?

We now explore the effect of changing the 'proportion observed', i.e. the second table in the spreadsheet, on the results.

(d) What does it mean when we say 'blood pressure is *missing completely at random*' (MCAR)?

(i) Change the proportions of observed data in the second table in the spreadsheet so that the 'observed data' (bottom table) are MCAR.

(*Hint:* if blood pressure is MCAR, then the proportion of observed data in each cell of the table cannot vary with either blood pressure or angina grade.)

(ii) Is the marginal estimate of the blood pressure distribution, calculated from the observed data (the third table in the spreadsheet), unbiased?

(iii) Is the overall average blood pressure estimate, calculated from the observed data, unbiased?

(e) What does it mean when we say 'blood pressure is *missing at random*' (MAR)?

(i) Change the proportions of observed data in the second table in the spreadsheet so that blood pressure is MAR given (fully observed) angina grade.

(ii) Is the marginal estimate of the blood pressure distribution, calculated from the observed data, unbiased?

(iii) Is the conditional estimate of blood pressure distribution given angina grade 2, calculated from the observed data, unbiased?

(iv) Is the conditional estimate of angina grade given blood pressure group 1, calculated from the observed data, unbiased?

(v) Is the 'MAR estimator' (bottom of spreadsheet) unbiased? Write down the formula used in this 'MAR estimator' and make sure you understand and can explain its rationale.

(f) What does it mean when we say 'blood pressure is *missing not at random*' (MNAR)? (sometimes 'not missing at random' is used instead).

(i) Change the proportions of observed data in the second table in the spreadsheet so that data are MNAR.

(ii) Is the marginal estimate of then blood pressure distribution, calculated from the observed data, unbiased?

(iii) Is the conditional estimate of the blood pressure distribution given angina grade 2, calculated from the observed data, unbiased?

(iv) Can you obtain an unbiased estimate of the overall average blood pressure?

(g) Change the proportions of observed data in the second table in the spreadsheet so that the reason for missing blood pressure ONLY depends on blood pressure (not angina grade). Is the estimate from the data of the conditional distribution of angina grade given blood pressure unbiased?

(h) On the basis of the observed data, can you decide if the missing data are MCAR, MAR, or MNAR? Why/why not? Can you set up a missing data mechanism where the data pattern of observed data is consistent with MCAR, but the data are in fact MNAR?

(i) What are the implications for the regression of a variable Y on a variable X when the reason for missing some values of X only depends on the values of X?

2. Generate your own data similar to Figure 1.2. Verify (i) empirically and (ii) theoretically that if income data are MAR given job type, the distribution of income given job type in is unbiased in the complete records, but the distribution of job type given income is biased.

3. Verify the results given in equations (1.12) and (1.13)

4. Sub-sample ignorability: In what practical settings might the sub-sample ignorability assumption be valid? By considering a simple situation, show that the sub-sample ignorable likelihood is an example of a partial likelihood.

2

The multiple imputation procedure and its justification

2.1 Introduction

In this chapter, we set out the multiple imputation (MI) procedure, initially from an intuitive standpoint in Section 2.2. We then give a more theoretical outline of MI from a Bayesian perspective in Sections 2.3 and 2.4, before going on to consider its frequentist properties in so-called *congenial* (in the sense defined below) settings in Section 2.5.

We discuss the choice of the number of imputations in Section 2.6. Section 2.7 considers some simple examples, deriving the frequentist variance of the MI estimator and relating it to the estimate obtained using Rubin's MI variance formula. More general settings, where the imputation model and substantive model are *uncongenial*, are discussed in Section 2.8. In Section 2.9 we discuss how to construct congenial imputation models. We conclude with a discussion in Section 2.10.

We do not provide a rigorous development. Instead, our aim is to highlight the main steps involved in justifying the MI procedure, together with how, and under what assumptions, these can be established. References are given for readers who wish to follow up the technical details. The principal goal is to draw attention to the aspects of the theoretical justification that have a bearing on the practical performance of MI, in particular to the several approximations that are employed. Understanding the role of these approximations sheds light on why MI works better in some settings than others, and on what we may do to improve its performance.

Rubin's original justification for MI is set out in Chapters 2–4 of Rubin (1987). Much of this is couched in the formalism of sample surveys from finite populations, in particular in terms of design (or randomization) based theory, although he extends the

Multiple Imputation and its Application, Second Edition.
James R. Carpenter, Jonathan W. Bartlett, Tim P. Morris, Angela M. Wood, Matteo Quartagno and Michael G. Kenward.

ideas to model-based inference. This was a natural framework for Rubin's exposition. At that time, the primary intended application was to missing data in surveys so that the aim was estimation of unknown observables rather than the unknown parameters of posited statistical models.

In this book, we are primarily concerned with the analysis of data arising from randomised experiments or from observational studies that do not arise from a classical survey design, and for which the analysis will involve conventional model-based techniques in a frequentist paradigm. We, therefore, focus on the model-based view of MI. In this context, in Section 2.8.3, we consider the pair of papers by Wang and Robins (1998) and Robins and Wang (2000), which together with Nielsen (2003) and Xie and Meng (2017), provide important additional insights on the justification of the MI variance rules in a broad range of settings. These are highly technical papers, and a more accessible exposition of some of this material is given in Chapter 14 of Tsiatis (2006).

While it is clear that the inference from an MI procedure may be improved in a number of settings, we will nevertheless see that the overarching picture is one of the remarkable robustness of the MI procedure, especially if appropriate consideration is given to choice of the imputation model (see Chapter 14). As Schafer (1999b) puts it, 'MI is not the only principled method for handling missing values, nor is it necessarily the best for any given problem, but it is often more practicable and close to the "best" method for a given problem', making it attractive.

2.2 Intuitive outline of the MI procedure

Suppose we have two continuous variables, $(\mathbf{Y}_1, \mathbf{Y}_2)$, and wish to estimate the regression of $\mathbf{Y}_1$ on $\mathbf{Y}_2$, but $\mathbf{Y}_2$ is missing at random (MAR) dependent on $\mathbf{Y}_1$. Then, as discussed in Section 1.7, the regression coefficients estimated from the complete records will be biased.

However, because $\mathbf{Y}_2$ is MAR given $\mathbf{Y}_1$, the complete records give valid, efficient inference for the regression of $\mathbf{Y}_2$ on $\mathbf{Y}_1$. This suggests the following procedure:

1. Fit the regression of $\mathbf{Y}_2$ on $\mathbf{Y}_1$ to the complete records:
$$Y_{i,2} = \alpha_0 + \alpha_1 Y_{i,1} + e_i, \quad e_i \overset{i.i.d.}{\sim} N(0, \sigma^2_{2|1}), \tag{2.1}$$
obtaining $\hat{\alpha}_0, \hat{\alpha}_1, \hat{\sigma}^2_{2|1}$.
2. Impute the missing values of $\mathbf{Y}_2$ using (2.1), obtaining a 'completed' dataset
3. Fit the substantive model, here the regression of $\mathbf{Y}_1$ on $\mathbf{Y}_2$, to the 'completed' data from step 2.

The problem with this strategy is that in step 3, the imputed values are given the same status as the actual observed values in fitting the substantive model. Further, as emphasised in Chapter 1, this strategy does not take into account that we can never recover the missing data; the best we can do is to estimate the distribution of the missing data given the observed, under a specific assumption about the missingness mechanism. This distribution is not represented by a single draw from the distribution of the missing data given the observed, especially one taken assuming the estimated values of $\alpha_0, \alpha_1, \sigma^2_{2|1}$ are known without error.

Instead, we need to draw multiple times from the distribution of the missing data given the observed, taking full account of the uncertainty, to create say K imputed, i.e. 'complete' datasets. As we shall see later, we need these draws to be (at least approximately) Bayesian for Rubin's variance formula to work. Then, if we fit our substantive model to each of these, the K results together reflect the additional uncertainty induced by the missing data, while correcting the bias caused by the missing data. Rubin's rules are a general procedure for summarising these K results to obtain point estimates, associated estimates of variance, and to construct confidence intervals and statistical tests.

Given a general data matrix $\mathbf{Y}$, write $\mathbf{Y}_O$ for the observed data and $\mathbf{Y}_M$ for the missing data. The general MI procedure is

1. For $k = 1, \dots, K$, taking full account of the uncertainty, impute each missing value from the posterior predictive distribution of the missing data given the observed, $f(\mathbf{Y}_M|\mathbf{Y}_O)$, to give K 'completed' (imputed) datasets.

2. Fit the substantive model to the kth imputed data set (which now contains no missing values), $k = 1, \dots, K$. This gives K estimates of the parameters of the substantive model, say $\hat{\boldsymbol{\beta}}_k$, and K estimates of their variance, $\widehat{\text{Var}}(\hat{\boldsymbol{\beta}}_k)_k$.

3. Combine these for inference using Rubin's rules.

We elaborate step 1 in detail in a simple setting in the worked example below, and focus on step 3.

We denoted the vector of parameters in our substantive model by $\boldsymbol{\beta}$, and in general, we may wish to apply Rubin's rules to all, or part, of this parameter vector. At this point, suppose we are interested in a scalar element which we denote by β with associated variance σ^2. Let the estimates from the imputed dataset k, obtained by fitting the substantive model to the 'completed' dataset exactly as we would do if there were no missing data, be $\hat{\beta}_k$, $\hat{\sigma}^2_k$.

Rubin's rules for inference are as follows: The MI estimate of β is

$$\hat{\beta}_{MI} = \frac{1}{K}\sum_{k=1}^{K}\hat{\beta}_k, \tag{2.2}$$

with variance

$$\hat{V}_{MI} = \hat{W} + \left(1 + \frac{1}{K}\right)\hat{B}, \tag{2.3}$$

where

$$\hat{W} = \frac{1}{K}\sum_{k=1}^{K}\hat{\sigma}^2_k \quad \text{and} \quad \hat{B} = \frac{1}{K-1}\sum_{k=1}^{K}(\hat{\beta}_k - \hat{\beta}_{MI})^2.$$

To test the hypotheses $\beta = \beta^0$, we refer

$$T = \frac{\hat{\beta}_{MI} - \beta^0}{\sqrt{\hat{V}_{MI}}}$$

to a t-distribution with v degrees of freedom, where

$$v = (K-1)\left[1 + \frac{\widehat{W}}{(1+1/K)\widehat{B}}\right]^2. \tag{2.4}$$

We use quantiles of the t_v distribution to construct confidence intervals for $\hat{\beta}_{MI}$.

Recall that the *information* on a parameter estimate is defined as the reciprocal of its variance; thus, if the variance is small (because the parameter is precisely estimated) the information about the parameter value is large. Denote the information about β in the complete data (were it is available) as I_C, and the information in the partially observed data as I_O. Then the percentage of information about β lost due to missing data is

$$\left(\frac{I_C - I_O}{I_C}\right) \times 100\%. \tag{2.5}$$

When there are no missing observations, then all the 'imputed' datasets are identical, so (2.5) is zero; when all observations are missing, as there is no information in the 'partially observed' data, it is 1.

From the definition of information, it follows that the information about β in the partially observed data is $I_O = 1/\widehat{V}_{MI}$. A reasonable estimate of the information in the complete data is $I_C = 1/\widehat{W}$, which intuitively makes sense as it is equal to (2.3) when the between-imputation variance is 0. Thus, (2.5) could be estimated by

$$\left(\frac{(1+1/K)\widehat{B}}{\widehat{W} + (1+1/K)\widehat{B}}\right) \times 100\%. \tag{2.6}$$

However, $\widehat{B}$ is poorly estimated and occurs in the denominator. Rubin (1987), p. 93 points out that a more accurate estimate of (2.5) is obtained by noting that minus the average second derivative of the log of the t_v distribution (i.e. the information) is $(v+1)\{(v+3)(\widehat{W} + (1+1/K)\widehat{B})\}^{-1}$. If, as above, we estimate the information in the complete data by $\widehat{W}^{-1}$, then a better estimate of the fraction of missing information is

$$\frac{\widehat{W}^{-1} - (v+1)\{(v+3)(\widehat{W} + (1+1/K)\widehat{B})\}^{-1}}{\widehat{W}^{-1}} = \frac{r + 2/(v+3)}{1+r}, \tag{2.7}$$

where

$$r = \frac{(1+1/K)\widehat{B}}{\widehat{W}}.$$

This is the expression which many software packages calculate.

Example 2.1 Simple example of MI for a marginal mean

Let $X_i = i$, $1 = 1, \ldots, 10$ and generate Y as

$$Y_i = 1 + X_i + e_i, \quad e_i \overset{i.i.d.}{\sim} N(0,1).$$

Table 2.1 Simple example of MI; imputed values shown in bold.

	Y	Y_O	Values imputed in imputation			
			1	2	3	4
	2.23	2.23	2.23	2.23	2.23	2.23
	3.72	3.72	3.72	3.72	3.72	3.72
	3.54	3.54	3.54	3.54	3.54	3.54
	6.09	6.09	6.09	6.09	6.09	6.09
	6.53	6.53	6.53	6.53	6.53	6.53
	5.63	.	**7.08**	**8.13**	**6.98**	**7.08**
	8.28	8.28	8.28	8.28	8.28	8.28
	10.64	.	**8.68**	**9.25**	**9.68**	**10.49**
	10.74	10.74	10.74	10.74	10.74	10.74
	10.58	.	**10.87**	**10.86**	**11.74**	**13.96**
Mean	6.80	5.88	6.78	6.94	6.95	7.27
SE	1.00	1.13	0.94	0.96	1.01	1.16

Suppose we wish to estimate the marginal mean of Y, but that we make Y MAR dependent on X, so that around half the observations on Y are missing if $X > 5$.

The resulting full set of 10 observations on Y are shown in the leftmost column of Table 2.1, and the observed values are shown in the second column. We see that the mean of the observed values is markedly below that of the full set of values, and the standard error is increased.

To impute the missing values, taking full account of the uncertainty, our imputation model is going to be the regression of Y on X,

$$Y_i = \beta_0 + \beta_1 X_i + e_i, \quad e_i \overset{i.i.d.}{\sim} N(0, \sigma^2).$$

Suppose we fit the model by least squares in the usual way, obtaining estimates $\hat{\beta}_0, \hat{\beta}_1, \hat{\sigma}^2$, and the estimated residuals $\hat{e}_i$, for $i \in 1, \dots, n$ the subjects with Y observed. Consider the Bayesian posterior distribution (see Appendix A) of $\beta_0, \beta_1, \sigma^2$, and choose priors so this is equivalent to the usual frequentist sampling distribution, so that a draw from the observed data posterior distribution of σ^2 can be obtained as

$$\frac{\sum_{i=1}^{n} \hat{e}_i^2}{(n-2)X^2}, \tag{2.8}$$

where $X^2 \sim \chi^2_{n-2}$, and

$$\begin{pmatrix} \beta_0 \\ \beta_1 \end{pmatrix} \sim N_2 \left[\begin{pmatrix} \hat{\beta}_1 \\ \hat{\beta}_2 \end{pmatrix}, \hat{\sigma}^2 \begin{pmatrix} n & \sum_{i=1}^{n} X_i \\ \sum_{i=1}^{n} X_i & \sum_{i=1}^{n} X_i^2 \end{pmatrix}^{-1} \right]. \tag{2.9}$$

To create the $K = 4$ imputed datasets shown in Table 2.1, we proceed as follows: for $k = 1, \dots, 4$:

1. draw σ_k^{2*} by drawing X^2 from χ^2_{n-2} and plugging into (2.8);
2. with $\sigma^2 = \sigma_k^{2*}$, draw $(\beta^*_{0,k}, \beta^*_{1,k})$ from distribution (2.9);
3. for each of the missing observations, impute them as

$$Y_{i,k} = \beta^*_{0,k} + \beta^*_{1,k} X_i + e^*_{i,k}, \quad e^*_{i,k} \sim N(0, \sigma_k^{2*}).$$

Notice that for imputation k, we draw from the posterior (estimated) distribution of the parameters and then impute the data; to create the second imputation, we draw new parameters and then impute the data. This is a vital part of the process, as it ensures that the imputed data is a Bayesian draw from the distribution of the missing data given the observed data.

Using this procedure, we obtain the four imputed datasets shown in the right columns of Table 2.1, with the imputed values shown in bold. Our substantive model is simply the marginal mean of $\mathbf{Y}$. The bottom two rows of Table 2.1 shows this for the full data, the observed data, and for each of the imputed datasets, together with the associated standard errors.

From (2.2), the MI estimate of the marginal mean is

$$(6.78 + 6.94 + 6.95 + 7.27)/4 = 6.99.$$

From (2.3), to calculate its standard error, we first calculate

$$\widehat{W} = (0.94^2 + 0.96^2 + 1.01^2 + 1.16^2)/4 = 1.042725,$$

and

$$\begin{aligned} \widehat{B} &= \{(6.78 - 6.99)^2 + (6.94 - 6.99)^2 + (6.95 - 6.99)^2 + (7.27 - 6.99)^2\}/3 \\ &= 0.0422, \end{aligned}$$

so that the standard error is

$$\sqrt{\widehat{V}_{MI}} = \sqrt{1.042725 + [(1 + 1/4) \times 0.0422]} = 1.05.$$

In this very simple setting, MI has reduced the bias, and the standard error of the imputation estimate is smaller than that of the complete records analysis while being larger than that of the original, full data (as must be the case). This is typical of what we should see in more general settings, subject to our (untestable) assumptions about the missingness mechanism and an appropriate choice of imputation model.

Notice that $\widehat{B}$ is an order of magnitude less than $\widehat{W}$. This will typically be the case and plays a role in some of the approximations later on.

If desired, we could calculate a confidence interval for the MI estimate of the mean using the t-distribution with degrees of freedom given by (2.4). From (2.6), we can calculate the percentage of missing information in this example as

$100 \times (0.0422/1.05^2) = 3.8\%$. That is, we estimate that we lost 3.8% of information compared to the hypothetical information we would have had with no missing data. □

There are three central points that make the MI procedure particularly attractive:

1. Rubin's rules are generic, requiring no substantive model specific or imputation-model specific calculations. This is a key attraction of MI.
2. MI gives good frequentist properties for a remarkably small number of imputations.
3. Rubin's rules should be applied to estimators which are normally (or at least asymptotically normally) distributed. For example for logistic regression, we apply them on the log-odds ratio scale, not the odds-ratio scale, and analogously for other generalised linear models and hazard ratios from survival analysis.

Key to MI is that, under the assumed missingness mechanism, we can obtain a valid estimate of the parameters of the imputation model from the observed data. Typically, assuming MAR, this is achieved by the multivariate regression of the partially observed variables on the fully observed ones or procedures that are approximately equivalent to this.

A key advantage of MI is that it can be applied in the same way whether the missing data are in the response of our substantive model, or its covariates, or any mixture of both. Further, MI lends itself to semi-automatic implementation. Given a substantive model, the user only has to specify the imputation model, and – given a method to fit this and impute the missing data – the computer can generate the imputed datasets, fit the substantive model to each and combine the results for inference using Rubin's rules. In practice, the greatest scope for error is inappropriate specification of the imputation model.

In the next sections, we consider the generic MI procedure from a more theoretical standpoint and then go on to outline the steps required for its justification.

2.3 The generic MI procedure

Suppose that our substantive scientific question means we are faced with a conventional estimation problem for a statistical model with a $(p \times 1)$ dimensional parameter vector $\boldsymbol{\beta}$. We call this the *substantive* model, and the aim is to make valid inferences about some or all of the elements of $\boldsymbol{\beta}$ from partially observed data. We assume that if no data were missing, so the data are *complete*, a consistent estimator of $\boldsymbol{\beta}$ is obtained as the solution to the estimating equation

$$\sum_{i=1}^{n} \mathbf{U}_i(\hat{\boldsymbol{\beta}}; \mathbf{Y}_i) = \mathbf{U}(\hat{\boldsymbol{\beta}}; \mathbf{Y}) = \mathbf{0}, \tag{2.10}$$

where the data represented by $\mathbf{Y}$ include both the outcome variable and covariates. Given complete data, we can calculate a consistent estimator of the covariance matrix of $\widehat{\boldsymbol{\beta}}$, denoted $\text{Var}(\widehat{\boldsymbol{\beta}})$, in the standard manner.

Suppose now that some data are missing and define $\mathbf{R}$ to be the matrix of binary indicator random variables, taking the value 0 if the corresponding element of $\mathbf{Y}$ is missing and 1 otherwise. Denote by $\mathbf{Y}_M$, the set of elements of $\mathbf{Y}$ that are missing, i.e. for which the corresponding element of $\mathbf{R}$ is zero. The complement of $\mathbf{Y}_M$ in $\mathbf{Y}$ is the observed data denoted by $\mathbf{Y}_O$. A consistent estimator of $\boldsymbol{\beta}$ from the observed (incomplete) data can then be obtained from the estimating equation:

$$\mathrm{E}_{f(\mathbf{Y}_M|\mathbf{Y}_O,\mathbf{R})}\{\mathbf{U}(\widehat{\boldsymbol{\beta}};\mathbf{Y}_O,\mathbf{Y}_M)\} = \mathbf{0}. \tag{2.11}$$

For the special case that $\mathbf{U}(\cdot)$ in (2.10) is the likelihood score function with the complete data, then the LHS of (2.11) similarly is the score function for the observed data. We call the conditional distribution over which the expectation is taken in (2.11), $f(\mathbf{Y}_M|\mathbf{Y}_O,\mathbf{R})$ the *conditional predictive distribution* of the missing data. Under the assumption of MAR , it is not necessary to condition on the missingness indicator, so $f(\mathbf{Y}_M|\mathbf{Y}_O,\mathbf{R}) = f(\mathbf{Y}_M|\mathbf{Y}_O)$.

A consistent estimator of the covariance matrix of $\widehat{\boldsymbol{\beta}}$ from (2.11) is obtained using Louis's formula (Louis, 1982) which expresses the information matrix for the observed data in terms of expectations over complete data quantities:

$$I_O(\boldsymbol{\beta}) = I_C(\boldsymbol{\beta}) - [\mathrm{E}\{\mathbf{U}(\widehat{\boldsymbol{\beta}};\mathbf{Y})\mathbf{U}(\widehat{\boldsymbol{\beta}};\mathbf{Y})^T\} - \mathrm{E}\{\mathbf{U}(\widehat{\boldsymbol{\beta}};\mathbf{Y})\}\mathrm{E}\{\mathbf{U}(\widehat{\boldsymbol{\beta}};\mathbf{Y})\}^T], \tag{2.12}$$

that is, the observed information is the complete information minus the missing information ($I_C(\cdot)$ is the information matrix based on the complete data). All expectations are taken over the conditional predictive distribution $f(\mathbf{Y}_M \mid \mathbf{Y}_O, \mathbf{R})$. Although (2.11) and (2.12) provide a general scheme for dealing with standard regression models when data are missing, their practical value varies greatly from problem to problem. The expectations require the calculation of so-called *incomplete data* quantities for which there do not exist sufficiently straightforward and general methods of calculation. In such settings, one-off solutions, often quite complex, are required. Away from standard regression problems, the situation may be even more intractable.

One view of MI is that it provides an alternative, indirect route, to solving this problem which, most importantly, uses in the analysis phase only *complete data* quantities, i.e. those that arise in the solution to (2.10) and the accompanying estimator of precision. In applications, such quantities are typically readily available from model fitting software. Crudely stated, MI reverses the order of expectation and solution in (2.11). Thus, the idea is to repeatedly:

1. draw $\mathbf{Y}_M^*$ from $f(\mathbf{Y}_M|\mathbf{Y}_O,\mathbf{R})$;
2. solve $\mathbf{U}(\beta;\mathbf{Y}_M^*,\mathbf{Y}_O) = \mathbf{0}$;

and combine the results in some way for inference.

Each $\mathbf{Y}_M^*$ is a *Bayesian* draw from the conditional predictive distribution of the missing observation, made in such a way that the set of imputations properly represent the information about the missing values that is contained in the observed data for the chosen model. Each draw of $\mathbf{Y}_M^*$ taken with $\mathbf{Y}_O$ gives a 'completed' dataset. Each of these is analysed using the method that would have been applied had no data been missing. The model used to produce the imputations, that is, to represent the conditional predictive distribution of the missing given the observed data, is called the *imputation* model. One great strength of the MI procedure is that these two models, substantive and imputation, can be fitted quite separately, and also considered, to some extent, separately – although certain relationships between them do need to be considered as we will see in Section 2.8.3 and throughout the rest of the book.

Thus, MI involves three distinct tasks:

1. The missing values are filled in K times to generate K complete datasets.
2. The K complete datasets are analyzed by using standard, complete data, procedures.
3. The results from the K analyses are combined to produce a single MI estimator and to draw inferences.

In more detail, the missing data are replaced by their corresponding imputation samples, producing K completed datasets. Denoting by $\widehat{\boldsymbol{\beta}}_k$ and $\widehat{\mathbf{V}}_k$ the estimate of $\boldsymbol{\beta}$ and its covariance matrix from the kth completed dataset, $k \in (1, \dots, K)$, the MI estimate of $\boldsymbol{\beta}$ is the simple average of the estimates:

$$\widehat{\boldsymbol{\beta}}_{MI} = \frac{1}{K}\sum_{k=1}^{K}\widehat{\boldsymbol{\beta}}_k. \tag{2.13}$$

We also need a measure of precision for $\widehat{\boldsymbol{\beta}}_{MI}$ that properly reflects the between- and within-imputation variance. Rubin (1987) provides the following simple expression for the covariance matrix of $\widehat{\boldsymbol{\beta}}_{MI}$. It can be applied very generally and uses only complete data quantities. Define

$$\widehat{\mathbf{W}} = \frac{1}{K}\sum_{k=1}^{K}\widehat{\mathbf{V}}_k \tag{2.14}$$

to be the average within-imputation covariance matrix, and

$$\widehat{\mathbf{B}} = \frac{1}{K-1}\sum_{k=1}^{K}(\widehat{\boldsymbol{\beta}}_k - \widehat{\boldsymbol{\beta}}_{MI})(\widehat{\boldsymbol{\beta}}_k - \widehat{\boldsymbol{\beta}}_{MI})^T \tag{2.15}$$

to be the between-imputation covariance matrix of $\widehat{\boldsymbol{\beta}}_k$. Then an estimate of the covariance matrix of $\widehat{\boldsymbol{\beta}}_{MI}$ is given by

$$\widehat{\mathbf{V}}_{MI} = \widehat{\mathbf{W}} + \left(1 + \frac{1}{K}\right)\widehat{\mathbf{B}}. \tag{2.16}$$

Apart from an adjustment of $1/K$ to accommodate the finite number of imputations used, this is a very straightforward combination of between- and within-imputation variability.

2.4 Bayesian justification of MI

Assume MAR and suppose we obtain K imputed datasets from a Bayesian predictive distribution $f(\mathbf{Y}_M|\mathbf{Y}_O)$, fit our substantive model to each and combine the results for inference using Rubin's rules.

Separate to this, assume that there exists a Bayesian model for the data for which

1. the posterior distribution of $\boldsymbol{\beta}$ given complete data has mean and variance identical to the point estimate and its variance estimate returned by fitting our substantive model to the complete data, and
2. the predictive distribution of $\mathbf{Y}_M|\mathbf{Y}_O$ matches the predictive distribution used by the imputation model.

If this is the case, we say the imputation model and the substantive model are congenial, in the sense introduced by Meng (1994), noting that Meng's original definition extends to broader settings.

In the Bayesian framework, the missing data, $\mathbf{Y}_M$, is equivalent to a set of additional parameters. Suppressing the parameters of the distribution of the observed data, $\mathbf{Y}_O$, the posterior distribution is therefore

$$f(\mathbf{Y}_M, \boldsymbol{\beta} \mid \mathbf{Y}_O).$$

Our focus is on $\boldsymbol{\beta}$, with $\mathbf{Y}_M$ being regarded as a nuisance. The posterior can be partitioned as follows:

$$f(\boldsymbol{\beta}, \mathbf{Y}_M \mid \mathbf{Y}_O) = f(\mathbf{Y}_M \mid \mathbf{Y}_O) f(\boldsymbol{\beta} \mid \mathbf{Y}_M, \mathbf{Y}_O),$$

so that the marginal posterior for $\boldsymbol{\beta}$ can be written

$$f(\boldsymbol{\beta} \mid \mathbf{Y}_O) = \mathrm{E}_{f(\mathbf{Y}_M|\mathbf{Y}_O)}\{f(\boldsymbol{\beta} \mid \mathbf{Y}_M, \mathbf{Y}_O)\}.$$

In particular, under regularity conditions which permit the order of integration to be exchanged, the posterior mean and variance for $\boldsymbol{\beta}$ can be expressed as

$$\mathrm{E}(\boldsymbol{\beta} \mid \mathbf{Y}_O) = \mathrm{E}_{f(\mathbf{Y}_M|\mathbf{Y}_O)}\{\mathrm{E}_{f(\boldsymbol{\beta}|\mathbf{Y}_M,\mathbf{Y}_O)}(\boldsymbol{\beta})\} \tag{2.17}$$

$$\begin{aligned}\mathrm{Var}(\boldsymbol{\beta} \mid \mathbf{Y}_O) = {} & \mathrm{E}_{f(\mathbf{Y}_M|\mathbf{Y}_O)}\{\mathrm{Var}_{f(\boldsymbol{\beta}|\mathbf{Y}_M,\mathbf{Y}_O)}(\boldsymbol{\beta})\} \\ & + \mathrm{Var}_{f(\mathbf{Y}_M|\mathbf{Y}_O)}\{\mathrm{E}_{f(\boldsymbol{\beta}|\mathbf{Y}_M,\mathbf{Y}_O)}(\boldsymbol{\beta})\}.\end{aligned} \tag{2.18}$$

The posterior mean and variance can then be approximated empirically. Let $\mathbf{Y}^*_{M,k}$ $k = 1, \ldots, K$, be draws from the Bayesian predictive distribution $f(\mathbf{Y}_M|\ \mathbf{Y}_O)$. Then, from (2.17)

$$\mathrm{E}(\boldsymbol{\beta} \mid \mathbf{Y}_O) \simeq \frac{1}{K}\sum_{k=1}^{K}\{\mathrm{E}_{f(\boldsymbol{\beta}|\mathbf{Y}^*_{M,k},\mathbf{Y}_O)}(\boldsymbol{\beta})\} = \hat{\boldsymbol{\beta}},$$

and from (2.3),

$$\text{Var}(\boldsymbol{\beta} \mid \mathbf{Y}_O) \simeq \frac{1}{K} \sum_{k=1}^{K} \text{Var}_{f(\boldsymbol{\beta}|\mathbf{Y}^*_{M,k},\mathbf{Y}_O)}(\boldsymbol{\beta})$$

$$+ \frac{1}{K-1} \sum_{j=1}^{K} \{\text{E}_{f(\boldsymbol{\beta}|\mathbf{Y}^*_{M,k},\mathbf{Y}_O)}(\boldsymbol{\beta}) - \widehat{\boldsymbol{\beta}}\}\{\text{E}_{f(\boldsymbol{\beta}|\mathbf{Y}^*_{M,k},\mathbf{Y}_O)}(\boldsymbol{\beta}) - \widehat{\boldsymbol{\beta}}\}^T.$$

To use this in practice, we need both Bayesian draws from the conditional predictive distribution, and a short cut to obtain the mean and variance of $\boldsymbol{\beta}$ over $f(\boldsymbol{\beta}|\mathbf{Y}_{M,k}, \mathbf{Y}_O)$. Without the latter, MI gains almost nothing in simplicity over a full Bayesian analysis. Thus, MI assumes that these can be approximated sufficiently well by the solution, and accompanying variance estimator, by solving the full data estimating equations (i.e. fitting the substantive model to the imputed data set in the standard way).

When the full data estimating equations are likelihood score equations this approximation follows from the asymptotic property of joint Bayesian posteriors known as the Bernstein–von-Mises theorem (Gelman *et al.*, 1995). This states that, under standard regularity conditions, as the sample size n increases, the joint posterior distribution tends to a multivariate normal. Moreover, as the sample size increases, the likelihood dominates the prior distribution and so the mode of the likelihood (the maximum likelihood estimator) and the inverse of the curvature of the likelihood (the information based covariance matrix) can be used to obtain the required moments. Additionally, the fact that after marginalising over $\mathbf{Y}_M$ only a relatively small marginal component of the full posterior is being approximated (i.e. that for $\boldsymbol{\beta}$, or more typically a subset of the elements of $\boldsymbol{\beta}$) potentially further improves the normal approximation.

We reiterate that two approximations are being used:

1. the asymptotic multivariate normal for the full data posterior, and
2. the estimator and covariance matrix from the full data estimating equations for the first two moments of this posterior.

Only when the substantive model gives rise to likelihood score equations does the second approximation have its usual justification. As usual, the approximations are not scale invariant. Thus, a scale should be chosen for the relevant elements of $\boldsymbol{\beta}$ that leads to the best approximation. For example quantities like odds-ratios and hazard-ratios should be log-transformed before the MI procedure is applied. In the same vein, Gelman *et al.* (1995) p. 95–96 give an instructive example on the variance of a normal distribution, showing that a log transformation leads to a better approximation than the original scale.

The above discussion makes it clear why we need to impute from the full Bayesian predictive distribution. In the congenial setting, provided we have a method for generating Bayesian posterior draws from the conditional predictive distribution of the missing data, we see that MI can be viewed as a three-step approximation to a full Bayesian analysis, in which, in the second part, we exploit the speed of computational algorithms for finding maximum likelihood estimates.

2.5 Frequentist inference

We now briefly discuss the additional considerations necessary for frequentist inference about $\boldsymbol{\beta}$, i.e. a valid estimate of the frequentist variance, the sampling distribution of pivotal quantities, and the resulting confidence intervals and tests. As before, we assume that the imputation model and substantive model are congenial.

We begin by considering inference for a single parameter, β, from the parameter vector $\boldsymbol{\beta}$. We suppose we have K imputations drawn from the Bayesian predictive distribution, resulting in K completed datasets, and fitted the substantive model to each, giving estimates $\hat{\beta}_k$, $k = 1, \dots, K$, with associated standard errors $\hat{\sigma}_k$ (of $\hat{\beta}_k$).

We assume that the sample size, n, is large enough that the approximations described in the previous section hold. Then the mean of $\widehat{\beta}_k$ is a consistent estimator of β, so we can set

$$\widehat{\beta}_{MI} = \frac{1}{K}\sum_{i=1}^{K} \widehat{\beta}_k.$$

We also calculate the terms

$$\widehat{B} = \frac{1}{K-1}\sum_{k=1}^{K} (\hat{\beta}_k - \hat{\beta}_{MI})^2,$$

which is the sample variance of $\hat{\beta}_k$ around $\hat{\beta}_{MI}$ and

$$\widehat{W} = \frac{1}{K}\sum_{k=1}^{K} \hat{\sigma}_k^2.$$

2.5.1 Large number of imputations

Suppose first that K is large, i.e. we have carried out a large number of imputations. Then $\widehat{W}$ will be a precise estimator of the first term in (2.3), and likewise $\widehat{B}$ will be a precise estimator of the second term in (2.3), so that, for practical purposes, denoting $\text{Var}(\hat{\beta}_{MI})$ by V_{MI}, we have

$$\widehat{V}_{MI} = \widehat{B} + \widehat{W}. \tag{2.19}$$

Implicit in the assumptions in the previous section is that n is large enough for $\hat{\beta}$ to be normally distributed if there are no missing data. Therefore, we can interpret the Bayesian posterior from a frequentist viewpoint, giving

$$\hat{\beta}_{MI} \sim N(\beta, \widehat{B} + \widehat{W}).$$

Thus, we can test the hypothesis that $\beta = \beta_0$ by comparing

$$\frac{\hat{\beta}_{MI} - \hat{\beta}_0}{\sqrt{\widehat{V}_{MI}}}$$

to a standard normal distribution, and construct a $100(1-\alpha)\%$ confidence interval as

$$(\hat{\beta}_{MI} - z_{1-\alpha/2}\sqrt{\hat{V}_{MI}},\ \hat{\beta}_{MI} - z_{\alpha/2}\sqrt{\hat{V}_{MI}}),$$

where z is standard normal and $\Pr(z_\alpha < \alpha) = \alpha$.

In practice, of course, we need to know if K is large enough for the above results to hold; the development below will enable us to judge this.

2.5.2 Small number of imputations

We suppose now that, as may often be the case, we have carried out a relatively small number of imputations, say $K = 5$. How should we modify the above procedure? We first show that an additional term is needed in the variance formula (2.19), and then that for inference we need to replace the normal reference distribution by a t distribution. Our arguments are not rigorous; for more details see Rubin (1987) p. 87–93.

The idea is to condition the results for infinitely large K – essentially the results above – on the first few imputations. We therefore define

$$\hat{\beta}_{MI,\infty} = \lim_{K\to\infty} \frac{1}{K}\sum_{k=1}^{K} \hat{\beta}_k = \lim_{K\to\infty} \hat{\beta}_{MI}$$

$$\hat{B}_\infty = \lim_{K\to\infty} \frac{1}{K-1}\sum_{k=1}^{K} (\hat{\beta}_k - \overline{\beta}_K)^2, \text{ where } \overline{\beta}_K = \frac{1}{K}\sum_{k=1}^{K} \hat{\beta}_k$$

and

$$\hat{W}_\infty = \lim_{K\to\infty} \frac{1}{K}\sum_{k=1}^{K} \hat{\sigma}_k^2.$$

The posterior for β is

$$\beta \sim N(\hat{\beta}_\infty, \hat{B}_\infty + \hat{W}_\infty). \tag{2.20}$$

Now suppose that we have only performed a finite number K of imputations. As above, denote the average of the corresponding K estimates of β by $\overline{\beta}_K$. The expected value of $\overline{\beta}_K$ is $\hat{\beta}_\infty$. The variability of $\overline{\beta}_K$ about $\hat{\beta}_\infty$ is $\hat{B}_\infty/K$. Therefore, if we substitute $\hat{\beta}_{MI}$, based on K imputations, as an estimator of $\hat{\beta}_\infty$ in (2.20) we need to increase the variance by $\hat{B}_\infty/K$, giving

$$\beta \sim N\{\hat{\beta}_{MI}, \hat{B}_\infty(K^{-1} + 1) + \hat{W}_\infty\}.$$

The extra term in the variance accounts for the increased uncertainty in the estimated mean of β when we take a finite number of imputations; it vanishes as K gets large.

Since, for a finite K, $\hat{B}$ is unbiased for $\hat{B}_\infty$, and likewise, $\hat{W}$ is unbiased for $\hat{W}_\infty$, we have

$$\beta \approx (\hat{\beta}_{MI}, \hat{B}(1 + K^{-1}) + \hat{W}). \tag{2.21}$$

Notice that we have dropped the 'N' from (2.21); since the variance parameters are estimated, the distribution can no longer be normal; instead, it is likely to be approximately t_ν, for yet-to-be-determined degrees of freedom ν. Note that the distribution will not be exactly t, because the variance estimator consists of the sum of two estimators; in this regard it resembles the distribution of the mean of observations from two groups with different variances – known as the Fisher–Behrens distribution.

Recall that if $Z_1, \dots, Z_K \overset{i.i.d.}{\sim} N(\mu, \sigma^2)$, $\frac{\overline{Z}-\mu}{\hat{\sigma}/\sqrt{n}}$ is distributed as t_{K-1}, because

$$\hat{\sigma}^2 = \frac{1}{K-1}\sum_{k=1}^{K}(Z_i - \overline{Z})^2 \sim \frac{\sigma^2\chi^2_{K-1}}{K-1}.$$

Thus, $\hat{\sigma}^2/\sigma^2$ has mean 1 and variance $2/(K-1)$.

Similarly, in our setting,

$$\frac{\hat{B}}{\hat{B}_\infty} \sim \frac{\chi^2_{K-1}}{K-1}, \tag{2.22}$$

with mean 1 and variance $2/(K-1)$. Next, notice that the MI variance estimator for finite K, divided by the same expression substituting the limiting values of the variance estimates can be written as

$$\frac{\hat{B}(1+K^{-1})+\hat{W}}{\hat{B}_\infty(1+K^{-1})+\hat{W}_\infty} = \frac{\left\{\frac{\hat{B}}{\hat{W}}(1+K^{-1})+1\right\}\hat{W}}{\left\{\frac{\hat{B}_\infty}{\hat{W}_\infty}(1+K^{-1})+1\right\}\hat{W}_\infty}. \tag{2.23}$$

Suppose we write $r = (\hat{B}/\hat{W})(1+K^{-1})$, and $A = \hat{B}/\hat{B}_\infty$. Then the above expression is

$$\left(\frac{\hat{W}}{\hat{W}_\infty}\right)\frac{r+1}{rA^{-1}(\hat{W}/\hat{W}_\infty)+1}.$$

Next notice that, in typical regression models with n observations and p parameters,

$$\frac{\hat{W}}{\hat{W}_\infty} \approx \frac{\chi^2_{n-p}}{n-p}, \tag{2.24}$$

so that the expected value of $\hat{W}/\hat{W}_\infty$ is 1 with variance $O(n^{-1})$. Since we are assuming n is large, we can say $\hat{W}/\hat{W}_\infty \approx 1$. Also assume that $\hat{B}_\infty/\hat{W}_\infty$ is $O(n^{-l})$, $l > 0$, so that $\hat{B}/\hat{W}$ has variance $O(K^{-1}n^{-l})$. This is a less plausible assumption but is more likely to be approximately true if there is relatively little missing information. Under this assumption, we can treat r as approximately constant, and to find the degrees of freedom ν of the approximating χ^2 distribution to (2.23), we need to consider the mean and variance of

$$f(A) = \frac{r+1}{r/A+1}. \tag{2.25}$$

Recalling from below (2.22) that A has a distribution with mean 1, variance $2/(K-1)$, we expand $f(A)$ about the mean of A to see

$$f(A) \approx f(1) + (A-1)f'(1),$$

where f' is the first derivative of f. It follows that $E\{f(A)\} \approx 1$ and

$$\text{Var}\{f(A)\} \approx \frac{2}{K-1}\left(\frac{r}{r+1}\right)^2,$$

so that the distribution of (2.23) can be approximated by the χ^2_ν distribution, where

$$\nu = (K-1)(1+r^{-1})^2 = (K-1)\left\{\frac{\hat{W} + (1+K^{-1})\hat{B}}{(1+K^{-1})\hat{B}}\right\}^2. \tag{2.26}$$

In line with intuition, we see that the smaller the between-imputation variance, the larger ν, and the greater the number of imputations, the larger ν. If desired, we can in applications perform K imputations, estimate (2.26), and increase the number of imputations till $\nu \approx 50$, say when the normal approximation is adequate for practical purposes.

Looking back to (2.21), one final step is needed, and this is to appeal to general results which allow us calibrate features of the posterior, such as credible intervals, from a frequentist repeated sampling perspective. Simply speaking, this allows us to interpret the posterior for β, with estimated mean $\hat{\beta}_{MI}$, as a sampling distribution for $\hat{\beta}_{MI}$, with population parameter value β. We therefore have that

$$\hat{\beta}_{MI} \sim \beta + t_\nu \sqrt{\hat{V}_{MI}}, \tag{2.27}$$

where $\hat{V}_{MI} = \hat{W} + (1 + 1/K)\hat{B}$ and ν is given by (2.26). We can use (2.27) to test hypotheses and form confidence intervals in the usual way.

Notice that in the above derivation we repeatedly use the fact that, if there is no missing data, the sample size n is large enough that the estimator of the quantity can be regarded as normally distributed. The case of small samples, so that with no missing data the estimator has a t-distribution, is considered by Barnard and Rubin (1999).

2.5.3 Inference for vector $\boldsymbol{\beta}$

Inference for vector $\boldsymbol{\beta}$ and finite K can be tackled along the same lines as above, as described by Li *et al.* (1991). They propose basing tests on the approximate pivot

$$F = (\hat{\boldsymbol{\beta}}_{MI} - \boldsymbol{\beta})^T \hat{\mathbf{V}}_{MI}^{-1} (\hat{\boldsymbol{\beta}}_{MI} - \boldsymbol{\beta}).$$

and referring $\{p(1+r)\}^{-1}F$ to an $F_{p,\nu'}$ reference distribution for the scaled statistic, where

$$\nu' = 4 + (t-4)\left[1 + \frac{(1-2t^{-1})}{r}\right]^2,$$

$$r = \frac{1}{p}\left(1 + \frac{1}{K}\right)\text{tr}(\mathbf{B}\mathbf{W}^{-1}), \text{ and}$$

$$t = p(K-1),$$

if $t > 4$, otherwise, $v' = t(1 + p^{-1})(1 + r^{-1})^2/2$. Here, r is the average relative increase in variance due to missingness across the components of $\boldsymbol{\beta}$. As expected, the limiting distribution of F, as $K \to \infty$, is the χ^2_p distribution. This procedure is applicable for any vector of parameters from the substantive model, or any linear combination of these. For inference about a scalar, this reduces in an obvious way to a t approximation for the ratio

$$\frac{\hat{\beta}_{MI} - \beta}{\sqrt{\hat{\mathbf{V}}_{MI}}}.$$

These results are derived under the strong assumption that the fraction of missing information for all elements of $\boldsymbol{\beta}$ are equal. In practice, this will not be true; nevertheless, Li *et al.* (1991) report a simulation study in this setting which finds that performance is good, albeit a little conservative. If in doubt, in many settings it is simplest to perform more imputations and use v' as a guide when variability in the denominator of the F can be assumed negligible. The case of small samples is considered by Reiter (2007).

2.5.4 Combining likelihood ratio tests

Meng and Rubin (1992) extend the MI combination rules to likelihood ratio statistics. To simplify the exposition, it is assumed that we wish to test the null hypothesis

$$H_0 : \boldsymbol{\beta}_2 = 0$$

for $\boldsymbol{\beta} = (\boldsymbol{\beta}_1, \boldsymbol{\beta}_2)^T$ with $\boldsymbol{\beta}_2$ of dimension $q < p$. Hence, under the null hypothesis, $H_0 : \boldsymbol{\beta} = (\boldsymbol{\beta}_1, 0)^T = \boldsymbol{\beta}_{H_0}$ say. From the kth completed dataset, we can obtain the unconstrained maximum likelihood estimate (MLE) $\hat{\boldsymbol{\beta}}_k$, and MLE under the null hypothesis, H_0, which we denote by $\boldsymbol{\beta}_{k,H_0}$. Denote the corresponding log likelihood ratio statistic from the kth set as

$$D_k = 2\{\ell(\hat{\boldsymbol{\beta}}_k) - \ell(\hat{\boldsymbol{\beta}}_{k,H_0})\}.$$

We can then define three averages over the imputation sets:

$$\overline{D}_{.} = \frac{1}{K}\sum_{i=1}^{K} D_k, \quad \overline{\boldsymbol{\beta}}_{.} = \frac{1}{K}\sum_{i=1}^{K} \hat{\boldsymbol{\beta}}_k, \quad \text{and} \quad \overline{\boldsymbol{\beta}}_{.,H_0} = \frac{1}{K}\sum_{i=1}^{K} \hat{\boldsymbol{\beta}}_{k,H_0}.$$

Finally, we define the average of the log likelihood ratios over the K imputed data sets *but with the parameters fixed at their average values*, that is

$$D_{\star} = \frac{1}{K}\sum_{i=1}^{K} 2\{\ell_k(\overline{\boldsymbol{\beta}}_{.}) - \ell_k(\overline{\boldsymbol{\beta}}_{.,H_0})\},$$

where the subscript k indicates that the log likelihood is evaluated using the kth imputed data set. The MI likelihood ratio statistic due to Meng and Rubin (1992) is

$$D_{\text{MI}} = \frac{D^*}{k(1 + r_*)}$$

for $r_* = (K+1)(\overline{D}_. - D_*)/\{q(K-1)\}$. The reference distribution for this is F_{q,v_*}, where

$$v_* = \begin{cases} 4 + (a-4)\{1 + (1 - 2/a)r_*^{-1}\}^2, & \text{if } a = q(K-1) > 4, \\ a(1 + 1/q)(1_1/r_*)^2/2, & \text{otherwise.} \end{cases}$$

However, this has seen limited use.

There is in addition a method for combining P-values over imputations, as developed by Li *et al.* (1991). This does not appear to be used widely in practice, and its behaviour appears such that it should only be used as a rough guide.

Practical settings lend themselves naturally to Wald tests, so that the above rules have not seen wide use in applications.

2.6 Choosing the number of imputations

MI is attractive because it can give valid inferences (that is, unbiasedness with confidence interval coverage as advertised) even for small values of K. In some applications, merely 3–5 imputations are sufficient to achieve acceptable properties. From the discussion above, we see that the information on $\hat{\beta}_{MI}$ based on K imputations, relative to that based on and infinite number, can be estimated by

$$\frac{I_K}{I_\infty} \approx \left\{ \frac{\widehat{W} + (1 + K^{-1})\widehat{B}}{\widehat{W} + \widehat{B}} \right\}^{-1} = \left\{ 1 + \frac{1}{K} \frac{\widehat{B}}{\widehat{B} + \widehat{W}} \right\}^{-1}.$$

Now, $\widehat{B}/(\widehat{B} + \widehat{W})$ is an estimate of the loss of information due to missing data, and from the discussion following (2.7), we have seen that a better estimate of this is

$$\gamma = \frac{r + 2/(\nu + 3)}{r + 1}.$$

Hence, the fraction of information lost for β using K rather than an infinite number of imputations is approximately $\gamma/(K + \gamma)$. The variance of an estimator based on an infinite number of imputations, divided by that based on K imputations, i.e. the relative efficiency of using K imputations, is approximately

$$\frac{I_K}{I_\infty} = \left(1 + \frac{\gamma}{K}\right)^{-1}, \tag{2.28}$$

as derived by Rubin (1987) p. 114. The efficiencies achieved for K versus an infinite number of imputations, for various γ, are shown in Figure 2.1.

On the basis of Figure 2.1, and the fact that MI inference works well for $K > 5$, it has been argued that a small number of imputations is sufficient for most applications.

While this is true, it is not the whole story. Figure 2.1 applies to estimation of β and does not carry over to other statistics, such as p-values (cf. for example, Carpenter and Kenward, 2008, Ch 4). If we want the error in estimating p-values to be small, say less

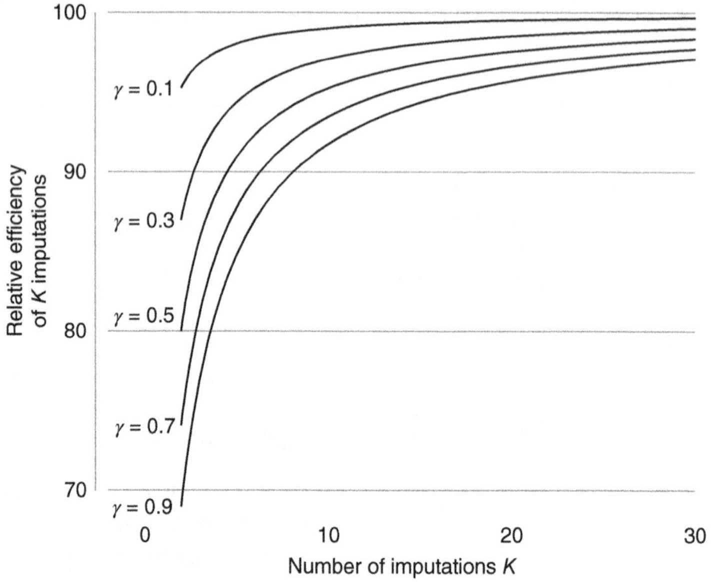

Figure 2.1 Relative efficiency (×100) from (2.28), for various values of K and γ.

than 0.005, then our experience is we will need to do at least $K = 100$ imputations. In a similar vein, Harel and Schafer (2003) report that the MI estimator of the fraction of missing information is considerably more noisy than the MI estimator of β.

We give more detailed practical guidance on this in Chapter 14. However, since computing time is cheap relative to data collection, in applications we would err towards too many imputations rather than too few. Nevertheless, especially in large datasets, where imputation will be slower, pausing after a small number of imputations to check both that the results are plausible and whether more imputations are really required is sensible.

2.7 Some simple examples

Rubin's MI variance rules, described above, are both extremely general and rely on a number of approximations. It is therefore interesting to examine them in some very simple settings, so simple in fact that imputation is strictly unnecessary. These settings allow us to derive exact expressions which add to our intuitive understanding of the procedure. We begin with arguably the simplest possible problem, the estimation of a simple mean under completely random missingness, then consider the situation with σ^2 unknown, and finally the general linear regression setting, again with σ^2 known.

2.7.1 Estimating the mean with σ^2 known by the imputer and analyst

Suppose that we have a sample of n observations $Y_1, \ldots, Y_n$, drawn identically from a normal distribution with mean μ and known variance σ^2. Suppose that we are missing n_M of the observations in a completely random way, and set $n_O = n - n_M$ to be the number actually observed, with the sets of indices for the observed and missing observations denoted by O and M respectively. Define $\pi_M = n_M/n$ to be the proportion missing. Our aim is to estimate μ together with an appropriate measure of precision.

Given the missing completely at random (MCAR) assumption and lack of other relevant information, the obvious approach for this is to use the MLE

$$\hat{\mu} = \overline{Y}_O = \frac{1}{n_O} \sum_{i \in \mathcal{O}} Y_i,$$

the simple average of the observed data, with variance σ^2/n_O. In spite of this simple and obvious solution, we are nevertheless going to approach this problem using MI.

For this, we need an appropriate imputation distribution for the missing data, which in turn requires a suitable posterior for the relevant parameters, in this case just μ. Further, we assume that whatever the distribution of the original data (in this case normal), the sample size is large enough for the posterior for μ to be approximately normal, and for the observed data to dominate the prior; that is the posterior mean and variance for $f(\mu \mid \mathbf{Y}_O)$ can be approximated by $\overline{Y}_O$ and σ^2/n_O, respectively. As discussed on p. 65, although the MI procedure is derived using a proper Bayesian argument, it relies on the data dominating any prior. It is in this sense not a *general* Bayesian procedure in terms of the use of informative priors. The elegant simplicity of the variance formula derives from the use of the limiting form of the posterior that is obtained as n increases.

Given such priors, the posterior for the missing set of observations is

$$\mathbf{Y}_M \mid \mathbf{Y}_O \sim \mathrm{N}\left[\overline{Y}_O \boldsymbol{I}_{n_M}; \sigma^2 \left(\boldsymbol{I}_{n_M} + \frac{1}{n_O} \mathbf{1}_{n_M} \mathbf{1}_{n_M}^T\right)\right],$$

for $\mathbf{1}_p$ the p-dimensional vector of ones. Hence, we can draw the ith of n_M values from the kth of K imputation sets by using

$$Y_{i,k}^* = Y_O + e_{i,k} + s_k, \quad i \in \mathcal{M}, \tag{2.29}$$

where $e_{ik} \sim N(0, \sigma^2)$, and $s_k \sim N(0, \sigma^2/n_O)$, noting that s_k is common to all draws from the kth imputation.

The mean is then estimated from each imputed dataset:

$$\begin{aligned} \overline{Y}_k &= \frac{1}{n}\left(\sum_{i \in \mathcal{O}} Y_i + \sum_{i \in \mathcal{M}} Y_{i,k}^*\right) \\ &= \overline{Y}_O + \pi_M(\bar{e}_{.,k} + s_k). \end{aligned} \tag{2.30}$$

If the analyst also knows the value of σ^2 (e.g. because the imputer and analyst are the same entity), the within-imputation variance can be set equal to σ^2/n in every imputed dataset and so $\widehat{W} = \frac{1}{K}\sum_{k=1}^{K}\frac{\sigma^2}{n} = \frac{\sigma^2}{n}$ (in this case the imputation model and analyst's full data procedure are congenial, cf. Section 2.8).

From these, we calculate the MI estimators of mean and precision using Rubin's rules. The MI estimator of μ is

$$\begin{aligned}\hat{\mu}_{MI} &= \frac{1}{K}\sum_{k=1}^{K}\overline{Y}_k \\ &= \overline{Y}_O + \pi_M(\bar{e}_{.,.} + \bar{s}_.)\end{aligned}$$

and the MI variance estimator of this is

$$\begin{aligned}\widehat{V}_{MI} &= \widehat{W} + \left(1 + \frac{1}{K}\right)\widehat{B} \\ &= \frac{\sigma^2}{n} + \left(1 + \frac{1}{K}\right)\left(\frac{1}{K-1}\right)\sum_{k=1}^{K}(\overline{Y}_k - \hat{\mu}_{MI})^2. \qquad (2.31)\end{aligned}$$

The advantage of this very simple setting is that we can explore directly the exact sampling properties of these. The necessary expectations need to be taken in proper order, that is over the imputation distribution first, and then over the data. Conditioning on the number of observed and missing observations, we find that the estimator, $\hat{\mu}_{MI}$ is unbiased, and has exact variance

$$\text{Var}(\hat{\mu}_{MI}) = \frac{\sigma^2}{n_O}\left(1 + \frac{\pi_M}{K}\right). \qquad (2.32)$$

Note how, as K increases, $\hat{\mu}_{MI}$ tends to $\overline{Y}_O$, and the expression in (2.32) tends to the exact variance of this, as we should expect. Our main goal however is to compare the finite (in terms of K) sampling properties of Rubin's variance estimator with the true variance (2.32). We can rewrite $\widehat{B}$ as

$$\frac{\pi_M^2}{K-1}\sum_{k=1}^{K}\{(\bar{e}_{.,k} - \bar{e}_{.,.})^2 + (s_k - \bar{s}_.)^2 + 2(\bar{e}_{.,k} - \bar{e}_{.,.})(s_k - \bar{s}_.)\}.$$

Noting that the third term inside the brackets has zero expectation (because the e_{ik} and s_k are uncorrelated), we get

$$\text{E}(\widehat{B}) = \frac{\pi_M\sigma^2}{n_O}.$$

Combining these gives

$$\text{E}(\widehat{V}_{MI}) = \frac{\sigma^2}{n} + \left(1 + \frac{1}{K}\right)\text{E}(\widehat{B}) = \frac{\sigma^2}{n_O}\left(1 + \frac{\pi_M}{K}\right),$$

and comparing this with $\text{Var}(\hat{\mu}_{MI})$, we see Rubin's variance estimator is unbiased in terms of finite K, given the large n approximation being used for the posterior. In fact, it is completely unbiased in a small sample sense (n and K) if we take a flat, improper, prior for μ.

This example illustrates that MI is not 'making up data'; no matter how many observations we might say are missing, MI gives a variance estimate that is bounded below by the variance of the mean of the observed data.

2.7.2 Estimating the mean with σ^2 known only by the imputer

We now consider the same setting but where the true value σ^2 is known only to the imputer, but not the analyst. In this case, the only change is that in the analysis of the imputed datasets, the analyst must estimate σ^2 in order to estimate the within-imputation variance. Specifically, the sample variance in imputation k is estimated by

$$S_k^2 = \frac{1}{n-1}\left(\sum_{i\in\mathcal{O}}(Y_i - \overline{Y}_k)^2 + \sum_{i\in\mathcal{M}}(Y_{i,k}^* - \overline{Y}_k)^2\right) \tag{2.33}$$

$$= \frac{1}{n-1}\left(\sum_{i\in\mathcal{O}}(Y_i - \overline{Y}_O)^2 + \sum_{i\in\mathcal{M}}(e_{i,k} - \bar{e}_{.,k})^2 + n(1-\pi_M)\pi_M(\bar{e}_{.,k} + s_k)^2\right).$$

In this case, the imputation model and analyst's full data procedure are no longer congenial. This is because given full data, the imputer's variance utilises the true value of σ^2, whereas the analyst's does not.

The MI point estimate of μ is as before, but the MI variance estimator is now

$$\widehat{V}_{MI} = \widehat{W} + \left(1 + \frac{1}{K}\right)\widehat{B}$$

$$= \frac{1}{nK}\sum_{k=1}^{K} S_k^2 + \left(1 + \frac{1}{K}\right)\left(\frac{1}{K-1}\right)\sum_{k=1}^{K}(\overline{Y}_k - \hat{\mu}_{MI})^2. \tag{2.34}$$

As the three components of (2.33) are independent, it follows that

$$\mathrm{E}(\widehat{W}) = \frac{\sigma^2}{n},$$

and so

$$\mathrm{E}(\widehat{V}_{MI}) = \mathrm{E}(\widehat{W}) + \left(1 + \frac{1}{K}\right)\mathrm{E}(\widehat{B}) = \frac{\sigma^2}{n_O}\left(1 + \frac{\pi_M}{K}\right).$$

Again, Rubin's variance estimator is unbiased, despite the aforementioned uncongeniality.

2.7.3 Estimating the mean with σ^2 unknown

Keeping the same basic setup we now assume, more realistically, that σ^2 is unknown both for the imputer and the analyst. We have the same prior for μ and take the (improper) prior for σ^2 to be proportional to σ^{-2}. This is the limiting form of the conjugate scaled inverse-χ^2 prior (see for example Gelman *et al.* 1995, Section 2.8, and Appendix B). It follows that the observed data posterior distribution for σ^2 has the form

$$\sigma^2 \mid \mathbf{Y}_O \sim \frac{(n_O - 1)S_O}{X^2} \tag{2.35}$$

for $X^2 \sim \chi^2_{n_O-1}$ and S_O the sample variance of the observed data:

$$S_O = \frac{1}{n_O - 1} \sum_{i \in \mathcal{O}} (Y_i - \overline{Y}_O)^2.$$

The imputation proceeds as before, except that it begins, for each k, by taking a draw, σ^{2*} say, from the posterior (2.35), which is used in the imputation of the data through (2.29), that is:

$$f(e_{i,k} \mid \mathbf{Y}_O, \sigma^{2*}) \sim N(0, \sigma^{2*}) \quad \text{and} \quad f(s_k \mid \mathbf{Y}_O, \sigma^{2*}) \sim N(0, \sigma^{2*}/n_O).$$

Again, because of the simplicity of the setup, we can derive exact properties of the MI quantities. The approach is exactly the same as above, except that expectations are taken in two steps, first conditional on the observed data $\mathbf{Y}_O$ and then with respect to this. As before it follows directly that $\hat{\mu}_{MI}$ is unbiased for μ. Its variance can be obtained as follows: first, we have

$$\text{Var}(\hat{\mu}_{MI} \mid \mathbf{Y}_O) = \frac{\pi_M}{n_O K^2} \sum_{k=1}^{K} \text{E}_\text{I}(\sigma^{2*} \mid \mathbf{Y}_O),$$

where the expectations are taken over the imputation distribution. Given that the mean of the inverse χ^2_v distribution is $(v-2)^{-1}$,

$$\text{E}_\text{I}(\sigma^{2*} \mid \mathbf{Y}_O) = \left(\frac{n_O - 1}{n_O - 3}\right) S_O,$$

and so

$$\text{Var}(\hat{\mu}_{MI} \mid \mathbf{Y}_O) = \left(\frac{n_O - 1}{n_O - 3}\right) \frac{\pi_M}{n_O K} S_O,$$

giving, as S_O is unbiased for σ^2:

$$\text{Var}(\hat{\mu}_{MI}) = \frac{\sigma^2}{n_O} + \left(\frac{n_O - 1}{n_O - 3}\right) \frac{\pi_M}{n_O K} \sigma^2.$$

The expectation of the MI variance estimator (2.31) is obtained using similar two-stage arguments. Omitting details, we find

$$\text{E}(\widehat{W}) = \frac{\sigma^2}{n} \left(\frac{n-3}{n-1}\right) \left(\frac{n_O - 1}{n_O - 3}\right),$$

and

$$\text{E}(\widehat{B}) = \frac{\pi_M}{n_O} \left(\frac{n_O - 1}{n_O - 3}\right) \sigma^2,$$

from which we get

$$\mathrm{E}(\hat{V}_{MI}) = \frac{\sigma^2}{n_O}\left(\frac{n_O - 1}{n_O - 3}\right)\left\{1 - \frac{2n_O}{n(n-1)} + \frac{\pi_M}{K}\right\}.$$

This bias in $\hat{V}_{MI}$ is then

$$\mathrm{E}(\hat{V}_{MI}) - \mathrm{Var}(\hat{\mu}_{MI}) = \frac{2\sigma^2}{n_O(n_O - 3)}\left\{1 - \frac{n_O(n_O - 1)}{n(n-1)}\right\}.$$

What is important here is the absence of K from this expression, implying that the bias does not depend on K, and so we do not need to rely on the number of imputations to ensure that the variance formula is working as we would wish. The bias that does exist disappears with increasing sample size n (assuming as usual, that the proportion of missing data is bounded), which is not an issue as we are anyway using large sample arguments to underpin the derivation on the MI procedure.

2.7.4 General linear regression with σ^2 known

Our final simple example is that of general linear regression where the imputer knows the value of σ^2. We can infer from the relationships between the previous two settings that the additional complication of an unknown variance does not have a profound impact on the basic development: it essentially adds an additional step to the imputation process and hence to the derivation of the properties of the statistics. Hence, by keeping the known variance assumption (for the imputer), we can keep the basic simplicity of the development without serious loss of generality.

Our aim is to estimate the parameters of a simple linear regression model:

$$f(\mathbf{Y} \mid \mathbf{X}) \sim \mathrm{N}_n(\mathbf{X}\boldsymbol{\beta};\ \sigma^2 \boldsymbol{I}_n), \tag{2.36}$$

for $\mathbf{X}$ and $(n \times p)$ matrix of covariates, and σ^2 known. It is assumed that some of the outcomes in $\mathbf{Y}$ are MAR dependent on $\mathbf{X}$, which is assumed to be completely observed. As with estimating the simple mean above, we do not need MI here, the obvious, unbiased, estimator is given by

$$\widehat{\boldsymbol{\beta}}_O = (\mathbf{X}_O{}^T\mathbf{X}_O)^{-1}\mathbf{X}_O{}^T\mathbf{Y}_O$$

for $\mathbf{Y}_O$ the observed outcomes and $\mathbf{X}_O$ the corresponding covariate matrix, with known covariance matrix $\mathbf{V}_O = \sigma^2(\mathbf{X}_O{}^T\mathbf{X}_O)^{-1}$. However, we again use MI for this, and it is instructive to see, in this simple setting, how this is related to the conventional approach.

Following the same basic steps as above, we assume that the large sample posterior for $\boldsymbol{\beta}$ is centred on the maximum likelihood estimator $\widehat{\boldsymbol{\beta}}_O$ with covariance matrix $\mathbf{V}_O$, that is,

$$\boldsymbol{\beta}^* \mid \mathbf{Y}_O \sim \mathrm{N}_p(\widehat{\boldsymbol{\beta}}_O;\ \mathbf{V}_O).$$

The imputation model can therefore we expressed, for the kth imputation,

$$\mathbf{Y}^*_{M,k} \mid \mathbf{Y}_O = \mathbf{X}_M(\widehat{\boldsymbol{\beta}}_O + \mathbf{b}_k) + \mathbf{e}_k$$

for $\mathbf{X}_M$ the covariate matrix for the missing outcomes, and

$$\mathbf{b}_k \sim N_p(\mathbf{0};\ \mathbf{V}_O) \quad \text{and} \quad \mathbf{e}_k \sim N(\mathbf{0};\ \sigma^2 \boldsymbol{I}_{n_M}).$$

The estimate of $\boldsymbol{\beta}$ from the kth imputation set is then

$$\boldsymbol{\beta}^*{}_k = (\mathbf{X}^T\mathbf{X})^{-1}\mathbf{X}_O{}^T\mathbf{Y}_O + (\mathbf{X}^T\mathbf{X})^{-1}\mathbf{X}_M{}^T\mathbf{Y}^*_{M,k}.$$

Using the fact that $\mathbf{Y}^*_{M,k}$ can be written

$$\mathbf{X}_M(\widehat{\boldsymbol{\beta}}_O + \mathbf{b}_k) + \mathbf{e}_k = \mathbf{X}_M\{(\mathbf{X}_O{}^T\mathbf{X}_O)^{-1}\mathbf{X}_O{}^T\mathbf{Y}_O + \mathbf{b}_k\} + \mathbf{e}_k$$

since $\mathbf{X}^T\mathbf{X} = \mathbf{X}_O^T\mathbf{X}_O + \mathbf{X}_M^T\mathbf{X}_M$, we see that $\boldsymbol{\beta}^*_{\mathbf{k}}$ can be written as a sum of $\widehat{\boldsymbol{\beta}}_O$ (which depends only on $\mathbf{Y}_O$) and terms involving the imputed random variables:

$$\boldsymbol{\beta}^*_{\mathbf{k}} = \widehat{\boldsymbol{\beta}}_O + (\mathbf{X}^T\mathbf{X})^{-1}\mathbf{X}_M{}^T(\mathbf{X}_M\mathbf{b}_k + \mathbf{e}_k).$$

It is then simple to average these over the imputation sets to obtain the MI estimator:

$$\widehat{\boldsymbol{\beta}}_{MI} = \widehat{\boldsymbol{\beta}}_O + (\mathbf{X}^T\mathbf{X})^{-1}\mathbf{X}_M{}^T(\mathbf{X}_M\overline{\boldsymbol{b}}_. + \overline{\boldsymbol{e}}_.),$$

using obvious notation.

To find the mean of $\widehat{\boldsymbol{\beta}}_{MI}$, we need to first take expectations over the imputation distribution (denoted I), given $\mathbf{Y}_O$ and then over $\mathbf{Y}_O$ itself, i.e.

$$\mathrm{E}(\widehat{\boldsymbol{\beta}}_{MI}) = \mathrm{E}_{\mathbf{Y}_O}\{\mathrm{E}_{\mathrm{I}|\mathbf{Y}_O}(\widehat{\boldsymbol{\beta}}_O)\}$$

which reduces to $\mathrm{E}_{\mathbf{Y}_O}(\widehat{\boldsymbol{\beta}}_O) = \boldsymbol{\beta}$. Hence, the MI estimator of $\boldsymbol{\beta}$ is unbiased. We also see that it tends to the ML (or ordinary least squares (OLS)) estimator as K increases. The latter property holds more generally for missing outcomes when estimation is based on score equations and the imputation model is congenial.

Similar arguments can be used to obtain the variance of $\widehat{\boldsymbol{\beta}}_{MI}$:

$$\mathrm{Var}(\widehat{\boldsymbol{\beta}}_{MI}) = \mathrm{E}_{\mathbf{Y}_O}\{\mathrm{Var}_{\mathrm{I}|\mathbf{Y}_O}(\widehat{\boldsymbol{\beta}}_{MI})\} + \mathrm{Var}_{\mathbf{Y}_O}\{\mathrm{E}_{\mathrm{I}|\mathbf{Y}_O}(\widehat{\boldsymbol{\beta}}_{MI})\},$$

which reduces to

$$\mathbf{V}_O + \frac{1}{K}\{\mathbf{V}_O - \sigma^2(\mathbf{X}^T\mathbf{X})^{-1}\}. \tag{2.37}$$

The matrix inside the braces is positive definite, so we see that the MI estimator is always less precise than the ML estimator $\widehat{\boldsymbol{\beta}}_O$, but the difference disappears as K increases. Again, we expect to see this in general for missing outcomes with ML estimation and a congenial imputation model.

Our final step is to compare the behaviour of the MI variance estimator (2.31) with this exact value in (2.37). For this, we need the expectation of

$$\widehat{\mathbf{V}}_{MI} = \frac{1}{K}\sum_{k=1}^{K}\sigma_k^{2*}(\mathbf{X}^T\mathbf{X})^{-1} + \left(\frac{K+1}{K}\right)\left(\frac{1}{K-1}\right)\sum_{k=1}^{K}(\boldsymbol{\beta}^*_k - \widehat{\boldsymbol{\beta}}_{MI})(\boldsymbol{\beta}^*_k - \widehat{\boldsymbol{\beta}}_{MI})^T \tag{2.38}$$

for σ_k^{2*} the residual variance from the analysis of the kth imputation set:

$$\sigma_k^{2*} = \frac{1}{n-p}\left\{(\mathbf{Y}_O - \mathbf{X}_O\beta_k^*)^T(\mathbf{Y}_O - \mathbf{X}_O\beta^*{}_k)\right.$$
$$\left. + (\mathbf{Y}_{M,k}^* - \mathbf{X}_M\beta_k^*)^T(\mathbf{Y}_{M,k}^* - \mathbf{X}_M\beta_k^*)\right\}.$$

By decomposing the two right-hand components separately, it can be shown that

$$\mathrm{E}_{\mathbf{Y}_O}\{\mathrm{E}_{\mathrm{I}|\mathbf{Y}_O}(\sigma_k^{2*})\} = \sigma^2,$$

and so the first term on the right-hand side of (2.38) is unbiased for

$$\sigma^2(\mathbf{X}^T\mathbf{X})^{-1}.$$

Noting that

$$\beta_k^* - \widehat{\beta}_{MI} = (\mathbf{X}^T\mathbf{X})^{-1}\mathbf{X}_M{}^T\{\mathbf{X}_M(\mathbf{b}_k - \overline{\mathbf{b}}_.) + (\mathbf{e}_k - \overline{\mathbf{e}}_.)\}$$

and using the independence of $\mathbf{b}_k$ and $\mathbf{e}_k$, it can also be shown that

$$\mathrm{E}_{\mathrm{I},\mathbf{Y}_O}\left[\left(\frac{1}{K-1}\right)\sum_{k=1}^{K}(\beta_k^* - \widehat{\beta}_{MI})(\beta_k^* - \widehat{\beta}_{MI})^T\right] = \mathbf{V}_O - \sigma^2(\mathbf{X}^T\mathbf{X})^{-1}.$$

Combining these two results, we have

$$\begin{aligned}\mathrm{E}_{\mathrm{I},\mathbf{Y}_O}(\widehat{\mathbf{V}}_{MI}) &= \sigma^2(\mathbf{X}^T\mathbf{X})^{-1} + \left(1+\frac{1}{K}\right)\left\{\mathbf{V}_O - \sigma^2(\mathbf{X}^T\mathbf{X})^{-1}\right\} \\ &= \mathbf{V}_O + \frac{1}{K}\left\{\mathbf{V}_O - \sigma^2(\mathbf{X}^T\mathbf{X})^{-1}\right\} \\ &= \mathrm{Var}(\widehat{\beta}_{MI}).\end{aligned} \tag{2.39}$$

The MI variance estimator is exactly unbiased for the true variance of $\widehat{\beta}_{MI}$.

Again, in this simple setting, we have been able to derive an exact result, which does not rely on asymptotics. This provides us with some insight into the behaviour of the MI variance estimator. For realistic problems, however, we must resort to asymptotic arguments, but interestingly we find that the structure observed here reflects the structure observed in the general case under congeniality when our substantive model is fitted by maximum likelihood. Specifically, let $\boldsymbol{I}(\beta)$ and $\boldsymbol{I}_O(\beta)$ be the expected Fisher information matrices for the complete data, here $\mathbf{Y}$, and observed data, here $\mathbf{Y}_O$, respectively. Then under congeniality and suitable regularity conditions, the MI variance estimator $\widehat{\mathbf{V}}_{MI}$ has a limiting distribution, as the sample size increases, that has mean equal to

$$\boldsymbol{I}_O(\beta)^{-1} + \frac{1}{K}\{\boldsymbol{I}_O(\beta)^{-1} - \boldsymbol{I}(\beta)^{-1}\}.$$

It is easy to see how this reduces to (2.39) for the simple regression example. This result is most succinctly derived in Nielsen (2003) but is also given by Wang and

Robins (1998). Another interesting feature of the MI variance estimator, as noted by both Wang and Robins (1998) and Nielsen (2003) is that the estimator is not actually consistent as the sample size increases; we also require $K \to \infty$. Nielsen (2003) shows that its limiting distribution is Wishart with $K - 1$ DF, with a mean that is shifted to the required value.

2.8 MI in more general settings

2.8.1 Proper imputation

In his original book, (Rubin, 1987, p119) defines the conditions for so-called 'proper' imputation in terms of the complete-data statistics which we denote, for a scalar problem, $\hat{\beta}_C$ and $\hat{V}_C$, the estimate of the parameter of the substantive model and associated variance, respectively, calculated using the *complete* data. Rubin gives three conditions that need to be satisfied to justify the frequentist properties of the MI procedure. These are expressed in terms of the MI quantities defined in Section 2.5 and are needed to derive more rigorously the results presented there. The first two conditions are expressed in terms of repeated sampling of the missing value process $\boldsymbol{R}$, given the complete data $\mathbf{Y}$ as fixed: first,

$$\frac{\hat{\beta}_{MI} - \hat{\beta}_C}{\sqrt{\hat{B}}} \overset{K\to\infty}{\sim} N(0,1)$$

and second, $\hat{W}$ is consistent for $\hat{V}_C$ as $K \to \infty$. The third condition is that as $K \to \infty$, $\hat{B}$ is of lower order than $\hat{W}$.

Rubin (1987) showed in some simple settings that imputations generated from a normal Bayesian model could be proper for estimation of means and gave a heuristic argument (Section 4.4) that imputations generated from an appropriate Bayesian model tend to be proper. As general guidance, he advocated choosing imputation models that are appropriate for the complete data statistics likely to be used, that is, for the types of analyses that will be performed on the imputed data. He pointed out that if the imputation model for the data is correctly specified, the model will be appropriate for all possible complete data statistics (i.e. all possible substantive models/analyses).

2.8.2 Congenial imputation and substantive model

Meng (1994) developed the concept of congeniality, a set of sufficient conditions that ensure validity of MI inferences and that tend to be more readily verifiable than Rubin's definition of proper imputation. When the imputation model (i.e. the conditional predictive model) and substantive model are the same, with the substantive model fitted using maximum likelihood, congeniality is satisfied and we can view MI as an approximate Bayesian procedure, with frequentist inference obtained by appealing to general asymptotic results which calibrate features of the posterior from a repeated sampling perspective.

The case where the imputation and substantive models are identical is however not very interesting, not least because as we noted previously, in this case MI reproduces (up to Monte-Carlo error) complete records estimates of the (common) model parameters. When there are missing values in covariates of the substantive model, some care is needed to ensure that the imputation model respects the structure and assumptions encoded by the substantive model. Examples which we consider later include imputation with survival data (Chapter 7), imputation when the substantive model includes non-linear terms, interactions or other derived variables (Chapter 6), and multi-level settings (Chapter 9). Failure to accommodate such complexities of the substantive model in the imputation model generally lead to the MI point estimator being biased.

An important practical question is whether the use of so-called auxiliary variables in the imputation model leads to uncongeniality. Auxiliary variables are variables included in the imputation process but that are not involved in the substantive model. Such variables may be included because they are thought to be predictive of the variables being imputed, which will lead to reduced uncertainty about missing values and hence more precise inferences. Moreover, if such variables are predictive of missingness, including them in the imputation model generally renders the MAR assumption more plausible (although see Thoemmes and Rose (2014) for a case where this is not the case).

By itself, inclusion of auxiliary variables in the imputation model does not automatically lead to uncongeniality. As a very simple example, consider bivariate normal data (X, Y), with some values in Y MAR given X. Suppose the analyst is interested in the marginal mean $E(Y)$, which given complete data they estimate with the sample mean and usual sample variance. To ensure MAR is satisfied, the imputation model needs to condition on X, whereas the analyst's substantive model ignores X completely. Suppose that the imputation model is a normal linear regression for $f(Y|X)$. Here the imputation model and substantive model are congenial. This is because the imputation model can be embedded in the bivariate normal model for $f(X, Y)$, and under this model, with complete data, the posterior mean and variance for $E(Y)$ matches the substantive model point estimator (the sample mean) and variance estimator (the usual sample variance).

More generally, however, inclusion of auxiliary variables can lead to uncongeniality. As an example, suppose a binary variable Y is MAR given continuous X_1 and X_2. The imputation model is a logistic regression for Y with X_1 and X_2 as covariates, while the substantive model is a logistic regression for Y with only X_1 as covariate. Unfortunately, in general the two logistic regression models cannot both be correctly specified because the logistic model is not collapsible. Therefore, the imputation and substantive models cannot be congenial.

2.8.3 Uncongenial imputation and substantive models

In practice, imputation and substantive models are often uncongenial, and there are a variety of different ways the uncongeniality can arise. For example, forms of estimation other than maximum likelihood are sometimes used, such as those employing generalized estimating equations. Or the imputation model may allow for certain interactions which the analysis model assumes do not exist. MI would lose much of its practical value if we were restricted to strict congeniality. In this subsection, we give a high-level overview of some of the technical results pertaining to Rubin's variance estimator and alternatives under uncongeniality, and in the following subsection give practical advice based on these.

Meng (1994) developed results which characterised certain uncongenial situations where MI confidence intervals would, despite the uncongeniality, have the desired coverage level. He also identified conditions under which the MI confidence intervals would have at least the nominal coverage level (i.e. conservative coverage). These results were subsequently extended by Xie and Meng (2017). To explore the potential bias in Rubin's variance estimator, consider a scalar parameter β. We assume that the complete data estimator $\hat{\beta}_C$ (and MI estimator $\hat{\beta}_{MI}$) are both consistent for the true parameter β, which is of course not guaranteed in general under uncongeniality. The true variance of the MI estimator $\hat{\beta}_{MI}$ can then be decomposed as

$$\begin{aligned}\text{Var}(\hat{\beta}_{MI}) &= \text{Var}(\hat{\beta}_{MI} - \hat{\beta}_C + \hat{\beta}_C) \\ &= \text{Var}(\hat{\beta}_{MI} - \hat{\beta}_C) + \text{Var}(\hat{\beta}_C) + 2\text{Cov}(\hat{\beta}_{MI} - \hat{\beta}_C, \hat{\beta}_C).\end{aligned}$$

It turns out that the first term on the right-hand side is consistently estimated by $\hat{B}$, even under uncongeniality, and the second term is similarly consistently estimated by $\hat{W}$. Thus, Rubin's variance estimator is consistent if and only if the covariance term is zero (Xie and Meng (2017)). Under uncongeniality, the covariance term may not be zero, causing bias in Rubin's variance estimator. It is however possible for the term to be zero even under uncongeniality. Meng (1994) showed that the covariance term is zero, such that Rubin's variance estimator is consistent, if and only if the complete data estimator $\hat{\beta}_C$ cannot be made more efficient by forming a new estimator $\lambda\hat{\beta}_{MI} + (1-\lambda)\hat{\beta}_C$ for some $\lambda \neq 0$. Based on this, Xie and Meng (2017) state 'if the analyst uses fully efficient complete-data estimators, such as MLE, then $\hat{V}_{MI}$ will be consistent as long as the imputer's model does not bring in "secret information" unused in forming the analyst's complete-data estimator'. An example where the imputation model contains such 'secret information' not used in the complete data estimator is reference-based MI for clinical trials (Section 10.5) and also certain settings with survey weights (Chapter 12).

Suppose now it is possible to make the complete data estimator $\hat{\beta}_C$ more efficient by mixing it with the MI estimator, such that Rubin's variance estimator $\hat{V}_{MI}$ is not consistent. Then provided the linear combination $\lambda\hat{\beta}_{MI} + (1-\lambda)\hat{\beta}_C$ is never more efficient than $\hat{\beta}_C$ for negative λ, Rubin's variance estimator is conservative Meng (1994). As noted by Meng (1994), the existence of such a negative λ would seem rather implausible, since this 'would imply weighting $\hat{\beta}_C$, which does not carry the imputer's extra information, by more than 100% and then giving a negative weight to $\hat{\beta}_{MI}$ to maintain consistency (e.g. $-30\%\hat{\beta}_{MI} + 130\%\hat{\beta}_C$)'.

More recently, Xie and Meng (2017) developed further results applicable in the important special case where the imputation and substantive models are nested.

Suppose first that the substantive model is nested within the imputation model, i.e. the substantive model makes stronger assumptions than the imputation model. An example of this could be that the imputation model allows for a possible interaction, or non-linear effect, which the substantive model does not allow. Then Xie and Meng (2017) show (Theorem 6) that Rubin's variance estimator is consistent, provided the 'analyst's procedure' satisfies a technical condition termed 'self-efficiency' (see below). The practical implication of this result is that the imputation model can be made more general than the substantive model(s) and Rubin's variance estimator can remain consistent. When instead the imputation model makes stronger assumptions than the substantive model, Xie and Meng (2017) show (Theorem 7), that Rubin's variance estimator is conservative, but this result requires the rather restrictive assumption that the fraction of missing information is the same for all parameters. These results suggest that, where feasible, the imputation model should be allowed to be flexible.

The requirement that the analyst's procedure, or in our terminology the fit of the substantive model, be *self-efficient* means, in the scalar setting, that the complete data estimator $\hat{\beta}_C$ has smaller mean squared error (MSE) than all linear combinations $\lambda\hat{\beta}_O + (1 - \lambda)\hat{\beta}_C$, where $\hat{\beta}_O$ denotes the estimator obtained from an incomplete version of the complete data. In the type of situations considered in this book, we will typically be dealing with self-efficient estimators, and we note that this extends the estimation procedures we might use for the substantive model beyond maximum likelihood. It is interesting that counterexamples to the appropriateness of the MI procedure often use estimation procedures that are not self-efficient. See for example Fay (1993) and Nielsen (2003) and the subsequent discussion in Meng and Romero (2003) and Xie and Meng (2017).

Wang and Robins (1998) and Robins and Wang (2000) approach the problem in terms of the properties of regular asymptotic linear estimators and compare the properties of MI estimators under both proper Bayesian and improper imputation schemes. The improper imputation is defined as repeated imputation using *fixed* consistent estimates of the parameters of the imputation model, that is, when new draws of these parameters are *not* made for each set of imputations. An advantage of this type of improper imputation is that they avoid the need to use computationally intensive methods, such as Markov chain Monte Carlo (MCMC), which are typically required by implementations of proper imputation. They show that although, for finite K, the 'improper' estimators are the more efficient, Rubin's variance estimator, (2.16) is an overestimate of the variability of these. A more accessible account of these developments is provided by Tsiatis (2006), Chapter 14. We note that von Hippel and Bartlett (2021) developed a formula similar to Rubin's rules to combine between- and within-imputation variances which is consistent when such improper imputation is used. von Hippel and Bartlett's variance estimator for improper MI, like Rubin's rules, relies on congeniality for its justification. A drawback compared to Rubin's rules is that it must be applied to the full vector of model parameters in the congenial joint model, whereas Rubin's rules can be applied element wise to whichever parameters are of interest.

Hughes *et al.* (2016) conducted a simulation study to examine the behaviour of the MI variance estimator and to compare it with two other approaches under uncongeniality or model mis-specification. The estimator derived in Robins and Wang (2000) and a 'full-mechanism bootstrap' approach (Efron, 1994); see below. They took as the substantive model a standard multivariable linear regression with four continuous covariates and one binary covariate. Only a single variable was partially observed, since the Robins and Wang variance estimator rapidly becomes very complex with more than one missing variable. In the simulation study, one of the continuous predictors was chosen for this, and the missingness mechanism was MCAR.

Briefly, the full-mechanism bootstrap involves imputing the incomplete dataset once, drawing a bootstrap sample, setting observations to missing under an assumed mechanisms, singly imputing this incomplete bootstrapped dataset, applying the analysis procedure to the imputed dataset, and storing the estimate. The resampling steps are repeated a large number of times as an estimate of the sampling distribution.

Several different uncongenial scenarios were explored, with rather large proportions missing, 40% and 60%. The scenarios were

1. domain analysis, in which the imputations were constructed from the whole dataset, but the substantive model was fitted to one category of the binary predictor;
2. when the true errors were heteroscedastic, but homoscedastic in the imputation model;
3. when an interaction was omitted from the imputation model that was present (although redundant) in the substantive model; and
4. non-normality of the true errors (both moderate and severe).

We summarise the results by focusing on the coverage of the 95% confidence intervals – the crucial operating characteristic in practice. With 60% average missingness, and a sample size of 1000, under scenarios (1) and (3) the coverage of the confidence intervals constructed using $\widehat{V}_{MI}$ was conservative (99% and 98%, respectively). This is in line with the theoretical results of Xie and Meng (2017), since in these scenarios, the imputation model was nested within the substantive model, by making stronger assumptions. Under (2) $\widehat{V}_{MI}$ was anti-conservative (92%). For moderate non-normality, the coverage was close to nominal (95%), but strongly anti-conservative under severe non-normality (86%). Interestingly, the use of a robust/sandwich estimate of variance in the complete data analysis step improved the coverage (93%). The Robins and Wang variance estimator led to a coverage closer to the nominal level in all scenarios (all 95% to two significant figure) except that of extreme non-normality, where it performed similarly to Rubin's variance estimator with robust variance (92%). With $n = 100$, results were similar for Rubin's variance estimator, but Robins and Wang's approach led to consistent under-coverage in all scenarios (ranging from 87% to 92%).

What should we conclude from these results? We know that when the imputation model is mis-specified, the confidence interval coverage in general will not be exactly at the nominal level. It is very comforting then to see that in the less-extreme scenarios, the coverage is conservative, and is only anti-conservative in the extreme examples (heteroscedasticity and extreme non-normality) that should be spotted anyway at the stage at which the imputation model is being formulated. In none of these scenarios is the imputation model 'richer' (in the sense used earlier) than the substantive model. As theory predicts, the Robins and Wang variance estimator provides better asymptotic coverage, although the consistent anti-conservative behaviour in the smaller sample size setting is worrying. We should note as well that these results have been obtained under very high missing data proportions (60%).

The problem with the Robins and Wang procedure is its lack of generality; it is far more problem-specific. To quote Hughes *et al.* (2016)

> A major disadvantage of the Robins and Wang method is that calculation of the imputation variance estimate is considerably more complicated than for Rubin's MI and full mechanism bootstrapping, with a greater burden placed on both the imputer and the analyst. To our knowledge, there is no generally available software implementing the Robins and Wang method. The analyst must make available derivatives of the estimating equations for use in calculation of variance estimates, and these become harder to calculate as the complexity of the analysis procedure increases. Also, the complexity of the calculations conducted by the imputer increases when there are multiple incomplete variables with a general missing data pattern. For this reason, our simulation scenarios were restricted to data missing in a single variable, as were the scenarios considered in the papers proposing the approach.
>
> The Robins and Wang method requires the data to be imputed under a single imputation model. Therefore, currently, it cannot be applied if imputation is conducted using [full conditional specification, (see Chapter 3)], a flexible and commonly used method of imputation[...] By contrast, calculation of the variance of an imputation estimator by Rubin's MI method [...] is straightforward for more complex missing data patterns and analysis procedures and can be applied when data are imputed using [full conditional specification].

More recently, combinations of MI with bootstrapping have been explored, where either bootstrapping is first performed followed by MI on each bootstrap sample, or missing data are multiply imputed first, and then bootstrapping is applied in each imputed dataset (Schomaker and Heumann (2018), Brand *et al.* (2019), Bartlett and Hughes (2020)). Bartlett and Hughes (2020) showed that, in order to obtain unbiased variance estimates under uncongeniality, one must first bootstrap and then multiply impute each bootstrap sample. Since combining bootstrapping with MI can lead to a large computational cost, they recommended a particular approach to bootstrapping followed by MI proposed by von Hippel and Bartlett (2021) which can give frequentist-valid inferences under uncongeniality but with a lower computational burden.

There are cases where Rubin's variance estimator can be biased downwards, giving anti-conservative inferences (Robins and Wang (2000)). Xie and Meng (2017) proved a remarkable result, that one can obtain at worst conservative inferences by forming the standard error of the MI estimate as the sum of the within-imputation standard error plus the between-imputation standard error. This contrasts with Rubin's standard error estimator, which is the square root of the sum of the corresponding variances. This alternative combination rule may prove attractive in settings where estimates have high precision, where accepting some conservatism in the standard error may be an acceptable price to pay to be assured of confidence validity.

The two main messages that we take from these various comparisons, and the theoretical results discussed earlier are

1. Sensible care must be taken in constructing an imputation model that properly represents the structure of the data under analysis and the substantive model;
2. Conservative behaviour of the inferences based on Rubin's rules is in most cases an acceptable price to pay for the exceptional simplicity, flexibility, and generality of the overall MI procedure.

As Rubin (2003) writes:

> In many fields, the collection of complete-data analyses that would be performed in the absence of missing data is often relatively fixed by tradition or the need to communicate clearly to an audience of non-statisticians and so these complete-data analyses [...] are not based on fully specified Bayesian or likelihood models. When confronted with missing data, it is a hopelessly daunting task to derive and implement new methods of data analysis, to validate their operating characteristics and to formulate ways to present them to an outside audience for each such situation compromised by the occurrence of missing data. For such problems, I believe that MI is a general solution because it allows the statistician to capitalize on what is already accepted–the complete–data analysis, and often avoid largely extraneous complications created by limited fractions of missing information.
>
> Also, MI allows the straightforward investigation of changes in the final completed-data inference resulting from changes in the assumed process for creating missing data, when there is a desire for such sensitivity analysis. In some cases, there will be a loss in efficiency, or in rare cases, even some validity, using MI, especially with large fractions of missing information, but this seems like a small price to pay relative to the practical benefits of MI in more realistic cases. [...] If statisticians do not provide solutions that are close to valid, users of data will not stop producing answers, but instead will turn to *ad hoc*, potentially entirely invalid methods, when approximately valid answers are readily available via MI. MI may not be the ideal solution for all missing data problems, but I now firmly believe it is as close as we have come to a general solution to them.

A further implication of these results is that when building an imputation model it is better to err on the side of over- rather than under-fitting. We see that the penalty for over-fitting, i.e. having a richer imputation model than strictly necessary, is some potential loss in efficiency, probably slight, while omitting key variables can lead to inconsistent estimators. This advice has long history in the MI literature. For example, Section 2.6 of Rubin (1996)

> The possible lost precision when including unimportant predictors is usually viewed as a relatively small price to pay for the general validity of analyses of the resultant multiply-imputed data base.

Collins *et al.* (2001) used a simulation study to compare restrictive 'minimal use of auxiliary variables' and inclusive 'liberal use of auxiliary variables' in the imputation model. Their conclusions are consistent with Rubin's advice: 'The simulation[s] showed that the inclusive strategy is much to be preferred'.

In more recent years, with the advent of datasets containing very large numbers of variables, such a strategy may not always be feasible or advisable. For recent work exploring imputation model choice with large numbers of variables, we refer readers to Hardt *et al.* (2012) and Zhao and Long (2016).

Our conclusion at this point is that within our model-based framework, we can make use of uncongenial imputation models when convenient, provided that they are not lacking an essential aspect of the analysis procedure, and we should at worst expect some conservatism in the long run properties of the MI based inferences.

2.8.4 Survey sample settings

Although we are not principally concerned in this book with the problems of applying MI in a survey sample context, we do touch on such issues when faced with estimators that require weighting. We summarise a few key points here before returning to the problem in Chapter 11. In the development so far in this chapter, it has been assumed that that the complete data have been generated through random sampling from some population model which forms the basis of our substantive model. The behaviour of MI has been considered under such conditions. When this is not the case, and the sampling of the data from the population is not simple, as with most survey samples, the justification for the MI procedure raises additional issues, in particular, a naive application of the Rubin's variance estimator is commonly inappropriate. One manifestation of this problem is the use of imputation procedures that are based on the entire sample, being applied to analyses applied to subsets of the data. Domain estimation is the common example of this. Again, a naive application of the MI variance in such settings will typically not be appropriate. Kott (1995) provides an early and clear description of the essential problem: the variance estimators derived from the sets of multiply imputed datasets do not follow from the actual sampling mechanism and so do not condition appropriately.

2.9 Constructing congenial imputation models

Consider the linear regression substantive model

$$f(\mathbf{Y} \mid \mathbf{X}) \sim N_n(\mathbf{X}\boldsymbol{\beta};\ \sigma^2 \boldsymbol{I}_n), \tag{2.40}$$

for $\mathbf{X}$ an $(n \times p)$ matrix of covariates, fitted using ordinary least squares in the usual way. Suppose that we have missing data in both response and covariates. Then, if we choose a distribution $g(\mathbf{X})$ for the covariates, the joint distribution for $(\mathbf{Y}, \mathbf{X})$ given by

$$f(\mathbf{Y}|\mathbf{X})g(\mathbf{X}) \tag{2.41}$$

gives an imputation model for the missing data which is congenial with the substantive model (2.8) fitted by ordinary least squares, in the sense described in Section 2.4. If both f and g are correctly specified, then this congenial imputation model is correctly specified. However, it maybe that g is mis-specified, in which case, the imputation model, though it remains congenial, will be mis-specified.

By specifying a distribution for the covariates in the substantive model, it is therefore always possible to derive a congenial imputation model. However, to use MI, we need to draw from the distribution of the missing data given the observed. In order to do this in a way that is consistent with (2.41), it is simplest to derive the distribution of the partially observed variables given the fully observed variables from (2.41), fit this and impute from it. This is because, under MAR, valid inference for the parameters of this distribution can be obtained from the observed data. For example, if $\mathbf{X}$ is continuous and g the p-variate multivariate normal distribution, this will be a multivariate normal regression model.

This works well when the distribution of the partially observed variables given the fully observed variables derived from (2.41) has a known form, or is well approximated by a known form. However, with non-linear relationships or interactions (Chapter 6), and in more complex settings (such as survival models, Chapter 7), this will generally not be the case. We then have a choice of either (i) approximating the joint distribution of the missing data given the observed with a distribution whose form we know, or (ii) using an appropriate MCMC sampler to fit (2.41) directly. We consider both approaches in Chapter 6.

Detailed practical guidance on choosing appropriate imputation models is given in Chapter 14. However, at this point, it is worth noting that – as the results of Hughes *et al.* (2012) show – the extensive discussion in this chapter of various issues surrounding Rubin's rules must be kept in proportion. In particular, we agree with Reiter (2017) that the greatest threat to materially invalid inferences from MI is from bias in the MI point estimator. To minimise the chances of this, we should ensure the imputation model choices we make are sensible in light of the types of variables involved and the types of analyses we plan, or can anticipate, will be performed on the imputed datasets.

2.10 Discussion

It is probably true that in many missing data settings, there are alternative approaches that can be taken, and these may be more efficient than MI, sometimes with a stronger justification in a strictly statistical sense. We have also seen that some care needs to be taken when using MI outside the congenial setting, for which a complete Bayesian framework exists, at least in principle. Following from this, it has also been argued that having put so much effort into sampling from an approximately correct Bayesian posterior, it would be more sensible to follow a fully Bayesian route altogether. This is certainly true in some examples. However, in practice any statistical analysis is surrounded by less mathematical issues, which must be carefully balanced in the full picture. More efficient analyses, or more subtle precision estimators, for example, often require extensive bespoke theoretical and computational developments. MI is extraordinarily general and flexible in this respect and can represent a very successful practical compromise, provided due care is given to the broad requirements that justify its use. When in doubt the frequentist operating characteristic of a particular MI setup can be checked through simulation, and there are many extant examples of this that we quote throughout the following chapters. We close this chapter with a quote from Zaslavsky (1994) (also quoted by Meng and Romero, 2003) which is an excellent expression of these main ideas:

> Because it may be so difficult to specify fully a Bayesian analysis, in many problems the best strategy can be to use a model-based Bayesian inference for the part that requires it, in particular the imputation of missing data, and to use frequentist methods, relying on estimates of means and variances and approximate normality for the rest of the inference. Multiple imputation is a device for such a combined approach[…] This strategy may engender uncongeniality of the analytic methods used in different parts of the inference, even though each is appropriate for its part of the inferential task, and even in cases in which the same organization carries out both parts of the analysis. Nonetheless, the mixed strategy is desirable when it is the most tractable valid approach.

Exercises

Some of the following exercises require use of basic multiple imputation commands in R or Stata. An overview of these are given in Appendix C. You may also find it helpful to refer to the book's website (see preface) and Chapter 14 which gives practical guidance on using multiple imputation.

1. For this question, you will need the two datasets: `ch2full.txt` and `ch2miss.txt`, available from the companion website. The variables needed for this question are shown in Table 2.2.

Table 2.2 Description of variables in the datasets `ch2full.txt`, `ch2miss.txt`.

Variable name	Missing any observations?	Details
`id`	No	Unique individual identifier
`sex`	No	Sex (0 = male, 1 = female)
`smok0`	Yes	Smoking status (1 = current smoker, 0 = non-smoker)
`x0`	No	A continuous variable measured at baseline
`y0`	No	A continuous variable measured at baseline
`y1`	Yes	`y0` measured at a follow-up time

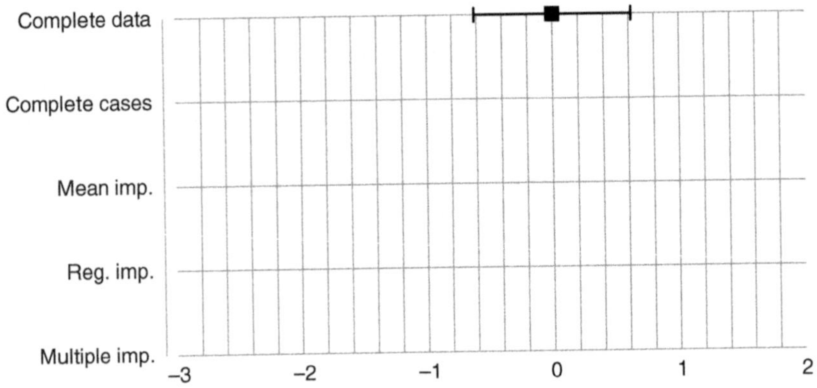

Figure 2.2 Fill in your estimates of the mean of `y1` *and its 95% confidence interval obtained from the different methods.*

(a) Using the full data, estimate the mean of `y1`, and check your results agree with Figure 2.2.

(b) Now open the dataset with missing values in `y1`. How many individuals have `y1` values missing?
Estimate the mean of `y1` in the complete records only, and plot it in Figure 2.2.

(c) Now, we will try mean imputation. Create a new variable `y1meanimp` in which the missing values in `y1` are replaced by the mean of the complete records.
Create plots of `y1meanimp` – histograms, scatter plots versus other variables, etc. How plausible are the values you have filled in?
Can you guess what the estimate of `y1`'s mean will be? Estimate the mean of `y1` again and fill in Figure 2.2.

(d) We will now fit a regression model, with `y1` as dependent variable, to the complete records. Then we will use the predicted values for missing `y1` to create a single imputed dataset. First, look at the other available variables and choose suitable variables for your regression model. Are any variables strongly associated with `y1`? Do any predict missingness in `y1`?
Once you have chosen the variables you will use to impute, fit a linear regression model with `y1` as the outcome and the variables you have chosen as covariates. Next, replace the missing values in `y1` with their predicted values from the fitted model.
Again, inspect the imputed data using plots, summaries, etc. Are these values more plausible than those based on simple mean imputation? Again, estimate the mean of `y1` and its 95% confidence interval and add these to Figure 2.2.

(e) Finally, we will try multiple imputation. Use MI to impute the missing values in `y1` 10 times, using a normal linear regression model, with the same covariates as you chose in the previous part. Refer to Appendix C and Chapter 14 for details of how to do this in `R` or Stata.
Fill in Figure 2.2 with your multiple imputation point estimate and confidence interval.

(f) Look at the different estimates of the mean of `y1` in Figure 2.2. Comment on your point estimates and confidence intervals (including their width). Which do you trust? Can you explain how the different analyses relate to each another?

2. Enter the data in Table 2.1 (recall from Example 2.1 that $X_i = i$ for $i = 1, \dots, 10$). Program the simple multiple imputation algorithm of Example 2.1 and use this to impute the missing values in Y for $K = 10, 20, 50, 100, 200, 500, 1000$ imputations.

(a) Plot the estimated mean of Y against the number of imputations and show it converges to ≈ 6.99. Verify this theoretically.

(b) Show by your simulations that the estimated standard error converges to ≈ 1.02. Why might we expect this to be greater than the SE of the mean of the complete data (1.00)?

(c) Show by your simulations that the fraction of missing information converges to $\approx 3\%$, and interpret this result.

(d) Do the mean, SE, and fraction of missing information converge at different rates? Discuss criteria for choosing the number of imputations.

3. **(a)** Consider a sample of size n from the bivariate normal distribution

$$\begin{pmatrix} Y_i \\ X_i \end{pmatrix} \overset{\text{i.i.d.}}{\sim} N\left[\begin{pmatrix} \mu_Y \\ \mu_X \end{pmatrix}, \begin{pmatrix} \sigma_Y^2 & \sigma_{YX} \\ \sigma_{YX} & \sigma_X^2 \end{pmatrix}\right],$$

and suppose some Y_i are missing at random given fully observed X_i. The substantive model (i.e. analyst's complete data procedure) is to estimate the mean, $E[Y] = \mu_Y$ by the sample mean, $\overline{Y} = \sum_{i=1}^{n} Y_i/n$, with its variance estimated by

$$\frac{1}{n(n-1)} \sum_{i=1}^{n} (Y_i - \overline{Y})^2.$$

Multiple imputation uses the linear regression model

$$Y_i = \alpha_0 + \alpha_1 X_i + e_i, \quad e_i \overset{i.i.d.}{\sim} N(0, \sigma^2_{Y|X}).$$

Are the MI model and substantive model congenial? Do you expect Rubin's variance estimator to be consistent? Do your answers depend on whether the marginal distribution of X is assumed to be normal?

(b) Suppose now that X and Z are two fully observed binary variables and again Y is partially observed. The MI model for Y is a linear regression of Y on covariates X, Z and their interaction XZ. The substantive model is a linear regression of Y on X and Z (i.e. omitting their interaction).

Are the imputation model and substantive model congenial? If the true value of the interaction parameter in the imputation model is 0, would you expect Rubin's variance estimator to be consistent?

(c) Consider the same setup as in the previous part, except now the imputation model does not include the XZ interaction, whereas the substantive model does.

Are the imputation model and substantive model congenial? Assuming again that in truth the interaction parameter is zero, would you expect Rubin's variance estimator to be consistent?

(d) Verify your answers using simulation.

4. (a) (hard) Consider a random variable Y with a t-distribution with n degrees of freedom with density

$$f(y;\mu) = \frac{\Gamma(\frac{n+1}{2})}{\sqrt{n\pi}\Gamma(\frac{n}{2})}\left(1 + \frac{(y-\mu)^2}{n}\right)^{-\frac{n+1}{2}}.$$

Show that the contribution of one observation to the information for the mean, μ, of Y is $(n+1)/(n+3)$. *Hint:* recall that, in a statistical model, the information is minus the expectation of the second derivative of the log-likelihood with respect to the parameter of interest (here μ) and that $\Gamma(n+1) = n\Gamma(n)$ with $\Gamma(0) = 1$.

(b) If $T = \sigma Y$, deduce the contribution of one observation to the information for the mean is $(n+1)/[(n+3)\sigma^2]$.

(c) Assuming that

$$T = \frac{\hat{\beta}_{MI} - \beta_0}{\sqrt{\hat{V}_{MI}}}$$

follows a t-distribution with degrees of freedom given by (2.4), deduce that a better estimate of the fraction of missing information is given by (2.7), i.e.

$$\frac{\hat{W}^{-1} - (\nu + 1)\{(\nu + 3)(\hat{W} + (1 + 1/K)\hat{B})\}^{-1}}{\hat{W}^{-1}}.$$

5. Consider outcome variable Y_i, covariate X_i and regression model $f(Y_i|X_i, \boldsymbol{\beta})$, for independent observations $i = 1, \ldots, n$. In this question, assume all missingness mechanisms are ignorable.

(a) Show that if Y_i is missing at random (given X_i) for individual i, their contribution to the observed data likelihood for β is 1.

(b) Now suppose that all the Y_i are observed, but some X_i are missing at random (given Y_i). Let the marginal density of X_i be $f(X_i)$. For an individual with X_i missing, their contribution to the observed data likelihood for β is

$$L_i = \int f(Y_i|X_i; \boldsymbol{\beta})f(X_i)\, dX_i.$$

Show that their contribution to the *score*

$$s_i(\boldsymbol{\beta}; Y, X_i) = \frac{\partial}{\partial \boldsymbol{\beta}} \log(L_i)$$

can be written as

$$\mathrm{E}_{f(X|Y)} \left\{ \frac{\partial}{\partial \boldsymbol{\beta}} \log f(Y_i|X_i; \boldsymbol{\beta}) \right\},$$

i.e. the expectation of the full data score contribution for individual i over the conditional distribution of the missing data given the observed data.

(c) Extend this result to show

$$\mathrm{E}_{f(\mathbf{Y}_M|\mathbf{Y}_O,\mathbf{R})}\{\mathbf{U}(\hat{\boldsymbol{\beta}}; \mathbf{Y}_O, \mathbf{Y}_M)\} = \mathbf{0},$$

for a score statistic $\mathbf{U}$ (cf. (2.11)).

6. Under the missing at random assumption, show Louis's formula, (2.12), for a score statistic $\mathbf{U}$ and a consistent estimator $\hat{\boldsymbol{\beta}}$.

7. Justification of Rubin's MI rules.

(a) From linear regression theory, why is (2.24) intuitively reasonable? Show that it implies that $\mathrm{E}[\hat{W}/\hat{W}_\infty]$ is 1, and $\mathrm{Var}[\hat{W}/\hat{W}_\infty]$ is $O(n^{-1})$.

(b) Assume that

$$\frac{\widehat{W}/\widehat{W}_\infty}{\widehat{B}/\widehat{B}_\infty}$$

approximately follows an $F_{n,K}$ distribution, and recall from above (2.24) that $r = (\widehat{B}/\widehat{W})(1 + K^{-1})$. Show that we need $\widehat{B}_\infty/\widehat{W}_\infty$ to be $O(n^{-l})$, $l > 0$ in order for r to be regarded as approximately constant.

(c) For the definition of $f(A)$ given by (2.25), and assuming r is approximately constant, show that $\mathrm{E}\{f(A)\} \approx 1$ and

$$\mathrm{Var}\{f(A)\} \approx \frac{2}{K-1}\left(\frac{r}{r+1}\right)^2.$$

(d) Deduce that (2.23) can be approximated by the χ^2_ν distribution, where

$$\nu = (K-1)(1+r^{-1})^2 = (K-1)\left\{\frac{\widehat{W} + (1+K^{-1})\widehat{B}}{(1+K^{-1})\widehat{B}}\right\}^2.$$

PART II

MULTIPLE IMPUTATION FOR SIMPLE DATA STRUCTURES

3

Multiple imputation of quantitative data

In this chapter, we describe and illustrate parametric multiple imputation for continuous data. In particular, we focus on situations where the joint distribution (possibly after appropriate transformation of one or more variables) of the data can be considered multivariate normal. We begin, in Section 3.1, with the simplest computational approach, appropriate when the missingness pattern is monotone. In general, this will not be the case, and Section 3.2 describes imputation based on the joint multivariate normal distribution. Another option, equivalent for multivariate normal data, is the full conditional specification (FCS) approach described in Section 3.3. We conclude with a brief review of software and a discussion in Sections 3.5 and 3.6.

3.1 Regression imputation with a monotone missingness pattern

Suppose we have $i = 1, \dots, n$ units, on each of which we seek to measure variables $Y_{i,j}, j = 1, \dots, p$. In other words, if no data are missing, then the dataset is rectangular, with dimension n by p. Let $\mathbf{Y}_j = (Y_{1,j}, \dots, Y_{n,j})^T$ be the n by 1 column vector of the observations on variable j.

As usual, our substantive model is a regression; specifically in this chapter a linear regression. Our response is thus one of the p variables, and we impute assuming that the remaining $p - 1$ covariates are potentially important for the substantive model; having done so, if desired we can fit the substantive model to a reduced set of variables. At its simplest, this means regressing the response on the constant alone, which estimates its marginal mean.

Multiple Imputation and its Application, Second Edition.
James R. Carpenter, Jonathan W. Bartlett, Tim P. Morris, Angela M. Wood, Matteo Quartagno and Michael G. Kenward.

In this section, we assume the missing data pattern is monotone, with $\mathbf{Y}_1$ fully observed and most missing observations on $\mathbf{Y}_p$. This is a common situation, for example, with longitudinal data, where missingness is often due to drop out and hence, once missing for a visit, patients do not come back for following visits. We assume data are missing at random (MAR) with a mechanism which means that each of the regressions of $\mathbf{Y}_j$ on $\mathbf{Y}_1, \dots, \mathbf{Y}_{j-1}, j = 2, \dots, p$ is validly estimated from the set of complete records on $\mathbf{Y}_1, \dots, \mathbf{Y}_j$. Suppose we fit each of these $(p-1)$ regression models, using the corresponding set of complete records for variables in each model, obtaining estimated vectors of regression coefficients $\hat{\boldsymbol{\beta}}_2, \dots, \hat{\boldsymbol{\beta}}_p$ and residual variances $\hat{\sigma}_2^2, \dots, \hat{\sigma}_p^2$. For example the vector $\boldsymbol{\beta}_3 = (\beta_{03}, \beta_{13}, \beta_{23})^T$, which are the parameters in the linear regression

$$Y_{i,3} = \beta_{03} + \beta_{13} Y_{i,1} + \beta_{23} Y_{i,2} + e_{i,3}, \quad e_{i,3} \overset{i.i.d.}{\sim} N(0, \sigma_3^2).$$

Then, to impute the dataset, we sequentially impute missing values of each $\mathbf{Y}_j$ (for $j = 2, \dots, p$) in turn using the following algorithm:

1. For variable j, suppose $i = 1, \dots, n_j$ individuals have $Y_{i,j}$ observed; the monotone assumption means they have $Y_{i,1}, \dots, Y_{i,j-1}$ observed. Using data from these n_j individuals, let $\mathbf{x}_{i,j} = (1, Y_{i,1}, Y_{i,2}, \dots, Y_{i,j-1})^T$ so that

$$Y_{i,j} = \mathbf{x}_{i,j}^T \boldsymbol{\beta}_j + e_{i,j}, \quad e_{i,j} \overset{i.i.d.}{\sim} N(0, \sigma_j^2). \tag{3.1}$$

   Fit this model, obtaining the ordinary least squares estimates of $\boldsymbol{\beta}_j, \sigma_j^2$, denoted $\hat{\boldsymbol{\beta}}_j, \hat{\sigma}_j^2$, respectively.

2. Then

   (a) draw z from the $\chi^2_{n_j - j}$ distribution and set

$$\sigma^{*2}_j = \frac{\hat{\sigma}_j^2 (n_j - j)}{z},$$

   and draw $\boldsymbol{\beta}^*$ from

$$N(\hat{\boldsymbol{\beta}}, \sigma^{*2}_j \mathbf{A}_j),$$

   where

$$\mathbf{A}_j = \left(\sum_{i=1}^{n_j} \mathbf{x}_{i,j} \mathbf{x}_{i,j}^T \right)^{-1}.$$

   (b) For each unobserved $Y_{i,j}$, $i = n_j + 1, \dots, n$, draw $e^*_{i,j} \sim N(0, \sigma_j^{2*})$ and impute by

$$(1, Y_{i,1}, \dots, Y_{i,j-1}) \boldsymbol{\beta}^* + e^*_{i,j}, \tag{3.2}$$

   so that all the missing values of $\mathbf{Y}_j$ are imputed. We note that for $j = 3, \dots, p$, there will be some units with $Y_{i,j}$ missing and with one or more of $Y_{i,2}, \dots, Y_{i,j-1}$ missing, and imputed at previous steps. These previously imputed values are used in (3.2) when imputing $Y_{i,j}$.

Performing steps 1 and 2 above for $j = 2, \dots, p$ gives the first imputed dataset; the whole sequence is repeated to generate successive imputed datasets. We call this sequential regression multiple imputation.

3.1.1 MAR mechanisms consistent with a monotone pattern

With a monotone missingness mechanism, we can regard missingness as withdrawal; if a unit (typically individual) i has $Y_{i,j}$ missing, the observations $Y_{i,j+1}, \dots, Y_{i,p}$ will be missing. Under MAR, we may envisage the probability that individual i withdraws at j, given observations up to that point, depends on the history $Y_{i,1}, \dots, Y_{i,j-1}$, $j = 2, \dots, p$. In other words, the conditional distribution of $Y_{i,j}, \dots, Y_{i,p} | Y_{i,1}, \dots, Y_{i,j-1}$ is the same whether or not $Y_{i,j}, \dots, Y_{i,p}$ are observed. If appropriate in the context, the fully observed variables can include group indicators, such as treatment in a randomized controlled study.

Example 3.1 Asthma study

We continue with the five-arm asthma clinical trial introduced in Chapter 1, p. 7. We consider the placebo arm. Clinic visits to record FEV_1 were scheduled at baseline, 2, 4, 8, and 12 weeks. The missingness pattern, which is monotone, is shown in Table 1.3. Histograms and Q–Q plots are consistent with the data following a multivariate normal distribution, so we can apply all the imputation algorithms discussed in this chapter.

In the placebo arm, let $\mathbf{Y}_1, \dots, \mathbf{Y}_5$ denote the lung function measurements at baseline, weeks 2, 4, 8, and 12. Note there were no missing observations at baseline and week 2. Using all the observed data for each $j = 3,4,5$ we regress of $\mathbf{Y}_j$ on $\mathbf{Y}_1, \dots, \mathbf{Y}_{j-1}$, giving the estimates in Table 3.1.

Using the above algorithm, we begin by imputing missing values on Y_3 (4 weeks):

1. Draw z from the χ^2_{71} distribution. Suppose we get 60.32, implying that the draw of σ^{*2} is $0.39^2 \times (74 - 3)/z = 0.39^2 \times 71/60.32 = 0.42^2$. Form $\mathbf{x}_{i3} = (1, Y_{i1}, Y_{i2})$, $i = 1, \dots, n_3$, of dimension (74×3). Draw $\boldsymbol{\beta}^*_3 = (\beta^*_{03}, \beta^*_{13}, \beta^*_{23})^T$ from the $N(\hat{\boldsymbol{\beta}}_3, 0.42^2\mathbf{A}_3)$ distribution where

$$\hat{\boldsymbol{\beta}}_3 = (0.52, 0.27, 0.44)^T$$

Table 3.1 Coefficient estimates from regressions on observed data in placebo arm of asthma study. There were no missing values on Y_1 (baseline) and Y_2 (week 2).

Response:	Regression on					Residual variance	n_j
	Intercept	Y_1	Y_2	Y_3	Y_4		
Y_3	0.52	0.27	0.44	—	—	0.39^2	74
Y_4	0.08	0.15	0.51	0.27	—	0.41^2	52
Y_5	0.49	−0.73	1.03	0.01	0.43	0.29^2	37

and

$$A_3 = \left(\sum_{i=1}^{74} \mathbf{x}_{i3}\mathbf{x}_{i3}^T \right)^{-1} = \begin{pmatrix} 0.15 & -0.06 & -0.01 \\ -0.06 & 0.07 & -0.05 \\ -0.01 & -0.05 & 0.06 \end{pmatrix}.$$

Suppose that this draw is equal to

$$\boldsymbol{\beta}^*{}_3 = \begin{pmatrix} 0.33 \\ 0.56 \\ 0.20 \end{pmatrix}.$$

2. Then, for each individual i, with missing data at week 4, draw the imputed value of $Y_{i,3}$ from

$$N(0.33 + 0.56Y_{i,1} + 0.20Y_{i,2}, 0.42^2).$$

To impute missing data at week 8, we proceed in a similar way, but now, for individuals i missing both Y_{i3} and Y_{i4}, we need the imputed data Y_{i3} in step 2. Lastly, we repeat the process again to impute missing values at week 12. Together this gives a single imputation of the whole dataset. The whole process is repeated to generate successive imputed datasets.

Applying this algorithm, we created 100 imputed datasets. For each we calculate the mean of $\mathbf{Y}_3, \mathbf{Y}_4, \mathbf{Y}_5$ and then combine the results using Rubin's rules. The results are shown in Table 3.2, where the top row shows the mean FEV_1 at each follow-up visits estimated using the 37 patients who completed, the second row shows the estimates using all available data at each visit (respectively, 90, 90, 74, 52, and 37 patients), and the third row shows estimates obtained by fitting a saturated repeated measures model with an unstructured covariance matrix using REstricted Maximum Likelihood (REML). We see that the complete records and all observed data estimates (which assume data are missing completely at random (MCAR)) are markedly higher at the end of the study than the REML estimates, which are valid under the assumption that data are MAR given earlier visits. As theory predicts, these agree very closely with the results using sequential regression MI. □

3.1.2 Justification

To see why this approach is valid, consider the joint distribution:

$$\begin{aligned} f(Y_{i,1}, Y_{i,2}, \dots, Y_{i,p}) = & f(Y_{i,p} \mid Y_{i,1}, \dots, Y_{i,p-1}) \\ & \times f(Y_{i,p-1} \mid Y_{i,1} \dots, Y_{i,p-2}) \times \cdots \times f(Y_{i,2}|Y_{i,1}) \times f(Y_{i,1}). \end{aligned} \quad (3.3)$$

With a monotone missingness pattern, the assumption of MAR means that each of the conditional distributions on the right-hand side can be validly estimated from the observed data. Putting these together gives a valid estimate of the joint distribution. Therefore, imputing from each of the conditionals in turn gives a valid imputation from the joint distribution.

Of course, in many applications, the missingness pattern will not be monotone. In that case, data may be MAR, although we cannot then assume that the same mechanism applies to all the units. Indeed, the concept of MAR for non-monotone missingness has been called into question by some authors (e.g. (Robins and Gill, 1997)). More reasonably, we might assume that MAR is a sufficiently good working assumption for the analysis. With non-monotone missingness one or more of the distributions on the RHS of (3.3) will not be validly estimated from corresponding regression (as there will be units where $Y_{i,j}$ is observed but one or more of $Y_{i,1}, \dots, Y_{i,j-1}$ will be missing). In this case, we need to model the joint distribution of the data explicitly in order to impute. We now describe how this is done.

3.2 Joint modelling

In this section, we make no assumptions about the missingness pattern, but assume that the missingness mechanism is ignorable, as defined in Section 1.4.4, so that we do not have to model it.

The imputation model, i.e. the joint model for the data, is then the multivariate normal model,

$$\mathbf{Y} \sim N(\boldsymbol{\beta}, \boldsymbol{\Omega}), \tag{3.4}$$

for

$$\mathbf{Y} = \begin{pmatrix} Y_{i,1} \\ Y_{i,2} \\ \vdots \\ Y_{i,p} \end{pmatrix} \quad \text{and} \quad \boldsymbol{\beta} = \begin{pmatrix} \beta_{0,1} \\ \beta_{0,2} \\ \vdots \\ \beta_{0,p} \end{pmatrix},$$

where $\boldsymbol{\Omega}$ is the unstructured $p \times p$ covariance matrix with $p(p+1)/2$ parameters.

We now describe an algorithm to impute under this multivariate model.

3.2.1 Fitting the imputation model

The Gibbs sampler is one possible approach to estimate the parameters in the joint imputation model (3.4) and impute the missing data. It is a special case of the more general Metropolis Hastings sampler; which is described in Appendix A. For a fuller description of Markov chain Monte Carlo (MCMC) methods in the context of missing data, and specifically fitting the multivariate normal model, see Schafer (1997).

We show in Appendix B how, if there were no missing data, we can take a flat, improper prior for the mean $\boldsymbol{\beta}$ of $\mathbf{Y}_i$ and a $\mathrm{W}(\nu, \mathbf{S}_p)$ prior distribution for the inverse of the covariance matrix $\boldsymbol{\Omega}^{-1}$, then the posterior distribution of $\boldsymbol{\beta}, \boldsymbol{\Omega}$ given $\mathbf{Y}$ can be written as the product of a normal distribution for $\boldsymbol{\beta}$ given $\boldsymbol{\Omega}^{-1}$ and a marginal Wishart distribution for $\boldsymbol{\Omega}^{-1}$. This can be expressed

$$\begin{aligned} \boldsymbol{\beta} \mid \mathbf{Y}, \boldsymbol{\Omega} &\sim N(\overline{\mathbf{Y}}, n^{-1}\boldsymbol{\Omega}), \quad \text{and} \\ \boldsymbol{\Omega}^{-1} \mid \mathbf{Y} &\sim \mathrm{W}\{n+\nu, (\mathbf{S}_p^{-1} + \mathbf{S})^{-1}\}, \end{aligned} \tag{3.5}$$

for $\overline{\mathbf{Y}} = (\overline{Y}_1, \dots, \overline{Y}_p)^T$, $\overline{Y}_j = n^{-1} \sum_{i=1}^{n} Y_{i,j}$ and

$$\mathbf{S} = \sum_{i=1}^{n} (\mathbf{Y}_i - \overline{\mathbf{Y}})(\mathbf{Y}_i - \overline{\mathbf{Y}})^T,$$

i.e. $\overline{\mathbf{Y}}$ and $(n-1)^{-1}\mathbf{S}$ are the sample mean and covariance matrix, respectively.

Now suppose we have missing data, and we write $\mathbf{Y} = (\mathbf{Y}_O, \mathbf{Y}_M)$. As described in Appendix A, the Gibbs sampler proceeds by drawing each parameter (or set of parameters) in turn, conditional on all the others and the data. Further, in the Bayesian framework, missing data are treated as parameters. We could take a prior for the missing data, and in subsequent chapters (for example chapter 10), we show this can be very useful in certain applications. For now, we assume the prior for the missing values is a flat improper one.

To initialize the Gibbs sampler, we choose starting values for (i) $\boldsymbol{\beta}$, (ii) $\boldsymbol{\Omega}$, and (iii) $\mathbf{Y}_O$. A natural choice is to estimate (i) and (ii) using the observed data. For (iii), we can draw a starting value for missing $Y_{i,j}$ by sampling with replacement from the observed values of the variable $\mathbf{Y}_j$. Denote these values by $\boldsymbol{\beta}^0, \boldsymbol{\Omega}^0$, and $\mathbf{Y}_M{}^0$. Form $\overline{\mathbf{Y}}^0$ as the sample mean calculated using $\mathbf{Y}_M{}^0, \mathbf{Y}_O$, and likewise calculate $\mathbf{S}^0$.

The algorithm then proceeds as follows: at iteration $r = 1,2,\dots,$

1. draw
$$\boldsymbol{\Omega}^{-1,r} \sim \mathrm{W}\{n+\nu, (\mathbf{S}_p^{-1} + \mathbf{S}^{r-1})^{-1}\};$$
2. draw
$$\boldsymbol{\beta}^r \sim N(\overline{\mathbf{Y}}^{r-1}, n^{-1}\boldsymbol{\Omega}^r);$$
3. Draw, as detailed below, $\mathbf{Y}_M{}^r \sim f(\mathbf{Y}_M \mid \boldsymbol{\beta}^r, \boldsymbol{\Omega}^r, \mathbf{Y}_O)$;
4. Update the sample mean $\overline{\mathbf{Y}}^r$ using $(\mathbf{Y}_M{}^r, \mathbf{Y}_O)$;
5. Update the sample matrix of sums of squares and cross products, $\mathbf{S}^r$ using $(\mathbf{Y}_M{}^r, \mathbf{Y}_O)$; We thus have $\boldsymbol{\beta}^r, \boldsymbol{\Omega}^r, \overline{\mathbf{Y}}^r, \mathbf{S}^r, \mathbf{Y}_M{}^r$ completing iteration r.
6. Return to step 1.

We next describe how to draw $\mathbf{Y}_M^r$. For each unit $i = 1, \dots, n$, with missing data, let $\mathbf{Y}_{Mi}$ denote the missing values and $\mathbf{Y}_{Oi}$ the observed data. We draw $\mathbf{Y}_{M_i}^r$ from the conditional normal distribution given $\mathbf{Y}_{Oi}$ calculated from the joint multivariate distribution at the current draws,

$$\mathbf{Y}_i \sim N_p(\boldsymbol{\beta}^r, \boldsymbol{\Omega}^T).$$

As we have, potentially, a different missingness pattern for each unit, the appropriate conditional will have to be derived for each unit in turn, as follows: re-order unit i's variables so that $Y_{i,1}, \dots, Y_{i,p_1}$ are observed and $Y_{i,p_1+1}, \dots, Y_{i,p}$ are missing.

Correspondingly re-order $\boldsymbol{\beta}, \boldsymbol{\Omega}$ and partition $\boldsymbol{\beta} = (\boldsymbol{\beta}_1^T, \boldsymbol{\beta}_2^T)^T$ where $\boldsymbol{\beta}_1^T = (\beta_1, \dots, \beta_{p_1})$, and $\boldsymbol{\beta}_2 = (\beta_{p_1+1}, \dots, \beta_p)$. Similarly partition

$$\Omega = \begin{pmatrix} \boldsymbol{\Omega}_{1,1} & \boldsymbol{\Omega}_{1,2} \\ \boldsymbol{\Omega}_{2,1} & \boldsymbol{\Omega}_{2,2} \end{pmatrix}.$$

Then, at the current values of $\boldsymbol{\beta}$, $\boldsymbol{\Omega}$, in the Gibbs sampler, draw $\mathbf{Y}_{Mi} = (Y_{i,p_1+1}, Y_{i,p_1+2}, \dots, Y_{i,p})^T$ using

$$N\{\boldsymbol{\beta}_2 + (\mathbf{Y}_{Oi} - \boldsymbol{\beta}_1)^T \boldsymbol{\Omega}_{1,1}^{-1} \boldsymbol{\Omega}_{1,2},\ \ \boldsymbol{\Omega}_{2,2} - \boldsymbol{\Omega}_{2,1} \boldsymbol{\Omega}_{1,1}^{-1} \boldsymbol{\Omega}_{1,2}\}. \tag{3.6}$$

This completes the Gibbs sampler for drawing from $f(\mathbf{Y}_M, \boldsymbol{\beta}, \boldsymbol{\Omega} | \mathbf{Y}_O)$, with prior $\mathrm{W}(\nu, \mathbf{S}_p)$. For MI we proceed as follows:

1. Start the sampler, and update it n_{burn} times to allow it to reach its stationary distribution:
2. Put the current draw of the missing data, $\mathbf{Y}_M{}^{n_{\text{burn}}}$, together with the observed data $\mathbf{Y}_O$ to form the first imputed dataset, denoted $\mathbf{Y}^1$.
3. Update the Gibbs sampler a further n_{between} times
4. Put the current draw of the missing data together with the observed data to form the second imputed dataset, $\mathbf{Y}^2$.
5. Repeat steps 3 and 4 to create successive imputed datasets $\mathbf{Y}^k$, $k = 3, \dots, K$.

We then fit the model of interest to each imputed dataset, obtaining K point estimates and associated standard errors, which are combined for inference using Rubin's rules.

To start the algorithm, we need values for $\overline{\mathbf{Y}}$ and $\mathbf{S}$. As already mentioned, the simplest approach is to estimate each component of these using all the available data. A more sophisticated approach is to use the expectation maximisation (EM) algorithm (Orchard and Woodbury, 1972, Dempster *et al.*, 1977) to estimate $\boldsymbol{\beta}, \boldsymbol{\Omega}$, then use these values to draw each unit's missing data from the appropriate conditional distributions, and then take these as starting values for the Gibbs sampler. Schafer (1997, p. 163) describes the appropriate EM algorithm in detail. The advantage of using the EM algorithm to provide initial values for the Gibbs sampler is (i) the Gibbs sampler starts from a converged state (or very close to it) so that limited burn in is needed; and (ii) it is obvious when the EM algorithm has not converged. If the EM algorithm fails to converge, this gives warning of a problem with the data. Such problems are much harder to detect from the output of the Gibbs sampler, which will continue to iterate whether or not the model is well specified.

Formal diagnostics for convergence of MCMC algorithms are discussed elsewhere (e.g. Gilks *et al.*, 1996), but for the multivariate normal model considered here, with starting values obtained from the observed data and of the order of 10 variables, we have found a burn-in of $n_{\text{burn}} = 1000$ iterations with $n_{\text{between}} = 500$ works well. The parameter chains should be checked for convergence, and more formal diagnostic tests may be appropriate. For larger datasets, the attraction of using the EM algorithm to obtain starting values increases, and more updates may be desirable, together with automating application of convergence diagnostics.

There are a number of other ways to obtain approximate samples from the Bayesian posterior distribution of $\boldsymbol{\beta}$, $\boldsymbol{\Omega}$. The most natural is to fit the multivariate normal model (3.4) to the observed data using maximum, or better restricted maximum, likelihood giving estimates $\hat{\boldsymbol{\beta}}$, $\hat{\boldsymbol{\Omega}}$ and create each imputed data set by

1. drawing $(\boldsymbol{\Omega}^{-1})^* \sim \text{W}\{n-p,(n\hat{\boldsymbol{\Omega}})^{-1}\}$;
2. drawing $\boldsymbol{\beta}^* \sim N(\hat{\boldsymbol{\beta}}, n^{-1}\boldsymbol{\Omega}^*)$
3. using $\boldsymbol{\beta}^*$ and $\boldsymbol{\Omega}^*$ to impute the missing data using (3.6).

Again, this has the advantage that lack of convergence of the REML algorithm is obvious and warns of difficulties with the data. As the sample size increases, this algorithm will give very similar results to the full Gibbs sampler.

Example 3.1 Asthma study *(ctd)*

Continuing with the asthma data, we apply the Gibbs sampler, with prior $\propto |\boldsymbol{\Omega}^{-1}|^{-(p+1)/2}$ to impute the placebo arm of the trial; we then calculate the sample means at each time point. Taking $n_{\text{burn}} = 5000$ and $n_{\text{between}} = 5000$, we created $K = 100$ imputations, then applied Rubin's rules to estimate the mean and standard error at each time point.

Figure 3.1 shows the chains for four of the parameters, which typical of what we would expect if the sampler has reached its stationary distribution at the end of the burn in and is mixing (i.e. moving around the posterior distribution) well. The resulting estimates are shown in the fifth row of Table 3.2. As expected, they are virtually identical to both the estimates from REML and sequential MI. □

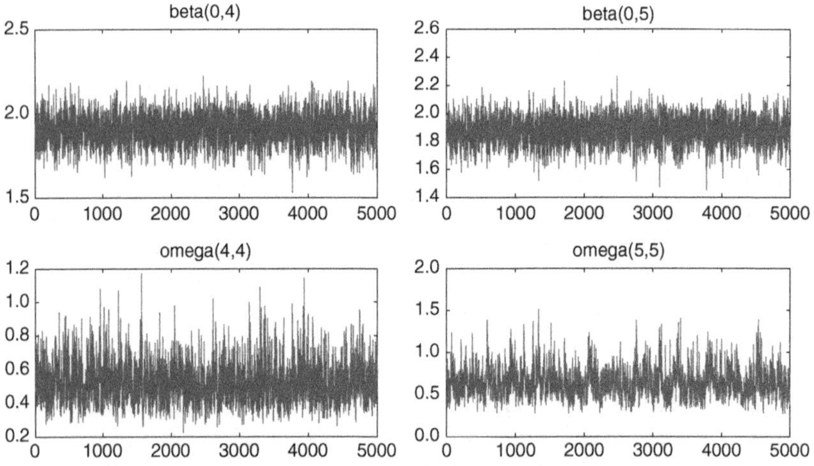

Figure 3.1 Post burn-in trace plots for β_{04}, β_{05} and corresponding elements of the covariance matrix $\boldsymbol{\Omega}_{44}, \boldsymbol{\Omega}_{55}$, from the Gibbs sampler.

Table 3.2 Results of multiple imputation for the placebo arm of the asthma study, using the different algorithms described in this chapter. Mean FEV_1 (litres) and standard error at each follow-up visit. Each method used 100 imputations.

Analysis	Mean FEV_1 (litres) measured at week				
	0	2	4	8	12
Complete records	2.11	2.14	2.07	2.01	2.06
	(0.09)	(0.09)	(0.10)	(0.10)	(0.09)
All observed data	2.06	1.97	1.98	2.04	2.06
	(0.06)	(0.07)	(0.06)	(0.08)	(0.09)
REML	2.06	1.97	1.94	1.91	1.88
	(0.06)	(0.07)	(0.06)	(0.08)	(0.09)
Sequential regression MI	2.06	1.97	1.94	1.92	1.88
	(0.06)	(0.07)	(0.06)	(0.09)	(0.09)
Joint MI(Jeffreys prior)	2.06	1.97	1.94	1.91	1.88
	(0.06)	(0.07)	(0.07)	(0.08)	(0.09)
FCS MI	2.06	1.97	1.94	1.91	1.87
	(0.06)	(0.07)	(0.07)	(0.09)	(0.10)

3.2.2 Adding covariates

Since, hitherto, the joint imputation model has just had the mean of each response on the right-hand side, we now give the additional Gibbs sampler step for a model with covariates.

As an illustration, suppose we have two response variables, so $\mathbf{Y}_i = (Y_{i,1}, Y_{i,2})^T$, and covariates $X_{i,1}, X_{i,2}, X_{i,3}$. Then our multivariate normal imputation model for $\mathbf{Y}_i$ given the covariates is

$$\begin{pmatrix} Y_{i,1} \\ Y_{i,2} \end{pmatrix} \sim \begin{pmatrix} \beta_{0,1} + \beta_{1,1}X_{i,1} + \beta_{2,1}X_{i,2} + \beta_{3,1}X_{i,3} + e_{i,2} \\ \beta_{0,2} + \beta_{1,2}X_{i,1} + \beta_{2,2}X_{i,2} + \beta_{3,2}X_{i,3} + e_{i,3} \end{pmatrix},$$

$$\begin{pmatrix} e_{i,2} \\ e_{i,3} \end{pmatrix} \sim N_2(\mathbf{0}, \mathbf{\Omega}). \tag{3.7}$$

In order to write the imputation model more succinctly, we introduce and illustrate the Kronecker product notation. Define the Kronecker product of two matrices, A (dimension I by J, elements a_{ij}) and B (dimension K by L) by $C = A \bigotimes B$, of dimension IK by JL where

$$C = \begin{pmatrix} a_{1,1}B & a_{1,2}B & \cdots & a_{1,J}B \\ a_{2,1}B & a_{2,2}B & \cdots & a_{2,J}B \\ \vdots & \vdots & \ddots & \vdots \\ a_{I,1}B & a_{I,2}B & \ddots & a_{I,J}B \end{pmatrix}.$$

Let $W_i = (1, X_{i,1}, X_{i,2}, X_{i,3})$ (1 for the intercept). Let $\boldsymbol{\beta}_1 = (\beta_{0,1}, \beta_{1,1}, \beta_{2,1}, \beta_{3,1})^T$ and $\boldsymbol{\beta}_2 = (\beta_{0,2}, \beta_{1,2}, \beta_{2,2}, \beta_{3,2})^T$. Let $\boldsymbol{\beta} = (\boldsymbol{\beta}_1^T, \boldsymbol{\beta}_2^T)^T$ (dimension 8×1) and $\mathbf{Z}_i = \boldsymbol{I}_2 \bigotimes W_i$ (dimension 2×8), i.e.

$$\mathbf{Z}_i = \begin{pmatrix} 1 & X_{i,1} & X_{i,2} & X_{i,3} & 0 & 0 & 0 & 0 \\ 0 & 0 & 0 & 0 & 1 & X_{i,1} & X_{i,2} & X_{i,3} \end{pmatrix}.$$

Then the multivariate normal imputation model is

$$\mathbf{Y}_i = \mathbf{Z}_i\boldsymbol{\beta} + \mathbf{e}_i, \quad \mathbf{e}_i \sim N(\mathbf{0}, \boldsymbol{\Omega}), \tag{3.8}$$

$i = 1, \ldots, n$.

We now consider the Gibbs sampler for sampling from the posterior distribution of the parameters $\boldsymbol{\beta}$, $\boldsymbol{\Omega}$, in (3.8). We initialize $\boldsymbol{\beta} = \mathbf{0}$, $\boldsymbol{\Omega} = \boldsymbol{I}$. Then at update step $r = 2, 3, \ldots$.

1. Given the current draw of $\boldsymbol{\Omega}$, assume an improper prior for $\boldsymbol{\beta}$ and draw the next $\boldsymbol{\beta}$ from the multivariate normal distribution

$$N\left[\left\{\sum_{i=1}^{n} Z^T\Omega^{-1}Z\right\}^{-1} \sum_{i=1}^{n}\{Z_i^T\Omega^{-1}\mathbf{Y}_i\}, \left\{\sum_{i=1}^{n} Z_i^T\Omega^{-1}Z_i\right\}^{-1}\right]. \tag{3.9}$$

2. Given the current draw of $\boldsymbol{\beta}$, choose $\mathrm{W}(n_p, S_p)$ prior for $\boldsymbol{\Omega}^{-1}$. Calculate the current residuals, $\mathbf{e}_i$. Then draw $\boldsymbol{\Omega}^{-1}$ from $\mathrm{W}(n + n_p, S_u)$, where

$$S_u = \left\{\sum_{i=1}^{n} \mathbf{e}_i\mathbf{e}_i^T + S_p^{-1}\right\}^{-1}.$$

   Note that if $\boldsymbol{\Omega}$ has dimension $p \times p$, then choosing $n_p = (p+1)$ and $S_p = \mathbf{0}$ gives a uniform prior on $\boldsymbol{\Omega}$.

3. For units with missing $\mathbf{Y}_i$, given current draws of $\boldsymbol{\beta}, \boldsymbol{\Omega}$, draw

$$\mathbf{Y}_i \sim N(\mathbf{Z}_i\boldsymbol{\beta}, \boldsymbol{\Omega});$$

   Should one of the responses be observed, we draw from the conditional normal distribution given the other response, as described in Section 3.2.

We can include categorical variables in the above approach too. If they are fully observed, we include dummy indicators for each level (bar the reference) as covariates in the imputation model (3.8).

3.3 Full conditional specification

If the missing data pattern is monotone, the sequential regression multiple imputation approach above is relatively simple to program within most statistical software packages, as it uses the linear regression command. One would also expect it to be a good approximation if the missingness pattern were close to monotone. Specifically, we may consider relaxing the requirement that all covariate values in the sequential regressions are observed. Following this line of thought leads to the approach of *imputation using chained equations* (ICE), which is now more commonly referred to as *FCS*. Early proponents were van Buuren *et al.* (1999) and, in the sample survey literature, Raghunathan *et al.* (2001). For a more recent review, see van Buuren (2007).

We first re-order the variables $\mathbf{Y}_1, \dots, \mathbf{Y}_p$ so that the missingness pattern is as close to monotone as possible. Then, to get started, we 'fill in' the missing values of each variable. Typically, this is done by drawing, with replacement, from the observed values of each variable. The algorithm is

For each $j = 1, \dots, p$ in turn

(a) regress *the observed part of* $\mathbf{Y}_j$ on all the remaining variables, whose missing values are set at their current imputed values;

(b) using the regression imputation algorithm above impute the missing values of $\mathbf{Y}_j$

Running through steps (a)–(b) for $j = 1, \dots, p$ is termed a *cycle*. Once we have gone through the first cycle, all the initial starting values have been replaced by the imputed values.

A number of cycles are run for the algorithm to 'converge', then the current values of $\mathbf{Y}_i$, $i = 1, \dots, n$, form the first imputed dataset. The algorithm is then run for some more cycles so that current imputed values are stochastically independent of the first imputation, and then second imputation is recorded. We proceed in this way until the desired number of imputed datasets has been created.

The name 'full conditional specification' was coined because each variable is imputed from its full conditional distribution on all the other variables.

3.3.1 Justification

We note that if the missingness pattern is monotone, then FCS is equivalent to sequential regression imputation. More generally, under the multivariate normal distribution, the joint distribution defines the unique conditional distributions, and vice versa. So the two specifications are compatible.

Now consider the relationship between FCS and the standard Gibbs sampler (Appendix A, also Gilks *et al.* (1996), Ch. 1). To implement a Gibbs sampler, we start with the joint distribution, work out the conditional distributions of each parameter given the remainder and the data, and then draw from each conditional in turn.

Suppose we have no missing data, and for illustration, $p = 2$. As discussed above, we have $f(\boldsymbol{\beta}, \boldsymbol{\Omega}|\mathbf{Y}) = f(\boldsymbol{\beta}|\boldsymbol{\Omega}, \mathbf{Y})f(\boldsymbol{\Omega}|\mathbf{Y})$. Thus, to fit the unstructured multivariate normal model using a Gibbs sampler at each iteration, we draw a covariance matrix, then a mean given this covariance matrix.

An alternative approach would be to consider the conditional distribution (regression) of Y_1 on Y_2, and Y_2 on Y_1 :

$$Y_{1,i} = \alpha_{1|2} + \gamma_{1|2} Y_{2,i} + \epsilon_{1,i}, \quad \epsilon_{1,i} \sim N(0, \sigma^2_{1|2}),$$
$$Y_{2,i} = \alpha_{2|1} + \gamma_{2|1} Y_{1,i} + \epsilon_{2,i}, \quad \epsilon_{2,i} \sim N(0, \sigma^2_{2|1}). \tag{3.10}$$

With a flat improper prior on all six parameters, we can draw from their posterior via the sampling distribution of the parameters (see the sequential regression imputation algorithm). Since the two conditional normal distributions define a unique joint normal distribution, this implies a draw from the posterior of $(\boldsymbol{\beta}, \boldsymbol{\Omega})$ given $\mathbf{Y}$. However, as we have drawn six parameters in (3.10), but the bivariate normal only has five parameters, we have sampled one parameter more than we need to; this is discarded before calculating $(\boldsymbol{\beta}, \boldsymbol{\Omega})$.

Now suppose we have $\mathbf{Y}_1$ and $\mathbf{Y}_2$ partially observed. To initialize the process, we fill in the missing values with some starting values. Once we have done this, given $\mathbf{Y}_1, \mathbf{Y}_2$ we can use the approach in the preceding paragraph to draw from the posterior of $(\alpha_{2|1}, \beta_{2|1}, \sigma^2_{2|1}; \alpha_{1|2}, \beta_{1|2}, \sigma^2_{1|2})$. Then, in turn, we can draw from the missing $\mathbf{Y}_1$ given $\mathbf{Y}_2$ and the current parameter draws, and vice versa. However, the FCS algorithm differs from this because each regression is only fitted using data from units whose response is observed.

These two points together mean the FCS algorithm is not a true Gibbs sampler; it has been described as a 'poor man's Gibbs sampler', see for example Section 5.6 of (Tanner, 1996).

However, the multivariate normal distribution has a special property: any conditional distribution implies no constraint on the parameters of the corresponding marginal distribution. For instance, for the bivariate normal, the distribution of $\mathbf{Y}_1 \mid \mathbf{Y}_2$ (which we can estimate by linear regression) does not restrict in any way, or give any information on, the marginal distribution of $\mathbf{Y}_2$. Hughes *et al.* (2014) and Liu *et al.* (2013) use this result to show that – with appropriate choice of priors – for the multivariate normal, FCS is equivalent to the Gibbs sampler for the joint distribution. Therefore, in the settings described in this chapter, there should be no inferential differences between results obtained from the two algorithms.

3.4 Full conditional specification versus joint modelling

There are few substantive reasons for choosing between a joint modelling approach and the FCS approach for the multivariate normal setting considered in this chapter. In general, FCS will be slower than Gibbs sampling for the joint model because of the existence of efficient algorithms for the latter, as discussed in Schafer (1997), Ch. 6. However, we have not experienced this as a practical issue with moderate datasets. FCS can be easily implemented because it avoids the need to define priors, has good easy-to-use software, and generally requires less iterations for convergence than the joint modelling approach. However, if we wish to include prior information, whether on the parameters or the distribution of the missing values, this is usually more natural and computationally straightforward through the joint modelling approach. Further, initializing the joint model using the EM algorithm acts as a useful check that the model is appropriate for the data.

An additional complication arises if the number of variables, p, is large relative to the number of observations, n. In this case, it may be useful to stabilize the covariance matrix using a ridge parameter. This is more naturally done using a joint-modelling approach, and we return to this in Chapter 7.

3.5 Software for multivariate normal imputation

Software is constantly changing; nevertheless, the packages we describe here are fairly well established, and will hopefully be available in a similar form for some time to come. Our choice reflects the packages we routinely use, and no criticism of other software is implied. Interested readers should also refer to issue 45 of the Journal of Statistical Software (2011) (http://www.jstatsoft.org/) which is devoted to software for multiple imputation.

Sequential regression imputation This can be readily programmed in any statistical software. It is available in SAS PROC MI. Note that the software first checks the missingness pattern is monotone and will not run if this is violated. If desired, a few non-monotone values can be imputed using a joint modelling approach in a preliminary step. In Stata, this approach is available via `mi impute monotone`.

Joint modelling approach Imputation with the multivariate normal model is available in R (`norm` package), based on Schafer's original stand-alone software of the same name. Details of the algorithm are presented in Schafer (1997). An EM algorithm is used to initiate the MCMC sampler.

The `norm` package is also the inspiration for multivariate normal imputation in SAS PROC MI (`proc mi`) and similar software in Stata (`mi impute mvn`). The windows stand-alone `REALCOM-impute` (Carpenter *et al.*, 2011a) also imputes using the joint multivariate normal model. It is available from www.bristol.ac.uk/cmm/ (accessed 24 Sept 2022). Stata routines for exporting and importing data to `REALCOM-impute` are available from https://missingdata.lshtm.ac.uk. There is also the `R` package `jomo` (see Chapter 9).

Full conditional specification This approach is implemented in SAS (`proc mi fcs`). In Stata, this approach is implemented via `mi impute chained`. In R, the most popular implementation is the `mice` package (van Buuren, 2007).

3.6 Discussion

In this chapter, we have outlined how to impute data which can be modelled using the multivariate normal distribution. If the multivariate normal distribution is not appropriate, for example because the data are skewed, one can transform the data to approximate multivariate normality, then impute, then transform back. In practice, this is usually done by looking at univariate summaries of the variables and transforming one or more of them as appropriate.

However, (Lee and Carlin, 2017) showed that how to impute a non-normal variable depends on the nature of the relationship between the variables of interest. If the relationship is linear in the untransformed scale, transforming can introduce bias. If the relationship is non-linear instead, it may be necessary to transform the variable first to capture this relationship.

In practice when using these methods, one should check for convergence of the stochastic algorithm. All the software packages allow output to be saved for this purpose, although with some it is easier than others. As with all statistical modelling, problems are likely to arise if variables are very highly correlated, and if the number of variables is large relative to the number of parameters.

Because, in practice, few examples involve only continuous variables, we need to consider as well imputation schemes for binary and categorical variables. We consider these now in Chapters 4 and 5.

Exercises

1. Suppose you have a dataset where the only variable with missing data is continuous. For which substantive models and missingness mechanisms would complete records analysis be valid? What about a MI analysis?

2. In this question, we use the data provided from the asthma study to replicate the results in Table 3.2, up to Monte Carlo error (cf Section 14.6).

   (a) Load the asthma data and retain only the placebo arm. Repeat the complete records analysis. Check your results agree with the complete records analysis row in Table 3.2.

   (b) Now repeat the same analysis for all the observed data. How do the results change from the previous analysis? Is this expected? Under which missingness mechanisms would you expect point estimates to broadly agree?

   (c) Now repeat the same analysis, but imputing the missing observations. Start with using FCS imputation. Do the mean estimates and standard errors vary? Would you expect them to and why? Would results differ if imputing with sequential imputation here and why?

   (d) Repeat the same analysis, using joint modelling (JM) imputation instead. Would you expect the two imputation strategies to lead to different results in these settings?

3. For this question, we use pseudo-data from a trial in which 750 patients with chronic obstructive pulmonary disease (COPD) were randomized to receive either 50 mg/day of fluticasone propionate or a placebo. Patients were followed up for three years, and here we consider their six monthly FEV_1 (litres) measures. Our substantive analysis model is a linear regression with FEV_1 measurement at three years as outcome and treatment arm and baseline FEV_1 as covariates. Our interest is mainly in the treatment effect parameter.

(a) Use a multivariate normal model to impute any missing value. In particular, include as outcomes of such a multivariate imputation model all six-monthly FEV_1 measurements, baseline body mass index (BMI), and the mean exacerbation rate (log-transformed). Repeat the imputation separately by treatment group and start by generating five imputations with 50 burn-in and between-imputation iterations. Note that several software packages can be used to fit a similar imputation model, including `norm2`, `jomo` and `Amelia` in `R`, `SAS PROC MI` and `mi impute mvn` in Stata.

(b) Fit the substantive analysis model and combine the estimates with Rubin's rules.

(c) Now increase progressively the number of iterations to 500 and then to 5000. Do the results substantially change? If possible with the software you are using, investigate the convergence of the sampler. Do you think 50 iterations were enough for this example?

(d) Now increase the number of imputations to 10 and finally to 50. Do you think this made a difference (cf Section 14.6)

4

Multiple imputation of binary and ordinal data

In this chapter, we extend the approaches described in Chapter 3 to handle first binary and then ordinal data. This extension allows imputation of a mix of continuous and binary/ordinal variables. We begin by considering the special case of a monotone missingness pattern in Section 4.1. We then consider the joint modelling approach, first using the multivariate normal assumption in Section 4.2 and then using a latent normal model and the general location model in Sections 4.3 and 4.4. Full conditional specification is described in Section 4.5. We conclude by discussing issues with over-fitting, the pros and cons of the various approaches, and software, in Sections 4.6–4.8 respectively.

4.1 Sequential imputation with monotone missingness pattern

The monotone data pattern is defined on p. 8, and its implications for the missingness mechanism are described on p. 107. A general justification of the sequential regression algorithm is given in Section 3.1.2.

Using the notation from Chapter 3, we suppose that $\mathbf{Y}_1$ is fully observed, and that the data are MAR with a monotone pattern. Suppose we apply the sequential imputation algorithm described on p. 106, and that as we work through $j = 2, \dots, p$, $\mathbf{Y}_j$ is the first binary variable. In essence, we replace linear regression with some sort of binomial regression, for example logistic regression. The details are as follows:

Multiple Imputation and its Application, Second Edition.
James R. Carpenter, Jonathan W. Bartlett, Tim P. Morris, Angela M. Wood, Matteo Quartagno and Michael G. Kenward.

1. For binary variable j, suppose $i = 1, \dots, n_j$ individuals have Y_{ij} observed. Using data from these n_j individuals, as before let $\mathbf{1}$ be a vector of n_j 1's and form $\mathbf{W} = (\mathbf{1}, \mathbf{Y}_1, \mathbf{Y}_2, \dots, \mathbf{Y}_{j-1})$, say, so that $\mathbf{W}$ is the $n_j \times j$ regression matrix with rows $\mathbf{W}_i$, $i \in 1, \dots, n_j$.
   Fit the model
$$\text{logit}\{\Pr(Y_{i,j} = 1)\} = \mathbf{W}_i \boldsymbol{\beta}_j, \tag{4.1}$$
   obtaining the maximum likelihood estimate $\hat{\boldsymbol{\beta}}_j$ with covariance matrix $\hat{\boldsymbol{\Sigma}}$ where $\boldsymbol{\Sigma} = (\mathbf{W}^T \hat{\mathbf{V}}^{-1} \mathbf{W})^{-1}$, and $\hat{\mathbf{V}}$ is a matrix with diagonal elements $\widehat{\text{Var}}(\mathbf{Y}_{i,j}) = \hat{\pi}_{i,j}(1 - \hat{\pi}_{i,j})$, and all off diagonal elements 0, where
$$\hat{\pi}_{i,j} = \frac{1}{1 + \exp(-\mathbf{W}_i \hat{\boldsymbol{\beta}}_j)}.$$
2. Then
   (a) draw $\boldsymbol{\beta}_j^*$ from $N(\hat{\boldsymbol{\beta}}_j, \hat{\boldsymbol{\Sigma}})$
   (b) For each unobserved Y_{ij} calculate
$$\eta_{i,j}^* = (1, Y_{i,1}, \dots, Y_{i,j-1}) \boldsymbol{\beta}_j^*, \tag{4.2}$$
   and draw Y_{ij} from the Bernoulli distribution with
$$\pi_{i,j}^* = \frac{1}{1 + \exp(-\eta_{i,j}^*)},$$
   so that all the missing values of $\mathbf{Y}_j$ are imputed. We note that for $j = 3, \dots, p$ there will be some units with $Y_{i,j}$ missing and with one or more of $Y_{i,2}, \dots, Y_{i,j-1}$ missing, and imputed at previous steps. These previously imputed values are used in (4.2) when imputing $Y_{i,j}$.

To impute a dataset with a monotone missingness pattern and a mix of binary and continuous data, we therefore begin by putting the variables in order to make a monotone missing pattern, with the fully observed variables first. Then we impute each partially observed variable in turn, conditional on previous variables, using steps 1 and 2 from p. 107 if the variable is continuous and steps 1 and 2 above if it is binary. The whole sequence is repeated to generate successive imputed datasets.

The above algorithm can be readily adapted for binomial data, assuming the denominators $m_{i,j}$ are known; we replace (4.1) with a binomial regression, and likewise impute from a binomial, instead of a Bernoulli, distribution in step 2(b). If the data are ordinal and satisfies the proportional odds model (McCullagh, 1980), then we replace (4.1) with ordinal logistic regression and impute from an ordinal logistic distribution in step 2(b).

In applications, for reasonably large j it is not uncommon to encounter difficulties with perfect or near-perfect prediction (see Section 4.6) for some parts of the dataset in model (4.1). In this case, the corresponding coefficient estimates in $\hat{\boldsymbol{\beta}}$ will be large in absolute magnitude, and the corresponding estimates of $\hat{\boldsymbol{\Sigma}}$ will also be large.

This allows drawn values of the corresponding components of $\boldsymbol{\beta}_j^*$ to be large and of *opposite sign* to $\hat{\boldsymbol{\beta}}_j$. This in turn means probabilities $\pi_{i,j}^*$ are close to the opposite of the fitted probabilities from (4.1), which leads to inappropriate imputations. We explore this issue further in Section 4.6, but note that it may be addressed by reducing the number of predictors in (4.1).

4.2 Joint modelling with the multivariate normal distribution

When we have a non-monotone missingness pattern, an attractive approach is to treat binary, binomial, and ordinal variables as continuous for the purpose of imputation, and then in the imputed data to round their imputed values to the nearest valid discrete value before continuing to fit the substantive model. If there are no missing observations in such variables, then treating them as continuous in a multivariate normal imputation implies that the distribution of other variables is conditioned on a linear function of them, just as when they are included as covariates in a regression imputation model. If, instead, we formally model fully observed binary variables using, say, the latent normal model described below, the results are likely to be indistinguishable in most applications.

If we adopt this approach, then we first apply the algorithm in Section 3.2 without modification to obtain the imputed datasets. Then we round the continuous imputed values for the discrete variables. Bernaards *et al.* (2007) consider the case of binary data and compare three ways this can be done:

1. *simple rounding*: round to the nearest of 0 or 1;
2. *coin flip*, and
3. *adaptive rounding*.

The *coin flip* algorithm is

1. if the imputed value, $Y_{i,j}$, is ≤ 0 return 0; if ≥ 1 return 1; otherwise
2. impute a binary response taking 1 with probability $Y_{i,j}$.

The *adaptive rounding* algorithm is

1. For binary variable j in imputed dataset $k = 1, \ldots, K$, let $\overline{\mathbf{Y}}_{j,k}$ denote the mean of the observed (binary) and imputed (continuous) values.
2. Construct the threshold $c_{j,k} = \overline{\mathbf{Y}}_{j,k} - \Phi^{-1}(\overline{\mathbf{Y}}_{j,k})\sqrt{\overline{\mathbf{Y}}_{j,k}(1 - \overline{\mathbf{Y}}_{j,k})}$
3. in imputed dataset k, re-code continuous imputed values of the binary variable $\mathbf{Y}_j$ according to the following rule: $Y_{i,j} \leq c_{j,k}$ becomes $Y_{i,j} = 0$, and $Y_{j,k} > c_{j,k}$ becomes $Y_{ij} = 1$.

The rationale for step 2 is the normal approximation to the binomial distribution, i.e.

$$\frac{\overline{\mathbf{Y}}_{i,j} - c_{i,j}}{\sqrt{\overline{\mathbf{Y}}_{j,k}(1 - \overline{\mathbf{Y}}_{j,k})}} = z_{i,j},$$

say where $\Phi(\,.\,)$ is the cumulative distribution function of the standard normal and we set $\Phi(z_{i,j}) = \overline{\mathbf{Y}}_{j,k}$.

Adaptive rounding is thus close to simple rounding, but now the threshold is adapted, as illustrated in Figure 4.1. Compared to simple rounding, the effect of this is that for $\overline{\mathbf{Y}}_j$ closer to 0 or 1, there will be more variability in the imputed binary values.

Horton *et al.* (2003) anticipate bias in parameter estimates when applying simple rounding. Bernaards *et al.* (2007) compare all three proposals in simulation studies looking at, among other things, bias and confidence interval coverage for a marginal (i.e. sample) proportion, odds ratio, difference in means of a continuous variable between groups defined by an imputed binary variable and coefficients in a logistic regression. The results show that coin flipping performs worst, and adaptive rounding has a slight edge over simple rounding. Focusing on the results from adaptive rounding, aside from the intercept in logistic regression when the outcome is rare (odds 0.07 and bias is over 50%), bias is below 12%, and often much smaller. Coverage for nominal 95% intervals is above 90% in all simulations, but furthest from the nominal level when estimating, with 50% of the data imputed, a marginal proportion whose true value is below 0.1.

Thus, when adopting this approach, adaptive rounding is the preferred method; this is likely to perform satisfactorily in applications if the underlying probability is between 0.1 and 0.9.

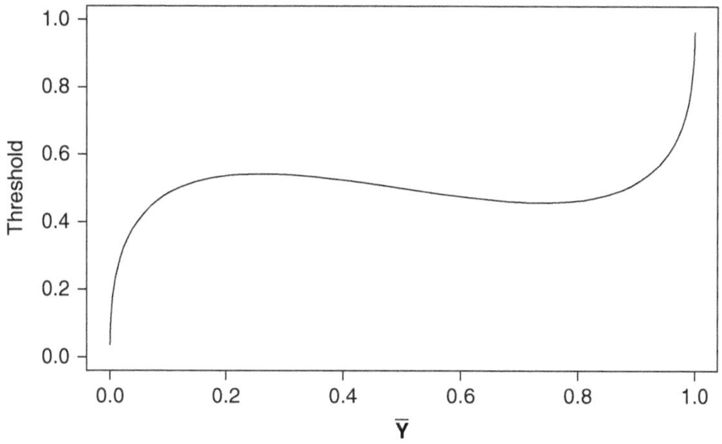

Figure 4.1 Adaptive rounding threshold, as $\overline{\mathbf{Y}}$ *varies.*

With binomial data, where each $Y_{i,j}$ is the number of successes out of say $m_{i,j}$ trials and $m_{i,j}$ is known, the most straightforward approach is to treat $Y_{i,j}$ as continuous, and round to the nearest integer in $0, \dots, m_{i,j}$. An alternative, analogous to the coin flip method above, is also possible. We treat $p_{i,j} = Y_{i,j}/m_i$ as the response in imputation, and then for missing $Y_{i,j}$ round the imputed $p_{i,j}$ to lie in $(0, 1)$ and then draw $Y_{i,j}$ from $\text{Bin}(m_{i,j}, p_{i,j})$. However, the simulation results discussed above for the coin flip approach with binary data provide little incentive to use it with binomial data.

While it is possible to see how to extend the adaptive rounding approach to ordinal data, given the relatively small advantage over simple rounding in the more difficult case of binary data, there appears no need in practice; simple rounding (back to the ordinal score) is likely to prove sufficient.

4.3 Modelling binary data using latent normal variables

While the rounding methods proposed in subsection 4.2 were shown to be preferable to complete records analysis under a general MAR missingness mechanism, coverage may still be unoptimal and some bias may appear, particularly with small (or large) event probabilities. An alternative approach is to use a latent normal variable, say $Z_{i,j}$, for each binary $Y_{i,j}$. We can define $Z_{i,j}$ so that for values for $Z_{i,j} \leq 0$, then $Y_{i,j} = 0$ and for $Z_{i,j} > 0$, then $Y_{i,j} = 1$. These latent normal variables and the other continuous variables can then be jointly modelled using the multivariate normal model, building on the approach set out in Section 3.2.

To describe how this approach works, consider a single binary variable **Y** and the probit regression on a constant:

$$\Phi^{-1}\{\Pr(Y_i = 1)\} = \beta, \quad i \in (1, \dots, n), \tag{4.3}$$

where $\Phi^{-1}(\,.\,)$ is the inverse cumulative density function of the standard normal. Let the latent normal variable $Z_i \sim N(\beta, 1)$ such that $Z_i > 0 \iff Y_i = 1$. Then[1]

$$\begin{aligned}\Pr(Y_i = 1) = \Pr(Z_i > 0) &= \Pr(Z_i - \beta > -\beta), \\ &= 1 - \Phi(-\beta), \\ &= \Phi(\beta). \end{aligned} \tag{4.4}$$

Equation (4.4) means that the latent normal formulation is equivalent to the probit model (4.3). The advantage is that it links in naturally with the multivariate normal imputation model introduced in Chapter 3, since we can model the latent Z's along with the continuous variables, subject only to restricting their variance to be 1.

The difference in the fitted probabilities from the probit and logit models is small; the linear predictor from a probit model is ≈0.6 that from the logit model. To illustrate this, Figure 4.2 shows a plot of $\Phi(0.6x)$ against $\text{expit}(x) = 1/\{1 + \exp(-x)\}$, where

[1] Recalling that $1 - \Phi(-x) = \Pr(Z > -x) = \Pr(Z < x) = \Phi(x)$.

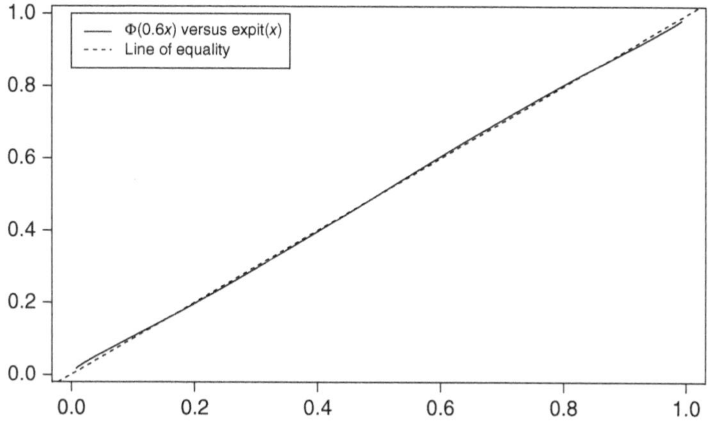

Figure 4.2 Plot of $\Phi(0.6x)$ versus expit(x) and line of equality, when x runs between −4 and 4.

expit(.) is the inverse of the logit(.) function. The minor departures from the line of equality are unlikely to be important in applications.

Albert and Chib (1993) give a Gibbs sampling algorithm for estimating β using the latent normal values explicitly. We first give this in the simplest case of fitting (4.3) (where it is of course not necessary) and then describe how it links in with the multivariate normal approach in the case of a binary and continuous variable. We proceed as follows: initialise $\beta^0 = 0$. At update step $r = 1, 2, \ldots$

1. For $i = 1, \ldots, n$
   (a) propose $Z_i^* \sim N(\beta^{r-1}, 1)$
   (b) if $Y_i = 1$ and $Z_i^* > 0$ or $Y_i = 0$ and $Z_i^* \leq 0$, accept the proposal, setting $Z_i^r = Z_i^*$; otherwise return to 1(a).
2. Since the variance of Z is fixed to be 1, we update β by drawing $\beta^r \sim N(\overline{Z}^r, 1/n)$, where $\overline{Z}^r = \sum_{i=1}^n Z_i^r/n$.

Now suppose we have two variables, continuous $\mathbf{Y}_1$ and binary $\mathbf{Y}_2$. Using the latent normal approach, the joint model is

$$Y_{i,1} = \beta_{0,1} + \epsilon_{i,1},$$
$$\Pr(Y_{i,2} = 1) = \Pr(Z_{i,2} > 0);\ Z_{i,2} = \beta_{0,2} + \epsilon_{i,2},$$
$$\begin{pmatrix} \epsilon_{i,1} \\ \epsilon_{i,2} \end{pmatrix} \sim N_2 \left[\mathbf{0}, \mathbf{\Omega} = \begin{pmatrix} \sigma_1^2 & \sigma_{1,2} \\ \sigma_{1,2} & 1 \end{pmatrix} \right]. \tag{4.5}$$

Notice the constraint that $\text{Var}(Z_{i,2}) = 1$. Beneath, we write $\mathbf{\Omega}_{1,1}$ to refer to the (1,1) element σ_1^2, $\mathbf{\Omega}_{1,2}$ to refer to $\sigma_{1,2}$, and so on. To use the latent normal algorithm, we have to draw from the conditional normal distribution of $Z_{i,2}$ given $Y_{i,1}$. The conditional normal distribution is given in Appendix B. Under model 4.5, this is

$$N\{\beta_{0,2} + (Y_{i,1} - \beta_{0,1})(\mathbf{\Omega}_{1,1})^{-1}\mathbf{\Omega}_{1,2}, 1 - \mathbf{\Omega}_{2,1}(\mathbf{\Omega}_{1,1})^{-1}\mathbf{\Omega}_{1,2}\}, \tag{4.6}$$

where in the bivariate model (4.5), both $\mathbf{\Omega}_{1,1} = \sigma_1^2$ and $\mathbf{\Omega}_{1,2} = \mathbf{\Omega}_{2,1} = \sigma_{1,2}$ are scalars. Model (4.5) has four free parameters, and the latent normal MCMC algorithm is now as follows: choose initial values $\beta_{0,1}^0, \beta_{0,2}^0, \mathbf{\Omega}^0$, for example using marginal sample estimates from the complete records. Then for update step $r = 1, 2, \ldots$

1. For $i = 1, \ldots, n$
   (a) Using $\beta_{0,1}^{r-1}, \beta_{0,2}^{r-1}, \mathbf{\Omega}^{r-1}$, draw a proposed latent normal $Z_{i,2}^*$ from the conditional normal (4.6) given $Y_{i,1}$.
   (b) if $Y_{i,2} = 1$ and $Z_{i,2}^* > 0$ or $Y_{i,2} = 0$ and $Z_{i,2}^* \leq 0$, accept the proposal, setting $Z_{i,2}^r = Z_{i,2}^*$; otherwise return to 1 (a).
2. Conditional on $(\mathbf{Y}_1, \mathbf{Z}_2^r)$, update the elements of $\mathbf{\Omega}$ to obtain $\mathbf{\Omega}^r$ as detailed below.
3. Draw $(\beta_{0,1}^r, \beta_{0,2}^r)$ from $N_2[(\overline{\mathbf{Y}}_1, \overline{\mathbf{Z}}_2^r)^T, n^{-1}\mathbf{\Omega}^r]$.

Comparing with the multivariate normal algorithm with no missing data in Section 3.2.1, the additional step we need is to draw the latent normals, conditional on continuous $\mathbf{Y}_1$ and binary $\mathbf{Y}_2$, which we do in step 1.

In fact, we can avoid the rejection step when drawing $Z_{i,2}$ in step 1. First, under the conditional normal distribution (4.6), we calculate the probability that $Z_{i,2} < 0$. Suppose this is p_i. Then if $Y_{i,2} = 0$ draw $u_i \sim \text{uniform}[0, p_i]$; otherwise, draw $u_i \sim \text{uniform}[p_i, 1]$. Lastly, set $Z_{i,j}^* = \Phi_{c,i}^{-1}(u_i)$, where $\Phi_{c,i}^{-1}$ is the inverse cumulative distribution function for the conditional normal (4.6).

Updating elements of Ω

The complication is that because $\mathbf{\Omega}$ has a constraint ($\mathbf{\Omega}_{2,2} = 1$) we cannot directly update with a draw from the Wishart distribution in step 2. Instead, we update $\mathbf{\Omega}$ elementwise, as proposed by Browne (2006), using the Metropolis–Hastings algorithm. In passing, notice that with more than two variables, we could bring together the continuous and binary variables into two groups A and B, respectively. We could then update $\mathbf{\Omega}_B$ elementwise (as below), and then update Ω_{AB} from the appropriate multivariate normal distribution and $\mathbf{\Omega}_A$ from the appropriate conditional Wishart (Mardia *et al.*, 1979). We do not pursue this further here.

Given $(\mathbf{Y}_1, \mathbf{Z}_1)$, the bivariate normal likelihood is

$$L(\beta, \mathbf{\Omega}) \propto |\mathbf{\Omega}|^{-n} \exp\left\{-\frac{1}{2}\sum_{i=1}^{n}(Y_{i,1} - \beta_{0,1}, Y_{i,2} - \beta_{0,2})\mathbf{\Omega}^{-1}(Y_{i,1} - \beta_{0,1}, Y_{i,2} - \beta_{0,2})^T\right\}. \tag{4.7}$$

At update step r, a generic Metropolis–Hastings sampler for updating element $\mathbf{\Omega}_{k,l}$ of $\mathbf{\Omega}$ is

1. draw a proposal $\boldsymbol{\Omega}^*_{k,l}$ from a symmetric proposal distribution;
2. check that $\boldsymbol{\Omega}$ is positive definite when $\boldsymbol{\Omega}_{k,l}$ is replaced by $\boldsymbol{\Omega}^*_{k,l}$. If not draw again, until it is.
3. accept $\boldsymbol{\Omega}^*_{k,l}$ with probability

$$\min\left(1, \frac{L(\boldsymbol{\beta}, \boldsymbol{\Omega}^*_{k,l}, \boldsymbol{\Omega}_{-k,l})p(\boldsymbol{\Omega}^*_{k,l}, \boldsymbol{\Omega}_{-k,l})}{L(\boldsymbol{\beta}, \boldsymbol{\Omega})p(\boldsymbol{\Omega})}\right), \tag{4.8}$$

   where L is given by (4.7) and $\boldsymbol{\Omega}_{-k,l}$ refers to elements of $\boldsymbol{\Omega}$ *excluding* the (k,l)th.
4. if $\boldsymbol{\Omega}^*_{k,l}$ is accepted, then set $\boldsymbol{\Omega}^r_{k,l} = \boldsymbol{\Omega}^*_{k,l}$, otherwise, retain $\boldsymbol{\Omega}^r_{k,l} = \boldsymbol{\Omega}^r_{k,l}$.

In (4.8), $p(\,.\,)$ is the prior distribution for $\boldsymbol{\Omega}$. We discuss options for this at the end of Appendix B.

There are a number of possible choices for the proposal distribution. Since we assume a symmetric proposal, we omit the Hastings ratio (Appendix A) from (4.8). Browne (2006) compared various options and found good performance with a normal proposal, centred at the current value, with component-specific variance $\gamma^2_{k,l}$, i.e. $\Omega^*_{k,l} \sim N(\boldsymbol{\Omega}_{k,l}, \gamma^2_{k,l})$. The value of $\gamma_{k,l}$ may be chosen adaptively during the burn in. To maximise the efficiency of the MCMC sampler, Browne (2006) suggest aiming for a ≈50% acceptance rate.

The `REALCOM-impute` program (Carpenter *et al.*, 2011a) uses the following by default:

1. for the (l,l) variance term, draw proposals from $N\,(\boldsymbol{\Omega}_{l,l}, \gamma^2_{l,l})$, where $\gamma_{l,l} = \boldsymbol{\Omega}_{l,l}\sqrt{2 \times 5.8/n}$, where the proposal standard deviation is given by Gelman *et al.* (1996);
2. for the (k,l) covariance term, draw proposals from $N\,(\boldsymbol{\Omega}_{k,l}, \gamma^2_{k,l})$, where $\gamma_{k,l} = 0.1\sqrt{\boldsymbol{\Omega}_{k,k}\boldsymbol{\Omega}_{k,l}}$.

For variance parameters, negative proposals are immediately rejected, and a new value drawn.

Imputing missing values

Thus far, we have assumed no missing data. Missing values are handled in the way described in Section 3.2.1. To initiate the MCMC sampler, we draw missing values on the variables by sampling at random from the observed values. Then we modify step 1 of the sampler as follows:

1. If binary $Y_{i,2}$ is missing, draw $Z^r_{i,2}$ from the conditional normal distribution given $Y_{i,1}$, (4.6). If $Z^r_{i,2} > 0$ set $Y^r_{i,2} = 1$, otherwise, set $Y^r_{i,2} = 0$.
2. If continuous $Y_{i,1}$ is missing, then in step 1(a) instead of drawing $Z^r_{i,2}$ from the conditional normal, draw it from the marginal normal $N\,(\beta^{r-1}_{0,2}, 1)$ Then accept or reject this draw usual in step 1(b).

Then draw $Y^r_{i,1}$ from the conditional normal given $Z^r_{i,1}$,

$$N\{\beta^{r-1}_{0,1} + (Z^r_{i,2} - \beta^{r-1}_{0,2})(\boldsymbol{\Omega}^{r-1}_{2,2})^{-1}\boldsymbol{\Omega}^{r-1}_{2,1}, \boldsymbol{\Omega}^{r-1}_{1,1} - \boldsymbol{\Omega}^{r-1}_{1,2}(\boldsymbol{\Omega}^{r-1}_{2,2})^{-1}\boldsymbol{\Omega}^{r-1}_{2,1}\}.$$

As discussed in Chapter 3, we (i) burn in the sampler for n_{burn} updates, and if satisfied that convergence has been achieved, then keep the current draws of the missing data to form the first imputed dataset, then (ii) update the sampler n_{between} times, and keep the current draws to form the second imputed dataset, and so on, until we reach desired number of imputed datasets, K.

A drawback of the probit model is that there are no sufficient statistics, and so implementing an EM algorithm is more awkward. Approximate starting values and a first test of the estimability of the model can be obtained by using the EM algorithm treating the binary responses as continuous, with 1 coded as 2.5 and 0 coded −2.5.

More than two variables; binomial data

Thus far, we have only considered two variables, one continuous and one binary. With p variables, the conditional normal distribution (4.6) is calculated from the p-variate normal. Now, $\boldsymbol{\Omega}_{1,2}$ is a vector, which we update element-wise using Metropolis Hastings steps as described above.

For binomial data, where $Y_{i,j}$ is the (possibly missing) number of successes out of a known $m_{i,j} > 1$ trials, the simplest approach is to use the variance stabilising transformation $Z_{i,j} = \arcsin(Y_{i,j}/m_{i,j})$ and treat $Z_{i,j}$ as normal responses in the imputation. Alternatively, one can draw a latent normal for each of the $m_{i,j}$ trials; these latent normals need to have covariance 0 to mimic the binomial being made up of $m_{i,j}$ independent draws. In practice, once the denominator of the binomial is greater than 3 or so, the discussion in Section 4.2 suggests the normal approximation followed by rounding will likely be adequate.

4.3.1 Latent normal model for ordinal data

Consider a single ordinal variable, Y_i, with M ordinal values, $m = 1, \dots, M$. Let $\pi_{i,m} = \Pr(Y_i = m)$, and let $\gamma_{i,m} = \Pr(Y_i \leq m) = \sum_{l=1}^{m} \pi_{i,m}$. The proportional probit model (McCullagh, 1980) is

$$\text{probit}(\gamma_{i,m}) = \Phi^{-1}(\gamma_{i,m}) = \alpha_m, \quad m = 1, \dots, M. \tag{4.9}$$

If we define $\alpha_0 = -\infty$ and $\alpha_M = \infty$, the above model implies

$$\pi_m = \int_{\alpha_{m-1}}^{\alpha_m} \phi(z)\, dz, \quad j = 1, \dots, M. \tag{4.10}$$

In other words, (4.9) is equivalent to a latent normal model, where $Z_i \sim N(0, 1)$ and

$$\begin{aligned} &Z_i \leq \alpha_1 \text{ if } Y_i = 1, \\ &Z_i \in (\alpha_{m-1}, \alpha_M] \text{ if } Y_i = m, m \in (2, \dots, M-1), \\ &Z_i > \alpha_{M-1} \text{ if } Y_i = m. \end{aligned} \tag{4.11}$$

If $M = 2$ so that Y_i is a binary variable, then this is equivalent to (4.3) and (4.4), because

- if $Z \sim N(\beta, 1)$ and $Y_i = 1 \iff Z_i > 0$ then

$$\Pr(Z > 0) = 1 - \Phi(-\beta) = \Phi(\beta)$$

  from (4.4), and

- if $Z \sim N(0, 1)$ and $Y_i = 1 \iff Z_i > -\beta$, then

$$\Pr(Z > -\beta) = 1 - \Phi(-\beta) = \Phi(\beta).$$

However, with $M > 2$, formulation (4.11) is easier to work with.

To estimate the cut points, $(\alpha_1, \dots, \alpha_{M-1})$ we could proceed as follows: choose initial values $(\alpha_1^0, \dots, \alpha_{M-1}^0)$, and then at update step $r = 1, 2, \dots$

1. for $i \in 1, \dots, n$
   (a) draw $Z_i^r \sim N(0, 1)$ and recalling $\alpha_0 = -\infty, \alpha_M = \infty$,

$$\text{if } Y_i = m, \text{accept } Z_i^r \text{ if } \alpha_{m-1}^{r-1} < Z_i^r \leq \alpha_M^{r-1}, \quad m \in (1, \dots, M)$$

   (b) if Z_i^r is rejected, return to 1(a)
2. for each parameter α_m, $m \in (1, \dots, M-1)$,
   (a) find unit m_L such that $Z_{m_L}^r$ is the largest latent normal Z_i^r with $Z_i^r < \alpha_m^{r-1}$.
   (b) find unit m_U such that $Z_{m_U}^r$ is the smallest latent normal Z_i^r with $Z_i^r > \alpha_m^{r-1}$.
   (c) sample α_m^r as a random draw from the interval $(Z_{m_L}^r, Z_{m_U}^r)$.

This update procedure is essentially due to Albert and Chib (1993) and Chib and Greenburg (1998). However, the parameters α_m only update slowly, especially if the dataset is large, as the update intervals in step 2(c) can be quite narrow.

Cowles (1996) proposed a Metropolis–Hastings algorithm for updating the parameters α_m, $l = 1, \dots, M-1$ which we now describe. Let $1[\,.\,]$ be an indicator for the event in brackets, so that $1[Y_i = m]$ is 1 when Y_i takes on the value m, and 0 otherwise. The likelihood is proportional to

$$L(\alpha_1, \dots, \alpha_M) = \prod_{i=1}^{n} \prod_{m=1}^{M} \pi_m^{1[Y_i=m]}, \tag{4.12}$$

and we proceed as follows: take an improper prior $\propto 1$ for each α_m. At update step $r = 1, 2, \dots$

1. for $m = 1$:
   (a) draw a proposal $\alpha^* \sim N(\alpha^{r-1}, \nu^2)$

(b) accept α^* with probability

$$\min\{1, L(\alpha^*, \alpha_2^{r-1}, \dots, \alpha_{M-1}^{r-1})/L(\alpha_1^{r-1}, \alpha_2^{r-1}, \dots, \alpha_{M-1}^{r-1}\}$$

(c) If α^* is accepted, set $\alpha_1^r = \alpha^*$, else $\alpha_1^r = \alpha_1^{r-1}$.

2. for $m = 2, \dots, (M-2)$

(a) draw a proposal $\alpha^* \sim N\,(\alpha_m^{r-1}, \nu^2)$

(b) accept α^* with probability

$$\min\left\{1, \frac{L(\alpha_1^r, \dots, \alpha_{m-1}^r, \alpha^*, \alpha_{m+1}^{r-1}, \dots, \alpha_{M-1}^{r-1})}{L(\alpha_1^r, \dots, \alpha_{m-1}^r, \alpha_m^{r-1}, \alpha_{m+1}^{r-1}, \dots, \alpha_{M-1}^{r-1})}\right\}$$

(c) If α^* is accepted, set $\alpha_m^r = \alpha^*$, else $\alpha_m^r = \alpha_m^{r-1}$.

3. for $m = (M-1)$

(a) draw a proposal $\alpha^* \sim N\,(\alpha_{M-1}^{r-1}, \nu^2)$

(b) accept α^* with probability

$$\min\{1, L(\alpha_1^r, \dots, \alpha_{M-2}^r, \alpha^*)/L(\alpha_1^r, \dots, \alpha_{M-2}^r, \alpha_{M-1}^{r-1})\}$$

(c) If α^* is accepted, set $\alpha_M^r = \alpha^*$, else $\alpha_M^r = \alpha_M^{r-1}$.

Following Gelman *et al.* (1996), we suggest taking $\nu^2 = 5.8/n$.

Continuous and ordinal variable

We now consider continuous $\mathbf{Y}_1$ and ordinal $\mathbf{Y}_2$. We can again use the latent normal structure to link into the multivariate normal model described in Section 3.2. The details are slightly different from the binary case, however. Let β_{01} be the mean of $\mathbf{Y}_1$, and $\boldsymbol{\Omega}$ the covariance matrix of $\mathbf{Y}_1, \mathbf{Z}_2$. Define $\alpha_0 = -\infty$ and $\alpha_M = \infty$. The latent normal model is

$$\begin{aligned} Y_{i,1} &= \beta_{0,1} + \epsilon_{i,1}, \\ \Pr(Y_{i,2} = m) &= \Pr(\alpha_{m-1} < Z_{i,2} < \alpha_m);\ Z_{i,2} = \epsilon_{i,2}, \quad m \in 1, \dots, M, \\ \begin{pmatrix} \epsilon_{i,1} \\ \epsilon_{i,2} \end{pmatrix} &\sim N_2 \left[\mathbf{0}, \boldsymbol{\Omega} = \begin{pmatrix} \sigma_1^2 & \sigma_{1,2} \\ \sigma_{1,2} & 1 \end{pmatrix}\right]. \end{aligned} \tag{4.13}$$

An MCMC algorithm for (4.13) has to update the following parameters: $\mathbf{Z}_2, \boldsymbol{\alpha}, \boldsymbol{\beta}, \boldsymbol{\Omega}$, given $(\mathbf{Y}_1, \mathbf{Y}_2)$, where $\boldsymbol{\alpha} = (\alpha_1, \dots, \alpha_{M-1})^T$. We set up the Gibbs sampler as follows:

1. update $(\mathbf{Z}_2, \boldsymbol{\alpha})$ given $(\boldsymbol{\beta}, \boldsymbol{\Omega}, \mathbf{Y}_1, \mathbf{Y}_2)$;
2. update $(\boldsymbol{\beta}, \boldsymbol{\Omega})$ given $(\mathbf{Y}_1, \mathbf{Y}_2, \mathbf{Z}_2, \boldsymbol{\alpha})$. This is simpler because given $\mathbf{Y}_1, \mathbf{Z}_2$, we do not need $\mathbf{Y}_2, \boldsymbol{\alpha}$.

Just as before, we draw from $f(\boldsymbol{\beta}, \boldsymbol{\Omega}|\mathbf{Y}_1, \mathbf{Z}_2)$ by noting $f(\boldsymbol{\beta}, \boldsymbol{\Omega}|\mathbf{Y}_1, \mathbf{Z}_2) = f(\boldsymbol{\beta}|\boldsymbol{\Omega}, \mathbf{Y}_1, \mathbf{Z}_2)f(\boldsymbol{\Omega}|\mathbf{Y}_1, \mathbf{Z}_2)$. We can use exactly the same approach for updating $(\mathbf{Z}_2, \boldsymbol{\alpha})$, since

$$f(\mathbf{Z}_2, \boldsymbol{\alpha}|\boldsymbol{\beta}, \boldsymbol{\Omega}, \mathbf{Y}_1, \mathbf{Y}_2) = f(\mathbf{Z}_2|\boldsymbol{\alpha}, \boldsymbol{\beta}, \boldsymbol{\Omega}, \mathbf{Y}_1, \mathbf{Y}_2)f(\boldsymbol{\alpha}|\boldsymbol{\beta}, \boldsymbol{\Omega}, \mathbf{Y}_1, \mathbf{Y}_2).$$

This gives the following MCMC sampler. Choose initial values $\mathbf{Z}_2^0, \boldsymbol{\alpha}^0, \boldsymbol{\beta}^0, \boldsymbol{\Omega}^0$. As usual let α_0 denote $-\infty$ and α_M denote ∞. Then at update step $r = 1, 2, \ldots$

1. conditional on $\boldsymbol{\beta}^{r-1}, \boldsymbol{\Omega}^{r-1}, \mathbf{Y}_1, \mathbf{Y}_2$ draw $\boldsymbol{\alpha}^r$, as described below;
2. conditional on $\boldsymbol{\alpha}^r, \boldsymbol{\beta}^{r-1}, \boldsymbol{\Omega}^{r-1}, \mathbf{Y}_1, \mathbf{Y}_2$, draw $\mathbf{Z}_2^r$ as follows: For each $i \in 1, \ldots, n$:
   (a) draw a proposed
   $$Z_{i,2}^* \sim N\{(Y_{i,1} - \beta_{0,1}^{r-1})(\boldsymbol{\Omega}_{1,1}^{r-1})^{-1}\boldsymbol{\Omega}_{1,2}^{r-1}, 1 - \boldsymbol{\Omega}_{2,1}^{r-1}(\boldsymbol{\Omega}_{1,1}^{r-1})^{-1}\boldsymbol{\Omega}_{1,2}^{r-1}\}; \quad (4.14)$$
   (b) recall $Y_{i,2}$ is ordinal so that $Y_{i,2} = m$, for some $m \in (1, \ldots, M)$. We thus accept $Z_{i,2}^*$ if $\alpha_{m-1} < Z_{i,2}^* \leq \alpha_m$.
   (c) if $Z_{i,2}^*$ is accepted, set $Z_{i,2}^r = Z_{i,2}^*$, else return to step 2(a).
3. conditional on $(\mathbf{Y}_1, \mathbf{Z}_2^t)$ update the elements of $\boldsymbol{\Omega}^{r-1}$ to obtain $\boldsymbol{\Omega}^r$, as described on p. 134.
4. Recalling $\beta_{0,2}$ is constrained to be zero, draw $\beta_{0,1}^r$ from the conditional normal distribution
   $$N\{\overline{\mathbf{Y}}_1 + \overline{\mathbf{Z}}_2^r(\boldsymbol{\Omega}_{2,2}^r)^{-1}\boldsymbol{\Omega}_{2,1}^r, n^{-1}(\boldsymbol{\Omega}_{1,1}^r - \boldsymbol{\Omega}_{1,2}^r(\boldsymbol{\Omega}_{2,2}^r)^{-1}\boldsymbol{\Omega}_{2,1}^r)\}.$$

Note the above has priors $\propto 1$ for all parameters except $\boldsymbol{\Omega}$.

As before, we can avoid the rejection step 2(b), as follows: for $Y_{i,2} = m$, use (4.14) to calculate $p_{iU} = \Pr(Z \leq \alpha_m)$ and $p_{iL} = \Pr(Z \leq \alpha_{m-1})$. Then, draw a uniform random number from the interval $[p_{iL}, p_{iU}]$, say u_i and set $Z_{2,i}^r = \Phi_Z^{-1}(u_i)$, where $\Phi_Z^{-1}(\,.\,)$ is the inverse cumulative normal distribution corresponding to (4.14).

Updating $\boldsymbol{\alpha}$

We amend the likelihood (4.12) to include information from $\mathbf{Y}_1$ through the conditional normal distribution derived from (4.13). Specifically, recalling that $\alpha_0 = -\infty$ and $\alpha_M = \infty$,

$$\Pr(Y_{i,2} = m) = \pi_{c,m,i} = \int_{\alpha_{m-1}}^{\alpha_m} \frac{1}{\sqrt{2\pi\sigma_c^2}} e^{-0.5(s-\mu_c)^2/\sigma_c^2}\, ds, \quad m \in (1, \ldots, M), \quad (4.15)$$

where at the beginning of update iteration r,

$$\mu_c = (Y_{i,1} - \beta_{0,1}^{r-1})(\boldsymbol{\Omega}_{1,1}^{r-1})^{-1}\boldsymbol{\Omega}_{1,2}^{r-1},$$
$$\sigma_c^2 = 1 - \boldsymbol{\Omega}_{2,1}^{r-1}(\boldsymbol{\Omega}_{1,1}^{r-1})^{-1}\boldsymbol{\Omega}_{1,2}^{r-1}.$$

At values $(\alpha_1, \dots, \alpha_M)$, we can then calculate

$$L_c(\alpha_1, \dots, \alpha_M) = \prod_{i=1}^{n} \prod_{m=1}^{M} \pi_{c,m,i}^{1[Y_i=m]}. \tag{4.16}$$

We then take (4.16) in place of (4.12) and update each element of $\boldsymbol{\alpha}$ using the Metropolis–Hastings steps described following (4.12) on p. 138.

Imputing missing data

We draw missing values after we have drawn $\boldsymbol{\alpha}^r$ and $\mathbf{Z}_2^r$, but before updating $\boldsymbol{\beta}, \boldsymbol{\Omega}$. For a missing ordinal observation, $Y_{i,2}$ say, at update r, we draw $Z_{i,2}^r$ from the conditional normal distribution (4.14), find the value of m such that $\alpha_{m-1} \leq Z_{i,2}^r \leq \alpha_m$ and impute $Y_{i,2} = m$.

For a missing continuous observation, we draw $Y_{i,1}^r$ from the conditional normal given $Z_{i,1}^r$:

$$N\{\beta_{0,1}^{r-1} + Z_{i,2}^r(\boldsymbol{\Omega}_{2,2}^{r-1})^{-1}\boldsymbol{\Omega}_{2,1}^{r-1}, \boldsymbol{\Omega}_{1,1}^{r-1} - \boldsymbol{\Omega}_{1,2}^{r-1}(\boldsymbol{\Omega}_{2,2}^{r-1})^{-1}\boldsymbol{\Omega}_{2,1}^{r-1}\}.$$

4.4 General location model

An alternative approach to a joint imputation model for continuous and categorical data is described in Schafer (1997), Ch. 9. It uses the general location model due to Olkin and Tate (1961). This separates the data into continuous and categorical variables, and then for each cell of the contingency table defined by the categorical variables, fits a separate multivariate normal model to the continuous variables. Since it is appropriate for categorical, not just binary, variables we discuss it more in depth in Section 5.4.

4.5 Full conditional specification

With binary data, full conditional specification proceeds as described in Section 3.3, but for binary variables, linear regression is replaced by logistic regression. As described before, it is preferable to first order the variables $\mathbf{Y}_1, \dots, \mathbf{Y}_p$, so that the missingness pattern is as close to monotone as possible. To initiate the algorithm, fill in the missing values of each variable, typically by drawing with replacement from the observed values of that variable. Then for each $j = 1, \dots, p$ in turn

1. using logistic regression for binary $\mathbf{Y}_j$ and linear regression for continuous $\mathbf{Y}_j$, regress *the observed part* of $\mathbf{Y}_j$ on all remaining $\mathbf{Y}$ variables, whose missing values are set at their current imputed values;

2. use the appropriate regression imputation algorithm (Section 3.1 for continuous data; Section 4.1 for binary data), impute the missing values of $\mathbf{Y}_j$.

As described on p. 119, we cycle through steps 1 and 2 for all p variables n_{burn} times, until we believe the algorithm has converged to the stationary distribution. We then keep the current imputed values to form the first imputed dataset. After n_{between} further cycles, chosen with a view to ensuring the imputed values are stochastically independent, the current values are kept to form the second imputed dataset. The algorithm is then updated a further n_{between} cycles between drawing each subsequent imputed dataset.

4.5.1 Justification

In Section 3.3.1, we cited Hughes *et al.* (2014) and Liu *et al.* (2013), who show that for multivariate normal data the FCS algorithm can be made equivalent to the corresponding joint modelling approach. One requirement for this result is that the parameter space of each conditional distribution is separate from the corresponding marginal distribution, so that parameters of the latter do not constrain, or provide any information about, the former.

We now explore this condition in the setting considered in this chapter. Suppose we have two variables, Y_1 continuous and Y_2 binary, drawn from the following distribution (which is a general location model):

$$\begin{aligned} f(Y_2) &\sim \text{Bernoulli}(\pi), \\ f(Y_1|Y_2 = 0) &\sim N(\mu_0, \sigma^2), \\ f(Y_1|Y_2 = 1) &\sim N(\mu_1, \sigma^2), \text{ so that,} \\ f(Y_1|Y_2) &\sim N(\mu_0 + Y_2(\mu_1 - \mu_0), \sigma^2). \end{aligned} \tag{4.17}$$

Typically, full conditional specification would use logistic regression for Y_2 on Y_1, and linear regression for Y_1 on Y_2.

Now consider the corresponding marginal distribution of Y_1 and the conditional of $Y_2|Y_1$:

$$\begin{aligned} f(Y_1) &\sim (1 - \pi) \times N(\mu_0, \sigma^2) + \pi \times N(\mu_1, \sigma^2), \\ f(Y_2|Y_1 = 1) &\sim \frac{\pi \times N(Y_1; \mu_1, \sigma^2)}{\pi \times N(Y_1; \mu_1, \sigma^2) + (1 - \pi) \times N(Y_1; \mu_0, \sigma^2)}, \end{aligned} \tag{4.18}$$

where (4.18) corresponds to a logistic regression model $\text{logit}(\pi) = \alpha_0 + \alpha_1 Y_1$ with $\alpha_0 = \log\{\pi/(1 - \pi)\} + (\mu_0^2 - \mu_1^2)/2\sigma$ and $\alpha_1 = (\mu_1 - \mu_0)/\sigma$.

Here the marginal distribution of Y_1 contains information about all the parameters of the conditional. For example if μ_0 and μ_1 are separated by more than 4σ there is a lot of information about $\pi, \mu_0, \mu_1, \sigma^2$ in the marginal $f(Y_1)$ distribution. This violates the condition of Hughes *et al.* (2014) for FCS to be equivalent to a joint MCMC sampler for (4.17).

In practice, this means an *end effect* can occur, where the distribution of the imputed data will vary slightly depending on whether the last step before imputing was regressing $\mathbf{Y}_1$ on $\mathbf{Y}_2$ or vice versa. Hughes *et al.* (2014) report a simulation which confirms this effect occurs, although it appears unlikely to be important in many applications.

4.6 Issues with over-fitting

More practically relevant is the potential for implicit or implicit over-fitting of models with a number of correlated binary variables. Consider the following example, which was also discussed by Carpenter and Kenward (2008), Ch. 5.

Example 4.1 Dental pain data

Three hundred and sixty-six subjects who had moderate or severe post-surgical pain following extraction of their third molar were randomised to receive a single dose of one of five increasing doses of test drug A, or active control C, or a placebo. The response was degree of pain relief, measured on an ordinal scale from 0 (none) to 4 (complete). This was measured before the extraction and 18 times in the 24 hours following extraction. In the latter part of the trial, many subjects withdrew, particularly in the low dose and placebo arms.

Here, we focus on pain relief 6 hours after randomisation. To illustrate imputation of binary data, we dichotomise the pain relief score to 0 if the original scale was 0, 1, 2, and 1 if the original scale was 3, 4. Thus, a response of 1 means some, or complete, pain relief.

Patients reported their degree of pain 0.25, 0.5, 0.75, 1, 1.5, 2, 3, 4, 5, and 6 hours after randomisation. For these analyses, we ignore subsequent measurements (which were increasingly missing). Five out of 366 patients had interim missing values and are excluded from this analysis. All patients were observed up to 1.5 hours. Subsequently, Table 4.1 shows the drop out pattern.

Table 4.1 Withdrawal pattern for dental data, for observations up to 6 hours after extraction. Unseen observations are denoted '·'. Five patients with interim missing data are excluded.

No. of patients	Hours after tooth extraction				
	2	3	4	5	6
212	✓	✓	✓	✓	✓
11	✓	✓	✓	✓	·
8	✓	✓	✓	·	·
10	✓	✓	·	·	·
33	✓	·	·	·	·
87	·	·	·	·	·
361 patients in total					

Table 4.2 Results of multiple imputation for the estimation of the treatment effects 6 hours after tooth extraction, without and with correction for perfect prediction. All parameter estimates are log-odds ratios versus the placebo (i.e. not adjusted for baseline).

Parameter	Observed data		Multiple imputation, with 50 imputations			
	$n = 212$		Without correction		With correction	
	Estimate	(se)	Estimate	(se)	Estimate	(se)
A, 450 mcg	−0.43	(0.92)	−1.03	(1.72)	−0.33	(0.92)
A, 900 mcg	0.43	(0.94)	−0.41	(2.05)	0.43	(0.92)
A, 1350 mcg	0.54	(0.94)	−0.27	(1.93)	0.60	(0.98)
A, 1800 mcg	1.46	(1.08)	0.46	(2.12)	0.99	(1.06)
A, 2250 mcg	1.23	(1.00)	0.80	(2.19)	1.42	(0.99)
C, 400 mcg	0.05	(0.89)	−0.53	(2.20)	0.35	(0.86)
Placebo, log(odds)	1.25		1.53		0.62	

At 6 hours, 179 out of 212 patients remaining had a response of 1. Further, patients often keep the same response for several visits. Indeed, 162 have the same response until withdrawal (152 always 0), and of the remainder 80% make only 1 transition.

Let $Y_{i,j}$ denote the binary response on subject $i = 1, \dots, 361$ at $j = 2, \dots, 6$ hours after the operation. As the missingness pattern is monotone, we use sequential imputation with logistic regression (Section 4.1) when imputing $\mathbf{Y}_j$. Further, preliminary investigation shows there is not enough information in the data to allow a general dependence on past time points. Instead, we impute using a simpler model. Let $\delta_{i,k} = 1$ if subject i is randomised to intervention group k, $k \in (1, \dots, 7)$. At each time $j = 2, \dots, 6$, hours, the imputation model is

$$\text{logit}\{\Pr(y_{i,j} = 1)\} = \sum_{k=1}^{7} \alpha_{j,k}\delta_{i,k} + \sum_{k=1}^{7} \beta_{j,k}\delta_{i,k}y_{i,(j-1)}, \tag{4.19}$$

in other words, for each treatment group, a different linear dependence on the previous observation on the logistic scale.

After imputing the missing data 6 hours after tooth extraction, we fit a logistic regression to estimate the treatment effects. Table 4.2 compares the results of a complete records analysis, and the usual sequential multiple imputation with $K = 50$ imputations. Looking first at the complete records analysis, there is little to choose between the treatments; the comparisons with significant p-values are between drug A at either 2250 mcg or 1800 mcg and drug A at 450 mcg, both with $p = 0.03$. The degree of pain relief increases with each increase in dose of A with the exception of the highest dose when there is a suggestion it falls back.

Turning to the usual sequential MI results in columns 4 and 5, we see quite substantial changes in the estimated log-odds ratios, against placebo, which no longer show any trend with dose. We also see an unexpected increase in the standard errors, suggesting MI is losing quite a lot of information. No comparisons are now significant.

These results are surprising, and turn out to be due to the problem of *perfect prediction*, which we discuss below. □

The problem of perfect prediction may arise when fitting any model to discrete data. With binary data, it occurs if the strata formed by the covariates create cells in which all the responses are either 1 or 0. In this case, the maximum likelihood estimate of the probability is either 1 or 0 and under logit or probit links the corresponding parameter estimates on the linear predictor scale tend to $\pm\infty$; the associated standard errors also become very large. Unfortunately, not all software packages will issue a warning when perfect prediction occurs.

This has implications for MI because these unstable parameter estimates and very large standard errors are used in the normal distribution from which, for each imputation, the parameters used to generate the imputed data are drawn (Section 4.5). This means that the parameters used to generate the imputed data give rise to imputation probabilities in the cell very different from those observed (i.e. 0 or 1). This in turn means that the models fitted to the resulting imputed data will have erratic parameter estimates and markedly inflated standard errors. This explains the results in columns 3 and 4 of Table 4.2.

This issue clearly affects the monotone imputation algorithm and the full conditional specification approach. It will also affect the joint latent normal approach, since if the probability in a cell is 1 or 0, the corresponding latent normal will diverge to $\pm\infty$.

White *et al.* (2010) have explored this issue further in the context of monotone imputation and FCS. They propose the following computationally convenient data-augmentation solution, and justify this approach by linking it to more general penalised regression procedures (Firth, 1993). Their algorithm is as follows. Suppose, in either the monotone imputation or the FCS algorithm, we are currently attempting logistic regression of observed binary $\mathbf{Y}_1$ on the remaining $\mathbf{Y}_2, \dots, \mathbf{Y}_p$, and perfect prediction is detected.

1. For each $j = 2, \dots, p$, calculate the sample mean and variance, respectively, $\overline{Y}_j, S_j^2$.
2. For each of $j = 2, \dots, p$ in turn, append four records to the data:

$$Y_1 = 1,\ \ Y_j = \overline{Y}_j - S_j, \text{ and for all } j' \neq j, Y_j = \overline{Y}_{j'},$$

$$Y_1 = 1,\ \ Y_j = \overline{Y}_j + S_j, \text{ and for all } j' \neq j, Y_{j'} = \overline{Y}_{j'},$$

$$Y_1 = 0,\ \ Y_j = \overline{Y}_j - S_j, \text{ and for all } j' \neq j, Y_{j'} = \overline{Y}_{j'},$$

$$Y_1 = 0,\ \ Y_j = \overline{Y}_j + S_j, \text{ and for all } j' \neq j, Y_{j'} = \overline{Y}_{j'},$$

   making a total of $4(p-1)$ additional records. Give each new record weight $w = p/4(p-1) \approx 1/4$ (all original observations have weight 1).

The weights are chosen to sum to p, the number of parameters in the imputation model for $\mathbf{Y}_1$ (including the constant).

The augmented data are then used to estimate the logistic regression and impute the missing values of $\mathbf{Y}_1$, as described in Section 4.5. The $4(p-1)$ additional records are then deleted, and the algorithm moves on to the next variable. The same approach is used in step 2 for each covariate Y_j, whether it is discrete or continuous. If the jth covariate is discrete, simply round to the nearest valid value. In general, this means results are not invariant to the choice of reference category for variables with more than two categories. However, this is unlikely to be a problem in most applications.

This procedure readily extends to more general logistic regression when the response has m levels, augmenting step 2 above to add two new records for each of the m levels, giving $m(p-1)$ new records in all, each with weight $w = p/(2(p-1)m) \approx 1/2m$.

White *et al.* (2010) report a simulation study with 500 observations and three variables: two binary and one continuous (the outcome in the substantive model). Probabilities are chosen so perfect prediction occurs in each simulated dataset. They compare ignoring perfect prediction with three methods that attempt to account for it: the above algorithm, using a Bayesian bootstrap (Rubin and Schenker, 1986) and using a penalised likelihood (Firth, 1993). All three methods that address perfect prediction have negligible bias, coverage within 1% of the nominal level and power within 2% of each other. However, ignoring perfect prediction and using standard FCS leads to marked bias and massive inflation of the standard error.

The above proposal does not apply naturally to the joint modelling setting. Instead, under the latent normal model for binary data, the simplest approach is to bound acceptable draws for the latent $Z_{i,j}$'s. A natural for the bounds is $\Phi^{-1}\{1/n\}$, $\Phi^{-1}\{(n-1)/n\}$. Draws outside these bounds are rejected, and this corresponds to a uniform prior of $[1/n, (n-1)/n]$ on the associated probabilities $\pi_{i,j}$. Alternative priors on can readily be incorporated if desired via rejection sampling. Briefly, if we wish to put a prior $f(\pi)$ on the fitted probabilities, then we (i) propose $Z_{i,j}$ in the usual way, (ii) calculate the corresponding π_{ij}, but (iii) impose an additional acceptance criterion, accepting $Z_{i,j}$ with probability $f(\pi_{i,j})/M$, where $M = \max_\pi f(\pi)$. For example, a natural choice for $f(\pi)$ is the Beta(1,1) distribution, the conjugate distribution for binomial data. If there are 0 out of n events, this gives a posterior with mean probability $1/(n+2)$; conversely if there are n out of n events, this gives a posterior with mean probability $n/(n+2)$.

For the ordinal regression model, priors to address over-fitting need to be included in the Metropolis–Hastings update step for the cut points, $\boldsymbol{\alpha}$.

Example 4.2 Dental data

Returning to the dental pain example, Table 4.2 columns 6 and 7, show the results of sequential regression imputation addressing perfect prediction using the proposal of White *et al.* (2010) described above. The results clearly show those obtained ignoring perfect prediction are wrong.

After addressing perfect prediction, all standard errors bar one are slightly smaller than the complete records analysis, as we would expect given the additional information from the patients who drop out early which is included in the imputation analysis. In addition, the log-odds ratios now increase steadily with each increasing dose of drug A, which is much more plausible.

In the complete records analysis, the contrasts of the 450 mcg dose of A with both the 1800 mcg and 2250 mcg doses were significant with $p = 0.03$. After imputation under MAR addressing perfect prediction, the contrast between the 450 mcg and 1800 mcg dose is less significant, $p = 0.09$, while that between the 450 mcg and 2250 mcg dose marginally gains significance, $p = 0.02$.

In fact, patients' pain profiles are characterised by relatively few changes between 0 and 1 (or vice versa) over time. A more appropriate imputation approach should take this into account, possibly in a non-parametric way as discussed in Chapter 7. □

4.7 Pros and cons of the various approaches

In practice, when using MI with a mix of binary and continuous data, unnoticed perfect prediction is the most likely pitfall. While some software attempts to detect perfect prediction, hence, triggering the data augmentation algorithm above, this detection is not failsafe. The usual maxim of careful exploratory data analysis before imputation therefore applies. Specifically in this setting, whether embarking on conditional or joint imputation, it may be useful to fit the conditional models using the complete records in a preliminary step to assess the chance of perfect prediction occurring in the imputation process. With FCS imputation, perfect prediction may arise in the imputation process, even though not present in the complete records, due to imputed values of the covariates.

As the dental pain data also illustrate, with binary data we may need to structure the FCS regression imputation models by carefully choosing the covariates we include. In the joint modelling framework, this corresponds to setting terms in the precision matrix, $\boldsymbol{\Omega}^{-1}$, to zero. For instance, in the dental pain example, suppose we impute separately in each treatment group, with Y_{j-1} only as a predictor for Y_j, $j = 2, \dots, 5$. The corresponding (symmetric) precision matrix has the following elements constrained:

$$\boldsymbol{\Omega}^{-1} = \begin{pmatrix} \gamma_{1,1} & \gamma_{1,2} & 0 & 0 & 0 \\ \gamma_{1,2} & \gamma_{2,2} & \gamma_{2,3} & 0 & 0 \\ 0 & \gamma_{2,3} & \gamma_{3,3} & \gamma_{3,4} & 0 \\ 0 & 0 & \gamma_{3,4} & \gamma_{4,4} & \gamma_{4,5} \\ 0 & 0 & 0 & \gamma_{4,5} & \gamma_{5,5} \end{pmatrix},$$

where γ_{ij} is the (i, j) element of $\boldsymbol{\Omega}^{-1}$ which is not simply the inverse of the (i, j) element of $\boldsymbol{\Omega}$.

While, as discussed in Section 4.5.1 above, with discrete data, the joint modelling approach has a stronger theoretical foundation, both in terms of a well-defined joint distribution and a valid MCMC sampler for imputing from this, in practice we have not found these issues important. Since the MCMC sampler for the joint model involves loops, if programmed in a high-level language, it will be slower than FCS, since the regression models used in the latter exploit efficient low-level code for their matrix calculations.

Lee and Carlin (2010) report a simulation study comparing FCS with joint multivariate normal imputation using adaptive rounding for discrete data. Their simulation study sampled datasets of 1000 individuals from a synthetic population of close to 1 million; the model of interest was linear regression of a continuous variable on six covariates: one continuous, one binary, three ordinal, and one categorical. The ordinal variables had five levels, and the categorical variable two levels. The continuous variables were skew, and best results were obtained when they were log-transformed before imputation and back transformed after imputation. A variety missing at random data mechanisms were explored; the most extensive had missing data on the continuous, two of the ordinal and the binary covariates. All mechanisms resulted in about 33% of values missing for each variable. Using adaptive rounding, they found no evidence that joint multivariate normal imputation performs less well than FCS; indeed, for a couple of parameters they report slightly better coverage than with FCS.

Similarly Demirtas *et al.* (2008) conclude joint multivariate normal imputation performs well even if multivariate normality does not hold; likewise Bernaards *et al.* (2007) (discussed above) report broadly good performance. Nevertheless, it is clear that for sparse data, this approach might break down and that, in general, multivariate normal imputations cannot be compatible with the distribution of the observed data (Yu *et al.*, 2007; van Buuren, 2007).

Drawing this together, research shows that in analyses where (i) the proportion of partially observed cases is less than $\approx 1/3$, and (ii) fitted probabilities from complete record regression models of partially observed binary variables on the other variables lie inside $(0.1, 0.9)$ joint normal imputation and using adaptive rounding is going to be indistinguishable from FCS.

Indeed, the results may be practically indistinguishable more broadly because in practice much of the information MI recovers is from the observed data on the additional, partially observed units it includes. With regards to the latent normal method, (Quartagno *et al.*, 2019) showed that it is possible to get good results, virtually identical, if not superior, to FCS in a wide range of scenarios, both in terms of coverage and bias. The only possible problem with this approach is that perfect prediction might make convergence difficult to achieve; this can be addressed by making use of more informative priors. A further advantage of joint normal imputation is that in large datasets (say with over 50 variables) it is more robust for semi-automatic use; in such cases, FCS often requires specification of reduced sets of covariates in the conditional models (Lee and Carlin, 2010). Joint latent normal modelling is also attractive for larger datasets as this naturally extends the multivariate normal approach to handle binary data. However, in smaller-scale situations FCS may have the edge. We note that we have not considered partially observed categorical data here—this is the subject of chapter 5.

As usual, there is no substitute for careful examination of the data before imputation, especially when there are a number of correlated binary variables with probabilities close to 0 or 1.

4.8 Software

For sequential imputation of monotone missing data, with a mix of binary and continuous variables, the linear and logistic model fitting software in most statistical packages can be used. Analysts need to be careful to create *proper* imputations, by sampling anew from the distribution of the regression coefficients before drawing each imputed dataset. Overfitting can be avoided by checking the results of each regression model are sensible before starting the imputation process.

For the joint multivariate normal approach, the same options discussed in Chapter 3 are available. Some packages include automatic rounding; however, for adaptive rounding, users will typically need to write their own post-imputation data step. An advantage of the multivariate normal approach is that it is more robust to perfect prediction errors. However, problems may arise if the variables are highly correlated, as the covariance matrix $\mathbf{\Omega}$ may be close to singular. This can often be successfully stabilised using a ridge parameter, as discussed in chapter 14, section 14.8.1.

The latent normal approach is available with `REALCOM-impute` and `jomo`. In `REALCOM-impute`, we can either treat all binary variables explicitly, or treat those where probabilities are not close to 0 or 1 using the normal distribution, with adaptive rounding, reserving explicit latent normal modelling for the remainder.

Turning to full conditional specification, all the packages mentioned in Chapter 3 can be used. Automatic detection and adjusting for perfect prediction using the approach described in Section 4.6, is implemented in Stata. Analysts should note that the detection of perfect prediction is not guaranteed.

4.9 Discussion

In this chapter, we have described how cross-sectional data, with a mix of binary and continuous outcomes, may be imputed. Of the various approaches, we will see that the attraction of the latent normal approach is that it allows a unified treatment of different data types and multi-level structure through the latent multivariate normal distribution. However, like the joint multivariate normal and FCS approach, the latent normal approach does not capture any higher-order associations in the binary data; it assumes that the binary observations arise from dichotomisation of a genuine (if unseen) normal variable. Thus, the imputed data will not contain the higher-order associations. If these are desired, then the general location model approach is needed, since this can allow a general model for the binary data (e.g. Bahadur, 1961; Bowman and George, 1995). However, unless inference concerning higher-order moments is the target of interest, the additional work to model such moments is of no practical value.

Exercises

1. This exercise uses pseudo-data from a trial of a treatment for dental pain. The trial randomised 366 subjects who had moderate or severe post-surgical pain following extraction of their third molar to receive one of five increasing doses of a test drug, or an active control, or a placebo. The outcome was degree of pain relief, measured on an ordinal scale from 0 (none) to 4 (complete). This was measured before the extraction and at multiple follow-up visits in the 24 hours following extraction. Our outcome of interest is pain relief 6 hours after randomisation. To illustrate the use of the imputation methods for binary data, we dichotomise the pain relief score to 0 if the original scale was 0, 1, 2, and 1 if the original scale was 3, 4. Our substantive analysis model is a logistic regression model with treatment as the only covariate.

   (a) Fit an imputation model where you include measurements at baseline, 0.25, 0.5, 0.75, 1, 1.5, 2, 3, 4, 5, and 6 hours after extraction. Possibly start with a simple logistic regression imputation with no adjustment for perfect prediction, as is possible to do with mi impute logit;

   (b) Now switch on the option for using augmentation to handle perfect prediction (option augment). How does this change the results?

   (c) When do you think it is most important to use a method robust to perfect prediction? What disadvantages can such a method have?

2. This exercise simulates data from a simple model to understand the results found by Hughes *et al.* (2014), who investigated whether a joint modelling rationale existed for FCS imputation in finite samples.

   (a) Design a simulation study where in each repetition you draw, for 100 individuals, a binary covariate X from a Bernoulli distribution with probability $p = 0.3$, a continuous covariate Z from a conditional normal distribution $N(5 + \beta X, \sigma^2 = 5)$ and a continuous outcome Y from a conditional normal distribution $N(4 + Z + 2\beta X, \sigma^2 = 4)$; try both with $\beta = 1$ and $\beta = 3$.

   (b) In each repetition, make a quarter of the observations for X and a quarter of those for Z as missing completely at random; justify your algorithm for doing this?

   (c) In each repetition, impute using FCS changing the order in which the univariate imputation models are fitted. Then fit the substantive model (linear regression of Y on X and Z) and store the estimates of the effect of Z when using data imputed using different orders;

   (d) Repeat for 1000 repetitions and summarise results. What is the absolute difference of the mean parameter estimates obtained using different orders and how does it vary for $\beta = 1$ and $\beta = 3$?

(e) Now repeat for X drawn from a standard normal distribution. Do you still see a similar absolute difference between the mean estimates? If not, why?

(f) Now impute using joint modelling imputation. How do the results compare?

(g) Do your conclusions agree with those of Hughes *et al.* (2014)? Do you think this is likely to be a problem in applications?

5

Imputation of unordered categorical data

Thus far, we have considered imputation of a mix of cross-sectional continuous and ordinal data. We have described and contrasted the different approaches that have been proposed in the literature and considered issues that are likely to arise in practice and how they might be addressed.

In this chapter, we consider unordered categorical data and imputing this alongside ordered and continuous data. Again, a number of approaches have been proposed in the literature, which we describe and contrast.

Section 5.2 describes how the multivariate normal approach may be used with categorical data. Section 5.3 outlines how the latent normal approach can be extended to include categorical data, while Section 5.4 describes the general location model, which has the richest potential structure. We discuss the full conditional specification (FCS) approach in this setting in Section 5.5, concluding with a discussion in Section 5.8.

5.1 Monotone missing data

Continuing with sequential imputation for data with a monotone missingness pattern from Section 4.1, recall we have p variables and suppose that as we work through $j = 2, \dots, p$ $\mathbf{Y}_j$ is the first unordered categorical variable. In essence, we replace logistic regression with multinomial logistic regression. Specifically,

1. For unordered categorical variable j, suppose $i = 1, \dots, n_j$ units have $Y_{i,j}$ observed. Using data from these n_j units, as before let $\mathbf{1}$ be a vector of n_j 1's and form $\mathbf{W} = (\mathbf{1}, \mathbf{Y}_1, \dots, \mathbf{Y}_{j-1})$ so that $\mathbf{W}$ is the $n_j \times j$ regression model with rows $\mathbf{W}_i$, $i \in 1, \dots, n_j$.

Multiple Imputation and its Application, Second Edition.
James R. Carpenter, Jonathan W. Bartlett, Tim P. Morris, Angela M. Wood, Matteo Quartagno and Michael G. Kenward.

2. Choose $m = 1$ as the base category. Let $\pi_{i,j,m} = \Pr(Y_{i,j} = m)$, $m = 1, \dots, M$. Fit the model
$$\log\left(\frac{\pi_{i,j,m}}{\pi_{i,j,1}}\right) = \mathbf{W}_i\boldsymbol{\beta}_{j,m}, \tag{5.1}$$
obtaining the maximum likelihood estimates $(\boldsymbol{\beta}_{j,2}, \dots, \boldsymbol{\beta}_{j,M})$ with covariance matrix $\hat{\boldsymbol{\Sigma}}$.

3. Then

   (a) draw $(\boldsymbol{\beta}^*_{j,2}, \dots, \boldsymbol{\beta}^*_{j,M})$ from
$$N((\hat{\boldsymbol{\beta}}_{j,2}, \dots, \hat{\boldsymbol{\beta}}_{j,M})^T, \hat{\boldsymbol{\Sigma}})$$

   (b) for each unobserved $Y_{i,j}$ calculate, for $m = 2, \dots, M$
$$\eta^*_{i,j,m} = (1, Y_{i,1}, \dots, Y_{i,j-1})\boldsymbol{\beta}^*_{j,m}. \tag{5.2}$$
   Then draw $Y_{i,j}$ from the multinomial distribution with probabilities
$$\frac{1}{1 + \sum_{i=2}^{M}\exp(\eta^*_{i,j,m})}(1, e^{\eta^*_{i,j,1}}, \dots, e^{\eta^*_{i,j,M}})$$
   so that all the missing values of $\mathbf{Y}_j$ are imputed. We note that for $j = 3, \dots, p$ there will be some units with $Y_{i,j}$ missing and with one or more of $Y_{i,2}, \dots, Y_{i,j-1}$ missing, and imputed at previous steps. These previously imputed values are included in (5.2) when imputing $Y_{i,j}$.

Going forward to the next variable in the sequence to be imputed, we will need to include the categorical variable $\mathbf{Y}_j$ as a covariate. This will typically mean including $(M - 1)$ dummy variables corresponding to the levels of $\mathbf{Y}_j$.

To impute a dataset with a monotone missingness pattern and a mix of unordered categorical, binary and continuous data, we therefore begin by putting the variables in order to make a monotone missing pattern, with the fully observed variables first. Then we impute each partially observed variable in turn, conditional on previous variables, using steps 1 and 2 from p. 107 if the variable is continuous, steps 1 and 2 from p. 125 if the variable is binary, and steps 1–3 above if it is unordered categorical.

The whole sequence is repeated to generate successive imputed datasets.

Perfect prediction, where one or more of the multinomial probabilities $\pi_{i,j,m}$ are estimated to be zero, occur with increasing frequency as the number of categories and number of categorical variables increases. Section 4.6 discusses the implication of perfect prediction for imputation and a data-augmentation approach – which can be used with categorical data – for addressing it in sequential imputation. To reduce problems with perfect prediction, it is usually good practice to reduce, as far as sensible in the context, the number of categories being imputed.

5.2 Multivariate normal imputation for categorical data

As with binary data, the joint multivariate normal model may be applied to categorical data. To illustrate, suppose we have two variables, $\mathbf{Y}_1$ continuous and $\mathbf{Y}_2$ categorical with M levels. The approach here, proposed among others by Allison (2002), is to create $M - 1$ dummy variables, indexing the categories. We re-order the categories if necessary so the most frequently occurring category is $m = 1$ and for $m = 2, \dots, M$ define dummy variables as follows:

$$Z_{i2m} = \begin{cases} 1 & \text{if } Y_{i,2} = m, \\ 0 & \text{otherwise.} \end{cases} \tag{5.3}$$

We then perform multivariate normal imputation, as described in Section 3.2, including $\mathbf{Y}_1, \mathbf{Z}_{2,2}, \dots, \mathbf{Z}_{2,M}$.

After creating the imputed datasets, we derive imputed values of the categorical variable $\mathbf{Y}_2$ from $\mathbf{Z}_{2,2}, \dots, \mathbf{Z}_{2,M}$ as follows:

$$\begin{aligned} Y_{i,2} &= 0 \text{ if all } Z_{i,2,2}, \dots, Z_{i,2,M} < 0.5, \\ Y_{i,2} &= m' \text{ if } Z_{i,2,m'} = \max_{m=1,\dots,M}(Z_{i,2,m}) > 0.5. \end{aligned} \tag{5.4}$$

There is no benefit in applying adaptive rounding (Section 4.2) before deriving the categorical variables (5.4), as this may distort the ordering (Figure 4.1). Notice that the model allows (linearised) chance of being in each category to be a different linear function of $\mathbf{Y}_1$, and indeed of all the other category indicators. Thus, if used with a number of categorical variables, each with two or more categories, over-parameterisation is likely to become an issue. A natural proposal is to fix the covariance of category indicators within the same categorical variable to be zero; e.g. in the example above $\text{Cov}(\mathbf{Z}_{2,m}, \mathbf{Z}_{2,m'}) = 0$, for all $m \neq m'$. As far as we are aware, this approach has not been extensively explored in the literature. Nevertheless, experience with binary data, discussed in Section 4.7, suggests it is likely to perform acceptably in many practical settings.

5.3 Maximum indicant model

A natural development of this approach is the maximum indicant model of Aitchison and Bennett (1970). The attraction of this approach is that it links naturally with the latent normal approach described for binary and ordinal data in Section 4.3.

To introduce this, suppose we have a single unordered categorical variable Y_i, $i \in 1, \dots, n$ taking values $m = 1, 2, 3$. We set up three independent latent normal variables:

$$\begin{aligned}
V_{i,1} &= \alpha_1 + \nu_{i,1},\\
V_{i,2} &= \alpha_2 + \nu_{i,2},\\
V_{i,3} &= \alpha_3 + \nu_{i,3},\\
\begin{pmatrix} V_{i,1}\\ V_{i,2}\\ V_{i,3}\end{pmatrix} &\sim N_3\left[\mathbf{0}, \begin{pmatrix} 0.5 & 0 & 0\\ 0 & 0.5 & 0\\ 0 & 0 & 0.5\end{pmatrix}\right].
\end{aligned} \tag{5.5}$$

We term the V's indicants. The variance of the indicants is set to 0.5 but could be potentially fixed to any number. The maximum indicant model has

$$Y_i = m \text{ if and only if } V_{i,m} > V_{i,m'} \text{ for all } m' \neq m.$$

Thus, if $Y_i = 2$ V_{i2} must be the maximum indicant, with $V_{i,2} > V_{i,1}$ and $V_{i,2} > V_{i,3}$.

In practice, model (5.5) is not fitted directly; instead, the following derivation is used. Define

$$\begin{aligned}
Z_{i,1} &= V_{i,1} - V_{i,3},\\
Z_{i,2} &= V_{i,2} - V_{i,3}.
\end{aligned}$$

Then

$$\begin{aligned}
Z_{i,1} &= \alpha_1 - \alpha_3 + \epsilon_{i1},\\
Z_{i,2} &= \alpha_2 - \alpha_3 + \epsilon_{i2},\\
\begin{pmatrix} Z_{i,1}\\ Z_{i,2}\end{pmatrix} &\sim N_2\left\{\mathbf{0}, \begin{pmatrix} 1 & 0.5\\ 0.5 & 1\end{pmatrix}\right\}.
\end{aligned} \tag{5.6}$$

Under this model,

$$\begin{aligned}
Y_i = 1 &\iff V_{i,1} > V_{i,2} \text{ and } V_{i,1} > V_{i,3},\\
&\iff Z_{i,1} - Z_{i,2} > 0 \text{ and } Z_{i,1} > 0.
\end{aligned}$$

Similarly, $Y_i = 2$ if and only if $Z_{i,2} > Z_{i,1}$ and $Z_{i,2} > 0$. Lastly,

$$\begin{aligned}
Y_i = 3 &\iff V_{i,3} > V_{i,1} \text{ and } V_{i,2} > V_{i,1},\\
&\iff Z_{i,1} < 0 \text{ and } Z_{i,2} < 0.
\end{aligned}$$

As (5.6) has one too many mean parameters, we define $\beta_{0,1} = \alpha_1 - \alpha_3$, and $\beta_{0,2} = \alpha_1 - \alpha_3$. In our context, it is convenient to further simplify (5.6) by setting the correlations to be zero.

In the case of M categories, the categorical variable Y_i, $i \in 1, \dots, n$, takes unordered categorical values $1, \dots, M$. For each Y_i, define $(M - 1)$ independent latent normal variables, $Z_{i,m} \sim N(\beta_{0,m}, 1)$ with

$$\begin{aligned}
Y_i = m &\iff \left\{\begin{matrix} Z_{i,m} > Z_{i,m'}, \text{ for } m' \neq m\\ \text{and } Z_{i,m} > 0\end{matrix}\right\}, \quad m = 1, 2, \dots, (M-1),\\
Y_i = M &\iff Z_{i,m} < 0 \text{ all } m = 1, \dots, (M-1).
\end{aligned} \tag{5.7}$$

We therefore have $M-1$ parameters, $\beta_{0,m}$, defining the $M-1$ probabilities. These sum to 1, as there are exactly $(M-1)$ possibilities in (5.7). Given values $\beta_1, \dots, \beta_m$, the probability of each possibility, and hence, each category can be calculated from the normal distributions of $Z_{i,1}, \dots, Z_{M-1}$.

For example, suppose we have three categories, and $\beta_{0,1} = \beta_{0,2} = 0$. Since Z_1 and Z_2 are independent, $\pi_3 = \Pr(Z_1 < 0 \;\&\; Z_2 < 0) = 0.25$. Further, as the chance of Z_1 being both greater than zero and greater than Z_2 is the same as the chance of Z_2 being both greater than Z_1 and greater than zero, we must have $\pi_1 = \Pr(Z_1 > Z_2 \;\&\; Z_1 > 0) = \pi_2 = \Pr(Z_2 > Z_1 \;\&\; Z_2 > 0) = 0.375$.

Unfortunately, in general calculation of the probabilities π_m implied by (5.7) requires numerical integration, typically by Gaussian quadrature, albeit only in one dimension because of the independence of the latent normals. However, when – as detailed below – we have a multivariate response model, with continuous variables alongside categorical ones, then conditioning on the continuous variables induces dependency among the latent $Z_{i,m}$, further complicating calculation of the probabilities. In practice, it often easiest to estimate them using Markov chain Monte Carlo (MCMC).

We now describe the MCMC algorithm to estimate the parameters, before going on to consider the multivariate response setting. Initialise $\beta^0_{0,m} = 0$, $m = 1, \dots, (M-1)$. At step $r = 1, 2, \dots$

1. for individual $i = 1, \dots, n$

   (a) draw
   $$\mathbf{Z}^*_i \sim N_{M-1}[(\beta^{r-1}_{0,1}, \beta^{r-1}_{0,2}, \dots, \beta^{r-1}_{0,M-1})^T, \boldsymbol{I}_{M-1}].$$

   (b) if $Y_i = m$, $m = 1, \dots, (M-1)$
   $$\text{accept } \mathbf{Z}^*_i \iff \begin{cases} Z^*_{im} > Z^*_{im'} & \text{for all } m' \neq m, \\ \text{and } Z^*_{im} > 0, \end{cases}$$

   (c) else if $Y_i = M$,
   $$\text{accept } \mathbf{Z}^*_i \iff Z^*_{im} < 0, \text{ for all } m = 1, \dots, M-1.$$

   (d) If $\mathbf{Z}^*_i$ is accepted, set $\mathbf{Z}^r_i = \mathbf{Z}^*_i$, otherwise return to (a).

2. Calculate $\overline{Z}^r_m = \sum_{i=1}^n Z^r_{i,m}/n$, $m = 1, \dots, (M-1)$. Draw
   $$(\beta^r_1, \beta^r_2, \dots, \beta^r_{M-1})^T \sim N_{M-1}\{(\overline{Z}^r_1, \overline{Z}^r_2, \dots \overline{Z}^r_{M-1})^T, \boldsymbol{I}_{M-1}/n\}.$$

For a unit with missing response, at update step r, we simply draw a latent normal in step 1, and then impute the missing response using the rule (5.7).

Along the same lines discussed when considering rejection sampling for ordinal data on p. 140, we can avoid the rejection sampling in step 1 above, which may speed up the computations.

5.3.1 Continuous and categorical variable

Now, suppose we have two variables: continuous $\mathbf{Y}_1$ and three-level unordered categorical $\mathbf{Y}_2$. We consider a three-level categorical variable below to keep the notation simple; the extension to M levels is direct. The joint model is

$$\begin{aligned}
Y_{i,1} &= \beta_{0,1} + \epsilon_{i,1},\\
\Pr(Y_{i,2}=1) &= \Pr(Z_{i,2,1} > Z_{i,2,2} \text{ and } Z_{i,2,1} > 0) \text{ where } Z_{i,2,1} = \beta_{0,2,1} + \epsilon_{i,2,1},\\
\Pr(Y_{i,2}=2) &= \Pr(Z_{i,2,2} > Z_{i,2,1} \text{ and } Z_{i,2,2} > 0) \text{ where } Z_{i,2,2} = \beta_{0,2,2} + \epsilon_{i,2,2},\\
\Pr(Y_{i,2}=3) &= \Pr(Z_{i,2,1} < 0 \text{ and } Z_{i,2,2} < 0),\\
\begin{pmatrix}\epsilon_{i,1}\\ \epsilon_{i,2,1}\\ \epsilon_{i,2,2}\end{pmatrix} &= N_3\left[0, \mathbf{\Omega} = \begin{pmatrix}\sigma_1^2 & \sigma_{1,2,1} & \sigma_{1,2,2}\\ \sigma_{1,2,1} & 1 & 0\\ \sigma_{1,2,2} & 0 & 1\end{pmatrix}\right].
\end{aligned} \tag{5.8}$$

Notice that, as before, the latent normal variables are marginally uncorrelated, with constrained variance. This means there are two parameters, $\beta_{0,2,1}, \beta_{0,2,2}$ defining the marginal probabilities that $\pi_{2,1} = \Pr(Y_{i,2} = 1)$, $\pi_{2,2} = \Pr(Y_{i,2} = 2)$ with $\pi_{2,3} = 1 - \pi_{2,1} - \pi_{2,3}$. Thus, we have one parameter for each of the two 'free' probabilities, and the model is not over-parameterised.

The MCMC algorithm for model (5.8) is as follows: Choose initial values $\boldsymbol{\beta}^0$, $\mathbf{\Omega}^0$. At update step $r = 1, 2, \ldots$

1. For $i = 1, \ldots, n$
   (a) draw $\mathbf{Z}_i^{*r} = (Z_{i,2,1}^{*r}, Z_{i,2,2}^{*r})^T$ from the conditional bivariate normal,

$$N\left\{\begin{pmatrix}\beta_{0,2,1}^{r-1}\\ \beta_{0,2,2}^{r-1}\end{pmatrix} + (Y_{i,1} - \beta_{0,1}^{r-1})(\mathbf{\Omega}_{1,1}^{r-1})^{-1}\begin{pmatrix}\mathbf{\Omega}_{1,2}^{r-1}\\ \mathbf{\Omega}_{1,3}^{r-1}\end{pmatrix},\right.$$
$$\left. I_2 - (\mathbf{\Omega}_{1,2}^{r-1}\mathbf{\Omega}_{1,3}^{r-1})^T(\mathbf{\Omega}_{1,1}^{r-1})^{-1}(\mathbf{\Omega}_{1,2}^{r-1}, \mathbf{\Omega}_{1,3}^{r-1})\right\}, \tag{5.9}$$

   (b) if $Y_{i,2} = m$, $m = 1, 2$

$$\text{accept } \mathbf{Z}_i^* \iff \begin{cases} Z_{i,m}^* > Z_{i,m'}^* & \text{for all } m \neq m',\\ \text{and } Z_{i,m} > 0, \end{cases}$$

   if $Y_i = 3$,

$$\text{accept } \mathbf{Z}_i^* \iff Z_{i,m}^* < 0, m = 1, 2.$$

   (c) If $\mathbf{Z}_i^*$ is accepted, set $\mathbf{Z}_i^r = \mathbf{Z}_i^*$, else return to 1(a).

2. Let $\mathbf{Z}_{2,m} = (Z_{1,2,m}, Z_{2,2,m}, \ldots, Z_{n,2,m})^T$, $m = 1, 2$. Given $\mathbf{Y}_1, \mathbf{Z}_{2,1}^r, \mathbf{Z}_{2,2}^r$ update $\mathbf{\Omega}^{r-1}$ elementwise, as described in Chapter 4, p. 134, subject to the constraints in (5.8). This gives $\mathbf{\Omega}^r$.

3. Calculate $\overline{\mathbf{Y}}_1 = \sum_{i=1}^n Y_{i,1}/n$, and $\overline{\mathbf{Z}}_{2,m}^r = \sum_{i=1}^n Z_{i,2,m}^r/n$, $m = 1, 2$. Draw

$$\begin{pmatrix}\beta_{0,1}^r\\ \beta_{0,2,1}^r\\ \beta_{0,2,2}^r\end{pmatrix} \sim N_3\left\{\begin{pmatrix}\overline{\mathbf{Y}}_1\\ \overline{\mathbf{Z}}_{2,1}^r\\ \overline{\mathbf{Z}}_{2,2}^r\end{pmatrix}, \mathbf{\Omega}^r/n\right\}.$$

Once again, an algorithm avoiding rejection sampling could in principle be derived, along the lines of what was presented in Chapter 4.

5.3.2 Imputing missing data

Suppose the categorical variable $Y_{i,2}$ is missing. Then at Step 1(a) of the MCMC algorithm for the joint model on p. 163, we draw $(Z^r_{i,2,1}, Z^r_{i,2,2})$ from the conditional normal distribution (5.9), and use rule (5.7) to impute $Y_{i,2}$.

Now suppose $Y_{i,1}$ is missing. Then we draw $(Z_{i,2,1}, Z_{i,2,2})$ from the marginal bivariate normal distribution

$$N_2\left[\begin{pmatrix}\beta^{r-1}_{0,2,1}\\ \beta^{r-1}_{0,2,2}\end{pmatrix}, \boldsymbol{I}_2\right],$$

accepting a draw, denoted $(Z^r_{i,2,1}, Z^r_{i,2,2})$ which satisfies the constraint implied by the observed value $Y_{i,2} = m$.

Given this, we draw $Y^r_{i,1}$ from the conditional normal distribution given $(Z^r_{i,2,1}, Z^r_{i,2,2})$, which has mean

$$\beta_{0,1} + (Z^r_{i,2,1} - \beta^{r-1}_{0,2,1}, Z^r_{i,2,2} - \beta^{r-1}_{0,2,2})\boldsymbol{I}_2 \begin{pmatrix}\boldsymbol{\Omega}^{r-1}_{1,2}\\ \boldsymbol{\Omega}^{r-1}_{1,3}\end{pmatrix},$$

and variance

$$\boldsymbol{\Omega}^{r-1}_{1,1} - (\boldsymbol{\Omega}^{r-1}_{1,2}, \boldsymbol{\Omega}^{r-1}_{1,3})\boldsymbol{I}_2(\boldsymbol{\Omega}^{r-1}_{1,2}, \boldsymbol{\Omega}^{r-1}_{1,3})^T.$$

Once we have drawn values for the missing data in step 1, we proceed to update the remaining parameters as before.

Summary

We have set out the MCMC algorithm for a joint model for a continuous and unordered three-category response using latent normal variables and the maximum indicant model. This extends directly to more than three categories. Through the latent normal structure, we can add additional binary or ordinal variables, categorical variables, and continuous variables. The latent normal model therefore provides a unified approach to the modelling different response types. The attraction of this approach is that it extends naturally to the multi-level setting, as we describe in Chapter 9, and other related structures.

5.4 General location model

An alternative model for multivariate normal and categorical data is the general location model of Olkin and Tate (1961). Suppose we have a continuous $(Y_{i,1}, Y_{i,2})$ and binary ($Y_{i,3}, Y_{i,4}$) variables. The binary variables define a contingency table with four cells:

	$Y_{i,3} = 0$	$Y_{i,3} = 1$	Total
$Y_{i,4} = 0$	n_1	n_2	$(n_1 + n_2)$
$Y_{i,4} = 1$	n_3	n_4	$(n_3 + n_4)$
Total	$(n_1 + n_3)$	$(n_2 + n_4)$	n

with corresponding probabilities π_g, $g = 1, \dots, 4$, $\sum_{g=1}^{4} \pi_g = 1$. Given that unit i belongs to cell g,

$$f(Y_{i,1}, Y_{i,2} | Y_{i,3}, Y_{i,4}) \sim N_2(\boldsymbol{\mu}_g, \boldsymbol{\Omega}_g). \tag{5.10}$$

In other words, conditional on unit i belonging to cell g, the continuous variables follow a multivariate normal model with cell-specific mean and covariance matrix.

A key difference with the latent normal model is that (5.10) allows the mean and variance of (Y_{i1}, Y_{i2}) to differ for each cell g of the contingency table defined by the binary (or in generality categorical) variables. By contrast, the latent normal model has a common covariance matrix. We anticipate few applications in which having a group-specific covariance matrix is important. In the latent normal setting, some flexibility can be introduced by including covariates in the covariance model (Browne, 2006). Model (5.10) with the assumption of a common covariance matrix across groups is the usual linear discriminant analysis model.

Schafer (1999b) has freely available software for fitting and imputing missing data under this model, using a MCMC approach described in Chapters 7–9 of Schafer (1997). Since, in general, the general location model has a saturated log-linear model for the categorical variables and given this a separate multivariate normal distribution for the continuous variables corresponding to each contingency table cell, both categorical and multivariate normal models usually need to be simplified before it is fitted. While it is strictly congenial with logistic and log-linear models (while the latent normal model is not), it does not extend so naturally to the multi-level setting if we wish to allow a full range of variable types at each level.

Example 5.1 Youth Cohort Study

This study was introduced in Chapter 1, Example 1.2. Here, we expand the substantive model to include the different ethnic groups, so it is a linear regression of General Certificate of Secondary Education (GCSE) educational score (between 0 and 84) on cohort, sex, parental social grouping (derived from questions answered by the students) and ethnicity.

As discussed in Chapter 1, the principal missing data pattern is missing parental social grouping; there are a few missing values of ethnicity, but because this variable has so many groups, it extremely time-consuming to impute these, for no practically relevant gain. We therefore restrict ourselves to the 54,872 cases where ethnicity is fully observed. The missingness pattern is shown in Table 5.1.

Table 5.1 Missingness pattern in the 62,578 Youth Cohort Study (YCS) records in which ethnicity is observed. Cohort and sex are fully observed.

Pattern frequency	Variable	
	GCSE score	Parental social grouping
54,872	✓	✓
6737	✓	·
673	·	✓
296	·	·

For multiple imputation, we use the latent normal model; virtually identical results are obtained with FCS. For student i, let $Y_{i,1}$ denote GCSE score and $Y_{i,2}$ be the three-level categorical variable identifying parental social grouping. The imputation model is

$$\begin{aligned}
Y_{i,1} &= \boldsymbol{\beta}_1^T\mathbf{X}_i + \epsilon_{i,1},\\
\Pr(Y_{i,2} = 1) &= \Pr(Z_{i,2,1} > Z_{i,2,2} \text{ and } Z_{i,2,1} > 0) \text{ where } Z_{i,2,1} = \boldsymbol{\beta}_2^T\mathbf{X}_i + \epsilon_{i,2,1},\\
\Pr(Y_{i,2} = 2) &= \Pr(Z_{i,2,2} > Z_{i,2,1} \text{ and } Z_{i,2,2} > 0) \text{ where } Z_{i,2,2} = \boldsymbol{\beta}_3^T\mathbf{X}_i + \epsilon_{i,2,2},\\
\Pr(Y_{i,2} = 3) &= \Pr(Z_{i,2,1} < 0 \text{ and } Z_{i,2,2} < 0),\\
\begin{pmatrix}\epsilon_{i1}\\ \epsilon_{i,2,1}\\ \epsilon_{i,2,2}\end{pmatrix} &= N_3\left[\mathbf{0}, \boldsymbol{\Omega} = \begin{pmatrix}\sigma_1^2 & \sigma_{1,2,1} & \sigma_{1,2,2}\\ \sigma_{1,2,1} & 1 & 0\\ \sigma_{1,2,2} & 0 & 1\end{pmatrix}\right].
\end{aligned} \tag{5.11}$$

Rather than put the dummy variables derived from the categorical variables identifying cohort, sex, and ethnic group as additional categorical responses in the imputation model, we include them as covariates in the matrix $\mathbf{X}$, which has 12 columns for, respectively, the constant, the four cohort contrasts, sex, and the six ethnic group contrasts. While for fully observed continuous variables, it is computationally simpler and quicker to include them in additional responses, rather than covariates, this is not the case for categorical variables, because of the rejection sampling required for the associated latent normal structure. We fitted (5.11) using the `REALCOM-impute` software, with a burn in of 1000 updates, and 10 imputation with 1000 further updates between each imputation.

The results are shown in Table 5.2. The left column shows the complete records analysis and the right column the results of multiple imputation (MI) under the assumption of missing at random (MAR) using the latent normal imputation model (5.11). Since, as discussed in Chapter 1, the key predictors of missing parental social group are GCSE score and ethnicity, parameter estimates in the model of interest are most likely to change for ethnicity, although other parameters may be more precisely estimated. Table 5.2 shows this is exactly what we find. Of particular note, the estimated coefficients for Black, Pakistani, and Bangladeshi ethnicity move

Table 5.2 Complete records analysis of the Youth Cohort Study data and analysis using multiple imputation. These results are based on five imputed datasets.

Variable	Complete records $n = 54,872$	Multiple imputation $n = 62,578$
Cohort90	Reference	
Cohort93	5.66 (0.20)	5.44 (0.20)
Cohort95	9.42 (0.22)	9.21 (0.20)
Cohort97	8.09 (0.21)	8.03 (0.20)
Cohort99	12.70 (0.22)	12.91 (0.21)
Boys	−3.44 (0.13)	−3.35 (0.13)
Managerial	Reference	
Intermediate	−7.42 (0.154)	−7.75 (0.16)
Working	−13.74 (0.17)	−14.32 (0.17)
White	Reference	
Black	−5.61 (0.57)	−7.16 0.51
Indian	3.58 (0.435)	2.97 (0.42)
Pakistani	−2.03 (0.58)	−3.63 (0.47)
Bangladeshi	0.27 (1.04)	−3.20 (0.74)
Other Asian	5.52 (0.68)	4.49 (0.63)
Other	−0.25 (0.70)	−1.32 (0.66)
Constant	39.66 (0.19)	39.09 0.18

further from the null, and the Bangladeshi estimate moves from non-significance in the complete records analysis to being statistically significant at the 0.1% level. We return to this example later in the book, when we carry out sensitivity analysis to the MAR assumption via MI in Chapter 10 and explore how to incorporate the survey weights that are provided with this study in Chapter 12. □

5.5 FCS with categorical data

With a mix of continuous, binary and categorical data, the FCS approach proceeds as described in Section 4.5, but we now use multinomial logistic (or multinomial probit) regression for each categorical variable in turn, as described in Section 5.1, conditioning on all the other variables as covariates. Note that when M-level categorical variables are included as predictors in the regression models that make up the FCS, then they need to be included as M-level categorical variables, in other words using $M - 1$ dummy indicators.

If the missingness pattern is monotone, then appropriately specified FCS will give the same distribution of the imputed data as the sequential regression imputation algorithm, once the former has converged. To see this intuitively, suppose we have ordered the p variables into a monotone missingness pattern. When imputing variable $j > 1$, variables $j' > j$ are always missing, so there is no information 'omitted' from sequential regression imputation that can be recovered by FCS.

Suppose now we have two categorical variables, $\mathbf{Y}_1, \mathbf{Y}_2$ of L and M levels, respectively, which define a two-way contingency table with LM cells. Let $\mu_{l,m}$ be the mean count for each cell. The log-linear model for the contingency table is

$$\log(\mu_{lm}) = \lambda + \lambda_l^1 + \lambda_m^2 + \lambda_{l,m}^{12}, \tag{5.12}$$

where (as usual for such models) to avoid over-parameterisation, $\lambda_1^1 = \lambda_1^2 = \lambda_{1.}^{12} = \lambda_{.1}^{12} = 0$, $l = 1, \dots, L; m = 1, \dots, M$. The parameters λ_l^1 are the log-odds of $\mathbf{Y}_1$ taking category l to $\mathbf{Y}_1$ taking category 1, when $\mathbf{Y}_2$ is 1. The parameters λ_{lm}^{12} are the $(L-1)(M-1)$ odds ratios in the contingency table.

Multinomial logistic regression of $\mathbf{Y}_1$ on $\mathbf{Y}_2$ (including $\mathbf{Y}_2$ as an M level categorical variable) estimates the log-odds λ_l^1 and the log-odds ratios $\lambda_{l,m}^{12}$. Likewise, multinomial logistic regression of $\mathbf{Y}_2$ on $\mathbf{Y}_1$ estimates the log-odds λ_m^2 and the log-odds ratios $\lambda_{l,m}^{12}$. Therefore, the two models are compatible with each other, and any imputed data are congenial with the usual log-linear model for the contingency table. Further, the multinomial logistic regression of $\mathbf{Y}_1$ on $\mathbf{Y}_2$ neither gives any information on the marginal distribution $\mathbf{Y}_2$ nor places any restriction on it. Using analogous arguments to those with the multivariate normal distribution, Hughes *et al.* (2014) use this to show that, with appropriate choice of priors, the saturated log-linear model fitted by the Gibbs sampler and the FCS sampler when each multinomial model has the full interaction of the categorical covariates, agree.

If we have three categorical variables, then FCS imputation, where in each multinomial regression the other two variables are included as categorical covariates (but their interaction is not included), corresponds to including all the two-way interactions in the log-linear model. In other words, it imputes data that are consistent with the partial association model which estimates odds ratios relating any two factors adjusting for the third. To impute under FCS allowing for heterogeneity in the odds ratios (in other words corresponding to the saturated log-linear model), we need to include the full interaction of the covariates in each of the imputation models. We discuss and illustrate this in Section 6.

Now consider the case of a continuous and categorical variable. Here, just as in the case of a continuous and binary variable discussed on p. 143, the conditional mean of the continuous variable given the categorical variable is a linear function of the category indicators. Likewise, the conditional distribution of the categorical variable given the continuous variable is linear on the logistic scale. However, as before, because the marginal distribution of the continuous variable does provide information about the parameters of the conditional distribution of the categorical variable given the continuous variable, FCS is not equivalent to a MCMC sampler for the joint model. Simulation studies reported by Hughes *et al.* (2014) suggest any discrepancy is unlikely to be important in applications.

5.6 Perfect prediction issues with categorical data

In Section 4.6, we considered the practical issues raised by perfect prediction with binary data. The same issues arise with categorical data; in fact they are more likely to arise, as there are more categories among which small probabilities may occur.

From a Bayesian perspective, if data are binary taking the conjugate Beta(1,1) prior addresses the issue, bounding probabilities away from 0 and 1. With discrete data, the analogue is the Dirichlet prior, with all parameters set equal to 1. While this can be formally included as a prior for all probabilities in the Bayesian joint model (as described in the context of the general location model in Schafer (1997, Chapter 7)), this is awkward for the maximum indicant model, at least if it is being fitted using the latent normal approach described here. A simple practically equivalent alternative is to restrict the latent normal variables interval $[C, D]$, where $C = -3$ and $D = 4$ seems appropriate for most applications. Note the asymmetry of the interval, because (apart from the top category) category probabilities are defined by the probability that the associated latent normal is both positive and greater than all the other latent normals. As part of the update process, a Monte-Carlo estimate of either the marginal or conditional unit-specific category probabilities can readily be estimated as a check on whether perfect prediction is close to occurring.

Under the FCS approach, provided perfect prediction is identified by the software, it is a simple matter to automatically apply the approximate data augmentation approach described on p. 144.

While we expect the performance of both adjustments above to be satisfactory, even with a relatively large number of categories, we are not aware of simulation studies, which have investigated this apart from in the binary case.

5.7 Software

There are a range of software packages for imputation with categorical data. Schafer's stand-alone `CAT` package uses a joint log-linear model, while the `MIX` package extends this to a mix of categorical and continuous data using the general location model; see Schafer (1999a). These have been ported to `R`. As discussed in Section 3.5, FCS is available in `Stata` (with function `mi impute chained`) and `R` (with package `mice`, van Buuren and Groothuis-Oudshoorn, 2011). Lastly, the maximum indicant approach is available with `REALCOM-impute` and with the `R` package `jomo`.

5.8 Discussion

In this chapter, we have outlined the main approaches in the literature for parametric MI with categorical data. We have seen that all approaches are consistent with a log-linear model with two-way interactions, and all may be extended to be consistent with the saturated log-linear model. The latent normal model extends the approach taken with binary data; the drawback is the relative difficulty of estimating the underlying category probabilities. This, though, is not of primary concern for imputation. When considering multilevel MI in Chapter 9, we will see the latent normal formulation is a key advantage, since it allows modelling and imputation of all types of the data at any level.

By contrast, the general location model, though potentially more general (because it allows for different variances of continuous variables in groups defined by categorical variables) does not extend so naturally to multilevel structure. Some of this flexibility can be included in the latent normal model through including covariates in the variance model (Browne, 2006).

Lastly, the FCS approach for categorical variables (including all the interactions in each regression imputation model) is equivalent to a joint saturated log-linear model. However, with a mix of variable types, this equivalence no longer formally holds, although this is unlikely to be a concern in practice.

Thus far, we have considered MI for a mix of continuous, ordinal, and categorical variables. Our imputation models have all allowed for linear relationships between the variables on the linear predictor (latent normal) scale, and are therefore (at least very close to) congenial with substantive models for cross-sectional data that seek to estimate these effects.

However, frequently we will be interested in non-linear relationships and interactions between variables. In such cases, the approaches described thus far will be inadequate; the imputed data will not have the non-linear relationships or interactions present. Further, frequently data are multilevel. In the next chapters, we therefore consider non-linear relationships including interactions (Chapter 6) and survival data (Chapter 7) before going on to full multilevel MI in Chapter 9.

Exercises

1. This exercise replicates and extends a simulation study originally presented in Quartagno *et al.* (2019).

(a) We begin with the scenario in Section 3.3.3 of the paper. For each replication, first generate a covariate X from a standard normal distribution for 300 participants, and then a second categorical covariate Z from a multinomial distribution with probabilities $0.2, 0.3, 0.4$, and 0.1. Finally generate the outcome from

$$Y \sim N(\beta_0 + \beta_1 I(Z = 2) + \beta_2 I(Z = 3) + \beta_3 I(Z = 4) + \beta_4 X$$

where category 1 is used as reference and I is the indicator function for the event in brackets. We initially set $\boldsymbol{\beta} = (\beta_0, \beta_1, \beta_2, \beta_3, \beta_4) = (0.1, 0.1, -0.2, 0.05, 0.1)$.

(b) Make 20% observations missing for Z with a MAR mechanism given the outcome. How did you choose the mechanism? Why is MAR?

(c) Impute using full conditional specification (FCS) and joint modelling (JM) and store the parameter estimates for different levels of Z.

(d) Repeat for 1000 replications and summarise the results. Are both methods approximately unbiased? What about coverage level and standard errors?

(e) Now repeat for $\boldsymbol{\beta} = (\beta_0, \beta_1, \beta_2, \beta_3, \beta_4) = (0.1, 0.1, -0.2, 0.05, 1)$. Do the results and the comparison between methods change? Can you suggest why?

2. In this exercise, we code the algorithm for the imputation of categorical variables using joint modelling imputation that was presented in this chapter.

(a) Code in your software language of choice into the algorithm for imputing a three-level categorical variable X from an imputation model with a single continuous covariate Y and the intercept.

(b) Simulate some data ($n = 100$) and apply the method. Does it work as expected? If you impute with your code, fit the substantive model of interest (e.g. linear regression of Y on X) and apply Rubin's rules, do you get approximately the correct parameter estimates?

(c) Increase the sample size to 1000 and 10,000 participants, respectively. What do you notice? What can you conclude about this method?

PART III

MULTIPLE IMPUTATION IN PRACTICE

6

Non-linear relationships, interactions, and other derived variables

In this chapter, we consider what changes need to be made to the imputation process when the substantive model contains non-linear terms, interactions, or other such derived variables. In Section 6.1, we introduce some of these settings and outline the problems caused by default imputation model specifications. In Section 6.2, we consider the special case where the derived variables are fully observed. We then consider the settings where the derived variables are partially observed, first, in Section 6.3, describing various simple methods for this situation. In Section 6.4, we describe more sophisticated MI approaches which construct imputation models for partially observed covariates compatible with the analyst's substantive model, which may include derived variables such as non-linear effects and interactions. We conclude in Section 6.5 by returning to some of the problems outlined in Section 6.1.

6.1 Introduction

It is common in applications for the substantive model to include squares, interactions, logarithms, ratios, or sums of variables. All of these examples have in common that they are functions derived from measured values. Some, such as squares, are calculated from just one variable. Others, such as ratios, interactions, and sums, are calculated from two (or more) variables. All but sums are non-linear functions of the 'original' variables. This feature in particular complicates multiple imputation.

Multiple Imputation and its Application, Second Edition.
James R. Carpenter, Jonathan W. Bartlett, Tim P. Morris, Angela M. Wood, Matteo Quartagno and Michael G. Kenward.

In this chapter, we describe why these *derived variables* complicate multiple imputation. In these situations, as we will see, the use of standard out-of-the-box imputation models will often induce bias. This is because in many cases specifying a congenial model for imputation requires more (and sometimes considerably more) effort than would be required in settings without derived variables.

We will suggest some simple and computationally convenient methods for imputation in these settings, and explain when they may be adequate and why they are often unsatisfactory. We subsequently introduce more general approaches to imputation of derived variables based on algorithms that effectively force congeniality/compatibility. We term these methods *substantive-model compatible* (SMC).

Ratios have a particularly interesting background in relation to MI, in part due to a 2007 paper (Hippisley-Cox *et al.*, 2007). The article published a new risk score ('QRISK') for cardiovascular disease in the United Kingdom. The substantive model was a Cox model, and several of the covariates used for prediction were incomplete. One of these was the ratio of total serum cholesterol to high-density lipoprotein (HDL). Approximately 70% of the values of this ratio variable were missing, though the breakdown according to its components was not clear. The authors used multiple imputation and reported the hazard ratio of 'total cholesterol/HDL' as 1.001 (95% CI 0.999, 1.002) in women and 1.001 (95% CI 0.999, 1.003) in men. The standard deviation of total-cholesterol/HDL was about 1.3. A series of rapid responses from the readers expressed disbelief because these precisely estimated hazard ratios contradicted what had been estimated from numerous previous studies. The authors rapidly responded. Their response included results based on a revised imputation model. Parameters were re-estimated with revised hazard ratios reported as 1.20 (95% CI 1.17, 1.22) in women and 1.25 (95% CI 1.23, 1.27) in men.

The QRISK example is particularly interesting. Unbiased parameter estimation is not typically the goal for a risk score, but the fact that the two imputation approaches estimated such different hazard ratios is concerning. While there was a large proportion of missing data (70%) in the cholesterol ratio, the initial method of multiple imputation moved the hazard ratio more than 70% of the way towards the null compared to the result given by the revised imputation procedure. This particular incident partially or wholly influenced lots of statistical research into how to use multiple imputation in practice. The statistical community's collective understanding of multiple imputation has been greatly advanced as a happy result.

The discussions in this chapter will mostly involve derived variables as covariates in the substantive model but for some situations we will consider derived variables as outcomes.

We will first describe some specific examples and explain why intuitive default multiple imputation approaches may lead to bias. In all cases, this is due to imputation model misspecification, which can be identified through uncongeniality between the substantive model and the imputation model. We next describe various solutions – some apply to specific problems and some apply to several of the problems – and explain why we see certain solutions as appropriate for certain problems.

6.1.1 Interactions

Suppose we have two covariates X_1 and X_2, which may be categorical or continuous. Their interaction is the product $X_1 \times X_2$ and is typically included in a substantive model with the two main effects terms producing the interaction also included, such that the linear predictor is

$$\beta_0 + \beta_1 X_1 + \beta_2 X_2 + \beta_3 X_1 X_2 + \dots$$

When we wish to use multiple imputation but X_1, X_2 or both are missing, our main task is to ensure that this is done so in a congenial manner. Using the term in a slightly less formal manner than in Chapter 2, we need to ensure not only that X_1–Y and X_2–Y relationships seen in the complete cases are preserved but also that $(X_1 \times X_2)$–Y relationships are preserved. Simply imputing $X_1, X_2 | Y$ using standard models and then forming the interaction acknowledges X_1–Y and X_2–Y relationships but implies that $(X_1 \times X_2)$–Y relationships are completely determined by these; it thus fixes the interaction term to be zero in the imputed data.

6.1.2 Squares

When a continuous covariate is included in a regression model, the assumption that its relationship to outcome through the linear predictor is linear may be strong. There are several approaches to relaxing the assumption of linearity, but perhaps the most common is to add the square X^2 to the regression model that already includes X. When X is incomplete, this leads to a problem similar to interactions: when we impute X, it is likely desirable that $(X_i^*)^2 = X_i^{2*}$. That is, for an individual with missing X_i, the value imputed for X_i^2 should be equal to the square of the value imputed for X_i. While this requirement alone would be simple enough to respect (by imputing X_i^* and squaring to form the imputed value of X_i^{2*}), attempting to do this in a congenial manner complicates matters.

To understand the difficulty, suppose we have two continuous variables, Y and X, and our substantive model is

$$Y_i = \beta_0 + \beta_1 X_i + \beta_2 X_i^2 + e_i, \quad e_i \overset{i.i.d.}{\sim} N(0, \sigma^2), \tag{6.1}$$

where, marginally, X_i is normally distributed. Suppose X is partially observed and Y is fully observed. Figure 6.1 shows 40 datapoints generated from this model with $X_i \sim N(0.5, 1)$ and $Y_i \sim N(0.2X_i + 2X_i^2, 1)$. Two datapoints have missing X_i, depicted by the hollow circles in the left panel. If we are to impute these values, we require a model for $X|Y$. The right panel transposes the axes for Y and X to depict X as the response and shows the fit of a *linear* regression model for $X|Y$ along with 10 imputed values for each missing X_i (represented by $\times$). It is clear that it is difficult to correctly specify the conditional distribution of $X|Y$ for this example using standard models. It is also clear that the mean function does not fit the data well and the imputed values do not sit well in the bivariate distribution.

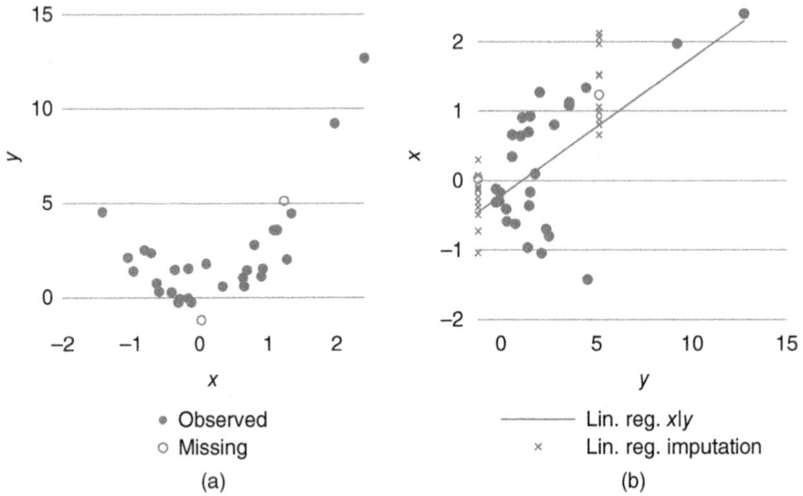

Figure 6.1 *(a) A strong quadratic relationship with two values of X_i missing (hollow circles). (b) Linear regression fit for $X|Y$ and 10 values imputed using linear regression imputation (crosses).*

6.1.3 Ratios

The use of a variable derived as the ratio of two other variables is reasonably common, particularly in medical research. Writing a ratio as $R = X_1 \times X_2^{-1}$ (instead of $R = X_1/X_2$) makes clear the close resemblance to interactions. However, there are some important differences. First, an interaction is rarely included in a regression model without the main effects of its components, while ratios are often included as a covariate without the component parts (for example, body mass index, total cholesterol to HDL, waist–hip ratio, and left ventricular ejection fraction). Second, both the denominator and numerator of a ratio can (at least to our knowledge) take only positive values. The latter point is an important constraint to respect for imputation.

In the special case that the ratio's component variables are observed or missing simultaneously, the multiple imputation task is greatly simplified: there is no information about the ratio in the cases with the numerator and denominator missing, meaning the ratio can be imputed and its individual components ignored.

In the general case that the components are not missing simultaneously, we clearly have some observed information on its value but the ratio itself is missing. Some method is needed that uses the observed information when just one component is missing. The most obvious approach is to impute the two components separately using standard imputation models and then construct the ratio from these. This intuitively attractive approach is, however, uncongenial and was primarily the reason for the unbelievable result in QRISK (Hippisley-Cox *et al.*, 2007).

6.1.4 Sum scores

In some studies, particularly surveys, missingness may occur in individual items or questions, while the substantive model may only depend on these *via* sums of scores (scale totals). In this setting, a sum score that depends on a number of individual items is missing as soon as just one of the items involved is missing, such that a complete records analysis, even if judged to be unbiased, may be quite inefficient (Plumpton *et al.*, 2016).

The instructions for compiling such scores typically include *ad hoc* rules for handling missing data. For example, they may state that the score cannot be calculated if more than half the items are missing, but can be summed in the usual way (and multiplied by the inverse of the proportion of observed items) if less than half are missing. Readers will by now realize that such *ad hoc* rules are likely to be introduce bias and misrepresent the uncertainty caused by missing data.

Multiple imputation is then a potentially attractive approach, but there are a number possible strategies one could adopt. One is to impute at the level of the sum/scale scores, rather than at the individual item level. If all items within a score are simultaneously missing, this is the appropriate approach. However, if many participants have just one or two items missing, the information on the remaining observed items is lost. To overcome this, one might impute at the individual item level. With a large number of items, a standard application of imputation using full conditional specification (FCS) may suffer from perfect prediction issues and be infeasible. This is particularly likely with sum scores made up of a number of binary variables.

To try and mitigate these issues, Plumpton *et al.* (2016) considered the complex scenario with many incomplete multi-item scales. To circumvent issues with perfect prediction, they proposed an imputation approach that imputes at the individual item level, but using a simplified set of covariates. Specifically, an individual item in a particular scale is imputed using the sum (scale) totals from the other components, plus any other items from the scale that the item being imputed belongs to. In the FCS approach, this can be implemented by generating variables for the sum (scale) totals and requesting the imputation function to passively update these variables as the algorithm iterates, and customizing the imputation model covariates as required. Plumpton *et al.* (2016) found through a case study-based simulation that their proposed simplified imputation performed adequately compared to a 'full' imputation model approach. Note that the approach was not proposed as the 'correct' solution *per se*, but as a compromise to handle bulky imputation models with issues such as perfect prediction. Whether the simplified imputation approach provides valid inferences depends on whether the assumption made by the simplified imputation model(s) is justified in the problem at hand; namely that the relationship between the value of each item that requires imputation and the items in other scales is captured *via* the sum totals from the other scales, conditional on the other covariates used.

6.1.5 Composite endpoints

Composite endpoints are frequently used in clinical trials where one of a number of outcomes could be used to define a 'bad' (or good) outcome. One such endpoint used extensively in cardiovascular trials is 'Major adverse cardiovascular events' (MACE) where a bad MACE outcome is one or more of non-fatal stroke, non-fatal myocardial infarction, cardiovascular death (Bonora *et al.*, 2020).

The way in which composite endpoints are constructed can lead to a strange problem: that the composite itself is missing not at random (MNAR) even when its components are missing completely at random (MCAR) (Pham *et al.*, 2021).

To understand the issue, consider a composite endpoint Y made up of two components Y_a and Y_b, where

$$Y = \begin{cases} 0 \text{ if } Y_a = 0 \text{ and } Y_b = 0, \\ 1 \text{ if } Y_a = 1 \text{ or } Y_b = 1. \end{cases}$$

Table 6.1 gives a dataset of six hypothetical observations. Suppose we wish to estimate the proportion of $Y = 1$. Half of the observations have Y_b missing completely at random. In this case, analysis of the complete cases for whom both Y_a and Y_b was observed is valid. Doing this, we correctly estimate the proportion with $Y_b = 1$ as 1/3.

However, we know that $Y_a = 1 \implies Y = 1$ and can use this to derive Y and increase the number of complete cases. Note that, if we do this, Y is missing-at-random (or perhaps observed-at-random) given Y_a. If we estimate the proportion with $Y = 1$ from *these* complete cases ignoring Y_a, we see bias because missingness now depends on the outcome. Doing this for the data in Table 6.1, we estimate the proportion with $Y = 1$ as 3/4, which is biased. Intuitively, we know that complete case analysis is biased when missingness depends on the outcome. The choice here presents a tension: By pretending that we cannot derive Y when $Y_a = 1$, we retain

Table 6.1 An example dataset with binary composite outcomes where Y_b is MCAR, along with the fraction of $Y = 1$.

	Components			Composite	
	Y_a	Full Y_b	Observed Y_b	Full Y	Observed Y
	0	0	0	0	0
	0	0	–	0	–
	0	1	1	1	1
	0	1	–	1	–
	1	0	0	1	1
	1	0	–	1	[**1**]
Fraction $Y = 1$:	1/3	1/3	1/3	2/3	3/4

The cell containing [**1**] indicates the outcome that is known despite Y_b being missing.

MCAR in the composite, but this involves throwing away observed information. If we derive $Y = 1$ from $Y_a = 1$, then we create an outcome-dependent missingness mechanism which leads to a more precise but biased complete records analysis.

Although we have said we will generally return to solutions later in the chapter, the solutions to the current problem can be described now. Pham *et al.* (2021) compared various MI approaches of increasing complexity in the context of randomized clinical trials. For each of the MI approaches, components are imputed and the composite passively formed. In the example of Table 6.1, the observed parts of Y_a would always be used for imputation. The first approach was to impute each incomplete component using other components and randomized arm as covariates in the imputation model; the second approach was to stratify imputation by randomized arm and impute using other components as covariates. The latter is similar to the former but with an implicit interaction between randomized arm and each component not being imputed. Because the composite is not a sum of its components, this is (strictly) necessary for congeniality.

The disadvantage of 'stratified' imputation occurs as the number of components increases. Strictly, imputation of each incomplete component should be stratified by randomized arm and all other components. This leads to very bulky imputation models that will simply not converge due to few individuals in some or many strata. Further, it seems fairly unlikely that (say) omitting a four- or five-way interaction would lead to appreciable bias. There is therefore a trade-off between the imputation model that would be correct with a large amount of data and one that works for the finite dataset at hand. In practice, this will sometimes lead to use of a reduced imputation model that incorporates main effects and some lower-order interactions, though this will depend on the context. See Pham *et al.* (2021) for more detailed discussion.

6.2 No missing data in derived variables

We now consider situations where the derived variables in the substantive model contain no missing values. One might presume that, since the derived variables are fully observed, imputation of the partially observed variables could proceed as in settings where the substantive model does not contain the derived variable. A simple example involving squared terms shows that this is not the case.

Suppose we have three continuous variables $Y_i, X_{i,1}, X_{i,2}$, with substantive model

$$Y_i = \beta_0 + \beta_1 X_{i,1} + \beta_2 X_{i,2} + \beta_3 X_{i,2}^2 + e_i, \quad e_i \overset{i.i.d.}{\sim} N(0, \sigma^2). \tag{6.2}$$

Recall from Chapter 1 that, in the absence of auxiliary variables, individuals with Y_i missing contribute no information to the analysis. Thus, suppose that $\mathbf{X}_1$ is partially observed, but that the other two variables are fully observed.

Suppose that $(Y_i, X_{i,1})$ are bivariate normal given $X_{i,2}$, with Y_i having conditional mean which is a linear function of $X_{i,2}$ and $X_{i,2}^2$, and $X_{i,1}$ having conditional mean a linear function of $X_{i,2}$ (but not $X_{i,2}^2$). This bivariate normal model implies that Y_i given

$X_{i,1}$ and $X_{i,2}$ is the model in equation (6.2). The imputation model is for $X_{i,1}$ given $Y_{i,1}$ and $X_{i,2}$, and from properties of the multivariate normal, this is

$$X_{i,1} = \gamma_0 + \gamma_1 Y_i + \gamma_2 X_{i,2} + \gamma_3 X_{i,2}^2 + e_i^*, \quad e_i^* \overset{i.i.d.}{\sim} N(0, \sigma^{2*}). \tag{6.3}$$

Note the presence of the $X_{i,2}^2$ term, which is due to its presence in the mean of $Y_{i,1}$. Thus, to impute the missing values in $X_{i,1}$ congenially with the substantive model of equation (6.2), we must include quadratic effects of $X_{i,2}$ in its imputation model, even if we do not think $X_{i,2}$ has a quadratic effect of $X_{i,1}$ marginal to $Y_{i,1}$.

This simple example demonstrates that, even in the case where they are fully observed, the presence of derived variables in the substantive model has implications for how to impute the partially observed covariates congenially with the substantive model.

In the example just considered, imputation by linear regression imputation for $X_{i,1}$ can be used. We now consider a case with two partially observed covariates, but again with the derived variable (again a quadratic in this case) fully observed.

Now suppose we have four continuous variables and substantive model

$$Y_i = \beta_0 + \beta_1 X_{i,1} + \beta_2 X_{i,2} + \beta_3 X_{i,3} + \beta_4 X_{i,3}^2 + e_i, \quad e_i \overset{i.i.d.}{\sim} N(0, \sigma^2), \tag{6.4}$$

now with $X_{i,1}$ and $X_{i,2}$ partially observed.

If $(Y_i, X_{i,1}, X_{i,2})$ are trivariate normal given a linear function of $X_{i,3}, X_{i,3}^2$, then $(X_{i,1}, X_{i,2})$ is bivariate normal with conditional mean a linear function of $Y_i, X_{i,3}, X_{i,3}^2$, and a congenial imputation model is

$$\begin{pmatrix} X_{i,1} \\ X_{i,2} \end{pmatrix} \sim \begin{pmatrix} \beta_{0,1} + \beta_{1,1} Y_i + \beta_{2,1} X_{i,3} + \beta_{3,1} X_{i,3}^2 + e_{i,1} \\ \beta_{0,2} + \beta_{1,2} Y_i + \beta_{2,2} X_{i,3} + \beta_{3,2} X_{i,3}^2 + e_{i,2} \end{pmatrix},$$
$$\begin{pmatrix} e_{i,1} \\ e_{i,2} \end{pmatrix} \sim N_2(\mathbf{0}, \mathbf{\Omega}). \tag{6.5}$$

Summarising, when a quadratic, and in general non-linear, relationship involving a fully observed variable is important in the substantive model, this non-linear relationship must be included in the linear predictor for each partially observed variable in the imputation model, whether a joint or FCS approach is adopted. In the FCS approach, it is straightforward to include these terms. For the joint model approach, we can use the multivariate normal model with covariates, as described in Section 3.2.2.

The above development has focused around simply including X^2 in the model. However, the extension to any non-linear function of fully observed variables, for example fractional polynomials, is immediate (Royston and Sauerbrei, 2008). When we discuss the full multi-level imputation model in Chapter 9, we will extend the imputation model to allow random coefficients. This then allows us to use the approach described by Verbyla *et al.* (1999); Welham (2010), in which cubic splines can be fitted by specifying a specific design matrix for the random effects.

6.3 Simple methods

In this section, we review the handling of derived variables which have missing values using imputation methods that are readily implemented using standard software.

6.3.1 Impute then transform

The simplest approach, sometimes termed *impute-then-transform*, ignores the presence of the derived variables entirely at the imputation stage (Von Hippel, 2009). The derived variables are generated once the imputed datasets have been finalized. This approach is not to be recommended as it produces bias even when data are MCAR (Von Hippel, 2009; Seaman *et al.*, 2012b; Tilling *et al.*, 2016). This is because standard choices of imputation model for the missing covariate values do not allow for the possibility of the non-linear/interaction effects contained in the substantive model.

The quadratic example in Section 6.1.2 (see Figure 6.1), given in equation (6.1) directly visualises this issue. A standard imputation model specification for X here, ignoring the presence of the X^2 term in the substantive model, would be a normal linear regression imputation model with Y as the sole covariate. However, we can see from Figure 6.1 that the true conditional distribution of $X|Y$ is bimodal. Imputing X from what would be the default imputation model specification does not allow for the non-linear association with Y correctly, leading to bias.

Seaman *et al.* (2012b) investigated the case of a linear regression model with quadratic effects through simulation, and empirically demonstrated the biases caused by an 'impute then transform' strategy. They similarly showed the approach led to bias in the case of a linear regression substantive model which contained an interaction between two covariates, one of which was partially observed.

In conclusion, imputing missing covariate values using models that might be appropriate when the substantive model does not contain derived variables and then re-generating the derived variables in the imputed datasets is not recommended.

6.3.2 Transform then impute/just another variable

An alternative approach proposed by Von Hippel (2009) is the so-called *transform-thenimpute* or 'just another variable' (JAV) (White *et al.*, 2011) method. Here the derived variable(s) is imputed as if it were JAV, ignoring the deterministic relationship between it and the variables from which it is derived.

To introduce this approach, consider again the quadratic model described in Section 6.1.2. Recall we have

$$Y_i = \beta_0 + \beta_1 X_i + \beta_2 X_i^2 + e_i, \quad e_i \overset{i.i.d.}{\sim} N(0, \sigma^2), \tag{6.6}$$

with X marginally normally distributed. The JAV approach proposes imputing X and $Z = X^2$ treating them as if they were unrelated variables; hence, the name 'JAV'.

Thus, the joint imputation model is

$$\begin{aligned} X_i &= \beta_{0,2} + \beta_{1,2} Y_i + e_{i,1} \\ Z_i &= \beta_{0,3} + \beta_{1,3} Y_i + e_{i,2} \\ (e_{i,1}, e_{i,2})^T &\overset{i.i.d.}{\sim} N_2(\mathbf{0}, \mathbf{\Omega}). \end{aligned} \tag{6.7}$$

Alternatively, using FCS we cycle between two linear regression imputation models:

$$\begin{aligned} X_i &= \gamma_{0,1} + \gamma_{1,1} Y_i + \gamma_{2,1} Z_i + e_{i,1}, \quad e_{i,1} \overset{i.i.d.}{\sim} N(0, \sigma_1^2) \\ Z_i &= \gamma_{0,2} + \gamma_{1,2} Y_i + \gamma_{2,2} X_i + e_{i,2}, \quad e_{i,2} \overset{i.i.d.}{\sim} N(0, \sigma_2^2). \end{aligned} \tag{6.8}$$

We see that the method can at best be approximate: first, because X and its square are deterministically related and this is ignored; second, because it is not possible that both X and $Z = X^2$ can be normally distributed given Y.

Seaman *et al.* (2012b) criticize this approach and show that it only gives valid point estimates for linear regression models when data are MCAR, and note that, even in this setting, the validity of Rubin's combination rules for the variance of an imputation estimator is not guaranteed. The intuition is as follows:

If data are MCAR, then the complete records analysis is a consistent estimator of population quantities. Specifically, marginal statistics such as means and cross-products are consistent for their population values when estimated from the complete cases. This means that using the complete cases gives consistent estimates of the sums of squares and cross-products from which the parameter estimates in (6.7) are derived. This in turn can be shown to imply that assuming data are MCAR, using the imputed data from the imputation model (6.7) results in estimates of sums of squares and cross-products from which the parameter estimates in (6.1) are consistently estimated, and hence, the parameter estimates of (6.1) are themselves consistently estimated.

Of course, if data are MCAR, then there is no need to use JAV for consistent estimation: a complete records analysis will suffice. The advantage of JAV under MCAR is thus the potential for recovery of more information, as reflected in smaller standard errors which, as usual, are derived using Rubin's combination rules. Unfortunately, Rubin's rules for the variance of a multiple imputation estimator assume a correctly specified imputation model (see Chapter 2). Since we know from (6.7) cannot be correctly specified, the variance estimator is not guaranteed to work with JAV, even assuming data are MCAR. The practical implication of this latter point should not be overstated, however, since Rubin's rules often work acceptably well, if slightly conservatively, in such settings.

If data are MAR, however, JAV generally gives biased, inconsistent, parameter estimates. This is because complete records give biased, inconsistent estimates of the marginal moments required to estimate the parameters in (6.7). In turn, this means that using imputed data from (6.7) gives inconsistent estimates of the parameters (6.1).

Seaman *et al.* (2012b) describe a series of simulation studies comparing passive imputation, predictive mean matching (PMM) and JAV. They initially consider linear regression, with 200 observations of a fully observed response on a partially observed covariate and its square under MCAR and MAR, when the marginal distribution of the covariate is normal, and lognormal, and the regression R^2 is 0.1, 0.5, and 0.8.

In line with theory, the bias of JAV is small or negligible when data are MCAR. Under MAR JAV is generally biased. Focusing on the quadratic parameter, when the marginal distribution of the covariate is normal, bias can decrease or increase with R^2, depending on the nature of the quadratic relationship. If the covariate is log-normal, bias is larger, and increases with increasing R^2. With logistic regression, under MCAR, the performance of JAV is markedly worse, with non-trivial bias (median absolute 23% bias across scenarios with marginal normal covariate; median absolute 66% bias across scenarios with marginal log-normal covariate). Bias is worse again under MAR; and now in 5/6 scenarios, it is worse than the impute then transform option, described earlier. Coverage can be very poor when bias is substantial.

The markedly varied and often disappointing performance of JAV, especially in logistic regression, means we cannot recommend this approach in general.

6.3.3 Adapting standard imputation models and passive imputation

In the presence of derived variables such as squares and interactions in the substantive model, a natural thought is whether we can somehow adapt what would be standard imputation model choices to accommodate their presence.

One such example is where the substantive model for an outcome Y includes effects of two covariates X and Z and their interaction $X \times Z$. If there are missing values in Y, it is straightforward to impute these congenially with the substantive model (at least if there are no auxiliary variables), since the imputation model for Y can be set as per the substantive model specification. It is less clear how the imputation models for X and Z should be specified such that they are congenial with the outcome model including the $X \times Z$ interaction. Tilling *et al.* (2016) considered settings where X and Z are binary, and the substantive model is either normal linear regression or logistic regression. The presence of the interaction term $X \times Z$ in the substantive model implies that, in the imputation model for X, the interaction $Y \times Z$ should be included as a covariate. Similarly, the interaction $Y \times X$ should be included in the imputation model for Z. This can be handled in the FCS imputation algorithm which, at each iteration, is able to impute the interaction terms based on the most recent values of the variables upon which they depend. Tilling *et al.* (2016) provide simulation results showing that this approach provides unbiased estimates under MAR missingness mechanisms in the scenarios considered.

In contrast, Seaman *et al.* (2012b) found in the setting of a normal linear regression substantive model with X and Z continuous and only X having missing values, including the $Y \times Z$ interaction in the imputation model for X did not generally result in unbiased estimates. Indeed, in some scenarios, this approach performed worse than omission of the $Y \times Z$ interaction in the imputation model.

For the earlier considered case of continuous outcome Y and covariate X, with the outcome depending quadratically on X, there is no way of modifying the imputation model for X parallel to that used for interactions that generally results in valid inference.

In conclusion, in some settings, it is possible to accommodate the presence of derived variables in the substantive modelby using standard imputation methods and adapting the imputation model covariates. Unfortunately, this does not offer a general solution to the problems.

6.3.4 Predictive mean matching

PMM is a method for imputing continuous variables that relaxes certain parametric assumptions, namely linearity and normality, involved in linear regression imputation. The idea is to fit an imputation model to create some measure of 'similarity' of observations with missing and observed data. For each observation with a missing value, this is imputed by using a non-missing value from a similar observation.

PMM is a general idea with several possible variations. We will outline the key steps here and note some flavours of the method available in software. The procedure is described here for a single incomplete variable Y, which could be an outcome or covariate in the substantive model, and complete variables $\mathbf{X}$. For each imputation,

1. Denote individuals with observed Y with the subscript *io* and with missing Y with the subscript *im*.
2. Fit the model
$$Y_{io} = \mathbf{X}_{io}^T \boldsymbol{\beta} + e_{io}, \quad e_{io} \overset{i.i.d.}{\sim} N(0, \sigma^2)$$
to obtain estimates of $\boldsymbol{\beta}$ and σ^2.
3. Take parameter draws σ^{2*} and $\boldsymbol{\beta}^*$ as with linear regression imputation.
4. For each i, estimate the predictive mean as either $\widehat{P}_i = \mathbf{X}_i^T \widehat{\boldsymbol{\beta}}$ or $P_i^* = \mathbf{X}_i^T \boldsymbol{\beta}^*$ (see below).
5. For each *im*, select d potential 'donors' as those minimising the distance:
   (a) $|\widehat{P}_{io} - \widehat{P}_{im}|$ (type 0);
   (b) $|\widehat{P}_{io} - P^*_{im}|$ (type 1); or
   (c) $|P^*_{io} - P^*_{im}|$ (type 2).

   These form the 'donor pool' (the naming convention here is due to the number of $*$ symbols above the Ps).
6. For each *im*, select one *io* at random from the d donors and impute $Y^*_{im} = Y_{io}$.

PMM is a computationally intensive method due to the step that involves searching for the d potential donors for each *im*.

In implementing PMM as described above, there are two key choices to be made: the matching type and the size of donor pool d. These were investigated by Morris *et al.* (2014a).

Heuristically, it is clear than type 0 matching does not acknowledge any parameter uncertainty in the imputation model and so will have poor properties as a component of a multiple imputation estimator. Since there is no draw of the parameters, the same k donors will always be selected; this leads to high variance of the estimator and low coverage of confidence intervals. Type 2 matching tends to have slightly lower coverage than type 1, whose coverage is generally closer to the nominal $(1 - \alpha)$. However, the type of matching is not often a choice for the user: type 2 is used by Stata's `mi impute pmm` command and SAS's `proc mi`. The `mice` package in R permits the user choice between types 1 and 2. Stata's `ice` command includes an option for the user to choose between types 0, 1, and 2.

The choice of d is not simple but can in most software implementations of PMM be controlled by the user. To understand the tension in making the choice, it is instructive to consider the two extremes of $d = 1$ and $d = n_{io}$. We consider these choices with type 0 matching to make the implications most extreme, despite the caution about type 0 matching above. Suppose we choose to use $d = 1$, so that for each im, we are searching for the single io that minimises $|\widehat{P}_{io} - \widehat{P}_{im}|$ (type 0 matching). This will always impute $Y^*_{im} = Y_{io}$ with the same io for each im over multiple imputations. This will create a between-imputation variance of 0, implying no uncertainty due to missing data and also causing Rubin's variance formula to underestimate the true variance. It is therefore clear that $d = 1$ is too small. Suppose we chose the opposite extreme of $d = n_{io}$. This effectively skips the regression and matching steps and imputes Y^*_{im} with a random Y_{im}, destroying any Y–X relationship in the observed data.

The ideal choice of d is then a trade-off between these two extremes and will in practice depend on the number of units with Y observed. Morris *et al.* (2014a) found that statistical properties of PMM tended to be reasonable with $d = 10$. If we have a dataset with millions of observed points, a larger value of d may be better.

In general, PMM may produce bias when the available donors are sparse around the correct value. Thus, an extreme missing-at-random mechanism can defeat PMM if it means there are no suitable donors in the region of the missing values. This is illustrated by example in Figure 6.2. We have 30 values of X, which take values of

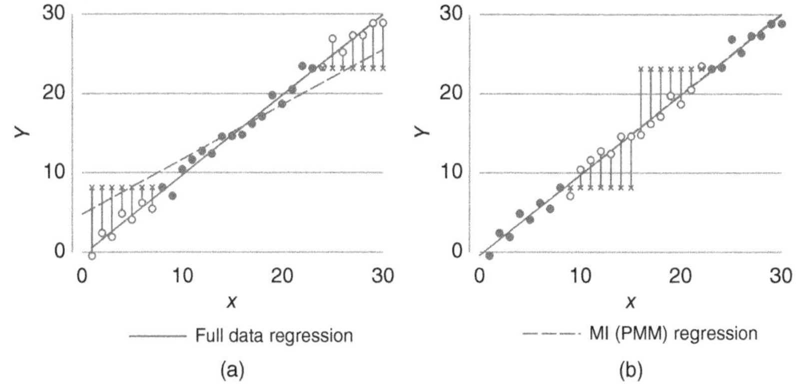

Figure 6.2 Predictive mean matching under two missing-at-random mechanisms. The mechanism in panel (a) is problematic, while the mechanism in (b) is not. Solid dots represent observed data; hollow dots represent true values of missing data; crosses represent a single value imputed using PMM.

1–30 in increments of 1. Y has a very close linear relationship to X (with a small amount of normally distributed random error) and is incomplete. The missingness mechanism in panel (a) is such that values of Y are missing in the tails of X, *i.e.*, in the smallest and largest values of X (missing at random). The solid dots represent observed data and the hollow dots represent units with Y missing. The solid line is the regression of Y on X in the full data. Suppose we use PMM to impute Y, here borrowing the single closest donor ($d = 1$). The closest match corresponds to units with the closest value of X. Imputed values are represented by crosses, and the grey lines link imputed values to their true values. Because of the missingness mechanism, there are no suitably large or small values of Y to 'borrow', and the PMM regression is biased (dashed line). The missingness mechanism in panel (b) is such that values of Y are missing in the center of the distribution of X, (also missing at random) and here we see no bias after PMM. The lesson is to beware of missing at random mechanisms that produce missingness in the tails of the distribution of the matching variables.

We have described PMM as a means of relaxing assumptions, particularly when non-linearity or non-normality may be issues, but a key attraction is that, by definition, it imputes observable values, since all imputed values are borrowed from observed values. If a variable is bounded such that it only takes positive values, PMM will preserve this feature in the imputed data. While this is superficially attractive, it is a mistake to believe that it justifies PMM's use: as explained in Chapter 1, the purpose of multiple imputation is not face validity of the imputed values but validity of inference Rubin (1996).

PMM is a popular method for multiple imputation, no doubt in part because it is the default imputation method for imputation of continuous variables in R's `mice` package. There are other (related) methods or aspects:

- 'Local residual draws' is a closely related method which, rather than borrowing an observed value of Y, borrows a residual $Y_{io} - \widehat{P}_{io}$ (Morris *et al.*, 2014a).
- The matching process need not be based on the predictive mean, but might, for example, be based on the Mahalanobis distance (Andridge and Little, 2010).
- The choice of a fixed donor pool, while simple, may be replaced with the use of a fixed predictive distance, or by allowing all *io* as donors but with donation probability inversely proportional to matching distance (Siddique and Belin, 2008).

6.3.5 Imputation separately by groups for interactions

In this subsection, we consider the case where the substantive model includes an interaction where one of the variables involved in the interaction is categorical. If this variable is fully observed, one approach is to perform imputation separately by groups defined by this variable.

Suppose the substantive model is

$$Y_i = \beta_0 + \beta_1 X_{i,1} + \beta_2 X_{i,2} + \beta_3 X_{i,1} X_{i,2} + e_i, \quad e_i \overset{i.i.d.}{\sim} N(0, \sigma^2), \tag{6.9}$$

with Y and X_1 continuous and X_2 binary.

If X_2 is fully observed, but Y and X_1 are partially observed then, since (6.9) fits a straight line for each group identified by X_2, we can impute as follows:

1. Divide the data into two groups by values of binary X_2.
2. Separately in each group, impute (Y, X_1) using a bivariate normal model or FCS equivalent (Chapter 3), creating K imputed datasets.
3. For $k = 1, \dots, K$ append the imputed datasets for the two groups, to give K imputed datasets.

This approach, of imputing separately in the groups defined by categorical variables in the interaction, is by far the simplest approach; clearly, we can have more than the two groups in the above discussion. The imputation groups may be defined by levels of a single categorical variable, or the interaction of categorical variables. The only requirement is that these variables be fully observed on each unit.

As this approach is straightforward, it will often be appropriate even when a few values of the categorical variables defining the imputation groups are missing. Since it is always permissible for the imputation model to be richer than the substantive model, it is also appropriate for when the substantive model does not have all possible interactions with the categorical variable. For example, if we add an additional variable (binary or continuous) X_3 to (6.9),

$$Y_i = \beta_0 + \beta_1 X_{i,1} + \beta_2 X_{i,2} + \beta_3 X_{i,1} X_{i,2} + \beta_4 X_{i,3} + e_i, \quad e_i \overset{i.i.d.}{\sim} N(0, \sigma^2) \tag{6.10}$$

the model does not have all possible interactions involving X_2, since it does not include $X_2 X_3$ as a covariate. However, if binary X_2 is fully observed and the other variables have missing data, the most sensible approach is again to impute separately in the two groups defined by X_2.

Example 6.1 Asthma study

We return to the asthma study, introduced in Chapter 1 and last considered in Chapter 3. Recall that we have two treatment arms (active and placebo), and lung function measured at baseline, and 2, 4, 8, and 12 weeks post-randomisation.

Let $Y_{i,1}, \dots, Y_{i,5}$ denote the lung function of patient i at baseline, 2, 4, 8, and 12 weeks. Let $T_i = 1$ if patient i is randomized to the active arm, and 0 otherwise. We focus on the estimated treatment effect, adjusted for baseline, at the final 12-week visit, that is

$$Y_{i5} = \beta_0 + \beta_1 Y_{i,1} + \beta_2 T_i + e_i, \quad e_i \overset{i.i.d.}{\sim} N(0, \sigma^2). \tag{6.11}$$

Baseline is fully observed, but only 37/90 patients in the placebo arm are present at 12 weeks, and only 71/90 in the active arm. The auxiliary variables are the lung function at the intermediate visits.

We could choose the six-variable normal distribution as our imputation model:

$$(Y_{i,1}, Y_{i,2}, Y_{i,3}, Y_{i,4}, Y_{i,5}, T_i)^T \sim N_6(\mu, \mathbf{\Omega}). \tag{6.12}$$

Note that, since binary T_i is fully observed, having it as a covariate or part of the normally distributed response makes no difference.

However, it turns out the covariance matrix varies between the treatment arms. In other words, the dependence of the 12-week measurement on earlier measurements is different in the two treatment arms. Our imputation model should reflect this. Thus, we should impute separately in the two treatment groups, using the unstructured multivariate normal model

$$(Y_{i,1}, Y_{i,2}, Y_{i,3}, Y_{i,4}, Y_{i,5})^T \sim N_5(\mu, \mathbf{\Omega}). \tag{6.13}$$

This is congenial with a full baseline–time–treatment interaction, which is richer than we require. However, following Section 2.8.3, having a richer imputation model than the substantive model is not expected to unduly affect the validity of the resulting inference.

Thus, this is an example where, although the model of interest (6.11) does not have an explicit interaction because the relationship between the auxiliary variables and response does vary by treatment group, imputing separately in the two groups is sensible.

Table 6.2 shows the results, obtained using $K = 1000$ imputations, where the model of interest is (6.11). Imputing with the interaction gives more appropriate imputations within each treatment group; as Figure 6.3 shows, this results in a larger treatment estimate. For a detailed analysis of these data, see Carpenter *et al.* (2013). □

Separate imputation in potentially distinct groups is therefore worth considering, even if the model of interest does not explicitly have an interaction. This approach only runs into difficulty when the numbers in the categories become small, for then we will need to borrow information across categories in order to fit the imputation model; in other words impose some constraints on the interaction model.

The simplest constraint is to have a common covariance matrix across some of the categories, while retaining a different mean structure. Taking the trial illustration above, one might have a common covariance structure across genetic sub-types within a treatment group, while allowing the mean structure to differ. In this case, in the clinical trial illustration, we would impute separately within each group, with genetic sub-type indicator as either an additional response, or a covariate, in the imputation model.

Table 6.2 Asthma data: estimates of 12-week treatment effect on FEV_1 (litres), adjusted for baseline, using complete records and imputing without, and with, a full treatment group interaction.

Analysis	Treatment estimate	Std. error	*p*-value
Complete records	0.247	0.100	0.0155
MI, imputation model (6.12)	0.283	0.093	0.0024
MI, imputation model (6.13)	0.335	0.106	0.0015

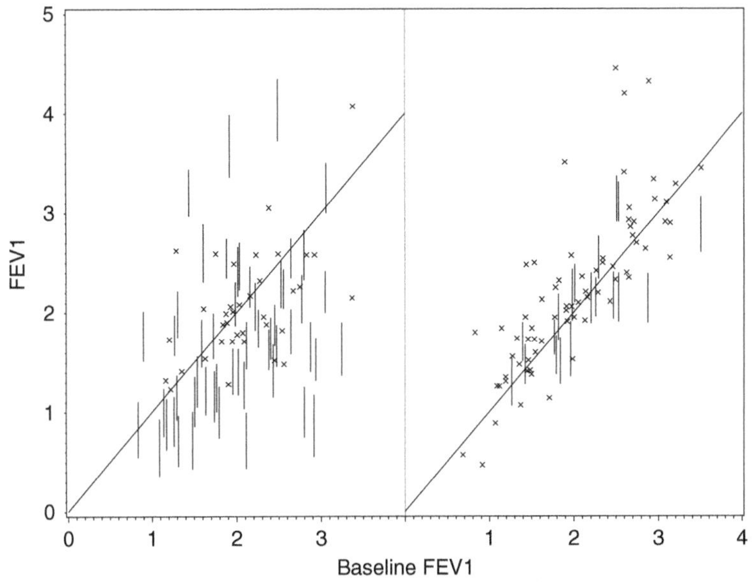

Figure 6.3 Plot of baseline FEV_1 (litres) versus 12 week FEV_1 (litres) by treatment group, under imputation model (6.13). For patients whose 12-week observation is missing, the inter-quartile range from $K = 1000$ imputations under randomized-arm MAR is shown. Left panel: placebo group, right panel: lowest active treatment group.

Beyond this, one may well wish to consider shrinkage, so that subgroups have a random covariance (or precision) structure, drawn from an inverse Wishart (or Wishart) distribution with common parameters across subgroups. This approach has been explored by Yucel (2011), and we return to it in the context of multilevel multiple imputation in Section 9.3.2.

To conclude this section, consider again (6.10), now supposing Y and X_3 have missing values, but X_1 and X_2 are fully observed. In other words, we have an interaction between a fully observed continuous and categorical variable. In this setting, paralleling the discussion in Section 6.2, the imputation model should have the interaction terms as covariates:

$$\begin{aligned}
Y_{i,1} &= \beta_{0,1} + \beta_{1,1}X_{i,1} + \beta_{2,1}X_{i,2} + \beta_{3,1}X_{i,1}X_{i,2} + e_{i,1} \\
X_{i,3} &= \beta_{0,2} + \beta_{1,2}X_{i,1} + \beta_{2,2}X_{i,2} + \beta_{3,2}X_{i,1}X_{i,2} + e_{i,2} \\
\begin{pmatrix} e_{i,1} \\ e_{i,2} \end{pmatrix} &\sim N_2(\mathbf{0}, \mathbf{\Omega}).
\end{aligned}$$

The corresponding FCS algorithm follows in the usual way. The extension to additional interactions involving fully observed variables is direct. In many cases, even if a small proportion of units are missing terms involved in the interaction, this will be sufficient.

Imputing in groups when group indicator has missing values

Consider again (6.10), where X_2 is now categorical, the other variables are continuous, and all variables have missing values.

If the context and complete records suggest it is plausible to assume that the probability X_2 is missing is independent of Y given the other covariates, X_1, X_3, then – as explained in Chapter 1 – omitting cases with missing X_2 does not bias the analysis. So one strategy is to do this, and then impute separately in groups defined by the remaining observed categorical X_2. This approach can often work quite well, particularly if there are predictive auxiliary variables which can be included in the imputation model (e.g. Carpenter and Plewis, 2011).

However, if a substantial proportion of categorical X_2 values are missing, this approach excludes a non-negligible proportion of the data and the associated information (which was likely to have been expensive to collect). In this case one of the more complex approaches described below is likely preferable, but the approach of the previous paragraph can still serve as a useful check on the plausibility of the results.

In summary, if either (i) we wish to investigate the possibility of interactions involving fully observed variables in our model of interest, or (ii) we would like to allow a different relationship between variables in the imputation model, in groups defined by a categorical covariate, we can use one of the approaches described above, with a preference for imputing in separate groups.

6.4 Substantive-model-compatible imputation

We have seen earlier in this chapter that when the substantive model contains derived variables such as non-linear effects or interactions, it is in many cases difficult to impute missing values of covariates using standard approaches in a way that leads to valid inferences. In this section, we describe a collection of related approaches which construct imputation models for partially observed covariates which impute compatibly (congenially) with the substantive model.

6.4.1 The basic idea

We first outline the basic idea of SMC imputation of missing covariate values. Consider once again the setting with a fully observed continuous outcome Y and partially observed continuous covariate X, where the substantive model of interest is

$$Y_i = \beta_0 + \beta_1 X_i + \beta_2 X_i^2 + e_i, \quad e_i \overset{i.i.d.}{\sim} N(0, \sigma^2).$$

The imputation distribution we must draw from to impute the missing X values is $f(X|Y)$. From the definition of conditional probability, we can express this distribution as

$$f(X|Y) = \frac{f(Y,X)}{f(Y)} = \frac{f(Y|X)f(X)}{f(Y)} \propto f(Y|X)f(X). \tag{6.14}$$

The substantive model specifies our assumptions for $f(Y|X)$. Equation (6.14) shows that once we additionally specify a model for the marginal distribution of X, we can derive the implied conditional distribution $f(X|Y)$ required for imputation. By construction, the resulting imputation model for X is compatible with the substantive model. By *compatible*, we mean that there exists a joint model for the data which yield the models for $f(Y|X)$ and $f(X)$ we have specified. For a more technical definition of compatibility, we refer readers to Bartlett *et al.* (2015b).

In the quadratic substantive model example, $f(Y|X)$ is the normal distribution density $N(\beta_0 + \beta_1 X + \beta_2 X^2, \sigma^2)$. For the marginal distribution of X, we could for example assume $X \sim N(\mu_X, \sigma_X^2)$. Unfortunately, even this seemingly most basic combination of assumptions means, as noted earlier in the chapter, that $f(X|Y)$ does not belong to a standard parametric distribution. This difficulty means the imputation model $f(X|Y)$ cannot be fitted directly using conventional regression commands, complicating the imputation process.

Instead, we can use the Markov chain Monte Carlo (MCMC) sampling approach (Appendix A). As usual, choose starting values for the parameters (β, σ^2), (μ_X, σ_X^2) and the missing X values. Then the MCMC sampler consists of the following steps:

1. Given the current draws for missing values of X and the observed values of Y and X, update the parameters of the linear regression substantive model $f_{Y|X}$, β, σ^2, as described in Section 3.1.

2. Given the current draw for (β, σ^2), (μ_X, σ_X^2) and Y_i, update each missing X_i as described below.

3. Given $\mathbf{X}$ (the observed part and the current draws for the missing observations), update the parameters, (μ_X, σ_X^2).

We next discuss two approaches for step 2: the first based on a Metropolis–Hastings step, and the other using rejection sampling. At the end of Section 6.4.8, we discuss pros and cons of the two approaches.

Metropolis–Hastings for drawing X

The first approach we consider are samples' missing X values using a Metropolis–Hastings step (Goldstein *et al.*, 2014). Under the Metropolis–Hastings approach, we need a proposal distribution for X_i; a natural choice is $X_i^\star \sim N(X_i, \tau^2)$, where $X_i^\star$ is the proposed new value, X_i the current value and τ^2 a fraction – e.g. a half – of the marginal variance of the observed $\mathbf{X}$. Then, given the current draw of (β, σ^2), (μ_X, σ_X^2), for each i with X_i missing in turn, we

1. propose a new value $X_i^\star$ drawn from $N(X_i, \tau^2)$. Note this is a symmetric proposal, so the Hastings ratio (see Appendix A) is 1.

2. Calculate $L(X_i^\star)$ and $L(X_i)$ where

$$L(x) = f_{Y|X}(Y|x; \beta, \sigma^2) f_X(x; \mu_X, \sigma_X^2). \tag{6.15}$$

Because the substantive model (6.1) is a linear regression , we have

$$f_{Y|X}(Y|x;\beta,\sigma^2) = \frac{1}{\sqrt{2\pi\sigma^2}} \exp\left\{-\frac{1}{2\sigma^2}(Y_i - \beta_0 - \beta_1 x - \beta_2 x^2)^2\right\} \quad (6.16)$$

and

$$f_X(x;\mu_X,\sigma_X^2) = \frac{1}{\sqrt{2\pi\sigma_X^2}} \exp\left\{-\frac{1}{2\sigma_X^2}(x-\mu_X)^2\right\}. \quad (6.17)$$

3. Accept the proposal with probability

$$\max\left\{1, \frac{L(X_i^\star)}{L(X_i)}\right\}; \quad \text{and} \begin{cases} \text{if accepted, set } X_i = X_i^\star; \\ \text{if rejected, retain the existing } X_i. \end{cases} \quad (6.18)$$

We have here considered a specific case of a normal linear regression substantive model with quadratic covariate effects. However, the approach is general in the sense that it can handle alternative substantive model types and other derived variables in the substantive model, such as interactions or more complex non-linear effects.

Rejection approach for drawing X

An alternative to the Metropolis–Hastings sampler is rejection sampling (Bartlett *et al.*, 2015b). If we can get a good bound, denoted κ below, this may prove more computationally efficient. It also has the attraction that, unlike the Metropolis–Hastings step above, each accepted draw is from the desired distribution.

As above, we draw each missing X_i value in turn conditional on all the other parameters. Like in Metropolis–Hastings, we have a proposal density from which we can easily draw, denoted $g(x)$. To use rejection sampling we must be able to bound, up to a constant of proportionality, the ratio of the target distribution to the proposal distribution. In the present setting, this is

$$\frac{f_{X|Y}(x|Y)}{g(x)} \propto \frac{f_{Y|X}(Y|x)f_X(x)}{g(x)}.$$

A natural choice of proposal distribution is $g(x) = f_X(x)$, so that to use rejection sampling we must be able to bound

$$\frac{f_{Y|X}(Y|x)f_X(x)}{f_X(x)} = f_{Y|X}(Y|x)$$

by a value κ not depending on x. Assuming we can do this, to generate a draw from $f_{X|Y}(x|Y_i)$, we draw $X^* \sim g(x)$ and accept the draw with probability

$$\frac{f_{Y|X}(Y_i|X^*)}{\kappa}.$$

If we do not accept the proposal, we repeat until a draw is accepted. The accepted value is a draw from the desired distribution $f_{X|Y}(X|Y_i)$.

In the normal linear regression substantive model case at hand, we have

$$\begin{aligned} f_{Y|X}(Y|x) &= \frac{1}{\sqrt{2\pi\sigma^2}} \exp\left\{-\frac{1}{2\sigma^2}(Y_i - \beta_0 - \beta_1 x - \beta_2 x^2)^2\right\} \\ &\leq \frac{1}{\sqrt{2\pi\sigma^2}} = \kappa. \end{aligned}$$

Notice that the preceding bound remains the same regardless of the way the covariates enter the linear predictor of the substantive model. As such, the approach described here automatically handles substantive models with covariates which are more complicated functions of the X variable(s), such as interactions and more complex non-linear effects.

Thus, we can draw $X^* \sim f_X(x)$ and accept with probability

$$\begin{aligned} \frac{f_{Y|X}(Y_i|X^*)}{\kappa} &= \frac{\frac{1}{\sqrt{2\pi\sigma^2}} \exp\left\{-\frac{1}{2\sigma^2}(Y_i - \beta_0 - \beta_1 x - \beta_2 x^2)^2\right\}}{\frac{1}{\sqrt{2\pi\sigma^2}}} \\ &= \exp\left\{-\frac{1}{2\sigma^2}(Y_i - \beta_0 - \beta_1 x - \beta_2 x^2)^2\right\}. \end{aligned}$$

In settings where the outcome variable Y is discrete, such as logistic regression, $f_{Y|X}(Y|x)$ is a probability, and as such is always less than or equal to 1. In this case, we draw $X^* \sim f_X(x)$ and accept with probability $f_{Y|X}(Y_i|X^*)$.

Thus far, we have considered the case that X is continuous. In cases where X is a categorical variable, the probabilities $P(X = x|Y_i)$ can be calculated (Bartlett and Taylor (2016) and Exercise 2) and thus direct sampling is straightforward.

Example 6.2 Simulation study

We use a simple simulation study to demonstrate the relative performance of the methods described above for a model with a quadratic effect of X.

The full data are generated from the following models:

$$\begin{aligned} i &\in (1, \ldots, 1000) \\ X_i &\sim N(0, 1) \\ Y_{i1} &= \beta_0 + \beta_1 X_i + \beta_2 X_i^2 + \epsilon_i, \quad \epsilon_i \sim N(0, \sigma^2) \end{aligned} \tag{6.19}$$

with $\sigma^2 = 3$ such that the coefficient of determination R^2 is 0.5. Missing data are then simulated under two missingness mechanisms:

1. MCAR: Pr(observe X_i) = 0.5
2. MAR: logit Pr(observe X_i) = $0.37 - 0.41Y_i$.

This means that the proportion of missingness is not fixed across simulation repetitions but varies randomly.

The estimands of interest are $\beta_0, \beta_1, \beta_2$ (parameters of the substantive model).

For each method of analysis, the substantive model is the true data-generating model for Y (6.19). The following methods of analysis are compared:

- Complete records analysis
- Impute then transform MI (also 'passive imputation'; see Section 6.3.1)
- Transform then impute MI (also 'JAV' imputation; see Section 6.3.2)
- SMC MI (implemented using rejection sampling; see Section 6.4.1).

$K = 10$ imputations were used for each MI method. The simulation procedure is repeated $n_{\text{rep}} = 1000$ times.

The main performance measure of primary interest is bias, defined as $E(\hat{\beta}) - \beta$ and estimated as

$$\frac{1}{1000}\sum_{j=1}^{1000}\hat{\beta}_j - \beta.$$

If two methods are unbiased, their precision is of interest, and is quantified by the empirical standard error (SE), defined as $\sqrt{\text{Var}(\hat{\beta})}$ and estimated as

$$\sqrt{\frac{1}{999}\sum_{j=1}^{1000}(\hat{\beta}_j - \overline{\beta})^2}.$$

The substantive model is (6.19), and so is correctly specified by all approaches; misspecification of methods arises through the missingness mechanism and/or the imputation model for X.

The results of the simulation study are given in Table 6.3.

We see that impute-then-transform MI is badly biased even under MCAR; clearly, this approach should be avoided. JAV is unbiased under MCAR but biased under MAR. Complete records analysis is unbiased under MCAR (as known). SMC MI performs best in terms of bias. Even when other methods are unbiased, SMC MI is at least as efficient. □

The approach we have outlined here is in some sense the 'natural' way for a Bayesian analysis to accommodate missing values in a covariate of a regression model. If we have additional fully observed covariates $\mathbf{Z}$, these can be conditioned-on: we specify the substantive model $f(Y|X, \mathbf{Z})$ and the model for the partially observed covariate $f(X|\mathbf{Z})$. We defer discussion of how to handle auxiliary variables to Section 6.4.5.

Now suppose that we have multiple partially observed covariates, as is commonly the case, by allowing X to be a vector $\mathbf{X} = (X_1, \ldots, X_p)$. To impute compatibly, we must now specify a joint model for $f(\mathbf{X}|\mathbf{Z})$. The approach used to specifying this joint model is the key feature distinguishing the three approaches to SMC imputation which we describe next.

Table 6.3 Results of simulation study with quadratic effect of X on Y.

Estimand value	Missingness	Complete records	Multiple imputation using … Impute then transform	JAV (Transform then impute)	SMC MI
			Bias		
$\beta_0 = 0$	MCAR	−0.003	0.435	−0.012	−0.002
$\beta_0 = 0$	MAR	−0.461	0.649	−0.076	0.000
$\beta_1 = 1$	MCAR	0.002	−0.023	0.012	0.002
$\beta_1 = 1$	MAR	−0.100	−0.066	0.267	−0.007
$\beta_2 = 1$	MCAR	0.003	−0.439	0.014	0.003
$\beta_2 = 1$	MAR	0.093	−0.473	0.271	0.005
			Empirical SE		
$\beta_0 = 0$	MCAR	0.094	0.080	0.082	0.080
$\beta_0 = 0$	MAR	0.092	0.089	0.111	0.085
$\beta_1 = 1$	MCAR	0.079	0.102	0.082	0.079
$\beta_1 = 1$	MAR	0.096	0.140	0.132	0.099
$\beta_2 = 1$	MCAR	0.056	0.044	0.059	0.053
$\beta_2 = 1$	MAR	0.079	0.056	0.103	0.069

Bias and empirical standard errors from 1000 repetitions are shown. Note: the Monte Carlo SE of bias can be computed by dividing empirical SE by $\sqrt{1000}$.

6.4.2 Latent-normal joint model SMC imputation

The first approach to specifying a joint model for $f(\mathbf{X}|\mathbf{Z})$ one could consider is a (conditional) multivariate normal model, as described in Section 3.2.2. When some of the partially observed covariates are binary or category, the extensions described in Section 4.3 and Chapter 5 can be used. The latent normal SMC imputation approach is implemented in the R package jomo (Quartagno *et al.*, 2019).

An advantage of the latent normal approach is that it readily extends to multi-level settings, as described further in Chapter 9. A potential limitation of the latent normal approach is that one cannot allow for higher-order relationships between the covariates in $\mathbf{X}$, since the multivariate normal implies linear dependence between the variables.

To illustrate the latent normal approach, we re-analyse the data example from Bartlett *et al.* (2015b). They considered data from $n = 383$ patients with mild cognitive impairment (MCI) from the Alzheimer's Disease Neuroimaging Initiative, following an earlier analysis by Jack Jr. *et al.* (2010). The analysis used a Cox proportional hazards model to investigate risk factors for time to conversion to Alzheimer's disease (AD) during follow-up. Table 6.4 shows the risk factors included, many of which had non-trivial rates of missingness. Bartlett *et al.* (2015b) found no evidence that missingness in the variables measured from cerebrospinal fluid (CSF)

Table 6.4 Baseline characteristics of $n = 383$ ADNI participants with mild cognitive impairment (MCI) at baseline.

Variable	Mean (SD) or number (%) among complete cases	Number (%) of missing values
$A\beta_{1-42}$ (ng/ml)	16.4 (5.5)	191 (49.9 %)
log(Tau) (log pg/ml)	4.50 (0.49)	194 (50.7 %)
log(P-tau) (log pg/ml)	3.44 (0.50)	190 (49.6 %)
Mother had AD	77 (25.3 %)	78 (20.4 %)
Father had AD	27 (9.3 %)	93 (24.3 %)
Intracranial volume (cm^3)	1475 (150)	43 (11.2 %)
Hippocampal volume (cm^3)	6.47 (1.04)	43 (11.2 %)
APOE4 positive	208 (54.3 %)	0 (0 %)

($A\beta_{1-42}$, Tau, P-tau) was related to the time to event or censoring or event indicator ($p = 0.48$), but there was some evidence ($p = 0.02$) that having a family history of AD was associated with a higher chance of having these variables measured. They also found evidence in a Cox model without the CSF variables included as covariates that hazard of conversion to AD depended on the family history variables and an interaction between these and an indicator of missingness of the CSF variables, which may suggest a complete records analysis will be biased.

The Cox model developed by Jack Jr. *et al.* (2010) contained each of the risk factors as covariates, including a quadratic effect of $A\beta_{1-42}$. Here, standard imputation models for the covariates would not be compatible with both the non-linear effect of $A\beta_{1-42}$ and also the non-linear Cox substantive model (see Section 7.1). Thus, using an approach which is by construction compatible with the substantive model is highly desirable.

Table 6.5 shows the estimates of the log hazard ratios from the Cox model based first on the $n = 127$ complete records. The next set of results are based on FCS imputation with 1000 imputations, using the impute then transform approach to handle the non-linear $A\beta_{1-42}$ effect. Since the substantive model was a Cox proportional hazards model, the event indicator and Nelson–Aalen cumulative hazard estimate were used as covariates in the imputation models (see Section 7.1.1). Binary variables were imputed using logistic regression and continuous variables using normal linear regression. The estimates from this approach differed materially for a number of the covariates compared to the complete records estimates. For the present discussion, we note the dilution of the quadratic $A\beta_{1-42}$ effect, which is what we would expect from using the 'impute then transform' approach. This then also leads to a biased estimate of the linear coefficient of $A\beta_{1-42}$. As expected, standard errors after MI were smaller than based on complete records.

The next column of estimates are from the latent normal SMC MI approach. The estimates are broadly similar to the FCS *impute then transform* ones, except for

Table 6.5 Estimated log-hazard ratios (SEs) for Cox proportional hazards model relating hazard of conversion to Alzheimer's disease to baseline risk factors.

Variable	Complete records	FCS impute Then transform	SMC-Latent	SMC-Factor	SMC FCS
$A\beta_{1-42}$ (ng/ml)	0.31 (0.18)	0.08 (0.10)	0.25 (0.14)	0.30 (0.15)	0.26 (0.16)
$A\beta^2_{1-42}$ (ng^2/ml^2)	−0.011 (0.005)	−0.004 (0.003)	−0.009 (0.004)	−0.010 (0.004)	−0.009 (0.005)
log(Tau) (log pg/ml)	−0.61 (0.47)	−0.20 (0.36)	−0.17 (0.35)	−0.06 (0.37)	−0.22 (0.37)
log(P-tau) (log pg/ml)	1.29 (0.51)	0.54 (0.38)	0.43 (0.37)	0.38 (0.40)	0.41 (0.39)
Mother had AD	−0.61 (0.32)	−0.10 (0.21)	−0.12 (0.21)	−0.13 (0.21)	−0.12 (0.21)
Father had AD	−1.07 (0.68)	−0.15 (0.32)	−0.16 (0.32)	−0.14 (0.33)	−0.17 (0.33)
Intracranial vol. (cm^3)	0.0005 (0.0010)	0.0014 (0.0007)	0.0014 (0.0007)	0.0013 (0.0007)	0.0014 (0.0007)
Hippocampal vol. (cm^3)	−0.64 (0.17)	−0.50 (0.10)	−0.53 (0.10)	−0.53 (0.10)	−0.53 (0.10)
APOE4 positive	−0.06 (0.30)	0.28 (0.21)	0.34 (0.21)	0.32 (0.21)	0.38 (0.21)

Estimates based on complete records ($n = 127$), FCS using impute then transform, and latent normal SMC MI (SMC-latent), factorised conditional model SMC MI (SMC-Factor) and SMC FCS. The Monte Carlo errors for the MI point estimates are of the order of 0.01 or less.

the linear and quadratic Aβ_{1-42} effects, which are much closer to the corresponding complete records estimates. This is to be expected because the SMC MI approach is accounting for the possibility of a quadratic Aβ_{1-42} effect in the imputation models for the partially observed variables.

6.4.3 Factorised conditional model SMC imputation

An alternative approach to specifying a model for $f(\mathbf{X}|\mathbf{Z})$ is to decompose it as a product of univariate conditional distributions:

$$f(\mathbf{X}|\mathbf{Z}) = f(X_1|\mathbf{Z})f(X_2|X_1,\mathbf{Z})\ldots f(X_p|X_1,\ldots,X_{p-1},\mathbf{Z}).$$

As with the FCS approach to MI, since the model for each partially observed variable is a univariate model, its type can be tailored to the type of variable accordingly. Variables of mixed type, including counts, can then be readily handled by specifying suitable univariate regression models.

Ibrahim *et al.* (2002) proposed adopting this approach to modelling $f(\mathbf{X}|\mathbf{Z})$ in a fully Bayesian analysis. Although they focused on a full Bayesian analysis rather than MI, the MCMC algorithm can naturally be used to produce multiple imputations of the missing values once the chain(s) has converged.

More recently, Erler *et al.* (2016) further investigated this approach and compared it with FCS MI in the setting of missing covariates in longitudinal data analysed using linear mixed models. In this setting, as discussed further in Section 9.4.1, it is difficult to set up imputation models for the covariates that are compatible with the linear mixed substantive model. Erler *et al.* (2016) showed in a data example and simulations that both FCS MI and the SMC factored-conditional approach can be unbiased, but for FCS only when the longitudinal outcome was appropriately conditioned-on by fitting a preliminary mixed model with only time as a covariate and generating predictions of the individual-specific random effects. Although the latter approach worked well in their simulations, it requires a high level of sophistication on the part of the user and is arguably somewhat *ad hoc* since it uses the data twice. In contrast, their proposed SMC factored-conditional Bayesian imputation approach ensures missing covariates are imputed compatibly with the substantive model automatically by construction.

The factored conditional approach is available in R *via* the `JointAI` package (Erler *et al.*, 2021). As well as single-level models, it also supports multi-level models (see Chapter 9). The approach is also implemented in the R package `mdmb` Grund *et al.* (2021) and the stand-alone software package `BLIMP` Keller (2022).

Table 6.5 shows results (SMC-Factor) for the ADNI Cox model analysis described previously using the JointAI package, based on 100,000 MCMC iterations. The estimates are broadly similar to those from the latent normal SMC MI approach (SMC-Latent), although there are some differences which are larger than can be explained by Monte Carlo error. For example, the linear coefficient of Aβ_{1-42} is somewhat larger and the coefficient of log(Tau) is somewhat smaller. Since both approaches impute compatibly with the same Cox proportional hazards substantive model, these differences are attributable to differences in the joint models being assumed for the covariates.

A potential drawback of the factored-conditional approach is that one must decide the ordering of the factorization. Erler *et al.* (2016) proposed choosing the ordering according to the amount of missingness (*i.e.*, starting with the marginal distribution of the most fully observed variable). They also reported that results were often good when using different factorizations, provided the conditional models used in each factorization were reasonable for the data. It is important to note that different factorizations do lead to different joint models for the covariates (in general), and so there is no guarantee that different choices will not affect the inferences obtained. However, the fact that one can choose the factorization and models used means in principle there is much greater flexibility in the joint models that can be specified for the covariates than in the latent normal approach.

In the ADNI data analysis, we ran a second analysis using the JointAI package where we specified the conditional models using a factorization which reversed the default ordering. The results (not shown) were virtually the same as those shown in Table 6.5 for SMC-Factor, supporting the conjecture that the order chosen may often not be crucial. This finding is in line with the findings of Grund *et al.* (2021).

6.4.4 Substantive model compatible fully conditional specification

The final SMC approach we describe avoids directly specifying a multivariate model for $f(\mathbf{X}|\mathbf{Z})$. The SMC FCS approach instead adapts the FCS idea whereby imputation models are specified separately for each partially observed covariate X_j (Bartlett *et al.*, 2015b).

Specifically, for covariate X_j, we specify a model for $f(X_j|X_{-j}, Z)$, where $X_{-j} = \{X_1, \dots, X_{j-1}, X_{j+1}, \dots, X_p\}$. Missing values in X_j can then be imputed from a model compatible with the substantive model by imputing from the distribution proportional to $f(Y|\mathbf{X}, \mathbf{Z})f(X_j|X_{-j}, Z)$. As described in Section 6.4.1, this distribution does not generally belong to a standard parametric family, and so Bartlett *et al.* (2015b) proposed the use of rejection sampling to generate the required draws, as described earlier in Section 6.4.1.

The SMC FCS approach is available in Stata (Bartlett and Morris, 2015) as `smcfcs`, available from SSC, and in R as the `smcfcs` package, available from CRAN. It is also implemented in the standalone BLIMP software package.

An advantage of SMC FCS compared to the SMC factored-conditional approach (Section 6.4.3) is that there is no need to choose an ordering among the partially observed variables $\mathbf{X} = (X_1, \dots, X_p)$ when specifying the models. A drawback is that, as with standard FCS, the theoretical foundation of SMC FCS is somewhat shaky; if the conditional models $f(X_j|X_{-j}, Z)$ across $j = 1, \dots, p$ are not mutually compatible, it is unclear what joint distribution (if any) the algorithm draws from. Nevertheless, as in the case of the standard FCS algorithm, empirical experience with SMC FCS thus far suggests generally good performance.

The last column of Table 6.5 shows estimates for the ADNI data using SMC FCS in R with $K = 1000$ imputations. The estimates are overall closest to those from the latent normal SMC MI approach. Comparing the results across all the MI approaches used, we see that the three SMC approaches give broadly similar inferences, while the FCS impute-then-transform approach gives somewhat different estimates, particularly for the $A\beta_{1-42}$ effects. As noted earlier, this is to be expected because the impute-then-transform approach does not impute the missing values of $A\beta_{1-42}$ compatibly with a quadratic effect in the substantive model. It is impossible from one data analysis or indeed simulations to say which of the three SMC MI approaches is to be preferred in general – they each make different assumptions about the joint distribution of the covariates of the substantive model. It is however reassuring that in this analysis, the three SMC MI approaches gave broadly similar results, suggesting that the most important point is that imputation of missing covariate values is done compatibly with the substantive model.

6.4.5 Auxiliary variables

Thus far, in this chapter, we have considered imputation of partially observed covariates and how their imputation models can be constructed to be compatible with the substantive model. As discussed in Chapter 2, an attractive feature of MI is the possibility of including auxiliary variables: variables $\mathbf{V}$ used in the imputation process which are not in the substantive model. For the SMC MI approaches described in this chapter, it is not immediately clear how such variables should be incorporated.

One approach is to include $\mathbf{V}$ in the outcome model at the imputation stage (i.e. as if they are covariates in the substantive model), but omit them when fitting the actual substantive model to the imputed datasets. This approach means the auxiliary variables are used in the imputation model(s) but not the substantive model. Often, this approach may be reasonable. However, we note that this approach does not generally lead to the imputation model (which includes the auxiliaries) being compatible with the substantive model which omits the auxiliaries, in the sense that the joint model which is compatible with the imputation model, and the outcome model which conditions on the auxiliaries, would not exactly imply the same model form for the outcome variable conditional on the covariates of interest (i.e. omitting the auxiliaries). For example, if a time-to-event outcome follows a Cox proportional hazards model conditional on two baseline covariates, it is not the case that the time-to-event outcome conditional on just one of the covariates is still a proportional hazards model.

An alternative approach that avoids the aforementioned issue would be to specify the joint imputation model as

$$f(Y, \mathbf{X}, \mathbf{V}|\mathbf{Z}) = f(\mathbf{V}|Y, \mathbf{X}, \mathbf{Z})f(Y|\mathbf{X}, \mathbf{Z})f(\mathbf{X}|\mathbf{Z}).$$

Whatever specification is used for $f(\mathbf{V}|Y, \mathbf{X}, \mathbf{Z})$ the resulting imputation model for $\mathbf{X}$ will be compatible with the substantive model for Y which does not include $\mathbf{V}$ as a covariate. Although certainly technically possible, thus far this approach does not appear to have been pursued in practice.

6.4.6 Missing outcome values

In some settings, there may be missing values in the outcome Y as well as covariates of the substantive model. This can be readily handled by the SMC MI approaches we have described, by simply imputing the missing Y values from the specified substantive model. Since the substantive model is often a standard regression model, this is typically straightforward. For example, the R package `smcfcs` will impute missing outcome values in the cases of linear, logistic, and Poisson substantive models.

6.4.7 Congeniality versus compatibility

Thus far in this chapter, we have used the terms 'congeniality' and 'compatibility' somewhat interchangeably. Strictly speaking, we should not do so. In this section, we briefly outline how the concepts are related.

Unlike our characterization in Section 2.4, Meng's (Meng, 1994) original definition of congeniality did not refer to a substantive model as such. Rather, his definition involved an analyst's (the person analyzing the imputed datasets) 'complete data procedure' (and indeed an incomplete data procedure, which for our purposes is not essential to include here). The analyst's complete data procedure, when applied to a dataset, gives a point estimate and variance estimate for some parameter(s). The analyst's complete data procedure is said to be congenial to the imputation model if there exists a Bayesian model for which the predictive distribution of the missing data given the observed matches that used by the imputation model and the posterior mean and variance of the parameter(s) given complete data match the analyst's complete data point estimate and variance, respectively. When congeniality is satisfied, MI using Rubin's rules is (essentially) equivalent to Bayesian inference for the parameter(s) under this Bayesian model.

Building on Liu *et al.* (2013), Bartlett *et al.* (2015b) gave the following definition for a set of conditional models to be compatible. Let $A = (A_1, \dots, A_p)$ be a vector of random variables, and B a further, possibly empty, vector of random variables. A set of conditional models $\{f_j(A_j|A_{-j}, B, \theta_j); \theta_j \in \Theta_j, j = 1, \dots, p\}$ is said to be compatible if there exists a joint model $g(A|B, \theta)$, $\theta \in \Theta$ and a collection of surjective maps $\{t_j : \Theta \to \Theta_j; j = 1, \dots, p\}$ such that for each j, $\theta_j \in \Theta_j$, and $\theta \in t_j^{-1}(\theta_j) = \{\theta : t_j(\theta) = \theta_j\}$,

$$f_j(A_j|A_{-j}, B, \theta_j) = g(A_j|A_{-j}, B, \theta).$$

Using the setup from earlier in the chapter, the substantive model is a model $f(Y|\mathbf{X}, \mathbf{Z}, \theta_1)$ and the imputation model is a model $f(\mathbf{X}|\mathbf{Z}, Y, \theta_2)$. Suppose these two models are compatible, with corresponding joint model $g(Y, \mathbf{X}|Z, \theta)$. A prior $f(\theta)$ is then specified and the missing data in $\mathbf{X}$ are imputed from the predictive distribution from $f(\mathbf{X}|\mathbf{Z}, Y, \theta_2)$ and the prior $f(\theta)$. Suppose further that the analyst's complete data procedure consists of fitting the model $f(Y|\mathbf{X}, \mathbf{Z}, \theta_1)$ using maximum likelihood, as would typically be the case. For typical default specifications of non-informative priors, the maximum likelihood estimates and corresponding variance estimates will match the complete data posterior mean and variance for θ_1, such that the imputation model and analyst's complete data procedure are congenial.

The preceding exposition is intended to make clear that, when, as is typically the case, the imputed datasets are analyzed by fitting a substantive model using maximum likelihood, congeniality between the imputation model and analyst's complete data procedure is essentially equivalent to compatibility between the imputation model and substantive model.

6.4.8 Discussion of SMC imputation

One advantage of SMC FCS is that it offers a solution to practical problems such as the following. Suppose that the substantive model is a regression of Y on X. X is missing at random and right-skewed taking only positive values (tumour size, for example). A congenial imputation model, normal linear regression of X on Y, may impute negative values of X – logically impossible – and the marginal distribution of imputed values may appear (marginally) normal. To avoid these two features and produce more satisfactory imputed values of X, we might take a preliminary transformation, for example $\ln(X)$, and then use linear regression imputation of $\ln(X)\,|\,Y$. However, this imputation model is uncongenial to the analysis model.

While we have tried to emphasize that reproducing missing values is not our aim and that congeniality is important, it is unsettling if the imputed data distribution is obviously different to the observed data, particularly if some imputed values could not exist. The latter in particular tells us that our imputation model is mis-specified. In the above example, it is clear that the negative values and normality of imputed values may simply reflect the use of normal linear regression imputation. SMC FCS offers a way to have our cake and eat it: a transformation can be taken that produces marginal normality; this transformed variable can be included in the proposal distribution; and the transformation can be inverted for the substantive model used as the basis of the rejection rule. This means that congeniality will be respected, but that the marginal distribution of imputed values will appear more reasonable, avoiding situations like negative imputed values.

When we have uncongeniality/incompatibility between the imputation model and the substantive model we know without recourse to any data that the imputation model and the substantive model cannot both be correct. When we specify an imputation model and substantive model that are congenial/compatible, this does not guarantee correct specification. That is, assuming the substantive model is correctly specified, congeniality/compatibility is a necessary but not sufficient condition for correct specification of the imputation model.

We note that our coverage is not exhaustive with respect to SMC MI methods. For example, Beesley and Taylor (2021) proposed an approach whereby missing covariates are imputed ignoring the outcome variable. Standard analysis of the resulting imputed datasets would then lead to biased estimates of the substantive model parameters. To fix this, a weighted analysis of the imputed datasets is performed, giving higher weights to imputed records where the imputed covariate values are more plausible given the individual's outcome value, the form of the substantive model, and (complete records) estimates of its parameters. An attractive feature of this approach is that one does not require specialist software to ensure the imputations are generated compatibly with the substantive model. Moreover, one set of imputed datasets could be used with a range of different substantive models, with the weights varying as the substantive model is changed.

6.5 Returning to the problems

Having described some solutions, it should be clear how to proceed with using multiple imputation for some of the problems outlined in Section 6.1, such as squares and interactions. For others, we now discuss some approaches in more detail. In several cases, it turns out that SMC FCS is a good solution.

6.5.1 Ratios

While ratios bear a resemblance to interactions, some different issues may arise as seen, for example, in QRISK (Hippisley-Cox *et al.*, 2007). In a paper that identified the main issues with the ratio in QRISK, Morris *et al.* (2014b) explored methods for imputing a ratio where the components are not missing simultaneously. Their main caution was that imputing the ratio's components as separate variables and then calculating the ratio could lead to catastrophic bias. This bias occurred when the distribution of the denominator was such that the left tail has values close to 0. It is then possible that missing values are imputed as small and close to 0. This leads to very large values of the ratio with high leverage in a regression model. Worse, if the imputation is not constrained to impute only positive values, the denominator may be imputed as small and negative rather than positive. For an incomplete observation with a missing value, if the posterior predictive distribution has mean 0, the denominator will be drawn as positive or negative at random, leading to high leverage of the imputed value.

No other method they considered was at risk of producing such high bias. In particular, taking a log-transformation of the numerator and denominator seemed to be a safe strategy. However, using a SMC MI approach has a better justification. We have since added SMC FCS to the simulation study reported in Morris *et al.* (2014b) and seen that it is at least as good as the other methods.

6.5.2 Splines

We have previously mentioned substantive models that contain a quadratic effect of a covariate. Often, when non-linear effects are posited, the analyst may use an approach that allows for more flexibility than simple polynomials. One such option is to use (restricted) cubic splines (Harrell, 2015). This assumes the covariate's effect on the outcome (on a suitable scale) can be described by a piece-wise cubic function with a specified number of knots at locations specified by the analyst.

The substantive model approaches to imputation we have discussed in Section 6.4 can in principle impute missing covariates compatible with such a substantive model. A possible practical limitation is whether software implementing these approaches can accommodate splines. To do so, they need to be able to calculate the basis functions involved in the linear predictor of the substantive model. At least for cubic spline models, where the basis function definitions are relatively simple, the `smcfcs` package in R can be used, through use of R's `I()` function; in Stata, this can be achieved through abs() to code the positive part function (which we will do in exercise 6.3).

6.5.3 Fractional polynomials

Fractional polynomial models are another alternative to simple polynomials for modelling possible non-linear effects of covariates. While 'conventional' polynomials would use increasing positive integers as powers of X, fractional polynomials involve fractional and negative powers of X, and in no particular order. A fractional polynomial regression model can be written as

$$f(Y) = \beta_0 + \sum_{d=1}^{D} \beta_d X^{p_d},$$

where X is a continuous variable taking only positive values. D denotes the *dimension* or *degree* of fractional polynomial for a given X: a model with $D = 1$ is described as a *first degree* or *dimension-1* fractional polynomial, or simply as 'FP1'. Values of p are typically chosen from $\{-2, -1, -0.5, 0, 0.5, 1, 2, 3\}$, where '$p = 0$' represents 'log($X$)', by choosing D, fitting the model with each in turn and selecting the value that maximizes the likelihood. Note that this description of how powers are selected is a clue that p should be regarded as a parameter to be estimated (with discrete rather than continuous space) rather than simply a 'transformation' of X. This is important for inference and for understanding the complexities of multiple imputation of incomplete X when using fractional polynomial models.

For $D > 1$, the same value of p can be 'repeated', but in fact this involves multiplying the second term by log(X). So for an 'FP2' model, we use the transformations

$$(X^{p_1}, X^{p_2}) \text{ for } p_1 \neq p_2,$$

$$(X^{p_1}, X^{p_1}\log(X)) \text{ for } p_1 = p_2.$$

Figure 6.4 depicts some fractional polynomial curves, where $Y = \beta_0 + \beta_1 X^3 + \beta_2 \log(X)$. Because there are two exponents for X, these are 'dimension-2'. It is apparent that, even with just these two powers, fractional polynomials are far more flexible than a quadratic function of X (though a quadratic function is one possible choice for a dimension-2 fractional polynomial model).

There are multivariable extensions to fractional polynomial models, where the exponents p can estimated for several continuous or ordered-categorical covariates. Royston and Sauerbrei (2008) advocate an approach for building and selecting multivariable models using fractional polynomials. The key idea is based on backwards elimination. This is an extension of the idea of variable elimination to higher-order-term elimination. For example a model including two FP exponents for X can be tested against a model excluding X on 4 df (2 df for each β and 2 for each p, since p is a parameter) and the decision to include or exclude X from the model is

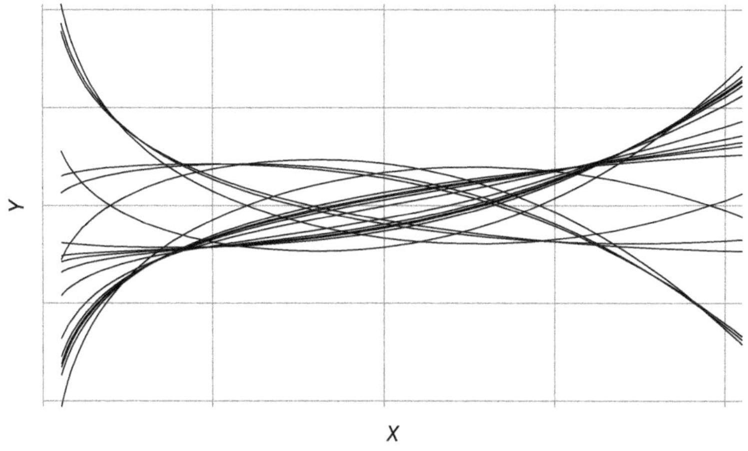

Figure 6.4 Some examples of 'FP2' fractional polynomial curves with powers $p_1 = 3, p_2 = 0$, *so* $Y = \beta_0 + \beta_1 X^3 + \beta_2 \log(X)$.

based on this test. If X is included, then the FP2 model can be tested against a model including X^1 on 3 df. If the FP2 is judged to provide a better fit, then the FP2 model is finally tested against the best fitting FP1 model to decide which form to include. This is a rough sketch and details can be found in Royston and Sauerbrei (2008).

Suppose now that X is incomplete, that we are willing to assume missing-at-random, and that we wish to use multiple imputation. There are various challenges when using multiple imputation with fractional polynomial models. First, X must take positive values and imputation must respect this. Second, even if the dimension of fractional polynomial is fixed, e.g. FP1, the uncertainty about p must be accounted for in imputation (recall that in the solutions outlined for multiple imputation of squares, the exponents were fixed in imputation and analysis). Third, the substantive model is not generally fixed before imputation but to be selected based on multiple imputation results. It is difficult to ensure congeniality with all models in the set of possible models.

Morris *et al.* (2015) proposed a procedure that approximates a congenial imputation model for an FP1 substantive model. For a single incomplete X:

1. Use the Bayesian bootstrap (or approximate Bayesian bootstrap) to draw a reweighted sample from the complete cases.

2. For exponents to be considered, for example $\{-2, -1, -0.5, 0, 0.5, 1, 2, 3\}$, fit a linear regression of X^p on Y. Include other covariates in this imputation model such that the imputation model is congenial to a substantive model that is a regression of Y on X^p and these other covariates.

3. Identify the value of p that returns the largest value of $\log(L) + J$ and denote this p^*. Here L is the likelihood and J is the Jacobian, which standardizes the likelihoods to permit comparison (as we have transformed from X to X^p).

The chosen p^* represents a draw from the posterior of P since it was the maximum from an ABB sample.

4. Using the incomplete dataset, impute missing values of X^{P^*} by standard linear regression imputation.

5. Finally, the imputed value X^* is obtained by inverting the transformation used to get X^{P^*}.

It is important that the procedure ensures draws of X^* are positive. This can be achieved by using, for example, a truncated normal distribution for imputation, or PMM (Morris *et al.*, 2015).

The above procedure performs univariate imputation and so can be embedded in an FCS procedure if multiple incomplete variables are to be imputed. This also handles imputation for multivariable fractional polynomial models if several of the covariates subject to fractional polynomial modelling are incomplete.

Unfortunately, the FP1 imputation method described above does not extend naturally to higher-dimension fractional polynomials. How to impute in a way that is congenial to higher-dimension fractional polynomials is an open question. A pragmatic solution is to note that, having chosen p, fractional polynomials models typically ignore uncertainty about p. It would therefore be consistent with this approach to use a similar approach to imputation: that is, impute using each possible pair of exponents, fit the analysis model, and use the pair with the highest likelihood after MI.

The Bayesian bootstrap

Use of the Bayesian bootstrap in the fractional polynomial procedure described above is a trick to obtain a draw p^* of p rather than having to take a parametric draw from the posterior distribution (Rubin and Schenker, 1986). The Bayesian bootstrap:

1. Draws and orders $(n-1)$uniform[0, 1] variables;

2. Calculates $p_1 = u_1, p_i = u_i - u_{i-1}, p_n = 1 - u_{n-1}$;

3. Resamples the n observations with replacement with probability $p_i, i = 1, \dots, n$.

Rubin (1981) shows this simulates the posterior distribution of a statistic $\theta = \theta(p_1, \dots, p_n, \mathbf{Y}_1, \dots, \mathbf{Y}_n)$ under the improper prior proportional to $\prod_{i=1}^{n} p_i^{-1}$; see also Lo (1986). The approximate Bayesian bootstrap draws weights from a scaled multinomial distribution (Rubin and Schenker, 1986).

For a univariable FP2 model, for example SMC FCS can be used where the substantive model is defined as the fractional polynomial model containing that pair of powers and then selection of the best fitting done by comparing likelihoods. As with any imputation method suitable for fractional polynomial models, the imputed values of X^* must be positive. This may be achieved by taking a log-transformation of X for the proposal distribution used by SMC FCS. An alternative may be to use PMM for the proposal distribution, but this is not yet implemented in software. Note that the SMC FCS approach sketched above is clearly computationally intensive, particularly with multivariable fractional polynomial models. It may be necessary to restrict the pairs of exponents considered.

6.5.4 Multiple imputation with conditional questions or 'skips'

Frequently in questionnaires, the answer to a particular question will determine the immediately succeeding questions. For example, for someone who reports that they are in paid employment (the 'skip question'), succeeding *conditional* questions may ask about the nature of the work and remuneration. For someone who reports that they are not in paid employment, such questions are not applicable. The interviewee will *skip* the conditional questions and possibly be asked a different set of conditional questions. For recent examples see He *et al.* (2010) and Drechsler (2011).

Imputation for data containing such conditional variables is structurally complex because conditional questions should only be imputed if the qualifying question (for example about paid employment) makes them applicable. As usual with imputation, careful consideration of the context is needed, on the one hand to avoid making the imputation model unduly complex, and on the other to avoid inappropriate imputation of important associations.

Example 6.3 Youth yohort study

General certificate of secondary education (GCSE) exam results from the Youth Cohort Study (YCS) illustrate how formulating imputation in terms of skips and conditional variables may be useful, even when the data are not actually presented in these terms but as a single variable: GCSE points score. We may imagine this was derived in answer to a series of questions along the lines of

(a) Did you obtain any GCSE at grade G or higher?

(b) If yes, in which subjects and with what grades? (If *no*, (b) is skipped.)

Each GCSE grade is given a point score, from $A/A^{\star} = 7$ through to $G = 1$. These are summed, and the score is capped at 84. Figure 6.5 shows the histogram of GCSE scores among pupils who had at least one pass at grade G or higher; 2468 of 64,045 (3.9%) did not obtain any GCSEs.

In the YCS data, only a small proportion of GCSE scores are missing. Given this, imputing assuming GCSE score has a normal distribution before rounding any negative imputed values to zero is likely to give similar results to more complex methods and is likely acceptable.

More generally, if a variable has a distribution with a spike at a particular value, then it is awkward to model and thus impute. Considering the variable as a binary skip indicator, plus a response for one value of the skip indicator, is a potentially attractive way around this problem, which connects to the literature on zero-inflated and, more generally, mixture models.

Thus, even when skips are not explicit in the way variables are constructed, the approaches described may be useful. □

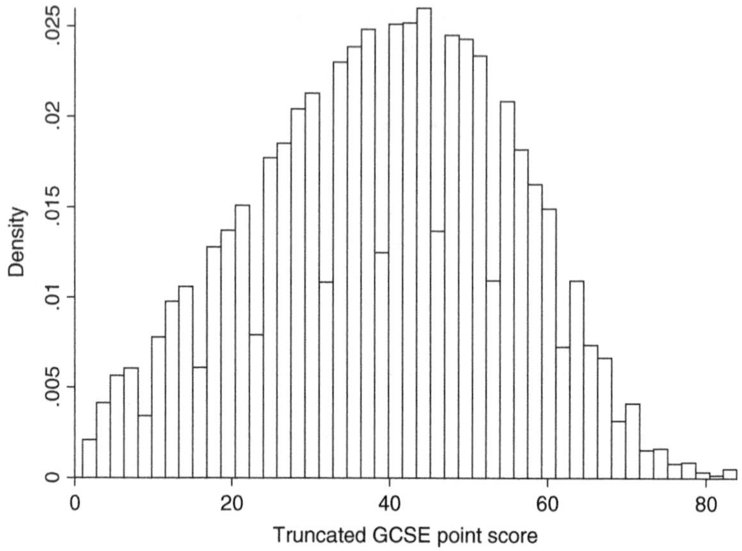

Figure 6.5 Histogram of GCSE points score, for pupils who obtained one or more GCSEs at grade G or above.

To explore this further, suppose the following linear regression is of interest:

$$Y_i = \beta_0 + \beta_1 X_{i,1} + \beta_2 X_{i,2} + \beta_3 (X_{i,2} X_{i,3}) + e_i, \quad e_i \overset{i.i.d.}{\sim} N(0, \sigma^2), \tag{6.20}$$

where Y, X_1, X_3 are continuous, and X_2 is a skip indicator for X_3, so that if the answer to the question coded in X_2 is 'no', $X_2 = 0$, and the information in X_3 is not asked for because it is not relevant or may not be defined. In the YCS example, X_2 would be whether any GCSE passes were obtained and X_3 would be the points score. The discussion below is general, so Y, X_1, X_3 can be variables, or groups of variables, of different types.

Framing the issue through (6.20), we see that skips are a special case of interactions; 'special' because we would usually include X_2, X_3 and X_2X_3, as covariates, but with a skip we do not include X_3: if $X_2 = 0$, it is not relevant. Thus, the consideration of interactions is directly relevant to skips. With a general missingness pattern, this points to the approaches described in Section 6.4. However, as described below, this may not always be necessary.

We note that, if X_2 is binary and X_3 is observed, X_2 cannot be missing. Thus, individuals either have $X_2 = 1$ observed and X_3 observed or missing, or have X_2 and X_3 missing. Particularly in settings where X_3 is undefined or does not make sense when $X_2 = 0$, those who in truth have $X_2 = 0$ do not have a 'missing' value of X_3. Thus, if we impute $X_2 = 0$ for an individual, there is no X_3 value required to be imputed. This special feature renders an FCS approach more attractive than a joint modelling approach, since some implementations of FCS have the ability to impute only in a subset of data rows, conditional on the value of another variable (here X_2). Keeping this in mind, we now discuss two cases.

Skip variable fully observed

If there are no missing values in the skip variable X_2, we can impute any missing values in X_3 among those with $X_2 = 1$ using a suitable imputation model for $f(X_3|Y, X_1, X_2 = 1)$ in an FCS approach. If the FCS software being used cannot restrict the imputation of missing values of X_3 to the subset with $X_2 = 1$, one can impute as normal, removing X_2 as a predictor from the imputation model for X_3, since there is no information to estimate the effect of X_2 on X_3 if X_3 is always missing when $X_2 = 0$. Moreover, since in FCS the imputation model at each iteration is only fitted to the subset of individuals with the target variable originally observed, only individuals with X_3 originally observed (who hence also have $X_2 = 1$) will inform the fit of the imputation model for X_3. Next, in the imputation models for other variables, by including X_2 and the X_2X_3 interaction as covariates but not the X_3 main effect, we ensure that the imputed values of X_3 among those with $X_2 = 0$ have no impact on the imputation process.

Alternatively, one can use a joint modelling approach, where we condition on X_2 since it is fully observed:

$$\begin{aligned}
Y_i &= \beta_{0,1} + \beta_{1,1}X_{i,2} + e_{i,1},\\
X_{i,1} &= \beta_{0,2} + \beta_{1,2}X_{i,2} + e_{i,2},\\
X_{i,3} &= \beta_{0,3} + e_{i,3},\\
(e_{i,1}, e_{i,2}, e_{i,3}) &\sim N_3(\mathbf{0}, \boldsymbol{\Omega}),
\end{aligned} \tag{6.21}$$

where note that we do not condition on X_2 in the model for X_3. Here we fit the imputation model and impute as usual, but then discard the imputed values for X_3 in those with $X_2 = 0$. Note that, when fitting this joint model, for those with $X_2 = 0$, the (unnecessarily) imputed value of X_3 will apparently be informing the imputation of any missing values in (Y, X_1), which seems somewhat undesirable. However, these imputed X_3 values are themselves simply draws conditional on $(Y, X_1, X_2 = 0)$, and so we would not anticipate this to adversely affect the resulting imputations.

Missing values in the skip variable

Now suppose we have missing values of X_2 (any missing X_2 for which we have observed X_3 are set equal to 1). In the FCS approach, we now additionally specify a model for $P(X_2 = 1|Y, X_1)$ to impute the missing values in X_2, omitting X_3 as a predictor from the imputation model.

In a joint modelling approach, we may extend model (6.21), including the binary skip indicator X_2 as a response through the latent normal structure:

$$\begin{aligned}
Y_i &= \beta_{0,1} + e_{i,1},\\
X_{i,1} &= \beta_{0,2} + e_{i,2},\\
\Pr(X_{i,2} = 1) &= \Pr(\beta_{0,3} + e_{i,3} > 0),\\
X_{i,3} &= \beta_{0,4} + e_{i,4},\\
(e_{i,1}, e_{i,2}, e_{i,3}, e_{i,4})^T &\sim N_4(\mathbf{0}, \boldsymbol{\Omega}), \quad \text{with } \boldsymbol{\Omega}_{3,3} = 1.
\end{aligned} \tag{6.22}$$

Because X_3 must be missing when imputing missing X_2, we constrain their dependence conditional on (Y, X_1) to be zero by setting the corresponding off-diagonal elements in the precision matrix (the inverse of the covariance matrix $\mathbf{\Omega}$) to zero: $\mathbf{\Omega}^{-1}_{3,4} = \mathbf{\Omega}^{-1}_{4,3} = 0$.

For each individual where the skip indicator X_2 is missing, that individual's variables will vary between imputed datasets: some will include imputed skip variables because X_2 was imputed to 1, others will not. While, with models like (6.20) this should not cause a problem, models fitted to, say, the subset of each imputed dataset for which $X_2 = 1$ will have different numbers of observations (sample size) for different imputations. This triggers an error for some software which applies Rubin's rules. Superficially, this looks like a computational issue: the substantive model can still be fitted to each imputed data set and Rubin's rules applied to combine the results.

However, this issue illustrates that the analysis of imputed data with skips may give rise to situations where the substantive model is fitted to a subset of the available data. As discussed in Chapter 2 and later in Chapter 11 section 11.4, this is a situation in which Rubin's rules will not, in general, hold, since the size of the dataset used to fit the substantive model changes from imputation to imputation and is smaller than the dataset used for imputation. The effect is that inferences are likely to be conservative; in most cases, the effect is likely of little practical consequence. We note that this issue also applies for subgroup analyses when the subgroup was partially observed.

Before leaving skips, note that both the FCS and joint modelling approaches extend directly when (i) there are more skip variables than just X_3, and (ii) there are more skip indicators than just X_2. For FCS, (i) when imputing skip indicators, we do not include corresponding conditional variables, and (ii) when imputing the conditional variables, we restrict ourselves to the subset of records defined by the observed and current imputed values of their skip indicator. For joint modelling, we simply constrain the covariance matrix so that that skip indicators are uncorrelated with the associated skip variables.

Exercises

1. **Interactions:** Simulate a dataset of size n =10,000 with variables $X_1 \sim Bern(0.5)$, $X_2|X_1 \sim Bern(0.25 + 0.5 \times X_1)$ and $Y|X_1, X_2 \sim N(X_1 + X_2 + X_1 \times X_2, 1)$. Make 50% of X_1 values MCAR and similarly make 50% of X_2 values MCAR.

   (a) **Impute then transform:** Apply FCS imputation to impute the missing values in X_1 and X_2, with $K = 10$. Specify logistic regression models for each, with X_2 and Y as covariates in the imputation model for X_1 and X_1 and Y as covariates in the model for X_2. Fit the linear regression substantive model with Y as outcome and covariates X_1, X_2, and $X_1 \times X_2$. What do you observe and are these in line with your expectations based on the chapter?

   (b) **Adapting standard imputation models:** Re-run the imputation process, but this time including an $X_2 \times Y$ interaction in the imputation model for X_1 and an $X_1 \times Y$ interaction in the imputation model for X_2. How do the resulting substantive model parameter estimates compare to the true values?

(c) **Transform then impute:** Re-run the imputation again using the transform then impute (just another variable) approach. That is, construct the interaction variable $X_3 = X_1 \times X_2$ in the dataset before imputation, and impute it, along with X_1 and X_2, as if it were just another variable. Moreover, tell your software to impute the partially observed variables using normal linear regression models, including main effects only of the variables in the imputation models. Re-estimate the substantive model parameters again, with X_1, X_2, and X_3 as covariates. How do they compare to the true values? Look at the imputed values in the first imputed dataset to check they look as you would expect. What would you expect to happen if instead of MCAR, X_1 had had values MAR, with missingness dependent on Y? If you wish, modify your code accordingly and see what happens.

(d) **Substantive model compatible imputation:** Use a substantive model compatible imputation approach to impute the missing values in X_1 and X_2, accounting for the normal linear regression substantive model which includes the main effects of X_1 and X_2 plus their interaction. How the resulting estimates compare to those obtained previously and with the true parameter values?

2. **Substantive model compatible imputation of discrete covariates:** In this exercise, we will derive expressions for how to directly sample (impute) missing values of a discrete covariate compatibly with a given substantive model.

   (a) Let X be a discrete covariate taking values $s = 1, \dots, S$. Let Y be the outcome, and $f(Y|X)$ denote the substantive model. Express the imputation distribution $f(X|Y)$ in terms of the substantive model $f(Y|X)$, a marginal model for $P(X = s)$ and a constant of proportionality k.

   (b) Use the fact that $\sum_{s=1}^{S} P(X = s|Y) = 1$ to derive an expression for k in terms of $f(Y|X = s)$ and $P(X = s)$.

   (c) Hence, derive an explicit expression for $P(X = s|Y)$ for $s = 1, \dots, S$.

3. **Imputation with splines:** In this exercise, we will explore through simulation the performance of an SMC MI approach to imputation of missing covariate values when the substantive modelinvolves a cubic spline.

   (a) For a dataset of size $n = 1000$, simulate a covariate $X \sim N(0, 4)$. Define the following cubic spline basis functions which are derived from X:

$$X_1 = X,$$
$$X_2 = X^2,$$
$$X_3 = X^3,$$
$$X_4 = (X - a)_+^3,$$
$$X_5 = (X - b)_+^3,$$
$$X_6 = (X - c)_+^3,$$

where $(a, b, c) = (-1, 0, 1)$ denotes three knot positions and $(.)_+$ denotes the positive part function. Simulate the outcome Y from

$$Y = \beta_0 + \beta_1 X_1 + \beta_2 X_2 + \beta_3 X_3 + \beta_4 X_4 + \beta_5 X_5 + \beta_6 X_6 + \epsilon$$

with $\boldsymbol{\beta} = (0, 1, 0.1, 0.2, -0.1, 0.4, 0.3)$. Plot Y against X to examine their relationship.

(b) Make 50% of the values of X missing completely at random. Then generate a single imputation of the missing values in X using a standard linear regression imputation model for $X|Y$. Re-plot Y against X using the imputed and observed X values. What do you conclude regarding the imputation model's performance?

(c) Delete the imputed values generated in the last part. Now create a new single imputation of the missing values of X using a SMC MI approach (e.g. SMC-FCS), accounting for the form of the cubic spline substantive model. Now re-generate the (Y, X) plot in the imputed data and compare with what you saw in the previous part.

7

Survival data

Thus far, we have described and illustrated the use of multiple imputation (MI) for a mix of continuous and discrete variables, linear, and non-linear relationships, and interactions. We have focused principally on settings where the substantive model is a linear or logistic regression model. In this chapter, we consider issues arising when performing imputation with survival/time-to-event data.

We begin in Section 7.1 by discussing the use of MI to handle missing covariates in time-to-event analyses. In Section 7.2, we describe MI approaches to imputing censored event times and follow this in 7.3 with a brief discussion on non-parametric or *hot-deck* MI. We then consider in 7.4 the problem of missing data and the use of imputation in prospective sub-study designs, specifically the case–cohort design. We conclude with a brief discussion in Section 7.5.

7.1 Missing covariates in time-to-event data

Time-to-event data, where units or individuals are followed till an event occurs, arise in almost all areas of scientific research. We consider the context of medical research, so unit i corresponds to individual i, who is followed up from entry into a study until either (i) the time to the event of interest or (ii) a censoring time – which typically occurs because the individual has not had the event of interest by the end of the study period. Let T_i be the time at which follow-up of individual i ends, with $D_i = 1$ indicating follow-up ends at the event of interest (so that T_i is the time-to-event), while $D_i = 0$ indicating that individual i is event-free when follow-up ends (so that T_i is the censoring time).

In time-to-event analyses, we typically aim to model the association between the time-to-event and covariates. These covariates can be measured at baseline, but may also be measured during the follow-up. Here, we only consider baseline covariates.

Multiple Imputation and its Application, Second Edition.
James R. Carpenter, Jonathan W. Bartlett, Tim P. Morris, Angela M. Wood, Matteo Quartagno and Michael G. Kenward.

In the case of partially observed time-varying covariates, a popular approach is based on a joint longitudinal and survival model to which we refer the reader to Rizopoulos (2012) and references therein.

We now consider how to impute missing values in covariates of our time-to-event substantive model. We begin in Section 7.1.1 by discussing various approaches which can be implemented using standard MI software, and which in some cases are approximately compatible with the time-to-event substantive model.

7.1.1 Approximately compatible approaches

In this section, we consider approaches for imputing missing covariate values which are in certain situations approximately compatible with the chosen substantive model for the time-to-event outcome.

Using the cumulative hazard

This approach was proposed by White and Royston (2009), from a consideration of the conditional distribution of covariates given the time-to-event, under Cox's well-known proportional hazards model. To describe the approach, suppose we have two covariates $X_{i,1},\ X_{i,2}$.

For a time-to-event distribution $f(t)$, $t \geq 0$, with cumulative distribution function $F(t)$, the survival function is $S(t) = \Pr(T > t) = 1 - F(t)$, the hazard is $h(t) = f(t)/S(t)$ and the cumulative hazard is

$$H(t) = \int_0^t h(s)\, ds = -\log\{S(t)\}.$$

The standard censoring assumption is that the event-time $\tilde{T}$ is conditionally independent of the censoring time C given the baseline covariates X_1, X_2. In this case, the log-likelihood for (T_i, D_i) given baseline covariates $X_{i,1},\ X_{i,2}$ is

$$\begin{aligned} &D_i \log f(T_i|X_{i,1}, X_{i,2}) + (1 - D_i) \log S(T_i|X_{i,1}, X_{i,2}) \\ &= D_i \log h(T_i|X_{i,1}, X_{i,2}) - H(T_i|X_{i,1}, X_{i,2}). \end{aligned} \tag{7.1}$$

We now suppose that the substantive model is the Cox proportional hazards model, which is ubiquitous in survival modelling. Under the proportional hazards model,

$$h(t|X_{i,1}, X_{i,2}) = h_0(t) \exp(\beta_1 X_{i,1} + \beta_2 X_{i,2}), \tag{7.2}$$

where β_1 and β_2 are log hazard ratio parameters and $h_0(t)$ is an arbitrary baseline hazard function. Under the Cox model $H(t|X_{i,1}, X_{i,2}) = H_0(t) \exp(\beta_1 X_{i,1} + \beta_2 X_{i,2})$, so (7.1) becomes

$$\begin{aligned} \ell(T_i, D_i, X_{i,1}, X_{i,2}, \beta) = {} & D_i[\log\{h_0(T_i)\} + \beta_1 X_{i,1} + \beta_2 X_{i,2}] \\ & - H_0(T_i) \exp(\beta_1 X_{i,1} + \beta_2 X_{i,2}). \end{aligned} \tag{7.3}$$

Suppose that $\mathbf{X}_1$ is partially observed, and $\mathbf{X}_2$ is fully observed. Denote the conditional density of $X_1|X_2$ by $f(X_1|X_2)$. Then we have that the conditional distribution required for imputation is

$$f(X_1|T,D,X_2) = \frac{f(T,D,X_1,X_2)}{f(T,D,X_2)} = \frac{f(T,D|X_1,X_2)f(X_1,X_2)}{f(T,D,X_2)}$$
$$= f(T,D|X_1,X_2)f(X_1|X_2)\left\{\frac{f(X_2)}{f(T,D,X_2)}\right\}. \quad (7.4)$$

Because the last term on the RHS of (7.4) is constant with respect to X_1, it follows from (7.3) that the log conditional distribution of X_1 given X_2 and (T_i, D_i) is, up to a constant of proportionality,

$$\log\{f(X_1|T,D,X_2)\} = \log\{f(X_1|X_2)\} + D[\log\{h_0(T)\} + (\beta_1 X_1 + \beta_2 X_2)]$$
$$- H_0(T)\exp(\beta_1 X_1 + \beta_2 X_2). \quad (7.5)$$

Suppose first that X_1 is binary, and that $\text{logit}\{P(X_1 = 1|X_2)\} = \eta_0 + \eta_1 X_2$. Then from (7.5), we have

$$\text{logit}\{P(X_1 = 1|T,D,X_2)\} = \text{logit } \Pr(X_1 = 1|X_2) + D\beta_1 - H_0(T)(e^{\beta_1} - 1)e^{\beta_2 X_2}$$
$$\approx \varsigma_0 + \varsigma_1 X_2 + \varsigma_2 D + \varsigma_3 H_0(T) + \varsigma_4 H_0(T) \times X_2, \quad (7.6)$$

for constants $\varsigma_0, \ldots, \varsigma_4$, provided $\text{Var}(X_2)$ is small. In other words, (7.6) is approximately the logistic regression of X_1 on $X_2, D, H_0(T)$ and the interaction of X_2 and $H_0(T)$. If X_2 is not present, then the logistic regression result is exact; otherwise, it is approximate, and the approximation is poorer, the larger the variance of X_2.

Now suppose that X_1 is continuous, specifically $X_1|X_2 \sim N(\alpha_0 + \alpha_1 X_2, \sigma^2)$. From (7.5), we have

$$\log f(X_1|X_2,T,D) \propto -\frac{(X_1 - \alpha_0 - \alpha_1 X_2)^2}{2\sigma^2} + D\beta_1 X_1 - H_0(T)e^{(\beta_1 X_1 + \beta_2 X_2)}. \quad (7.7)$$

The term $\exp(\beta_1 X_1 + \beta_2 X_2)$ means that (7.7) is not normal, nor any common distribution. However, it turns out (White and Royston, 2009) that if $\text{Var}(X_1)$ and $\text{Var}(X_2)$ are small, then (7.7) is approximately a linear regression on $D, H_0(T), X_2, H_0(T) \times X_2$.

The implication is that the conditional distribution of covariates is approximately linear (or linear on the logistic scale for binary variables) if we include the baseline cumulative hazard, and the censoring indicator D and the interaction of the baseline cumulative hazard with the covariates. Whether a joint modelling or full conditional specification (FCS) approach is adopted, as described in Section 6.4, this becomes increasingly difficult, and potentially numerically unstable, with increasing numbers of variables in the imputation model. As all the interactions may well not be important in every dataset, preliminary variable selection based on the complete records may be appropriate.

At the imputation stage, we do not know the baseline cumulative hazard function $H_0(t)$. White and Royston (2009) suggested a number of approaches for estimating it. If for example, it were reasonable to assume the hazard, conditional on covariates, is constant, then $H_0(t) \propto t$, and so T can be used in the imputation process rather than $H_0(T)$. The second approach proposed was to use the Nelson–Aalen estimate of the marginal cumulative hazard. Third, they considered an FCS approach where the Cox substantive modelis fitted at each iteration, the current estimate of $H_0(t)$ extracted from the fit, and this is used as a covariate in the imputation model(s) for the partially observed covariates.

Example 7.1 Simulation study

White and Royston (2009) report simulations studies with a single covariate (binary, then continuous) and also two covariates. We briefly review results for the latter here and refer readers to the paper for full details.

In the two covariate study, event times were drawn from an exponential distribution with hazard $h(t) = \lambda \exp(\beta_1 X_1 + \beta_2 X_2)$, where $\lambda = 0.002$, and (X_1, X_2) are bivariate normal, mean zero, variance 1 and correlation ρ. Censoring times were independently drawn with exponential hazard, again with $\lambda = 0.002$, giving about 50% censoring. Only X_1 was allowed to be missing; missing completely at random (MCAR) and missing at random (MAR) mechanisms dependent on X_2 were explored and around 50% of the $\mathbf{X}_1$ values were missing.

As only one variable had missing data, there was only one imputation model, a linear regression for missing $\mathbf{X}_1$ values. The following methods were compared.

Imputation from model regressing X_1 on

1. $X_2, D, \log(T)$;
2. X_2, D, T, (appropriate for the exponential hazard);
3. X_2, D, T^2, (appropriate for a Weibull hazard with shape parameter $\kappa = 2$);
4. $X_2, D, \hat{H}(T)$, where $\hat{H}(T)$ is the Nelson–Aalen estimate of $H(T)$;
5. $X_2, D, \hat{H}(T), X_2 \times \hat{H}(T)$ ($\hat{H}(T)$ again the Nelson–Aalen estimate), and
6. $X_2, D, \hat{H}_0(T)$, where $H_0(T)$ is re-estimated only on the first two cycles of the FCS algorithm, by fitting the Cox proportional hazards model to the current observed and imputed data and then extracting the baseline cumulative hazard.

Method 4 approximates baseline cumulative hazard $H_0(T)$ by $H(T)$, and this may cause bias with larger effects. For method 6, the results showed that re-estimating the baseline hazard at each cycle of the FCS algorithm did not materially change the results.

With data MCAR, focusing first on β_1, bias towards the null is present and increases slowly with increasing β_1, β_2, ρ. Bias is least for method 4 (maximum −5% when $\beta_1 = \beta_2 = \rho = 0.5$), but similar for all methods with maximum of 10% for method 3 when $\beta_1 = \beta_2 = \rho = 0.5$. Including the interaction (method 5) gives no detectable benefit The difference between empirical and imputation standard errors is smallest with method 4, with a maximum of 11% too high when $\beta_1 = \beta_2 = \rho = 0.5$. Power was weaker for method 3, but otherwise comparable.

Still focusing on β_1, under MAR, the same pattern is observed; methods 4 and 5 give the least bias, of around −10% when $\beta_1 = \beta_2 = \rho = 0.5$. For the standard error, MI estimates are again larger than empirical estimates, but now method 5 is best with a maximum of 12% too high when $\beta_1 = \beta_2 = \rho = 0.5$; methods 1 and 4 peak at 15–16.% Confidence interval coverage ranged between 94–97%.

Turning to β_2, bias was much smaller and comparable across all methods, with a maximum of +5% when $\beta_1 = \beta_2 = \rho = 0.5$. Overall, method 4 was better than, or as good as, the other methods in all scenarios. Methods 4 also performed well for agreement between MI and empirical standard errors, with a maximum difference of 9%; however, there was less to choose between methods here as the maximum difference across all methods was an overestimation by 11%.

In summary, White and Royston (2009) concluded that method 4, using the Nelson–Aalen estimate of the cumulative hazard, $H(T)$, and the censoring indicator as covariates is the 'best method in general'. □

Time-to-event data as transformed normal

An alternative approach is to transform the event time to approximate normality and then include the resulting variable in the imputation model as normally distributed. We may use any appropriate order-preserving transformation, fit the imputation model, and then back-transform afterwards. A further attraction of this approach is that we do not have to model the censoring indicator directly. Instead, if unit i is censored at T_i, we put a prior of 0 on $[0, T_i]$ and an improper prior on (T_i, ∞), and set T_i to be missing. This can readily be accommodated in principle in the joint modelling and FCS approaches outlined in the earlier chapters.

This approach will work well if (i) we can find a good normalising transformation for the event time data, and (ii) the relationships between the normalised event time data and the other variables are appropriately modelled. Unfortunately, the second point is harder in general because if the proportional hazards assumption holds and the log-hazard is linear in the covariates, the log-hazard for transformed survival time will not be linear in the covariates.

Thus, in practice, this approach is likely to be satisfactory if event times are approximately log-normal, but could introduce bias otherwise. This approach is equally applicable to the FCS setting; the transformed event time is modelled using linear regression conditional on the other covariates. Censored times contribute the appropriate cumulative distribution to the log-likelihood. Such models are often referred to as *Tobit* models and can be fitted in most software packages.

Time-to-event data as categorical

One way around the issues raised by transformation of the event time is to discretise the time-to-event variable into a categorical variable and include this derived categorical variable in the imputation model. This could be done either as an ordinal variable or as an unordered categorical variable. The latter is preferable because it does not impose a linear relationship between the event time and the other variables; instead it allows an interaction between them. Thus, the hazard is not constrained to vary linearly with time, so a range of event time distributions can be approximated. This approach has been adopted more generally for modelling survival data in a multi-level setting (Steele *et al.*, 2004). Censored event times are then handled via a prior on the categorical variable. Suppose the derived categorical time-to-event variable has $m = 1, \ldots, M$ categories, and unit i is censored at the time interval corresponding to category m_i'. Then we set unit i's event time to be missing, but put a prior of 0 on all categories $\leq m_i'$ and an uninformative (uniform) prior across the remaining categories. Imputation of any missing event times then proceeds in the same way as imputing a missing categorical variable (Chapter 5); imputation of other variables conditional on event times likewise follows the approaches described in Chapters 3–4.

This is a natural approach if the time-to-event data are already grouped, for example to the nearest week, month, or year. If the time-to-event data are not grouped, it makes sense to group them over regions of approximately constant hazard. This could be assessed prior to imputation using the non-parametric Nelson–Aalen estimate of the cumulative hazard. However, if the number of categories becomes large relative to the number of observations, it will be computationally demanding, and possibly unstable.

Again, this method could in principle be applied using FCS, using multinomial logistic regression for the categorised event time, and handling censored observations through an appropriate unit-specific prior.

Example 7.2 Cancer registry data

Nur *et al.* (2010) describe the application of MI for missing covariates in relative survival analysis for colorectal cancer patients. The data consist of all adults (15–99 years) resident in the north-west of England who were registered in the North-West Cancer Intelligence Service with malignant, invasive colorectal cancer diagnosed during 1997–2004. A total of 29,563 records were linked to hospital episode statistics on co-morbidity and treatment, and available for analysis.

Unfortunately, a substantial proportion of patients were missing important covariates on stage at diagnosis (40%), morphology (12%), and grade (25%). The proportion of missing values rose with age, deprivation, and non-surgical treatment. Vital status and survival time were also strongly associated with missingness. A complete records analysis (CRA) was reduced to 16,233 cases, 55% of the total.

Data were imputed using FCS, and follow-up time was categorized as 0–6 months, 6–12 months, yearly up to 5 years, and > 5 years; over each of these periods, the hazard is approximately constant. The three FCS imputation models included all the other variables in the substantive model, together with vital status, follow-up time categorised as above, and two interactions: deprivation and follow-up time; and age and follow-up time. Stage and grade imputed with ordinal logistic regression; unordered categorical (multinomial logistic) regression was used for morphology. Ten imputed datasets were created.

A relative survival model was fitted to the complete records and imputed data, where the relative survival $R(t)$ is defined as

$$R(t) = \frac{S_c(t)}{S_r(t)},$$

where $S_c(t)$ is the survivor function for the cancer cases in the registry, and $S_r(t)$ is the survivor function for the general population, taken from life tables stratified by age, sex, and calendar period. The excess hazard ratio (EHR) for patient i is modelled using an additive risk model,

$$h_i(t) = h_0(t) + \exp(\mathbf{x}_i^T \boldsymbol{\beta}),$$

for a background hazard $h_0(t)$ estimated from life tables, and a patient with covariates $\mathbf{x}_i$. Roughly speaking, the adjusted EHR for a factor x estimated by such models, can be thought of as the probability of dying from cancer when one has factor x, divided by the probability when x is absent.

Table 7.1 shows the results. Here, morphology types A–C are, respectively, adenocarcinoma, mucinours and serous, and other; site A–C are, respectively, colon, rectosigmoid, and rectum. These data are clearly not MCAR, and the probability of missing data is associated with the outcome. MAR is therefore a good working approximation, especially given the number of predictors in the model. We see that the analysis of the imputed data recovers information from the partially observed records, resulting in narrower confidence intervals. In addition, the estimated EHRs with age are markedly higher, the estimated EHRs with deprivation are slightly higher, while the excess hazard of stages III and IV though still dominating the model are markedly reduced. □

7.1.2 Substantive model compatible approaches

In following Section 6.4, we now consider approaches which construct imputation models for the partially observed covariates which are compatible with the time-to-event substantive model.

Again, we consider the case of a Cox proportional hazards model. The second term in the log likelihood contribution from the Cox model (7.3) implies that, excluding a couple of special cases outlined below, the conditional distribution of covariates given survival time will not follow any common distribution. Thus, following the developments in Section 6.4, a more complex approach is needed to ensure we impute compatibly with the time-to-event substantive model. As in Section 6.4, we can take up either a joint model or an FCS type approach.

Joint model approach

For a joint imputation model approach, the natural route is to factorise the joint distribution of the variables as $f(T, D, X_1, X_2) = f(T, D|X_1, X_2)f_{1,2}(X_1, X_2)$. Suppose that (X_1, X_2) are marginally bivariate normal so that $f_{1,2} = N_2(\boldsymbol{\mu}, \boldsymbol{\Omega})$. An MCMC sampler

Table 7.1 Adjusted excess hazard ratio (EHR) of death in the first year following diagnosis, estimated from complete records and after MI with 10 imputations using FCS (from Nur *et al.*, 2010).

Covariate	Complete records (16,223 cases)				MI (29,563 cases)		
	EHR	95% CI			EHR	95% CI	
Stage: 1				Reference			
2	3.56	2.69	4.72		2.56	2.17	3.02
3	10.20	7.72	13.48		7.02	5.86	8.40
4	26.39	19.60	35.53		16.53	13.80	19.80
Morphology: type A				Reference			
B	1.03	0.94	1.13		1.02	0.95	1.10
C	1.17	0.61	2.24		0.99	0.75	1.30
Grade: I				Reference			
II	1.18	1.07	1.30		1.22	1.14	1.30
II/IV	2.04	1.82	2.28		1.94	1.77	2.14
Site: A				Reference			
B	0.82	0.73	0.91		0.90	0.84	0.97
C	0.76	0.70	0.82		0.88	0.85	0.92
Sex: male				Reference			
female	0.93	0.88	0.99		0.95	0.91	0.98
Age group: 15–44				Reference			
45–54	1.08	0.77	1.53		1.29	1.04	1.60
55–64	1.40	1.02	1.91		1.75	1.44	2.11
65–74	1.99	1.47	2.69		2.38	1.97	2.88
75–84	2.72	2.01	3.69		3.56	2.95	4.29
85–99	3.97	2.87	5.49		5.41	4.45	6.57
Deprivation: 1 (least)				Reference			
2	0.99	0.85	1.15		1.05	0.97	1.14
3	1.12	0.97	1.29		1.16	1.07	1.26
4	1.20	1.05	1.39		1.24	1.14	1.34
5	1.29	1.13	1.47		1.37	1.27	1.47
Charlson index: 0				Reference			
1	1.41	1.21	1.65		1.20	1.08	1.34
2	1.46	1.14	1.87		1.31	1.13	1.53
>3	2.06	1.25	3.41		2.45	1.84	3.26

Details of categorical variables are in the text.

can then proceed by choosing initial values for the missing values of $(\mathbf{X}_1, \mathbf{X}_2)$, and then iterating steps 1–3:

1. Given the observed values and current draws for missing values, of $\mathbf{X}_1, \mathbf{X}_2$, update the parameters $\boldsymbol{\beta}$ of the proportional hazards model (7.2) and update the cumulative hazard, $H_0(t)$, as discussed below.

2. Given the observed values and current draws for missing values of $\mathbf{X}_1, \mathbf{X}_2$, update the parameters of $f_{1,2}(\boldsymbol{\mu}, \boldsymbol{\Omega})$. Since $f_{1,2}$ is a bivariate normal, we can use the approach described in Chapter 2 for this.

3. Given the current draw for $\boldsymbol{\beta}$, the baseline hazard, and $(\boldsymbol{\mu}, \boldsymbol{\Omega})$, for each $i = 1, \dots, n$, if one or both of $(X_{i,1}, X_{i,2})$ is missing, then draw new values as described below.

For step 1, for a full Bayes approach, we need an MCMC algorithm for the Cox proportional hazards model. This is beyond the scope of this book; see, for example Clayton (1991). Alternatively, we may approximate this by fitting the Cox model using the usual maximum partial likelihood, drawing $\boldsymbol{\beta}$ from the approximate bivariate normal sampling distribution of the maximum partial likelihood estimators, $N(\hat{\boldsymbol{\beta}}, \text{Var}(\hat{\boldsymbol{\beta}}))$ and then extracting a revised estimate of the baseline hazard. However, this is strictly improper, and this may result in reduced confidence interval coverage, although as all the remaining uncertainty is acknowledged, this error is likely to be small.

For step 3, we work in turn through units (indexed by i), where one, or both, of $(X_{i,1}, X_{i,2})$ is missing, as follows:

1. Propose new values $(X^\star_{i,1}, X^\star_{i,2})$ by drawing from the bivariate normal distribution whose mean is the current values $(X_{i,1}, X_{i,2})$ and whose variance is $\tau\hat{\Sigma}$, where $\hat{\Sigma}$ is the sample variance of the observed $(\mathbf{X}_1, \mathbf{X}_2)$ and τ can be adapted during the burn-in of the sampler to maximise the acceptance rate; alternatively, $\tau = 0.5$ may be a reasonable choice.

   (a) If one of $X_{i,1}$ or $X_{i,2}$ is observed, draw a proposal for the other from the marginal normal corresponding to the bivariate proposal in 1. Again, write $(X^\star_{i,1}, X^\star_{i,2})$ for what is now the pair of observed and drawn values.

2. Accept the proposed values $(X^\star_{i,1}, X^\star_{i,2})$ with probability

$$\min\left\{1, \frac{L(X^\star_{i,1}, X^\star_{i,2})}{L(X_{i,1}, X_{i,2})}\right\},$$

where

$$L(x_1, x_2) = \exp\{\ell(T_i, D_i, x_1, x_2; \boldsymbol{\beta}\} f_{12}(x_1, x_2; \boldsymbol{\mu}, \boldsymbol{\Omega}), \tag{7.8}$$

and ℓ is given by (7.3).

Since it is derived without approximation from the joint distribution, the imputation model described is compatible with the Cox proportional hazards model. Should the substantive model be parametric, we simply replace ℓ in (7.8) by the corresponding parametric log-likelihood. The attractive aspect of this approach is that, as described in Chapter 6, we can extend to the case of binary and categorical covariates, together with any interactions and non-linear transformations, if present. The joint model approach described is implemented in R in the `jomo` package Quartagno and Carpenter (2023).

SMC-FCS approach

The SMC-FCS approach, described previously in Section 6.4.4, was adapted to the Cox model by Bartlett *et al.* (2015b).

The first step in each cycle of the SMC-FCS algorithm is to fit the substantive model – here a proportional hazards Cox model – to the observed and current imputed values of the data. This gives maximum partial likelihood estimators $\hat{\beta}$ and associated covariance matrix $\text{Var}(\hat{\beta})$. We then approximate a draw from the Bayesian posterior by (i) drawing $\boldsymbol{\beta}$ from $N(\hat{\boldsymbol{\beta}}, \text{Var}(\hat{\beta}))$, and then at the drawn value of $\boldsymbol{\beta}$ extracting the estimate of $H_0(t)$.

Now, consider the SMC-FCS rejection sampling step for variable X_1, conditional on the others. Define the proposal distribution $g(\ .\ )$ for X_1 given X_2 as described in Section 6.4.4, and consider the proposal $X_{i,1}^{\star}$ for the ith individual missing X_1. Following the derivation in Section 6.4.1, at the current value of $\boldsymbol{\beta}$, this is accepted with probability

$$\frac{S(T_i|X_1^{\star}, X_2; \boldsymbol{\beta}, H_0(t))}{\max_{X_1} S(T_i|X_1, X_2; \boldsymbol{\beta}, H_0(t))} \tag{7.9}$$

if $D_i = 0$, and

$$\frac{f(T_i|X_1^{\star}, X_2; \boldsymbol{\beta}, H_0(t))}{\max_{X_1} f(T_i|X_1, X_2; \boldsymbol{\beta}, H_0(t))} \tag{7.10}$$

if $D_i = 1$. For a censored observation, $D_i = 0$, since the maximum of the survivor function is 1, from (7.9), the acceptance probability is

$$S(T_i|X_{i,1}^{\star}, X_{i,2}; \boldsymbol{\beta}, H_0(t)). \tag{7.11}$$

For an uncensored individual, we have

$$\begin{aligned}\max_{X_1} f(t) &= \max_{X_1}[h(t)\exp\{-H(t)\}] \\ &= \max_{X_1}[h_0(t)\exp\{(X_1\beta_1 + X_2\beta_2) - H_0(t)\exp(X_1\beta_1 + X_2\beta_2)\}],\end{aligned} \tag{7.12}$$

which takes its maximum when

$$(X_1\beta_1 + X_2\beta_2) - H_0(t)\exp(X_1\beta_1 + X_2\beta_2) \tag{7.13}$$

takes its maximum in X_1. Differentiating with respect to X_1 and solving shows (7.13) is at a maximum in X_1 at $\log H_0(t) = -(X_1\beta_1 + X_2\beta_2)$. Substituting into (7.12), we see this is bounded by

$$h_0(t)\exp[-\{1 + \log H_0(t)\}].$$

Thus, when $D_i = 1$, we accept $X^\star_{i,1}$ with probability

$$\begin{aligned}\frac{f(T_i|X_1^\star, X_2; \boldsymbol{\beta})}{\max_{X_1} f(T_i|X_1, X_2; \boldsymbol{\beta})} &= h_0(t)\exp[(X^\star_{i,1}\beta_1 + X_{i,2}\beta_2) \\ &\quad -H_0(t)\exp\{X^\star_{i,1}\beta_1 + X_{i,2}\beta_2\}] \times \frac{e^1 H_0(t)}{h_0(t)} \\ &= H_0(t)\exp[1 + (X^\star_{i,1}\beta_1 + X_{i,2}\beta_2) \\ &\quad -H_0(t)\exp\{X^\star_{i,1}\beta_1 + X_{i,2}\beta_2\}].\end{aligned}$$

As with the joint modelling approach described above, this approach extends to allow interactions and non-linear transformations of the covariates. The SMC-FCS approach for imputing missing covariates with Cox substantive models is available in `smcfcs` in R and Stata.

Bartlett *et al.* (2015b) compared through simulation studies the SMC-FCS approach to the cumulative hazard approach developed by White and Royston (2009), described earlier in Section 7.1.1. Survival times were simulated with hazard function $h(t|X_1, X_2) = 0.002\exp(\beta_1 X_1 + \beta_2 X_2)$ with $\beta_1 = \beta_2 = 1$. Censoring times were generated from an exponential distribution with hazard 0.002. The covariate X_1 was simulated from a Bernoulli distribution with probability 0.5, and $X_2|X_1 \sim N(X_1, 1)$. Values in X_1 and X_2 were made (independently) missing completely at random, with probability of observation 0.7. Simulations with $n = 1000$ subjects and also with $n = 100$ subjects were performed. For each simulated dataset, a complete-records analysis was first performed. Next, missing values in X_1 and X_2 were imputed using FCS using logistic and linear regression imputation models, respectively, with the event indicator and Nelson–Aalen cumulative hazard estimate as covariates. The SMC-FCS approach was then also applied, assuming a logistic model for $X_1|X_2$ and a normal linear model for $X_2|X_1$.

Table 7.2 shows the results from the 1000 simulations. The results from the complete records analysis are consistent here, since missingness is completely at random. However, with $n = 100$ the complete records analysis showed some upward finite sample bias for both β_1 and β_2. In accordance with the results of White and Royston (2009), FCS with the cumulative hazard method resulted in somewhat biased estimates, with the bias larger for the coefficient corresponding to the continuous covariate, although confidence interval coverage for both β_1 and β_2 was approximately 95%. SMC-FCS, like the complete records analysis, showed some slight upward bias, but was somewhat more efficient. Of interest was that the confidence intervals had correct coverage, despite the fact that the implementation ignores uncertainty in the baseline hazard function.

For $n = 1000$, the complete records analysis was essentially unbiased. The biases of FCS were larger than for $n = 100$, which is due to the fact that the finite sample bias, which acted in the opposite direction to the bias caused by the approximation used in the FCS approach, had largely disappeared. Consequently, confidence interval coverage was below the nominal 95% level, with coverage for β_2 particularly poor at 47%. In contrast, SMC-FCS was unbiased and had correct confidence interval coverage.

Table 7.2 Cox proportional hazards outcome model simulation results.

Parameter	Complete records		FCS		SMC-FCS	
	Mean (SD)	Cov	Mean (SD)	Cov	Mean (SD)	Cov
$n = 100$						
$\beta_1 = 1$	1.04 (0.47)	95.6	0.94 (0.36)	96.5	1.02 (0.41)	94.7
$\beta_2 = 1$	1.05 (0.26)	95.6	0.89 (0.17)	94.0	1.05 (0.21)	94.8
$n = 1000$						
$\beta_1 = 1$	1.000 (0.129)	95.2	0.902 (0.107)	89.1	1.002 (0.114)	95.0
$\beta_2 = 1$	1.007 (0.070)	94.8	0.861 (0.049)	45.7	1.006 (0.058)	95.1

Empirical mean (SD) of estimates of $\beta_1 = 1$ and $\beta_2 = 1$ from 1000 simulations, using complete records analysis, multiple imputation of X_1 and X_2 using FCS with the event indicator and Nelson–Aalen marginal baseline cumulative hazard function as covariates (FCS), and SMC-FCS. Empirical coverage of nominal 95% confidence intervals is also shown (Cov). Monte Carlo errors in means and SDs are no more than 0.02 for $n = 100$ and 0.005 for $n = 1000$.

The SMC-FCS approach with a Cox substantive model has been extended in a number of directions. Bartlett and Taylor (2016) extended the approach to the case of competing risks data. Here the analyst specifies a separate Cox model for each cause-specific hazard function, and missing covariates are imputed from imputation models compatible with these. Keogh and Morris (2018) extended the SMC-FCS approach to the setting where the covariates' effects are allowed to vary over time.

7.2 Imputing censored event times

In this section, we consider the use of MI to impute censored event times. We first consider why one might want to do this, given that the standard machinery of survival analysis can already accommodate censoring. Standard survival analysis approaches rely on a type of independent or censoring at random assumption. Specifically, we have three kinds of censoring mechanisms, respectively, paralleling MCAR, MAR, and MNAR:

1. Time-to-event data are said to be censored completely at random (CCAR) when the time to censorship is completely independent of the event time. This typically happens when censoring is caused by the cessation of study follow-up, provided each unit's entry into the study is independent of its event time.

2. Time-to-event data are said be censored at random (CAR) if *conditional on covariates in the survival model*, such as treatment or exposure group, the censoring time is independent of the event time.

3. Time-to-event data are said to be censored not at random (CNAR) if, even given covariates, the censoring time is dependent on the event time.

Mechanisms 1 and 2 are often referred to as 'non-informative', 'independent', or 'ignorable' while mechanism 3 is often referred to as 'informative'.

If we believe censoring is at random conditional on the covariates in our substantive survival model, there is nothing to be gained by imputing censored event times. MI is however useful if event times are plausibly CAR, conditional on a number of variables, $X_1, \dots, X_p$, but we wish to estimate either the marginal survival distribution, or a survival regression with a subset of the covariates. Just as in the standard regression setting, discussed in Chapter 1, fitting the model to the observed data with no covariates (i.e. a marginal summary), or with only a subset of the p covariates, gives invalid results – because we are not conditioning on all the variables required for CAR to hold. In addition, as in the regression setting, we may also have additional (auxiliary) variables predictive of event time, which we might wish to include to improve our prediction of censored event times, but which we do not wish to include in our substantive model.

The strategy is to use MI to impute the censored event times, including in the imputation model all the covariates necessary for CAR as well as those not involved in the CAR mechanism but nevertheless predictive of survival. We proceed as follows:

1. Use a time-to-event model with all p covariates as an imputation model and impute the censored event times, creating K 'completed' datasets with no censored observations;
2. fit the substantive model to each imputed dataset;
3. combine the results for inference using Rubin's rules.

As usual, the imputation model needs to contain the covariates needed for (i) CAR to hold and (ii) that are in the substantive model, compatible with any interactions, or non-linear relationships, among covariates in the substantive model. We also need to be careful that we apply Rubin's rules to quantities with at least approximately normal sampling distributions.

The algorithms described thus far in this chapter all include steps for updating the coefficients of the survival model, which in turn allow the calculation of an estimate of the survivor function $\hat{S}(t|\boldsymbol{\beta}, X_1, \dots, X_p)$. At each iteration of the algorithm, immediately following this update step, impute the censored event times as follows:

1. for each censored unit i, censored at T_i, calculate
$$p_i = 1 - \hat{S}(T_i|\boldsymbol{\beta}, X_{i,1}, \dots, X_{i,p}),$$
2. draw $u_i \sim \text{uniform}[p_i, 1]$, and
3. impute the censored event time, say T_i^*, as the solution of $u_j = 1 - \hat{S}(T_i^*|\boldsymbol{\beta}, X_{i,1}, \dots, X_{i,p})$.

This ensures that each imputed event time is greater than the time at which the unit was censored.

If we wish to do sensitivity analyses with respect to the CAR assumption, we will need to impute censored event times with a hazard modified from the CAR estimate. We discuss this in Chapter 10, Section 10.3.3.

Next we consider non-parametric MI, and then discuss a non-parametric approach to MI for survival data proposed by Hsu *et al.* (2006).

7.3 Non-parametric, or 'hot deck' imputation

Thus far, we have only discussed parametric imputation models, that is choosing, estimating, and imputing from a parametric statistical model for the distribution of the missing data given the observed data. Here, we briefly consider non-parametric imputation also known as 'hot deck' imputation – we explain the name below.

To describe the approach, suppose we have $Y_1, \dots, Y_{p'}$ fully observed discrete variables, and $Y_{p'+1}, \dots, Y_p$ partially observed variables of any type. Then the p' discrete variables form G exclusive subgroups of the data, indexed by $g = 1, \dots, G$, each with n_g members, where $\sum_{g=1}^{G} n_g = n$, the sample size. We further assume that within each group, one or more units have all of the remaining $p - p'$ variables observed. Within each group, we order the observations so that $i = 1, \dots, n_{g_O}$ units are fully observed, and $i = (n_{g_O} + 1), \dots, n_g$ are partially observed.

Non-parametric imputation proceeds independently within each group g as follows:

1. Sample with replacement, n_{g_O} times from the fully observed units $i \in (1, \dots, n_{g_O})$, with probability $1/n_{g_O}$, to form the donor pool,
$$\{\mathbf{Y}_1^\star, \dots, \mathbf{Y}_{n_{g_O}}^\star\}.$$
2. For each unit $i = (n_{g_O} + 1), \dots, n_g$, with missing data, draw a donor from the donor pool $\{\mathbf{Y}_1^\star, \dots, \mathbf{Y}_{n_{g_O}}^\star\}$ with equal probability with replacement. Impute missing values of $\mathbf{Y}_i$ with values from this donor.

These two steps give an imputed group g, with no missing data. Applying the same algorithm for each group $g = 1, \dots, G$ gives a complete imputed dataset.

Repeating the whole process gives a series of imputed datasets, $k = 1, \dots, K$. The substantive model is then fitted to each imputed data set in turn, and the results combined for inference using Rubin's rules. This algorithm was proposed by Rubin and Schenker (1986).

The term 'hot-deck' imputation arose when data were stored on punched cards. A deck of cards were 'hot' because it was currently being processed; for a unit with missing data, we select a card from the current 'hot deck' and substitute it (i.e. impute from it).

The double resampling in the above algorithm approximates the Bayesian bootstrap (Rubin, 1981). The non-parametric imputation algorithm above is therefore a version of the Bayesian bootstrap; see Chapter 6, page 218. This reflects uncertainty in estimating the resampling probabilities p_i within each group g.

Rubin and Schenker (1986) showed the validity of Rubin's rules in this context for constructing a confidence interval for large n and fixed K. They also showed the consistency of the variance estimator as sample size and number of imputations tend to infinity. However, Kim (2002) considers non-parametric imputation for the sample mean and shows that the MI variance formula underestimates the variance with the bias of order n^{-2}. In the context of the sample mean, Kim gives a formula for a reduced donor group size to compensate for this. Rao and Wu (1988) discuss related points in the context of survey sampling.

However, non-parametric imputation is attractive in very large datasets, such as a census, where parametric imputation is likely to prove cumbersome. Thus, in practice, the principal concern is not likely to be the validity of Rubin's rules, but instead how to form appropriate donor groups – in other words deciding on the groups within which units are exchangeable. In our motivating discussion, we avoided this issue by assuming that the fully observed variables were categorical and using their values to form groups. More generally, one might consider using Malahanobis distance or kth nearest neighbours. An alternative is to use the propensity score (Rosenbaum and Rubin, 1983). Simply speaking, one uses logistic regression to estimate the probability of data being missing, and then forms donor groups from units with similar probabilities. This is discussed more fully in, for example Lavori *et al.* (1995).

The key advantage of non-parametric imputation is that it is compatible with all interactions and complex relationships within the data, and these do not have to be specified. Unfortunately, this advantage will not be realised if the matching itself introduces bias. Assuming that it does not, however, the remaining disadvantage is that it is inefficient relative to parametric imputation. One can look at it in terms of a bias-variance trade off. If we form valid donor pools, then non-parametric imputation will be unbiased, but the parameter estimates will be less precise than a correctly specified parametric imputation model.

In very large datasets, such as census data, there is a lot of information to form donor pools and precision is not a major concern; thus non-parametric imputation is attractive. Conversely, in smaller studies, such as those considered in this book, parametric imputation is most likely preferable. For an application in imputing health records, including consideration of issues raised by MNAR data, see Siddique and Belin (2008). Andridge and Little (2010) give a good overview, highlighting the diversity of approaches to non-parametric imputation and the lack of consensus on how to obtain inferences from the completed dataset.

7.3.1 Non-parametric imputation for time-to-event data

As the proportional hazards model is semi-parametric, with the baseline hazard unspecified, it is natural to consider non-parametric imputation. Hsu, Taylor, and Murray consider this in a series of articles (Taylor *et al.*, 2002, Hsu *et al.*, 2006,2007, Hsu and Taylor, 2009); we outline their approach. As discussed in Section 7.2, the aim is to impute censored event times using auxiliary variables, thus increasing the plausibility of CAR, and then estimate either the marginal survival distribution or the marginal effect of a subset of covariates.

For unit $i = 1, \dots, n$, we have as before data T_i and D_i, where T_i is the survival time if $D_i = 1$ and T_i is the censoring time if $D_i = 0$. We denote the ith unit's covariates by the p by 1 column vector $\mathbf{X}_i = (X_{i,1}, \dots, X_{i,p})^T$, so that each unit's data are $(T_i, D_i, \mathbf{X}_i)$. The algorithm is then as follows:

1. Sample the n units with replacement and form the corresponding bootstrap dataset
$$\{(T_i, D_i, \mathbf{X}_i)^\star\}_{i=1,\dots,n}.$$
2. Use the bootstrap data to estimate an appropriate metric defining the distance $d(i,j)$ 'between' unit i and j, as discussed below.
3. For each unit i with censored event time,
   (a) identify the set of N nearest neighbours using the distance metric,
   (b) using the set of data from the nearest neighbours, calculate the Kaplan–Meier estimate of the survivor function, $\hat{S}_i$, and
   (c) use $\hat{S}_i$ to impute the unseen event time, $\widetilde{T}_i$ for unit i, subject to $T_i^* \geq T_i$, the censoring time.

Steps 1–3 create a single imputed dataset; we repeat the whole process to obtain K imputed datasets. Repeating step 1 as part of each imputation is important, as discussed on p. 245, to ensure appropriate between-imputation variability for the MI variance estimator. Using the Kaplan–Meier estimate in step 3, the procedure will always impute an event time from one of the observed event times among the nearest neighbours, unless the last observation time among the nearest neighbours is censored, in which case occasionally a censored time may be imputed.

The metric is derived as follows:

(i) fit the proportional hazards model to the bootstrap data generated in Step 1, using all the available covariates, giving parameter estimates $\hat{\boldsymbol{\beta}}$;

(ii) using $\hat{\boldsymbol{\beta}}$, calculate each unit's risk score, i.e. their linear predictor, $Z_i = \mathbf{X}_i^T \hat{\boldsymbol{\beta}}$;

(iii) calculate $d_i^S = (Z_i - \overline{Z})/\hat{\sigma}_Z$, where $\overline{Z}$ and $\hat{\sigma}_Z$ are, respectively, the sample mean and standard deviation of the Z_i's; and

(iv) define $d^S(i,j) = (d_i^S - d_j^S)^2$.

Within the current bootstrap dataset, we then construct the donor pool for unit i as the $j = 1, \dots, N$ 'nearest neighbours' as measured by $d^S(i,j)$. If the covariates have missing values, one option is to generate a single imputed data set using one of the approaches of Section 7.1 in order to generate a working data set to calculate the distances.

In applications, Hsu *et al.* (2006) show performance can be further improved by, in step (i), additionally fitting a second model with time to censoring, rather than event time, as the outcome. This is simply achieved by changing the event indicator from D_i to $1 - D_i$. Then for unit i, we can analogously define d_i^C, and $d^C(i,j)$ (C for censoring). We can then choose the N nearest neighbours for unit i in terms of

$$\sqrt{w_S d^S(i,j) + w_C d^C(i,j)}, \tag{7.14}$$

where w_S and w_C are non-negative weights that sum to 1, and typically $w_S = w_C = 0.5$.

As Hsu *et al.* demonstrate, the advantage of this procedure is that it induces a form of double robustness: if either the model for the time-to-event or the censoring time is correct, then in large samples, the survival estimate from this procedure will be have good properties because conditional on the two risk scores, event and censoring times will be independent. In smaller samples, bias may occur because within the neighbourhood, censoring and event time may not be independent. In moderate sample sizes (n =300–500), their simulation study demonstrates small bias and good coverage if both time-to-event and time-to-censoring models are correct. If not, there is some bias, but this can be alleviated if in (7.14), instead of weighting d^S and d^C equally, we up-weight the model that is correct. The simulation studies suggest that $N = 10$ is a reasonable choice for the number of nearest neighbours. The non-parametric imputation approach for time-to-event data developed by Hsu *et al.* is implemented in the R package `InformativeCensoring`.

Hsu *et al.* (2007) describe the application of this approach to interval censored survival data. Here, the model required to determine the distances and to impute survival times within sets of nearest neighbours is no longer the proportional hazards/Kaplan–Meier model, but the non-parametric model for the interval censored data (Peto, 1973). Further, with interval-censored data, they report that using linear interpolation to smooth the estimated survivor function before imputing reduces bias. This is because interpolation compensates for the fact that survivor functions estimated from interval-censored data inevitably have fewer, larger, jumps than the underlying survival curve. Again, a simulation study shows good performance.

In applications, Monte Carlo error is likely to be larger than with parametric imputation methods, so a greater number of imputations may be desirable, say $K = 100$.

7.4 Case–cohort designs

In this section, we consider missing data and imputation in the case–cohort design as described by Keogh *et al.* (2018). A case–cohort design is one of the main approaches for carrying out a sub-study within a prospective cohort; another common design is the nested-case–control study. Sub-studies are generally used to reduce costs by measuring expensive covariates only on individuals with the outcome of interest (the 'cases') and a subset of the non-cases. In a case–cohort study a random sample of individuals from the full cohort is selected at the start of follow-up – the 'subcohort' – and the case–cohort sample is this sub-cohort plus all the cases from the rest of the cohort. Borgan and Samuelsen (2013) provides a useful overview of this design, which is increasing in its use (Sharp *et al.*, 2014). This section describes how multiple imputation for handling missing covariates in full-cohort studies can be adapted for case–cohort studies.

7.4.1 Standard analysis of case–cohort studies

Before discussing various motivations and options for performing MI in case–cohort studies, we first describe the standard approach to their analysis. We assume that interest lies in modelling how the hazard depends on covariates X_1, X_2, and Z. The variable(s) X_1 is only measured in the sub-study, and is thus missing by design. X_2 and Z are measured in the full cohort.

The substantive model is a Cox proportional hazards model

$$h(t|X_1, X_2, Z) = h_0(t)\exp(\beta_{X_1}X_1 + \beta_{X_2}X_2 + \beta_Z Z).$$

If we consider only the sub-cohort data (i.e. not including the data on cases outside the sub-cohort), since the missingness (in X_1) is by design and is completely at random, we could fit the substantive model Cox model to only the sub-cohort data. This complete records analysis would be valid, but not fully efficient, since it does not exploit the additional information in the cases which are not in the sub-cohort.

The standard approach to estimating the parameters of the Cox substantive model exploits the information in the cases which are not in the sub-cohort by including these additional cases in Cox's partial likelihood, as we now describe. Let $\tau_1, \tau_2, \ldots, \tau_J$ denote the unique event times in the full cohort, assuming no ties for simplicity. The analysis of the full-cohort data would maximise the partial likelihood,

$$L_{\text{full-cohort}} = \prod_{j=1}^{J} \frac{e^{\beta'_{X_1}X_{1i_j}+\beta'_{X_2}X_{2i_j}+\beta'_Z Z_{i_j}}}{\sum_{k\in\mathcal{R}_j} e^{\beta'_{X_1}X_{1k}+\beta'_{X_2}X_{2k}+\beta'_Z Z_k}},$$

where i_j is the index of the individual who has the event at time τ_j ($j = 1, \ldots, J$) and $\mathcal{R}_j$ denotes the set of individuals at risk in the full cohort at time τ_j. In the analysis of the case–cohort study we have data on all cases, and so the product remains over all J cases. However, we do not have access to the covariate information of all individuals in the risk set $\mathcal{R}_j$. We do however have access to the covariate information for a random subset of these, and we can use this in the denominator of the partial likelihood expression. That is, we use the modified partial likelihood equation:

$$L_{\text{substudy}} = \prod_{j=1}^{J} \frac{e^{\beta'_{X_1}X_{1i_j}+\beta'_{X_2}X_{2i_j}+\beta'_Z Z_{i_j}}}{\sum_{k\in\mathcal{R}^*_j} e^{\beta'_{X_1}X_{1k}+\beta'_{X_2}X_{2k}+\beta'_Z Z_k}},$$

where $\mathcal{R}^*_j$ denotes the subset of individuals at risk at time τ_j who are in the sub-study plus the case at time τ_j if that case is outside the sub-cohort. L_{substudy} is a pseudo–partial likelihood, thus a sandwich estimator or appropriate alternative should be used for standard errors (Borgan and Samuelsen, 2013).

7.4.2 Multiple imputation for case–cohort studies

There are two general types of missing data relevant to case–cohort designs:

- **Missing by design:** Covariates measured only in the sub-study (X_1) are missing by design in the remainder of the full cohort.
- **Sporadic missing data:** Covariates which are measured in the full cohort are commonly subject to sporadic missingness (X_2), and it may be reasonable to make the assumption that data are missing at random.

Depending on what data are available to the analyst and what assumptions they are willing to rely on, MI can potentially handle both types of missingness.

As originally framed, the analyst only has access to data from members of the sub-study – the sub-cohort plus any cases not in the sub-cohort. Here we may contemplate using MI to handle sporadic missingness in X_2.

Alternatively, the analyst may have access to all of the observed data from the full cohort plus the measurements of X_1 from the sub-study. Here we might consider using MI to impute both the sporadic missingness in X_2 and the values in X_1 missing by design. A final possibility is that the analyst has access to the sub-study data plus information on (T, D) in the full cohort.

In the following subsections, we describe different MI methods suitable for these different settings.

7.4.3 Full cohort

If we have information on all the observed data from the full cohort plus the measurements of X_1 from the sub-study, we may choose to impute the missing (by design) values of X_1 plus any sporadic missing values in X_2, in a so-called 'full-cohort' approach. While we would not expect major efficiency gains for the coefficient of X_1, we may expect gains for the others.

In this case the setup falls within that considered earlier in Section 7.1. Since in the observed full cohort dataset X_1 is missing by design, with missingness dependent on the fully observed (T, D), the missingness is at random provided any sporadic missingness in X_2 is MAR. As such, we could adopt either an approximately compatible approach as described in Section 7.1.1 or a SMC type approach such as SMC-FCS, as described in 7.1.2. The Cox model is then fitted to the entire cohort in the imputed datasets and estimates and variances combined using Rubin's rules in the usual way. Keogh and White (2013) investigated the approximately compatible approach and a version of SMC MI, showing that an MI analysis using full cohort data can lead to important gains in efficiency compared with the traditional sub-study analysis.

7.4.4 Intermediate approaches

Typically, the subcohort may be a rather small proportion of the full cohort. In this case, one may be wary about using the full-cohort MI approach, since it involves imputing (and subsequently analysing) a very large fraction of missing values. In particular, one may be concerned that even relatively minor misspecification in the imputation model may lead to non-trivial biases.

An alternative to alleviate such concerns is to generate the imputed datasets using the full cohort but only fit the substantive model to the sub-study data. This approach will only rely on correct specification of the imputation model for X_1 only in so far as there are sporadic missing values in X_1 in the sub-study. The drawback is of course that it will not be as efficient as the full cohort approach. Indeed, it would only be expected to be more efficient than an approach (to be described next) that only uses data from the sub-study in so far as uncertainty about the imputation model parameters is reduced through fitting it to the full cohort. Since this intermediate approach fits the imputation model to the same observed full cohort data, its validity rests on the same missingness assumptions as the full cohort approach.

7.4.5 Sub-study approach

Now suppose we use or only have access to data from the sub-study. Suppose further for simplicity there are no sporadic missing values in X_1 within the sub-study. The task therefore is to impute the sporadic missing values in X_2. The imputation distribution for X_2 is $f(X_2|T,D,X_1,Z,S=1)$, where $S=1$ denotes that an individual belongs to the sub-study. Since $P(S=1|T,D,X_1,X_2,Z)=P(S=1|D)$, it follows that $f(X_2|T,D,X_1,Z,S=1)=f(X_2|T,D,X_1,Z)$. That is, we should fit and impute from a full population model for X_2 given the other variables. This justifies the following adapted versions of MI when values in X_2 are sporadically MAR in the sub-study.

Approximately compatible MI

The approximately compatible MI approach described in Section 7.1.1 requires an estimate of the cumulative baseline hazard $H_0(t)$, which we typically approximate by an estimate of the marginal cumulative hazard $H(t)$. In settings where information on (T,D) is available for the full cohort, one could simply use the Nelson–Aalen estimate from the full cohort. If not, one could use the Nelson–Aalen estimate obtained using the subcohort only. A drawback to this route is that it does not exploit information in the cases which are not in the subcohort. To address this, Keogh *et al.* (2018) proposed using a weighted estimator of $H(t)$ that uses information from cases not in subcohort and the subcohort sampling fraction:

$$\hat{H}_{CC}(t)=\frac{n_S(0)}{n}\sum_{\tau_k\le t}\frac{d(\tau_k)}{n_S(\tau_k)},$$

where $d(\tau_k)$ is the number of events at time τ_k (in our setting, $d(\tau_k)=1$), $n_S(\tau_k)$ is the number at risk in the sub-cohort at time τ_k, and n is the total number in the cohort. This exploits the fact that (in expectation) the ratio of the number at risk in the full cohort to the number at risk in the sub-cohort is approximately constant over time $(n/n_S(0))$, which is implied by the random sampling into the sub-cohort. The practical feasibility of using this estimator is increased by the fact that $\hat{H}_{CC}(t)$ is proportional to $\sum_{\tau_k \leq t} \frac{d(\tau_k)}{n_S(\tau_k)}$, which is approximately equal to $\hat{H}^*_{CC}(t) = \sum_{\tau_k \leq t} \frac{d(\tau_k)}{n_{cc}(\tau_k)}$, where $n_{cc}(\tau_k) = n_S(\tau_k)$ if the case whose event time is τ_k is in the sub-cohort and $n_{cc}(\tau_k) = n_S(\tau_k) + 1$ otherwise. This means that $\hat{H}^*_{CC}(t)$ can be obtained directly by applying the Nelson–Aalen estimator to the sub-study data.

Substantive model compatible MI

With missing values in X_2, the substantive model compatible approach requires us to specify and fit a model for $f(X_2|X_1, Z)$ (note that this is in the full cohort/population) and to estimate $H_0(t)$. In general $f(X_2|X_1, Z, S = 1)$ will not equal $f(X_2|X_1, Z)$, and similarly the cumulative baseline hazard will differ in the sub-study from the full cohort. Because of this, one cannot apply SMC MI approaches to only the sub-study data without modification.

For the covariate model $f(X_2|X_1, Z)$, we can obtain valid estimates by fitting the model to only those individuals in the sub-cohort (i.e. excluding those cases not in the sub-cohort). For the cumulative baseline hazard $H_0(t)$, within each iteration of the SMC MI algorithm, we can make use of a modified Breslow estimator (Borgan and Samuelsen, 2013):

$$\hat{H}_0^{CC}(t) = \frac{n_S(0)}{n} \sum_{\tau_k \leq \tau} \frac{1}{\sum_{l \in S_k} \exp(\hat{\beta}_{X_1} X_{1,l} + \hat{\beta}_{X_2} X_{2,l} + \hat{\beta}_Z Z_l)},$$

where S_k denotes the set of sub-cohort members who are at risk at time τ_k, and the regression coefficients are calculated at their current values. This estimator uses the sub-cohort sampling fraction $\frac{n_S(0)}{n}$, which is typically known. These modifications for case–cohort studies are available in the R package `smcfcs`.

Example 7.3 ARIC study cohort

Keogh *et al.* (2018) applied the previously described MI approaches to data from the ARIC Study cohort to investigate the association between death due to cardiovascular disease and the traditional risk factors of systolic blood pressure (mmHG), total and HDL cholesterol (mmol/l), smoking and body mass index (BMI), with adjustment for sex, age, race, and education level. The cohort comprises 15,792 individuals, and there were 1089 cardiovascular deaths over the course of follow-up. A case–cohort study was created by sampling a sub-cohort of 650 individuals reflecting a real example (Sanders *et al.*, 2014). Measurements of total and HDL cholesterol were set to be missing outside of the sub-study, creating missingness by design. Missingness by chance was introduced in systolic blood pressure, smoking status, BMI, race, and education level; the probability of missingness depended on sex and age, and 10% missing data was generated conditionally independently in each variable in the full cohort.

Age, systolic blood pressure, total cholesterol, HDL cholesterol, and BMI are continuous variables and were assumed to have linear effects on the log hazard. The remaining variables were treated as categorical. Table 7.3 shows estimates for the resulting Cox model based on the full cohort, a complete records case–cohort, the

Table 7.3 Results from applying MI methods to the ARIC cohort with case–cohort sub-study, to investigate the association between the variables listed and the hazard for death due to cardiovascular disease. The estimates (standard errors) are log hazard ratios.

	Complete-data full cohort	Complete records case–cohort	MI full cohort approach		MI substudy approach		MI intermediate approach	
			MI-approx	SMC-FCS	MI-approx	SMC-FCS	MI-approx	SMC-FCS
Male	Reference							
Female	−0.481	−0.796	−0.436	−0.453	−0.508	−0.481	−0.282	−0.502
	(0.073)	(0.188)	(0.072)	(0.071)	(0.139)	(0.140)	(0.140)	(0.140)
*Education: 1	Reference							
Education: 2	−0.149	0.323	−0.119	−0.090	0.066	0.026	0.062	0.052
	(0.092)	(0.274)	(0.096)	(0.101)	(0.208)	(0.214)	(0.214)	(0.218)
Education: 3	−0.426	0.136	−0.373	−0.369	−0.093	−0.097	−0.080	−0.114
	(0.097)	(0.288)	(0.101)	(0.103)	(0.211)	(0.215)	(0.221)	(0.233)
Non-smoker	Reference							
Current smoker	0.641	0.735	0.609	0.622	0.584	0.609	0.595	0.610
	(0.067)	(0.178)	(0.071)	(0.070)	(0.140)	(0.141)	(0.143)	(0.141)
White race	Reference							
Non-white race	0.434	0.456	0.508	0.498	0.363	0.319	0.365	0.355
	(0.072)	(0.201)	(0.077)	(0.080)	(0.159)	(0.159)	(0.161)	(0.166)
SBP (mmHG)	0.015	0.008	0.015	0.015	0.012	0.013	0.013	0.013
	(0.002)	(0.004)	(0.002)	(0.002)	(0.004)	(0.003)	(0.004)	(0.004)
BMI (kg/m^2)	0.040	0.060	0.037	0.038	0.042	0.042	0.040	0.042
	(0.006)	(0.019)	(0.006)	(0.006)	(0.014)	(0.014)	(0.014)	(0.014)
Total chol (mmol/l)	0.055	0.055	0.037	0.043	0.026	0.028	0.028	0.028
	(0.030)	(0.066)	(0.043)	(0.050)	(0.052)	(0.052)	(0.052)	(0.052)
HDL chol (mmol/l)	−0.453	−0.427	−0.637	−0.600	−0.473	−0.458	−0.477	−0.464
	(0.102)	(0.275)	(0.134)	(0.110)	(0.187)	(0.187)	(0.187)	(0.187)

*Education levels: 1 = Primary, 2 = Secondary, 3 = Vocational/University.

approximately compatible MI approach, and SMC-FCS. For the two MI approaches, results are presented based on the full cohort, sub-study, and intermediate versions, as described previously.

The log hazard ratio estimates are broadly similar across the different analyses. The MI full cohort approach gives standard errors that are typically less than half those obtained in the complete records case–cohort analysis, with the gain in efficiency being somewhat less for the two cholesterol variables, which are missing by design in the full cohort. The MI sub-study and intermediate approaches give smaller but still substantial gains in efficiency. The following explanatory variables are statistically significantly associated with an increased hazard for CVD death ($p < 0.05$) in all analyses: being male, older age, smoking, non-white race, higher BMI. The following additional explanatory variables are statistically significantly associated with an increased hazard in the full cohort analysis and in all MI analyses, but not in the CRA: lower level of education (not in MI-approx and MI-SMC in the sub-study and intermediate approaches), higher SBP, lower HDL cholesterol. □

7.5 Discussion

In this chapter, we have considered issues raised in the analyses of survival/time-to-event data where MI may be usefully applied. Principal among these issues is that both time-to-event and censoring information need to be appropriately included when imputing missing values of covariates. Failure to do so can severely bias effect estimates towards the null, as was partly the case in Hippisley-Cox *et al.* (2007); see also related discussion in Sterne *et al.* (2009).

Exercises

The aim of this exercise is to appreciate the difference compatibility can make in survival models and to understand how compatible imputation models can be implemented.

We will use data from the German Breast Cancer Study Group (GBSG) (see Royston and Sauerbrei (2008) p. 262–3). The GBSG breast cancer dataset can be downloaded from https://mfp.imbi.uni-freiburg.de/book#dataset_tables, which includes the dataset in `.csv`, `dta`, `sas7bdat` and `.xls` formats.

The data describe recurrence-free survival (the earlier of death or disease recurrence) in 686 women with primary breast cancer. There are 299 events for this outcome. The aim is to produce a useful prognostic model.

Thus, we focus on fitting a Cox survival model on the seven covariates: age (years), meno (post-menopausal binary status), grade (tumour grade 1, 2, or 3), nodes (number of nodes), pgr (progesterone receptor, fmol/l), tam (binary indicator for treatment of tamoxifen), and size (tumour size, mm).

1. Since the data are largely complete, for the purpose of illustration, we will first induce approximately 20% missing at random data in size, grade, nodes, and pgr, dependent on age as follows:

  (a) Generate a variable `age2` equal to age if `age` is 35–70 years; equal to 35 if age is less than 35 years; equal to 70 if age is greater than 70 years.

  (b) For `meno` and `pgr`, make

$$P(R) = \text{expit}(0.07 \times (50 - \text{age2}) - 1.5)$$

  and draw missingness indicators for meno and pgr separately as Bernoulli random draws with the specified probability. Use the missingness indicator variables generated to set observed values to missing.

  (c) For `grade`, `nodes` and `size`, make

$$P(R) = \text{expit}(0.07 \times (\text{age2} - 50) - 1.7)$$

  and draw a single missingness indicator for the three variables simultaneously as a Bernoulli random draw with the specified probability. Again, use the missingness indicator variable generated to set observed values to missing.

  (d) The probability of missingness as a function of age is given in Figure 7.1.

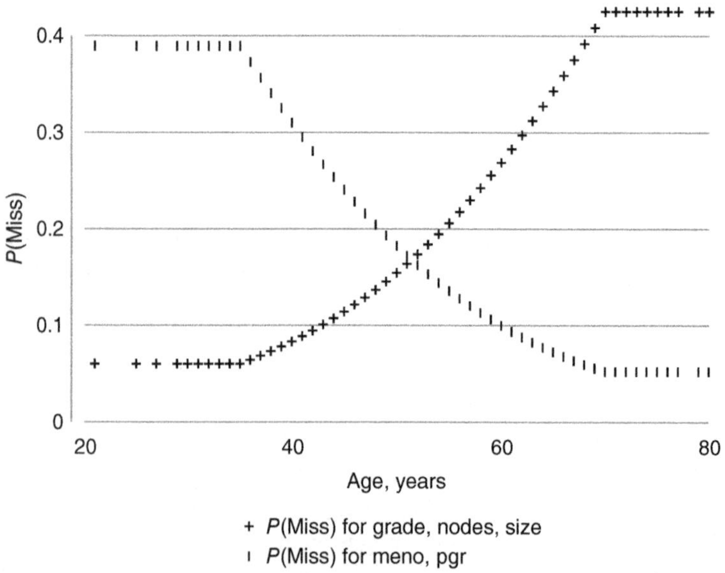

Figure 7.1 Probability of missingness for covariates as a function of age.

2. **Complete records analysis**: Fit the Cox regression model for time to death or disease recurrence on the seven covariates, using a CRA. Note the number of individuals included in this analysis.

3. **Imputation omitting the survival outcome**: Use FCS MI to multiply impute grade nodes pgr size and meno 10 times. Carefully select an appropriate imputation model for each variable, but do not include the survival outcome (both time-to-event and censoring indicator) in the imputation models. Now fit the Cox regression model of interest to the MI data and obtained the pooled results. How have results changed compared with complete cases? Do the results fit with what you expected?

4. **Imputation including the survival outcome**: Now re-do the imputation with a model that includes the survival outcome through the Nelson–Aalen estimator and the censoring indicator. As before, perform the MI analysis model of interest. How have the results changed compared with complete cases and those from an MI approach with the outcome omitted? Do the results fit with what you expected?

5. **MI analysis using SMC-FCS**: Using the Stata package `smcfcs` or R package `smcfcs`, perform a multiple imputation analysis using SMC-FCS, to fit the same Cox model above. How are the results different?

8

Prognostic models, missing data, and multiple imputation

> The impact of missing data on out-of-sample prediction performance is uniformly understated in the statistical and clinical literature
>
> — Fletcher Mercaldo and Blume (2018)

8.1 Introduction

This chapter discusses the approaches to handling missing data when the aims of an analysis involve *prediction*. To be clear about this context, the aim of the analysis is not to produce some multivariable model reporting 'risk factors' but to develop and validate a prognostic model or rule that might be implemented in medical practice to enhance decision-making by producing accurate predictions about patients' prognoses.

This practical context is important to bear in mind for several reasons. The majority of chapters in this book focuses on parameter estimation, and in chapter 1, we detailed what we regard as attractive properties of an estimator, such as (asymptotic) unbiasedness for one or more parameters of interest. For the purposes of prediction, we also wish to evaluate the quality of predictions that result from the use of a particular multivariable rule or model. Interest is in measures of predictive performance, in particular when applied to data outside of the development sample. To have any hope of realising the claimed predictive performance at the point of implementation, we must either ensure that at this point all predictors will be measured, or alternatively have a method for handling missing data that is *implementable* at that point.

Multiple Imputation and its Application, Second Edition.
James R. Carpenter, Jonathan W. Bartlett, Tim P. Morris, Angela M. Wood, Matteo Quartagno and Michael G. Kenward.

8.2 Motivating example

The QRISK®-3 risk prediction model, described in Hippisley-Cox *et al.* (2017), calculates an individual's risk of developing cardiovascular disease over the next 10 years. The model has been developed by doctors and academics working in the UK National Health Service based on routinely collected data from thousands of general practices (GPs) across the United Kingdom who have freely contributed data to the QResearch database for medical research. A 2 : 1 split-sample approach was used to develop the model (development sample) and validate it (validation sample).

Due to the nature of the data collection, there were up to 70% of missing values for some predictor variables. Consequently, multiple imputation was used to impute the missing values in risk predictors in the development (training) sample, and also separately in the validation sample. For clinical implementation of the tool, the QRISK-3 algorithm has built-in methods for substituting missing values of risk factors using age-, sex-, and ethnicity-specific population average values. Notably, this substitution approach for implementation is different from the multiple-imputation approach used for model development and validation, and to our knowledge has not yet been validated. The QRISK-3 developers distinguish between 'actual' QRISK-3 cardiovascular disease scores, which are calculated where all values needed to calculate the score are available, and 'estimated' QRISK-3 cardiovascular disease scores, which are calculated not only using the available data but also using substituted values based on ethnicity, age, and sex.

8.3 Missing data at model implementation

As illustrated in the motivating example above, the role of missing data in prognostic modelling needs consideration at model development and validation. To decide how to handle missing data, we need to consider different scenarios at model implementation:

1. **Complete data at implementation** denotes the context in which there would be no missing data in risk predictors for individuals when the model is used to make predictions;
2. **Incomplete data at implementation** denotes contexts in which there would be missing data in risk predictors for some individuals when the model is used to make predictions.

It is necessary to be clear about the presumed implementation context when we consider how to handle missing data during the development and validation of a model. First, because any model developed must be *implementable*. If it is not, either the model cannot be implemented, or it has to be modified to be implemented. In the latter case, a model's *advertised* performance may not then quantify the performance of the model as actually implemented (*model performance* will be discussed in Section 8.6). As a simple example, suppose we are faced with an incomplete dataset for model development and validation but would have complete data at implementation. Suppose the model is developed and validated using the complete records. The performance estimated at validation will then not in general match the group (everyone) for whom it would be implemented, unless data at both model development and model validation are missing completely at random (MCAR). Tsvetanova and colleagues' review of the literature found such mismatches to be extremely common in practice (Tsvetanova *et al.*, 2021), as in the QRISK-3 example of Section 8.2.

Prior to Section 8.8, we will assume that there will be complete data at implementation, or at least that the goal is to develop a prediction model which anticipates the full set of predictors to be available. In Section 8.8, we then consider how things change when incomplete data at implementation are anticipated.

8.4 Multiple imputation for prognostic modelling

Suppose for a moment that we have a pre-specified prognostic model for the distribution of the outcome given a set of predictors, and we have some missingness in the predictors (and possibly outcomes) in the development dataset. We then seek to use multiple imputation (MI) to provide unbiased and precise estimates of the parameters in the prognostic model, on the basis that that is what we would seek to obtain had the development data been complete. As such, the considerations described in the book thus far apply. In particular, we should impute missing predictors using imputation models that condition on the outcome variable. If the substantive model is non-linear or contains non-linear covariate effects, missing values in the predictors should be imputed compatibly with the substantive model, as described in Chapters 6 and 7.

After performing MI, we obtain from Rubin's rules an estimate $\hat{\beta}_{MI}$. To predict the outcome for future individuals, remembering that for now we assume that predictors for new individuals will be complete, we simply calculate the model predicted outcome using $\hat{\beta}_{MI}$.

8.5 Model building

In practice, the form of the prognostic model is rarely, if ever, pre-specified. Model building or selection is used in order to arrive at a model with good prognostic performance. Where a large number of potential predictors are available, our model building process may also need to consider the potential cost or difficulty of measuring each potential predictor.

8.5.1 Model building with missing data

Model building may include variable selection, tests for interactions, selecting shapes of relationships (e.g. fractional polynomials) and penalisation. Following Wood *et al.* (2008), we outline several model building approaches which could be used when some data are missing. Many of the procedures involve hypothesis tests for use on multiply imputed data, as described in Chapter 2, including Wald tests and Meng and Rubin's likelihood-ratio tests (Meng and Rubin, 1992), see Section 2.5.

Model building in complete records

The single complete records development dataset, consisting of individuals with non-missing values for all potential predictors, may be used for model building. An alternative approach uses available cases (*i.e.*, individuals with non-missing values for the predictors under current consideration) at each stage of the model building process. Using complete records or available cases may fail to detect important predictors due to loss of power and, when missing data are not MCAR, may select unimportant variables due to biased regression estimates.

Model building in a single stochastic or deterministic imputation

A single imputed dataset may be used for variable selection, not only maintaining the convenience of dealing with a single dataset but also reducing inefficiency caused by excluding individuals in the complete records approach and missing data biases. However, model building is then performed under the assumption that the imputed data were actually fully observed, resulting in estimated standard errors being too small and an increased chance of accepting noise variables. For a stochastic imputation, it is very possible that different model builds would result from different single imputations.

Model building in each imputation then summarise

Rather than choosing one imputed dataset for model building, the procedure can be performed separately in a number of imputed datasets. This approach may select a range of different models across imputed datasets, but this can be overcome by applying pragmatic rules for summarising across the imputations. For example, in a variable selection, we could select predictors that appear in any, at least half or in all the imputation-specific models. Bear in mind that selecting variables appearing in all or any imputation-specific models is dependent on the number of imputations used, and this approach may not be useful for large K.

Model building based on MI combination rules

Model building can be conducted interactively within the Rubin inferential framework, *i.e.*, decision rules are applied to the pooled parameter estimates and tests based on these. For example, in the backwards selection approach, we first fit a model which includes all candidate predictors. We then remove the predictor which has the highest p-value. With multiply imputed datasets, we can calculate a p-value for each predictor from this full model based on Rubin's rules. We then remove the predictor with the largest Rubin's rule p-value and proceed to fit the simpler model in each imputed dataset, pooling as usual with Rubin's rules. A potential practical difficulty with this approach is that for large datasets and large K, the computational cost may be prohibitive, but such concerns are reduced given increasing computational capacity.

Model building in the stacked dataset

Another possible method is to apply model building to one large 'stacked' dataset. Briefly, the K imputed datasets (i.e. observed and imputed data) are 'stacked' on top of each other as though they were one large dataset. Models can then be fitted to this single stacked dataset. The resulting estimator is asymptotically equivalent to the MI estimator $\hat{\beta}_{MI}$ (Wang and Robins, 1998), and so variable selection can legitimately be based on the stacked data estimated coefficients. However, the naive standard errors obtained from fitting the model to the stacked data are too small – they ignore the fact that some data have been imputed, and that the sample size is only n, not $K \times n$. To account for this, Wood *et al.* (2008) investigated using a weighted fit of the model to the stacked data. For large datasets with relatively small amounts of missingness, fitting models to the stacked data with each observation assigned a weight of $1/K$ can be used. Wood *et al.* (2008) also motivated and investigated use of some alternative weighting schemes which account for the fraction of missing data, but found that these could lead to inflated type I error rates. As such, at least for the step-wise variable selection, which was the subject of their investigation, Wood *et al.* (2008) recommended that variable selection decisions be made using the 'Model building based on combined results across multiple imputations' approach described in the preceding paragraph.

8.5.2 Imputing predictors when model building is to be performed

When variable or model selection is to be performed on a single set of multiply imputed datasets, it is clear from our earlier developments that the imputation model(s) used should be sufficiently flexible to accommodate the various potential analyses. In particular, all variables that are to be included in the model building process as potential predictors should be included in the imputation models. Following Chapter 6, if the model building process will include decisions about the necessity of interactions or non-linear effects, in principle, the imputation model should allow for the possibility of those interactions and non-linear effects that will be investigated. It is clear however that this prescription may not always be feasible in practice if a large number of such effects are to be investigated. Thus in a particular setting, pragmatic decisions may need to be taken to simplify the imputation model specification.

8.6 Model performance

In this section, we consider the assessment of model performance for a prognostic model developed using MI. Model performance is generally quantified through a measure defined from the predicted and observed outcomes, for example mean squared prediction error (MSPE), calibration measures, R^2-type measures, or measures of discrimination. The multiple imputation procedure presents specific challenges for such assessments (Marshall *et al.*, 2009; Wood *et al.*, 2015).

8.6.1 How should we pool MI results for estimation of performance?

When MI is used for model development and validation, it is not immediately obvious how the results should be pooled for estimation of model performance. Let $\hat{\beta}_k$ denote the estimated model parameters from imputation k and let X_i^k denote the possibly partially imputed predictor vector for individual i in imputation k. Suppose the chosen prediction model provides predictions $h(\beta, X)$ for some function $h(\ .\ ,.\ )$. Let $\mathbf{Y} = (Y_1, \ldots, Y_n)$ denote the observed outcomes (for simplicity assumed here to be fully observed) and $\hat{\mathbf{Y}} = (\hat{Y}_1, \ldots, \hat{Y}_n)$ denote the predicted outcomes in the development data. We then assess model performance by some function $V(\mathbf{Y}, \hat{\mathbf{Y}})$, such as MSPR, R^2 or the area under the receiver operating characteristic (ROC) curve.

Wood *et al.* (2015) investigated various approaches to quantifying the performance of the prognostic model fitted to multiply imputed datasets, depending on whether performance is assessed separately in each imputed dataset, or alternatively predictions (or linear predictors) are first pooled across datasets and then performance assessed using these. To estimate the performance of the model when complete data will be available at implementation, Wood *et al.* (2015) recommended that the performance measure be estimated within each imputation, and these performance measures are then pooled using Rubin's rules. That is, within imputation k, we obtain

$$\hat{V}_k = V(\mathbf{Y}, \hat{\mathbf{Y}}^{(k)}),$$

where $\hat{\mathbf{Y}}^{(k)} = (h(\beta^{(k)}, X_1^{(k)}), \ldots, h(\beta^{(k)}, X_n^{(k)}))$ denotes the vector of predicted outcomes in imputation k, based on the imputation specific estimates $\hat{\beta}_k$ and each individual's predictor vector in imputation k, X_i^k. We then pool these imputation-specific estimates of model performance using Rubin's rules:

$$\hat{V}_{MI} = \frac{1}{K} \sum_{k=1}^{K} \hat{V}_k. \tag{8.1}$$

This approach thus treats the performance measure as a parameter or estimand and applies Rubin's rules to its estimate and associated variance. As such, the 'true' value of the estimand being targeted by this approach is that which would be obtained in the (infinite) population based on the true parameter value β and the true predictor values of the individuals in this population.

8.6.2 Calibration

Measures of calibration quantify the agreement between the observed and predicted outcomes. These are well described by van Calster *et al.* (2019). Calibration plots are popular graphical displays, whereby average observed outcomes are plotted against grouped predicted outcomes. Ideally, the average observed outcome would equal the average predicted outcome, and this creates a line of equality on such a plot. With complete data, these are often constructed by first grouping individuals based on deciles of the predicted outcome and then plotting the mean observed outcome in each group against the mean predicted outcome in that group. Alternatively, to avoid the arbitrariness of choosing, e.g. deciles, smoothers (e.g. lowess) can be used to show how the mean observed outcome varies a function of the predicted mean. To formally assess whether the model's calibration is good, one can regress the observed outcome against the predicted outcome and test whether the intercept differs from 0 and the slope differs from 1 (their values under the hypothesis of perfect calibration).

With multiply imputed data, the calibration plot in each imputed dataset can be constructed and, if desired, these could be overlaid on a single plot (Wood *et al.*, 2015). The calibration intercept and slope can be readily estimated in each imputed dataset, which can then be pooled using Rubin's rules.

8.6.3 Discrimination

Measures of discrimination quantify the ability of a model to distinguish/separate individuals in relation to their observed outcome. The greater the separation, the more likely the model will identify individuals at highest or lowest risk and be more clinically useful. Measures of discrimination include the area under the receiver operating characteristic (AUROC) curve for binary outcomes and the C-index for survival outcomes.

The true AUROC and C-index are bounded and take values between 0.5 and 1. It is possible to transform estimates of such measures to an unbounded scale (e.g. using a logit-transformation) before pooling with Rubin's rules, and finally transforming back to the unbounded scale. Performing a normalising transformation will produce the most appropriate confidence intervals, especially for measures close to the boundaries. For estimates away from the boundaries, simply pooling the AUROC or C-index using Rubin's rules is a sensible pragmatic approach.

8.6.4 Model performance measures with clinical interpretability

Other measures such as sensitivity, specificity, net reclassification index (Pencina *et al.*, 2012), and numbers need to screen to prevent a case are used to quantify the clinical relevance of a model or of new biomarkers. Again, since these can be viewed as well-defined population estimands, we recommend that such measures be estimated separately in each imputed dataset and then combined using Rubin's rules. As for the AUROC and C-index, depending on the measure, it may be appropriate to apply Rubin's rules after a suitable transformation.

8.7 Model validation

In the previous section, we outlined the measures commonly used to assess model performance. In prognostic modelling, rigorous model evaluation (often termed *validation*) is required to assess the performance of a model when applied to data in which it was not developed, especially in small samples. The aim is to account for any over-fitting and obtain an 'honest' assessment of model performance for future individuals. In this section, we consider first how internal model validation can be performed when MI has been used to impute incomplete predictors. We then consider external validation.

8.7.1 Internal model validation

If we use the same set of data to develop the model and assess its performance, our estimates of model performance are generally optimistic. A simple example of this is the standard R^2 measure in linear regression, which is biased upwards relative to the true proportion of explained variation. Various techniques have been developed to obtain honest assessments of model performance when a model is developed using a given dataset, including sample-splitting, cross-validation, and bootstrapping-based methods (Hastie *et al.*, 2009; Steyerberg, 2019).

A variety of approaches have been proposed and investigated for performing internal validation in combination with MI for incomplete predictors, as described, for example by Musoro *et al.* (2014), Wood *et al.* (2015), Wahl *et al.* (2016), and Carroll (2022). Here we outline two broad approaches, but note that at the time of writing there is no clear consensus on what is the best approach. For simplicity, we describe possible methods for a split-sample approach to validation, whereby we split the data into a development subset and a validation subset. The performance of the model developed on the development subset is evaluated on the validation subset.

First, we could apply MI to the entire dataset before splitting. The prediction model can then be developed using the development subset of the imputations. The performance of the resulting model can then be evaluated in each imputation, using only the validation subset records, and the performance measure estimates averaged across imputations. The potential issue with this approach is that, to some extent, the development subset data has affected the validation subset, since the imputation model fit used to impute missing predictors in the validation subset has been influenced (typically to a large extent) by the data in the development subset. As such, we are no longer evaluating the model's performance in an independent set of data to that which was used to develop the model. This is a form of data leakage.

A second approach is to perform MI entirely separately in the development and validation subsets. This obviates the issue of the imputation of missing data in the validation subset being influenced by data in the development subset, and therefore seems preferable to the first approach outlined. An outstanding concern here is that the evaluation of model performance in the validation subset is contingent on the reliability of the imputation of missing predictors in the subset, which may be more suspect in small subsets. For example, if the imputation models used are mis-specified, the performance estimated in the validation subset will not reflect the model's performance at implementation, when predictors (are assumed thus far) will be complete.

8.7.2 External model validation

Before considering whether to use a prognostic model in practice, ideally one should evaluate its performance in the population in which it is to be employed. Often, the latter is related but not identical to the population from which the data used to develop the prognostic model were obtained (Steyerberg, 2019). As such, the model's performance at implementation in the target population may not be as good as in the population in which the model was developed.

Thus, suppose we have external validation data on predictors and outcome from the target population. If we anticipate complete predictors at implementation, and the predictors are complete in the external validation dataset, external validation is straightforward: given our developed model, we evaluate its performance in the external validation data. The fact that missing data had to be accommodated at the model development stage does not change the process at validation. In reality, even if complete data are anticipated in the future at implementation, it may well be the case that the external validation data are incomplete. In this case, performing MI separately in the external validation dataset, followed by evaluation of the developed model across the imputed datasets, would seem a reasonable approach.

8.8 Incomplete data at implementation

In reality, we may anticipate missing values in the predictors at the implementation stage. In this section, we first describe the potential role of MI in this setting and then describe a number of alternative approaches which may be preferable.

8.8.1 MI for incomplete data at implementation

If some predictors will be incomplete at implementation, MI may still be an attractive approach for handling missing data at the model development stage, as described previously. However, if predictors may be incomplete at implementation, we must consider how the missing values will be handled at the implementation stage. This is so because the end users will require some approach for accommodating missing predictors in order to predict outcomes. Moreover, if we want to evaluate how well the model will perform in practice at implementation, we need to evaluate the performance of the combination of the developed model and whatever method we choose to handle incomplete predictors at implementation (Tsvetanova *et al.*, 2021; van Smeden *et al.*, 2020).

In principle, we might consider using MI at the implementation stage to handle missing predictor values. First, note that at the implementation stage the outcome variable will always be missing for the individual whose (future) outcome we are predicting. Consider then an individual at the implementation stage, who is missing one or more predictors, plus (necessarily) their outcome. The imputation model fitted to the development data could then be used to create multiple imputations of the individual's incomplete predictors and missing outcome. Hoogland *et al.* (2020) suggested that a difficulty here if full conditional specification (FCS) MI is used is that an

FCS imputation model cannot be used when more than one variable is missing for an individual, which is the case here since the outcome is always missing and at least one predictor is missing. In fact, as per the FCS algorithm, we can initialise the missing values first, then iteratively impute the missing predictors and outcome, using sufficient iterations for the imputations to have converged to their joint distribution. In the resulting imputed datasets, the individual's outcome could be predicted, and the predictions averaged across imputations. Hoogland *et al.* (2020) suggested that the imputed outcomes that would be generated should be discarded, but if the imputation model used for the outcome is the same as the chosen prediction model, one could quite legitimately use the imputed outcomes themselves to form the prediction, for example by calculating their mean across imputations.

As noted by Hoogland *et al.* (2020), most imputation packages do not return the imputation model fits to the user, rendering the preceding approach difficult to apply in practice. An approach which overcomes this, proposed by Janssen *et al.* (2009), involves appending the data from the new individual for whom we want to impute and predict for to the original development dataset. MI is then re-run on the resulting augmented dataset, resulting in multiple imputations of the incomplete predictors for the new individual. A further alternative explored by Hoogland *et al.* (2020) is to fit the conditional models required for imputing incomplete predictors for a new individual to the multiply imputed development datasets.

A major disadvantage of the approaches which involve refitting imputation models at the point of prediction for a new individual is the potentially high computational burden and issues with data sharing and privacy. Thus, in practice simpler approaches for handling incompleteness in predictors at the implementation stage are typically used, such as simple mean imputation or conditional mean imputation. While such approaches (particularly simple mean imputation) are likely to lead to a degradation in prediction performance relative to what could have been achieved had predictors been complete, the critical issue is that we obtain assessments of model performance which incorporate how we plan to deal with incomplete predictors at implementation. That is, if simple mean imputation is proposed to be used at implementation, we should similarly use simple mean imputation to impute missing values in the validation data when evaluating model performance.

Ideally, to evaluate the performance of the model as it would be implemented using a simplistic approach to incomplete predictors, we should use a validation dataset representative of the target population. Specifically, if the amount and patterns of missing data in the dataset used to assess performance are not reflective of what missingness will be realised at implementation, our assessment of model performance will not be valid. In particular, if a prognostic model is rolled out for implementation, levels of missingness at implementation may be expected to be lower than in the development dataset, since a clinician is more likely to measure the set of predictors knowing that these are the required inputs for the prognostic model available to them (Sperrin *et al.*, 2020; van Smeden *et al.*, 2020). Such a feedback loop means that predicting the future missingness levels and patterns at implementation, and hence the future model performance, is difficult.

8.8.2 Alternatives to multiple imputation

If data are incomplete at both model development and implementation stages, it may be preferable to avoid using MI altogether (Sperrin *et al.*, 2020).

Simple mean imputation and missing category methods

One of the simplest and most commonly used approaches to handling missing data in general is to replace missing values in continuous variables by the mean of the observed values and for categorical variables to add a new 'missing' category. We know that these approaches rarely lead to valid inferences for the parameters of a substantive model. However, as noted earlier, in the prognostic modelling context, our objective is instead to predict well the outcome, rather than to accurately estimate parameters of a model. As such, one could use these approaches to handle incomplete predictors at the model development and validation stages. One would anticipate that use of mean imputation would degrade prediction performance somewhat relative to more sophisticated approaches. However, as indicated earlier, if we evaluate the performance of the combination of the model with the chosen approach for handling incomplete predictors at implementation, and the resulting performance is deemed acceptable, then this approach may be a pragmatic and defensible solution.

Missing data indicators

The use of missing indicators is not generally advisable for parameter estimation, but it is far more attractive in the context of prognostic and diagnostic research. Sperrin *et al.* (2020) advocated for more widespread use of missing indicators in the prognostic modelling context, where we are not concerned with bias or interpretation of individual coefficients but with producing accurate outcome predictions in the target population.

The idea is to use the response indicator $R_{i,j}$ for individual i and incomplete variable j as a predictor of outcome. An incomplete variable $X_{i,j}$ is set to an arbitrary value (such as $X_{i,j} = 0$) when missing and an interaction between X_j and $R_{i,j}$ is included in the model. This may be done for more than one j. Including missing indicators may lead to better prognostic performance than, for example trying to impute the missing values. This is because missingness of covariates itself may be prognostic for the outcome.

In response to Sperrin *et al.* (2020), a commentary by van Smeden *et al.* (2020) was generally supportive but highlighted some potential problems. The difficulty, as outlined earlier, is that at the implementation stage, the levels and patterns of missingness are likely to be different to those at the development stage. This is not least because, at implementation, the users of the prognostic model may be aware of what predictors the model requires, and this may influence what is measured, thus changing the prognostic information in the missing indicators. In contrast, a prognostic model implemented as part of an electronic health records system may be expected to have less of an impact on measurement processes. In conclusion, while incorporating missingness indicators into prognostic models offers potential for both handling missingness and improving prediction, its use in practice requires careful consideration and monitoring over time once deployed.

Pattern sub-models

A promising strategy for prediction models with incomplete predictors in the development, validation, and implementation data is termed the *pattern submodels* approach (Fletcher Mercaldo and Blume, 2018). Rather than constructing and evaluating a single prediction model including all predictors of interest, several prediction models are constructed, one for each subset of observed predictors. For example in a setting with three predictors X_1, X_2, X_3, where X_1 is always observed but X_2 and X_3 are incomplete, there are four observation patterns. Either X_1 alone is observed, X_1, X_2 are observed, X_1, X_3 are observed, or X_1, X_2, X_3 are observed. There then exist three potential incomplete-data sub-models with predictor sets $(X_1), (X_1, X_2), (X_1, X_3)$, as well as the complete records model with predictor set (X_1, X_2, X_3). These models are fitted on individuals with the relevant missing data pattern.

The pattern submodels approach is closely linked to the missing indicator method but is more general. To see this, suppose that we have only two predictors, X_1, X_2, of which only X_2 has missing values. The missing indicator method then involves imputing X_2 at some arbitrary value and including an interaction of X_2 with the pattern indicator (which here is the same as the missingness indicator). By also including an interaction of X_1 with the pattern indicator, we effectively have a model when X_2 is observed and another when it is missing. The latter contains a constant for X_2, the choice of which changes only the model intercept and so is equivalent to a model that includes X_1 only, *i.e.*, the variable observed under that pattern. The extra step here was to interact the missing indicator with the fully observed variable X_1 as well as the partially observed variable X_2.

Like the other simple methods described above, the pattern submodels approach does not require any imputation of missing predictors. Moreover, any prognostic information contained in the missingness pattern is automatically accommodated by virtue of fitting outcome models separately by missingness pattern. The difficulty lies, however, as with the other simple methods described earlier, that the prognostic value of missingness patterns in the development dataset may not transport well to the target population at implementation. Nonetheless, in settings where the levels and patterns of missingness are anticipated to be stable between development and implementation, this may be less of a concern. A further potential difficulty is that of sparsity. If many predictors are incomplete, there may be many distinct missingness patterns, some of which may contain few individuals. This may lead to computational difficulties in fitting some of the models and even if not, potentially poor prediction performance if many of the models are imprecisely estimated.

An alternative related approach proposed by Marshall *et al.* (2002) is to use a fitted prediction model, developed, for example by using MI to handle incomplete predictors in the development data, to derive the implied distribution of the outcome conditional on particular subsets of the predictors. To predict for a new individual with a given subset of predictors observed, one uses the derived model for that particular predictor subset combination. It turns out that this approach is closely related to imputation of the incomplete predictors by their best linear prediction given the complete predictors. Note that unlike the pattern sub-model approach, this approach does not condition on the missingness pattern in the outcome model, and so does not exploit any prognostic information that may be contained in the missingness pattern.

Exercises

1. Suppose you have developed a prognostic model and, during development, used multiple imputation to handle incomplete predictor data. The prognostic model uses multivariable logistic regression. At implementation, data are anticipated to be incomplete. Write out how you would use multiple imputation to make a prediction at implementation in a way that matches its use at the model development and evaluation.

- **(a)** Start by assuming there is one missing value for one person.
- **(b)** Describe how you would draw one imputation.
- **(c)** Now describe how to extend this procedure to multiple missing values.
- **(d)** Suppose you repeat the above step and draw K imputations. How would you combine the imputations: by averaging imputed values X^*; averaging linear predictions βX^*; or averaging predictions on the probability scale? Justify your choice.

2. There are numerous publications describing prognostic and diagnostic models; see for examples the reference list of Wynants *et al.* (2020).

Choose one article describing a prognostic or diagnostic model with missing predictor values. If you do not have one in mind, we suggest Tanboğa *et al.* (2021), Li *et al.* (2020), or Ryan *et al.* (2020).

Answer the following questions, justifying your answers:

- **(a)** Is it clear, or implicit, whether the intended implementation context is one in which everyone has complete data or in which data may be incomplete? Why?
- **(b)** What is the description given for handling of missing data?
- **(c)** Suppose you were given the data used by the authors. Would you know how to implement their methods for handling missing data at model development and validation? If not, what extra information would be needed to resolve ambiguity?
- **(d)** Does the article provide sufficient information that you would know how to handle a missing predictor value to produce a prediction for an individual? As above, what extra information might you need?

9

Multi-level multiple imputation

In this chapter, we consider the imputation of data with a multi-level, or equivalently a hierarchical, structure.

We extend our joint imputation model for a mix of discrete and continuous response types to the multi-level setting in Section 9.1 and describe the Markov chain Monte Carlo (MCMC) algorithm for fitting this model in Section 9.2. We illustrate this with the analysis of a dataset of paediatric hospital admissions from Kenya. Next, Section 9.3 sketches out how the approach described here can be extended to more complex data structures, including random level 1 covariance matrices and cross-classified structures. In Section 9.4, we introduce alternative imputation strategies for multi-level data, focusing on the full conditional specification (FCS) approach. Then Section 9.5 explores the challenges posed by a specific type of multi-level data, namely individual participant data from multi-centre studies, for example, individual participant data meta-analyses.

We conclude with a review of software for multi-level multiple imputation (MI) in Section 9.6 and an overall discussion in Section 9.7.

9.1 Multi-level imputation model

Multi-level data structures arise when the observations on individual units (typically individuals) cannot be considered independent but instead are correlated because they are nested within groups or clusters of various kinds. For example, in educational research, children are nested in classes within schools within educational authorities. In medical research, individual participants may be nested within general practices within health authorities. Goldstein (2010) considers the analysis of multi-level data from a wide range of settings. The following is a typical educational example, which we use to highlight the issues raised by missing data in a multi-level setting.

Multiple Imputation and its Application, Second Edition.
James R. Carpenter, Jonathan W. Bartlett, Tim P. Morris, Angela M. Wood, Matteo Quartagno and Michael G. Kenward.

Example 9.1 Class size data

Blatchford *et al.* (2002) report a study on the effects of class size on educational attainment among children in their first year of education in England. Each child's literacy and numeracy skills were assessed when they started school, and at the end of their first school year, known as the reception year. After adjustment for key confounders, the study found a non-linear effect of class size on attainment, with falling attainment associated with class sizes above 25.

Our analyses here are merely illustrative. The version of the dataset we explore below was derived from the original; we restrict the analysis to a complete subset of 4873 pupils in 172 schools. School sizes vary greatly in these data, and this is reflected in the number of pupils each school contributes to the analysis, which ranges from 1 to 88. The dataset is thus multi-level, and here we set aside class and focus on children at level 1 belonging to schools at level 2.

Our model of interest regresses literacy score at the end of the first year on literacy score measured when the children started school, adjusting for eligibility for free school meals and gender. The pre- and post-reception year (i.e. first school year) literacy scores were normalised as follows: for each test, the children's results were ranked. Then for observation in rank order i, where n children sat the test, the normalised result was calculated as the inverse normal of $i/(n+1)$.

Let j denote school and i denote pupil. Our first illustrative model of interest is

$$\begin{aligned} nlitpost_{i,j} &= \beta_{0,i,j} + \beta_1 nlitpre_{i,j} + \beta_2 gend_j + \beta_3 fsmn_j, \\ \beta_{0,i,j} &= \beta_0 + u_j + e_{i,j}, \\ u_j &\overset{i.i.d.}{\sim} N(0, \sigma_u^2), \\ e_{i,j} &\overset{i.i.d.}{\sim} N(0, \sigma_e^2), \end{aligned} \tag{9.1}$$

where the u_j are independent of the e_{ij}, *nlitpost* and *nlitpre* are, respectively, numerical post- and pre-reception year measures of attainment in literacy, and *gend* and *fsmn* are, respectively, indicators for boys and eligibility for free school meals.

Model (9.1) is a simple multi-level model known as a *random intercept* model. While the effect of the covariates *nlitpre*, *gend*, and *fsmn* is common across schools, we can think of every school, $j = 1, \dots, J$ having a school-specific intercept $\beta_0 + u_j$. These are normally distributed with mean β_0 and variance σ_u^2.

Additionally, we consider a second substantive model:

$$\begin{aligned} nlitpost_{i,j} &= \beta_{0,i,j} + \beta_{1,i,j} nlitpre_{i,j} + \beta_2 gend_j + \beta_3 fsmn_j, \\ \beta_{0,i,j} &= \beta_0 + u_{0,j} + e_{i,j}, \\ \beta_{1,i,j} &= \beta_1 + u_{1,j}, \\ \begin{pmatrix} u_{0,j} \\ u_{1,j} \end{pmatrix} &\overset{i.i.d.}{\sim} N\left(\begin{pmatrix} 0 \\ 0 \end{pmatrix}, \begin{pmatrix} \sigma_{u,0}^2 & \rho_{u,0,1}\sigma_{u,0}\sigma_{u,1} \\ \rho_{u,0,1}\sigma_{u,0}\sigma_{u,1} & \sigma_{u,1}^2 \end{pmatrix} \right), \\ e_{i,j} &\overset{i.i.d.}{\sim} N(0, \sigma_e^2). \end{aligned} \tag{9.2}$$

Table 9.1 Class size data: parameter estimates (standard errors) from fitting models (9.1) and (9.2) to full and reduced data (using restricted maximum likelihood).

Parameter	Estimates (standard errors) from				
	Full data Model (9.1) ($n = 4873$)	Full data Model (9.2) ($n = 4873$)	Full data Single level ($n = 4873$)	Complete records Model (9.1) ($n = 3132$)	Complete records Model (9.2) ($n = 3132$)
β_0 (intercept)	0.088 (0.040)	0.076 (0.041)	0.065 (0.017)	0.016 (0.041)	0.006 (0.041)
β_1 (nlitpre)	0.733 (0.010)	0.745 (0.016)	0.662 (0.012)	0.712 (0.013)	0.720 (0.018)
β_2 (gender)	−0.058 (0.018)	−0.055 (0.018)	−0.086 (0.022)	−0.024 (0.023)	−0.027 (0.023)
β_3 (fsmn)	−0.068 (0.027)	−0.059 (0.027)	−0.095 (0.030)	−0.038 (0.031)	−0.033 (0.031)
$\sigma^2_{u,0}$	0.237	0.244	—	0.216	0.215
$\rho_{u,0,1}$	—	−0.036	—	—	−0.037
$\sigma^2_{u,1}$	—	0.020	—	—	0.022
σ^2_e	0.372	0.357	0.573	0.369	0.353

This is a simple example of a model known as *random intercept and slope* model or *random coefficient* model. Such a model would be more appropriate if the effect of *nlitpre* on *nlitpost* varied across schools.

Parameter estimates from fitting (9.1) and (9.2) (using restricted maximum likelihood) are shown in columns 2 and 3 of Table 9.1, respectively. Focusing on model (9.1) first, the total variance is estimated as $\hat{\sigma}^2_u + \hat{\sigma}^2_e = 0.237 + 0.372 = 0.609$, of which $100 \times 0.237/0.609 = 39\%$ is between schools (i.e. between level 2 units). Estimates from the single-level model, where σ^2_u is constrained to be 0, equivalent to a standard least squares regression, are shown in column 3. Now the level 1 (residual) variance estimate increases to 0.573.

Comparing the fixed-effect estimates, we see that when the (substantial) component of variability between schools is omitted from the analysis, the gender coefficient changes by more than one standard error. This is consistent with stronger gender differences in the larger (presumably urban) schools, which – as they contribute more pupils to the analysis – have a larger effect on the coefficients in the single-level (standard least squares regression) analysis.

Parameter estimates from model (9.2) are similar to those from model (9.1), both in terms of fixed effects and of common random variance components. However, the residual variance is estimated to be lower because a larger (though relatively limited) proportion of the variability is explained by the random slope.

We now make the data missing according to the following mechanism:

$$\text{logit}\{\Pr(\text{observe } nlitpre_{i,j})\} = 1.5 + 0.5 \times nlitpost_{i,j} - fsmn_j - gend_j. \tag{9.3}$$

This mechanism implies that we are more likely to see *nlitpre* for girls with higher *nlitpost* who are not eligible for free school meals. Using these probabilities, we generate 4873 random numbers from a uniform distribution on [0, 1] and make each child's *nlitpre* observation missing if these are less than their probability implied by (9.3). This results in 3313 complete cases. Fitting the multilevel substantive models to these, we see that the effect of gender, and of eligibility for free school meals, are diluted so that they are no longer significant (columns 5 and 6, Table 9.1).

After describing multi-level imputation below, we return to this example to illustrate its application. □

9.1.1 Imputation of level-1 variables

We know from the basic principles behind MI that the imputation model is derived from the conditional distribution of the missing data given the observed, congenial with the substantive model. This implies, in multi-level examples like the one above, that the conditional distribution of a missing observation will depend on any other variable with which it is correlated. For example, in a simple clustered setting, one observation from a cluster is correlated with all other observations in the same cluster, and the imputation model should take this into account. To achieve this, we need to introduce the multi-level dependency structure into the imputation model. If we ignore such structure, the variance and covariance properties of the imputed data will not match those of the actual data. The implications of ignoring multi-level structure in imputation for the resulting analysis can be hard to predict. It depends on which parameter is being estimated, in particular whether the information on the estimator comes principally from within- or between-cluster information, on the actual design, and on the size of the correlations in the data.

Suppose we have $i = I_1, \ldots, I_J$ level 1 units observed on each of $j = 1, \ldots, J$ level 2 units. With two partially observed continuous variables, $Y_{1,i,j}$, $Y_{2,i,j}$ and fully observed variables $Y_{3,i,j}$, $Y_{4,i,j}$, a possible joint random intercepts imputation model is

$$\begin{aligned}
Y_{1,i,j} &= \beta_0 + u_{1,j} + \beta_1 Y_{3,i,j} + \beta_2 Y_{4,i,j} + e_{1,i,j},\\
Y_{2,i,j} &= \beta_5 + u_{2,j} + \beta_6 Y_{3,i,j} + \beta_7 Y_{4,i,j} + e_{2,i,j},\\
\begin{pmatrix} u_{1,j} \\ u_{2,j} \end{pmatrix} &\overset{i.i.d.}{\sim} N(\mathbf{0}, \mathbf{\Omega}_2),\\
\begin{pmatrix} e_{1,i,j} \\ e_{2,i,j} \end{pmatrix} &\overset{i.i.d.}{\sim} N(\mathbf{0}, \mathbf{\Omega}_1), \text{independent of } (u_{1,j}, u_{2,j})^T.
\end{aligned} \tag{9.4}$$

Comparing with (9.1), we see that (9.4) is a joint random intercepts model for $Y_{1,ij}$ and $Y_{2,ij}$, where the fully observed variables are covariates and the partially observed variables responses. As discussed in Chapter 2, assuming missing at random (MAR), we obtain valid estimates of the parameters by fitting this model to the observed data and can then, as outlined above, impute missing data from the appropriate conditional distribution.

Thus, if only $Y_{1,i,j}$ is missing for level 1 unit i belonging to level 2 unit j, it will be imputed from the conditional normal given $(Y_{2,i,j}, Y_{3,i,j}, Y_{4,i,j})$; if only $Y_{2,iji}$ is missing it will be imputed from the conditional normal given $(Y_{1,i,j}, Y_{3,i,j}, Y_{4,i,j})$, and if both are missing, they will be imputed from the bivariate normal given $(Y_{3,i,j}, Y_{4,i,j})$.

If we additionally assume a bivariate normal random intercepts model for $(Y_{3,i,j}, Y_{4,i,j})$, then $Y_{1,i,j}, Y_{2,i,j}, Y_{3,i,j}, Y_{4,i,j}$ have a joint random intercepts model:

$$
\begin{aligned}
Y_{1,i,j} &= \beta_1 + u_{1,j} + e_{1,i,j}, \\
Y_{2,i,j} &= \beta_2 + u_{2,j} + e_{2,i,j}, \\
Y_{3,i,j} &= \beta_3 + u_{3,j} + e_{3,i,j}, \\
Y_{4,i,j} &= \beta_4 + u_{4,j} + e_{4,i,j}, \\
\begin{pmatrix} u_{1,j} \\ u_{2,j} \\ u_{3,j} \\ u_{4,j} \end{pmatrix} &\overset{i.i.d.}{\sim} N(\mathbf{0}, \boldsymbol{\Omega}_2) \perp \begin{pmatrix} e_{1,i,j} \\ e_{2,i,j} \\ e_{3,i,j} \\ e_{4,i,j} \end{pmatrix} \overset{i.i.d.}{\sim} N(\mathbf{0}, \boldsymbol{\Omega}_1),
\end{aligned} \tag{9.5}
$$

where '$\perp$' denotes independence.

While model (9.5) is computationally slightly easier to fit than (9.4), with multi-level data (9.4) is more flexible, because we can extend it to allow $Y_{3,i,j}$ and $Y_{4,i,j}$ to have random coefficients at level 2. This aspect is useful when the covariate is observation time, and data are observed irregularly. More generally, a typical multi-level model of interest will have a number of covariates with random coefficients at level 2, and this should be reflected in the imputation model. This again points to including fully observed variables as covariates in the form of (9.4). If the random coefficients are for partially observed variables instead, this makes it more complicated to achieve a congenial imputation model (cf Section 9.1.3).

Looking at (9.5), we see that while the mean of $Y_{1,i,j}, Y_{2,i,j}, Y_{3,i,j}, Y_{4,i,j}$ varies across level 2 units, the covariance, $\boldsymbol{\Omega}_1$, is common across all level 2 units. This means that the conditional distributions of any of the Y's given the others is the same across all level 2 units. This will not in general be true. Looking at (9.4), we see that if we extend the model to allow $Y_{3,i,j}$ and $Y_{4,i,j}$ to have random coefficients at level 2, then the conditional distribution of $(Y_{1,i,j}, Y_{2,i,j})$ given $(Y_{3,i,j}, Y_{4,i,j})$ varies by level 2 units: this is the distributional implication of introducing random coefficients at level 2. Nevertheless, the level 1 covariance matrix of $(Y_{1,i,j}, Y_{2,i,j})$ remains constant across level 2 units. If this is inappropriate, we may wish to allow the level 1 covariance matrix, $\boldsymbol{\Omega}_1$, to vary across level 2 units. We discuss this computationally more demanding option in Section 9.3.2. We will see, though, in Section 9.1.3, that the only way to guarantee full congeniality with a substantive model whenever the model of interest includes random coefficients on partially observed variables is to use substantive model compatible imputation.

Example 9.1 Class size study *(ctd)*

Returning to the class size example, we now compare multi-level and single-level imputation for the missing *nlitpre* values (under missingness mechanism (9.3)). Having previously fitted the substantive model (9.1) to the partially observed data, we impute using the multi-level multiple imputation `R` package jomo with imputation model (9.5), which allows different means for the variables across schools, but imposes a common correlation through $\mathbf{\Omega}_1$. Thus, as discussed in the preceding paragraphs, this would not be appropriate if our model of interest had random coefficients, as it is the case, for example for (9.2). In the latter case, we would need an imputation model of the form of (9.4), with only the partially observed variable as response, and the fully observed variables as covariates with random level 2 coefficients as supported by the data.

However, substantive model (9.1) has only random intercepts, so an imputation model as (9.5), which treats all the variables as responses, is appropriate. This model can potentially allow for missing data in each variable (though in this case there is only missing data in *nlitpre*). The two continuous variables come first, each having its own intercept, random at the school level, and residual. The two binary variables we treat as unordered categorical with two levels each. Thus, each level is associated with a single latent normal in exactly the way described in Chapter 4. Taking *fsmn*, this is shown by the notation

$$\text{fsmn:}\, \pi_{c,3,i,j} \,:\, Y_{c,3,i,j} = \beta_{c,0,3} + u_{c,0,3,j} + e_{c,0,3,i,j}.$$

This indicates that the probability that $fsmn_{\,i,j}$ takes the value c is derived from the latent normal $Y_{c,3,i,j}$, which is modelled with a random intercept at the school level and a residual at the pupil level which is constrained to have variance 1. The index '3' identifies this as the third of the four responses, and the index '0' identifies terms associated with the 'constant' (i.e. fixed parameter, level 2 and 1 residuals). Additional fully observed auxiliary variables could be included on the RHS for each response variable if desired.

We use the `R` package jomo, which by default assumes a weakly informative inverse-Wishart prior over positive-definite inverse covariance matrices at levels 1 and 2. We fit this model with a burn in of 2000 and impute 20 datasets updating the MCMC sampler 500 times between each. We also create imputations ignoring the multi-level structure, effectively simply taking a linear regression model of *nlitpre* on the other variables as the imputation model. With single-level imputation, we still fit the multi-level model of interest, (9.1) to the imputed data. Table 9.2 shows the results.

By correctly taking into account the hierarchical nature of the data, multi-level MI gives point estimates close to the original, fully observed, data but with slightly increased standard errors (reflecting the lost information in the partially observed data). By contrast with single-level multiple imputation, the school-level variance is dramatically underestimated, while the pupil-level variance is overestimated. This has a direct impact on the standard errors of the linear model parameters. For coefficients that correspond to effects that are wholly, or largely, between-cluster, such as the intercept, the standard errors will be too small from single-level MI analysis. By contrast, those estimated largely from within-subject information, i.e. those that vary mainly within-clusters, in this example gender, eligibility for free school meals and pre-reception attainment, will have standard errors that are too large. This is exactly the same impact that we see when a single-level substantive model is wrongly used for clustered data, albeit in a diluted form: the effect comes only from the

Table 9.2 Class size data: parameter estimates from original data, and with 20 imputations using multi-level MI and single-level MI.

Parameter	Estimates (std. errors) from		
	Full data multilevel model ($n = 4873$)	Multilevel MI	Single level MI
β_0	0.088 (0.040)	0.102 (0.041)	0.117 (0.036)
β_1	0.733 (0.010)	0.731 (0.012)	0.648 (0.014)
β_2	−0.058 (0.018)	−0.050 (0.022)	−0.075 (0.023)
β_3	−0.068 (0.027)	−0.077 (0.029)	−0.108 (0.032)
σ_u^2	0.237	0.239	0.141
σ_e^2	0.372	0.376	0.435

inappropriate variance structure of the imputations not from an inappropriate variance structure applied to the entire dataset. There is also an impact on the estimates themselves. We see that the gender and free school meal coefficients are over-estimated (in absolute magnitude). This is because the effect of gender and free school meals is larger in the schools with more pupils (which are typically urban), which dominate the single-level imputation model. More discussion of this example is given in Carpenter *et al.* (2012), and also Carpenter *et al.* (2011a) where imputation of the class size variable is also discussed. □

9.1.2 Imputation of level 2 variables

We now consider the more general setting, where the multi-level model of interest has covariates at level 1 and level 2. The latter are covariates that are constant for all level 1 units within a level 2 unit. For example, if level 1 is pupils and level 2 is classes, then characteristics of the class teacher (age, experience, etc.,) are constant for all pupils in the class. In general, data can be missing at both levels 1 and 2, and we wish to impute respecting the multi-level structure. We show how the multi-level imputation model described above can be extended to achieve this.

Example 9.2 Improving medical records

Ayieko *et al.* (2011) report the results of a cluster randomised trial involving eight hospitals to evaluate the effectiveness of a multi-faceted intervention to improve admission to paediatric care in Kenyan district hospitals. Overall, the results showed marked benefit of the intervention, including improved completion of admission tasks, improved uptake of guideline recommended therapeutic practices and a reduction in inappropriate drug dosage.

Within this study was embedded the evaluation of a structured Patient Admission Record (PAR) form, designed to both systematize and improve the completion of essential paediatric admission information. This PAR form was made available to staff in all eight hospitals. Here, we give an illustrative analysis of how the completeness of paediatric admission records is affected by the use of this form, and some other relevant factors described below. A full analysis is given by Gachau *et al.* (2020) and Tuti *et al.* (2016).

Our analysis takes as a response the percentage completion of the desired admissions tasks and explores variation in this by use of the PAR form, child's gender, whether the hospital was one of the four randomised to receive the multi-faceted intervention (hospitals numbered 1–4), the admitting clinician's gender and years of experience, and attendance of the admitting clinicians at short, ad hoc refresher training sessions (termed continuing medical education (CME) training) which were available in the four intervention hospitals.

For our analyses here, we use the data which were collected every six months as part of hospital performance surveys. Each of these surveys sought to review 400 paediatric admission records from children admitted with an acute medical diagnosis in the preceding six months. This resulted in data from 8349 admissions, handled by 396 admitting clinicians in 8 hospitals, as shown in Table 9.3.

Table 9.3 also shows the proportion of missing observations. While around 6% of children did not have their sex recorded, most of the missing information is at the clinician level. Since each clinician was responsible for the admission of a number of children, this results in a complete records analysis of only 6775 out of 8349 (81%) of the available cases. Moreover, preliminary analyses suggest clinician-level data may not be missing completely at random (MCAR).

Table 9.3 Summary of data used for analysis of effectiveness of the PAR form. Denominators for proportions exclude admissions with missing values. Right column: proportion of total child-level or clinician-level records which are missing that variable. Hospitals 1–4 were randomised to receive a multi-faceted intervention to improve admission of paediatric care.

		Hospital								
		1	2	3	4	5	6	7	8	% missing
No of admissions		1197	1210	1188	1007	798	798	1116	1035	
Mean completion	(%)	89	72	88	83	32	49	63	75	0
PAR use	(%)	97	82	96	92	22	52	60	97	0
Female child	(%)	42	39	41	39	44	38	44	41	6
Female clinician	(%)	76	60	52	70	64	92	58	54	14
Median years experience		0.5	0	0	4	3	3	0	0	20
Cont. med. ed.	(%)	46	20	35	59	Not offered				9

Let i index child, j clinician, and k hospital and '1[.]' denote an indicator random variable for the event in brackets. Our first multi-level model of interest is the following:

$$\begin{aligned}
\text{completion}_{i,j,k} = {} & \beta_0 + u_{j,k} + v_k + \beta_1 1[\text{PAR use}_{i,j,k}] + \beta_2 1[\text{Female child}_{i,j,k}] \\
& + \beta_3 1[\text{Female clinician}_{j,k}] + \beta_4 \text{ years experience}_{j,k} \\
& + \beta_5 1[\text{Intervention hospital}_k] + \beta_6[\text{Clinician takes CME}_{j,k}] \\
& + \beta_7 1[\text{PAR use}_{i,j,k}] \times 1[\text{Clinician takes CME}_{j,k}] + \epsilon_{i,j,k}, \\
v_k \sim {} & N(0, \sigma_v^2), \\
u_{j,k} \sim {} & N(0, \sigma_u^2), \\
e_{i,j,k} \sim {} & N(0, \sigma_e^2).
\end{aligned} \tag{9.6}$$

Additionally, we consider a second possible model of interest that differs from the first by including a random slope for PAR use:

$$\begin{aligned}
\text{completion}_{i,j,k} = {} & \beta_0 + u_{0,j,k} + v_k + (\beta_1 + u_{P,j,k})1[\text{PAR use}_{i,j,k}] + \beta_2 1[\text{Female child}_{i,j,k}] \\
& + \beta_3 1[\text{Female clinician}_{j,k}] + \beta_4 \text{ years experience}_{j,k} \\
& + \beta_5 1[\text{Intervention hospital}_k] + \beta_6[\text{Clinician takes CME}_{j,k}] \\
& + u_{P,j,k} 1[\text{PAR use}_{i,j,k}] \times 1[\text{Clinician takes CME}_{j,k}] + \epsilon_{i,j,k}, \\
v_k \sim {} & N(0, \sigma_v^2), \\
\begin{pmatrix} u_{0,j,k} \\ u_{P,j,k} \end{pmatrix} \sim {} & N(0, \Sigma_u), \\
e_{i,j,k} \sim {} & N(0, \sigma_e^2).
\end{aligned} \tag{9.7}$$

We return to this example after describing an appropriate multi-level imputation model. □

We now describe the extension of the imputation model (9.4) to include level 2 variables. As usual, we begin by considering continuous variables, which we model with the normal distribution, before extending the discussion to other data types via the latent normal structure described in Chapters 4 and 5. Let $j = 1, \dots, J$ index level 2 units, and $i = 1, \dots, I$ index level 1 units nested within level 2. For notational simplicity, we assume there are I level 1 units for each level 2 unit, but this is not required for any of what follows.

We suppose that in the multi-level dataset at hand, there are p_1 partially observed level 1 variables observed on level 1 unit i nested within level 2 unit j, which we denote by the $p_1 \times 1$ column vector $\mathbf{Y}_{i,j}^{(1)}$. We also suppose there are f_1 fully observed level 1 variables, including the constant, which we use as level 1 covariates in our imputation model and thus denote by the $1 \times f_1$ row vector $\mathbf{X}_{i,j}^{(1)}$. In general, we will allow each of these f_1 variables, $(X_{i,j,1}^{(1)}, \ldots, X_{i,j,f_1}^{(1)})$ to predict each of the p_1 level 1 variables observed on unit i, j: $(Y_{i,j,1}^{(1)}, \ldots, Y_{i,j,p_1}^{(1)})$, so there will be $f_1 p_1$ level 1 regression coefficients.

Further, let $\mathbf{Z}_{i,j}^{(1)}$ denote the $(1 \times q_1)$ row vector of covariates with random coefficients at level 2, including the constant. Typically, but not necessarily, a subset of the covariates $\mathbf{X}_{i,j}^{(1)}$ will have random coefficients at level 2 so that $\mathbf{Z}_{i,j}^{(1)}$ is a subset of $\mathbf{X}_{i,j}^{(1)}$. For each of the p_1 level 1 responses on unit i, j there are q_1 random effects; there are thus $p_1 q_1$ random effects for each level 1 unit i, j.

Using similar notation, let $\mathbf{Y}_j^{(2)}$ denote the $(p_2 \times 1)$ column vector of partially observed level 2 variables on unit j. Again, we also suppose there are f_2 fully observed level 2 variables, including the constant, which we use as level 2 covariates in our imputation model and denote by the $1 \times f_2$ row vector $\mathbf{X}_j^{(2)}$.

We note that some of the level 1 covariates included in $\mathbf{X}_{i,j}^{(1)}$ may be 'level 2 covariates' – that is, constant across all level 1 units i belonging to the same level 2 unit j. However, the reverse is not allowed: level 2 covariates must take a single value for each level 2 unit, j.

The general form of the multivariate normal model we use for imputation is then

$$
\begin{aligned}
\mathbf{Y}_{i,j}^{(1)} &= (\boldsymbol{I}_{p_1} \otimes \mathbf{X}_{i,j}^{(1)})\boldsymbol{\beta}^{(1)} + (\boldsymbol{I}_{p_1} \otimes \mathbf{Z}_{i,j}^{(1)})\boldsymbol{u}_j^{(1)} + \boldsymbol{e}_{i,j}^{(1)}, \\
\mathbf{Y}_j^{(2)} &= (\boldsymbol{I}_{p_2} \otimes \mathbf{X}_j^{(2)})\boldsymbol{\beta}^{(2)} + \boldsymbol{u}_j^{(2)}, \\
\boldsymbol{u}_j &= (\boldsymbol{u}_j^{(1)T}, \boldsymbol{u}_j^{(2)T})^T, \quad \boldsymbol{u}_j \sim N(\mathbf{0}, \boldsymbol{\Omega}_2), \\
\boldsymbol{e}_{i,j}^{(1)} &\sim N(\mathbf{0}, \boldsymbol{\Omega}_1). \qquad (9.8)
\end{aligned}
$$

As introduced above, the superscript (1) indicates level 1, and (2) level 2. The column vector $\boldsymbol{\beta}^{(1)}$ has $p_1 f_1$ elements, and the column vector $\boldsymbol{u}_j^{(1)}$ has $p_1 q_1$ elements. The column vector $\boldsymbol{\beta}^{(2)}$ has $p_2 f_2$ elements and the column vector $\boldsymbol{u}_2^{(2)}$ is simply the residuals at level 2 and thus a column vector of p_2 elements. $\boldsymbol{I}_p$ denotes the $(p \times p)$ identity matrix, and the symbol $\otimes$ is the Kronecker product. For example, if $\mathbf{X} = (X_1, X_2, X_3)$, then

$$
\boldsymbol{I}_3 \otimes \mathbf{X} = \begin{pmatrix} X_1 & X_2 & X_3 & 0 & 0 & 0 & 0 & 0 & 0 \\ 0 & 0 & 0 & X_1 & X_2 & X_3 & 0 & 0 & 0 \\ 0 & 0 & 0 & 0 & 0 & 0 & X_1 & X_2 & X_3 \end{pmatrix}.
$$

Thus, for example, the notation $(\boldsymbol{I}_{p_1} \otimes \mathbf{X}_{ij}^{(1)})\boldsymbol{\beta}^{(1)}$ is a concise way of writing that the mean of each of the p_1 responses from unit i, j is a different linear function of $\mathbf{X}_{i,j}^{(1)}$.

The multi-level imputation model (9.8) allows us to naturally handle irregular observation times, and if desired impute at a specific observation time for all individuals. Under model (9.8), if i indexes observation time, then we have an unstructured covariance matrix for all observations at a particular time, and the longitudinal correlation comes through the random structure at level 2. With random intercepts alone, we have an exchangeable structure (correlation is constant across time); if we include time as random at level 2, we allow the correlation to decline as time between observations increases, while the marginal variance may increase with time. If we have a dummy variable indexing time, random at level 2, we obtain an unstructured longitudinal covariance matrix. In applications, ideally the covariance structure in the imputation model should be consistent with that in the model of interest. In practice, unless the number of level 2 units is sufficiently large an unstructured covariance over time may be poorly estimated, and random intercepts and slopes will likely give adequate flexibility.

9.1.3 Accommodating the substantive model

As we said towards the end of Section 9.1.1, the imputation models presented thus far were built to be compatible with a multi-level substantive model when variables included in such model with a random effect were fully observed. When the random slope variables are partially observed, additional complications arise. To understand why, note that in order for the substantive and joint imputation models to be compatible, it should be possible to derive one from the other by conditioning appropriately. For example, if we take an imputation model such as (9.5) and condition on Y_2, Y_3, and Y_4, from simple laws of conditional probabilities of multivariate normal distributions we find (letting $\omega_{i,j}$ denote the (i,j) element of $\Omega_1+\Omega_2$) that

$$
\begin{aligned}
&E[Y_{1,i,j} | Y_{2,i,j}, Y_{3,i,j}, Y_{4,i,j}] \\
&= (\beta_1 + u_{1,j}) + \begin{pmatrix} \omega_{1,2} \\ \omega_{1,3} \\ \omega_{1,4} \end{pmatrix}^T \begin{pmatrix} \omega_{2,2}^2 & \omega_{2,3} & \omega_{2,4} \\ \omega_{3,2} & \omega_{3,3}^2 & \omega_{3,4} \\ \omega_{4,2} & \omega_{4,3} & \omega_{4,4}^2 \end{pmatrix} \begin{pmatrix} Y_{2,i,j} - (\beta_2 + u_{2,j}) \\ Y_{3,i,j} - (\beta_3 + u_{3,j}) \\ Y_{4,i,j} - (\beta_4 + u_{4,j}) \end{pmatrix}.
\end{aligned}
$$

Hence, the effect of Y_2, Y_3, and Y_4 on the mean of the outcome depends on the variance-covariance elements only, which are common across studies under the homoscedastic imputation model (9.5). For this reason, imputation model (9.5) is compatible with a random intercept substantive model, such as (9.1), but not with a random slope substantive model as (9.2), when the effect of either Y_2, Y_3, or Y_4 differs between level-2 units (here, clinicians).

In order to achieve perfect compatibility, as discussed in Chapter 6 where we considered interactions and non-linearities, one solution is to factor the joint distribution of the outcome and the covariates:

$$
f(Y_1, Y_2, Y_3, Y_4) = f_1(Y_1 | Y_2, Y_3, Y_4) f_{2,3,4}(Y_2, Y_3, Y_4). \tag{9.9}
$$

This way the conditional distribution of the outcome of the substantive model given the covariates, $f_1(Y_1 | Y_2, Y_3, Y_4)$ can be made to match the substantive model itself, for example (9.1) or (9.2). Not only does this allow for the inclusion of random slopes but also for polynomial effects, interactions, and non-linear models (e.g. Cox proportional hazards), all situations in which finding a compatible joint model is otherwise difficult, if not impossible. Since this method requires the choice of a substantive model in advance of imputation and guarantees the compatibility of this model with the imputation model, it is a Substantive Model Compatible imputation strategy, and we henceforth refer to it as substantive model compatible (SMC)-joint modelling (JM).

9.2 MCMC algorithm for imputation model

We now describe a general MCMC algorithm for fitting the multivariate multi-level imputation model (9.8).

We have the following parameters: $\boldsymbol{\beta}^{(1)}, \boldsymbol{\beta}^{(2)}$, the random effects $\boldsymbol{u}_j^{(1)}, \boldsymbol{u}_j^{(2)}$, the level 1 residuals $\boldsymbol{e}_{i,j}^{(1)}$ and the covariance matrices $\boldsymbol{\Omega}_2, \boldsymbol{\Omega}_1$.

Taking an improper prior for the coefficients $\boldsymbol{\beta}$, and Wishart priors for the inverse covariance matrices, at update step r, we update each of these in turn, conditional on all the others, as follows:

1. draw $\boldsymbol{\beta}^{(1)}$ from the $f_1 p_1$ variate normal distribution with mean

$$\left[\sum_{i,j} (\boldsymbol{I}_{p_1} \otimes \mathbf{X}_{i,j}^{(1)})^T (\boldsymbol{\Omega}_1)^{-1} (\boldsymbol{I}_{p_1} \otimes \mathbf{X}_{i,j}^{(1)})\right]^{-1}$$

$$\times \left[\sum_{i,j} (\boldsymbol{I}_{p_1} \otimes \mathbf{X}_{i,j}^{(1)})^T (\boldsymbol{\Omega}_1)^{-1} \{\mathbf{Y}_{i,j}^{(1)} - (\boldsymbol{I}_{p_1} \otimes \mathbf{Z}_{i,j}^{(1)}) \boldsymbol{u}_j^{(1)}\}\right],$$

and covariance matrix

$$\left[\sum_{i,j} (\boldsymbol{I}_{p_1} \otimes \mathbf{X}_{i,j}^{(1)})^T (\boldsymbol{\Omega}_1)^{-1} (\boldsymbol{I}_{p_1} \otimes \mathbf{X}_{i,j}^{(1)})\right]^{-1}.$$

2. We now focus on the update step for $\boldsymbol{\beta}^{(2)}, \boldsymbol{u}_j^{(1)}$, conditional on all the other parameters.

   If there were no level 1 model, then $\boldsymbol{\beta}^{(2)}$ would be drawn from the $p_2 f_2$ variate normal distribution with mean:

$$\left[\sum_{j} (\boldsymbol{I}_{p_2} \otimes \mathbf{X}_{j}^{(2)})^T (\boldsymbol{\Omega}_2^{(2)})^{-1} (\boldsymbol{I}_{p_2} \otimes \mathbf{X}_{j}^{(2)})\right]^{-1} \sum_{j} (\boldsymbol{I}_{p_2} \otimes \mathbf{X}_{j}^{(2)})^T (\boldsymbol{\Omega}_2^{(2)})^{-1} \mathbf{Y}_j^{(2)},$$

   and covariance matrix

$$\left[\sum_{j} (\boldsymbol{I}_{p_2} \otimes \mathbf{X}_{j}^{(2)})^T (\boldsymbol{\Omega}_2^{(2)})^{-1} (\boldsymbol{I}_{p_2} \otimes \mathbf{X}_{j}^{(2)})\right]^{-1}.$$

   Likewise, if there were no level 2 model, then $\boldsymbol{u}_j^{(1)}$ would be drawn from the $p_1 q_1$ multivariate normal distribution with mean

$$\left[\sum_{i} (\boldsymbol{I}_{p_1} \otimes \mathbf{Z}_{i,j}^{(1)})^T (\boldsymbol{\Omega}_1)^{-1} (\boldsymbol{I}_{p_1} \otimes \mathbf{Z}_{i,j}^{(1)}) + (\boldsymbol{\Omega}_2^{(1)})^{-1}\right]^{-1}$$

$$\times \left[\sum_{i} (\boldsymbol{I}_{p_1} \otimes \mathbf{Z}_{i,j}^{(1)})^T (\boldsymbol{\Omega}_1)^{-1} \{\mathbf{Y}_{i,j}^{(1)} - (\boldsymbol{I}_{p_1} \otimes \mathbf{X}_{i,j}^{(1)}) \boldsymbol{\beta}^{(1)}\}\right],$$

and covariance matrix

$$\left[\sum_i (\boldsymbol{I}_{p_1} \otimes \mathbf{Z}_{i,j}^{(1)})^T (\boldsymbol{\Omega}_1)^{-1} (\boldsymbol{I}_{p_1} \otimes \mathbf{Z}_{i,j}^{(1)}) + (\boldsymbol{\Omega}_2^{(1)})^{-1}\right]^{-1}.$$

However, in the two-level response model, we have a covariance between the $p_1 q_1 \times 1$ vector $\boldsymbol{u}_j^{(1)}$ and the $p_2 f_2 \times 1$ vector of level 2 residuals $\mathbf{Y}_j^{(2)} - (\boldsymbol{I}_{p_2} \otimes \mathbf{X}_j^{(2)})\boldsymbol{\beta}^{(2)}$.

In fact, the model specifies

$$\begin{pmatrix} \boldsymbol{u}_j^{(1)} \\ \mathbf{Y}_j^{(2)} - (\boldsymbol{I}_{p_2} \otimes \mathbf{X}_j^{(2)})\boldsymbol{\beta}^{(2)} \end{pmatrix} \sim N\left[\mathbf{0}, \boldsymbol{\Omega}_2 = \begin{pmatrix} \boldsymbol{\Omega}_2^{(1)} & \boldsymbol{\Omega}_2^{(1,2)} \\ \boldsymbol{\Omega}_2^{(2,1)} & \boldsymbol{\Omega}_2^{(2)} \end{pmatrix}\right], \qquad (9.10)$$

where $\boldsymbol{\Omega}_2^{(2,1)}$ is of dimension $p_2 f_2 \times p_1 q_1$.

This suggests the following strategy:

(a) draw $\boldsymbol{\beta}^{(2)}$ from its marginal distribution set out above, and hence calculate $\{\mathbf{Y}_j^{(2)} - (\boldsymbol{I}_{p_2} \otimes \mathbf{X}_j^{(2)})\boldsymbol{\beta}^{(2)}\}$.

(b) calculate, using (9.10), the conditional normal distribution of $\boldsymbol{u}_j^{(1)} | \{\mathbf{Y}_j^{(2)} - (\boldsymbol{I}_{p_2} \otimes \mathbf{X}_j^{(2)})\boldsymbol{\beta}^{(2)}\}$.

(c) Amend the update step for $\boldsymbol{u}_j^{(1)}$, replacing the marginal update step given above (starting from the marginal $\boldsymbol{u}_j^{(1)} \sim N(\mathbf{0}, \boldsymbol{\Omega}_2^{(1)})$) to that derived by starting from the conditional normal distribution of $\boldsymbol{u}_j^{(1)} | \{\mathbf{Y}_j^{(2)} - (\boldsymbol{I}_{p_2} \otimes \mathbf{X}_j^{(2)})\boldsymbol{\beta}^{(2)}\}$.

Write $\boldsymbol{u}_j^{(2)} = \{\mathbf{Y}_j^{(2)} - (\boldsymbol{I}_{p_2} \otimes \mathbf{X}_j^{(2)})\boldsymbol{\beta}^{(2)}\}$. Then, recalling level 2 units are independent, we have

$$\begin{aligned} \boldsymbol{u}_j^{(1)} | \boldsymbol{u}_j^{(2)} &\sim N[\boldsymbol{u}_j^{(2)T} \{\boldsymbol{\Omega}_2^{(2)}\}^{-1} \boldsymbol{\Omega}_2^{(2,1)}, \boldsymbol{\Omega}_2^{(1)} - \boldsymbol{\Omega}_2^{(1,2)} \{\boldsymbol{\Omega}_2^{(2)}\}^{-1} \boldsymbol{\Omega}_2^{(2,1)}], \\ &= N[\boldsymbol{\mu}_j^{1|2}, \boldsymbol{\Omega}_2^{1|2}], \text{ say.} \end{aligned}$$

3. Thus, draw each $\boldsymbol{u}_j^{(1)}$ in turn from the $p_1 q_1$ multivariate normal distribution with mean

$$\left[\sum_i (\boldsymbol{I}_{p_1} \otimes \mathbf{Z}_{i,j}^{(1)})^T (\boldsymbol{\Omega}_1)^{-1} (\boldsymbol{I}_{p_1} \otimes \mathbf{Z}_{i,j}^{(1)}) + (\boldsymbol{\Omega}_2^{(1|2)})^{-1}\right]^{-1}$$
$$\times \left[(\boldsymbol{\Omega}_2^{(1|2)})^{-1} \boldsymbol{\mu}_j^{(1|2)} + \sum_i (\boldsymbol{I}_{p_1} \otimes \mathbf{Z}_{i,j}^{(1)})^T (\boldsymbol{\Omega}_1)^{-1} \{\mathbf{Y}_{i,j}^{(1)} - (\boldsymbol{I}_{p_1} \otimes \mathbf{X}_{i,j}^{(1)})\boldsymbol{\beta}^{(1)}\}\right],$$

and covariance matrix

$$\left[\sum_i (\boldsymbol{I}_{p_1} \otimes \mathbf{Z}_{i,j}^{(1)})^T (\boldsymbol{\Omega}_1)^{-1} (\boldsymbol{I}_{p_1} \otimes \mathbf{Z}_{i,j}^{(1)}) + (\boldsymbol{\Omega}_2^{(1|2)})^{-1}\right]^{-1}.$$

4. Calculate
$$e_{i,j} = \mathbf{Y}_{i,j}^{(1)} - (I_{p_1} \otimes \mathbf{X}_{i,j}^{(1)})\beta^{(1)} - (I_{p_1} \otimes \mathbf{Z}_{i,j}^{(1)})u_j^{(1)},$$
and form $u_j = (u_j^{(1)T} u_j^{(2)T})^T$.

5. Draw $(\mathbf{\Omega}_2)^{-1}$ from $\mathrm{W}(v_u, \mathbf{S}_u)$, where $v_u = J + v_{up}$, (J is the number of level 2 units),
$$\mathbf{S}_u = \left[\sum_j u_j u_j^T + \mathbf{S}_{up}^{-1}\right]^{-1},$$
and the prior for $(\mathbf{\Omega}_2)^{-1}$ is $\mathrm{W}(v_{up}, \mathbf{S}_{up})$.

6. Draw $(\mathbf{\Omega}_1)^{-1}$ from $\mathrm{W}(v_e, \mathbf{S}_e)$, where $v_e = IJ + v_{ep}$, (IJ is the total number of level 1 units),
$$\mathbf{S}_e = \left[\sum_{i,j} e_{i,j} e_{i,j}^T + \mathbf{S}_{ep}^{-1}\right]^{-1},$$
and the prior for $(\mathbf{\Omega}_1)^{-1}$ is $\mathrm{W}(v_{ep}, \mathbf{S}_{ep})$.

We note that the multi-level imputation model (9.8) naturally extends from two levels to any number of levels, including allowing coefficients to be random at the different levels. Likewise, the fitting procedure described above extends to any number of levels without requiring any additional conceptual development.

9.2.1 Ordered and unordered categorical data

Thus far, we have only considered continuous data. We handle binary, ordinal, or categorical data using the latent normal approach described in Chapters 4 and 5, which we can use at both levels 1 and 2.

Thus, for an M-level categorical level 1 variable, there will be $(M - 1)$ uncorrelated latent normal variables at level 1, each with variance constrained to 1, and constrained to be uncorrelated with the other $M - 2$ latent normals. Each of these may have a random intercept at level 2, and these intercepts may be correlated, although in applications with relatively few level 2 units, we may need to restrict some of these correlations to zero in order to avoid over-parameterization at level 2. We return to this point in Section 9.5.

For level 2 discrete variables, the associated latent normals may in principle be correlated with the level 2 random effects associated with level 1 variables.

As mentioned above, and discussed in more detail in Chapters 4 and 5, the latent normal structure for handling categorical variables imposes constraints on elements of the covariance matrices. When fitting the model using MCMC, this means we can no longer update the inverse covariance matrices using a draw from a Wishart distribution, as described in steps 6 and 7 on p. 298. Instead, we need to update the elements of the covariance matrix individually using an appropriate Metropolis–Hastings (MH) step. This proceeds exactly as described in Chapter 4.

9.2.2 Imputing missing values

As described in Chapter 3, missing continuous responses are imputed from the appropriate conditional normal distribution, conditional on current parameter values and other data for the unit. With discrete data, again as described in Chapters 4 and 5, for each missing value, we first draw the latent normal from the appropriate conditional distribution, and then draw the corresponding discrete variable value.

9.2.3 Substantive model compatible imputation

The substantive model-compatible imputation model (9.9) can be fitted with a similar MCMC; in the absence of missing data, the algorithm is identical and repeated for the two parts in which the imputation model (9.9) is factored. However, while missing data in the outcome of the substantive model are similarly easily handled, missing data in the covariates have to be imputed taking into account the effect that the new imputed values have on the likelihood of the substantive model. In Section 6, we have seen how to do this with rejection sampling within a FCS imputation strategy. However, here we impute using a full MCMC i.e. via a Metropolis–Hastings step. As an example, for an individual i from cluster j with a single missing value, in Y_2, and with available measurements for the outcome of the substantive model Y_1 and the other two covariates Y_3 and Y_4, the algorithm would first calculate the mean and variance of the normal distribution from which to draw the proposed imputation. The most natural choice for the proposal distribution is the marginal joint distribution of the three covariates Y_2, Y_3, and Y_4. Specifically, let $\omega_{i,j}$ denote the (i,j) element of the covariance matrix and use the standard conditional normal distribution formula to calculate

$$E[Y_{i,2}|Y_{i,3},Y_{i,4}] = E[Y_{i,2}] + u_{i,j,2} + \begin{pmatrix}\omega_{2,3} & \omega_{2,4}\end{pmatrix}\begin{pmatrix}\omega^2_{3,3} & \omega_{3,4}\\ \omega_{4,3} & \omega^2_{4,4}\end{pmatrix}\begin{pmatrix}Y_{i,3} - E[Y_{i,3}] - u_{i,j,3}\\ Y_{i,4} - E[Y_{i,4}] - u_{i,j,3}\end{pmatrix},$$

$$\mathrm{Var}[Y_{i,2}|Y_{i,3},Y_{i,4}] = \omega^2_{2,2} - \begin{pmatrix}\omega_{2,3} & \omega_{2,4}\end{pmatrix}\begin{pmatrix}\omega^2_{3,3} & \omega_{3,4}\\ \omega_{4,3} & \omega^2_{4,4}\end{pmatrix}\begin{pmatrix}\omega_{2,3}\\ \omega_{2,4}\end{pmatrix}.$$

However, choosing the current value of $Y_{i,2}$ as the mean makes the acceptance step simpler to implement. In particular, after drawing a value $Y^*_{i,2}$ from a normal distribution with mean $Y_{i,2}$ and variance $\mathrm{Var}[Y_{i,2}|Y_{i,3},Y_{i,4}]$, the proposed imputation would be accepted with probability:

$$p = \min\left(1, \frac{L(Y^*_{i,2})}{L(Y_{i,2})}\right),$$

where

$$L(Y^*_{i,2}) = f(Y_{i,1}|Y^*_{i,2},Y_{i,3},Y_{i,4};\theta_y)f(Y^*_{i,2},Y_{i,3},Y_{i,4};\theta_x)$$

is the likelihood of the full imputation model with the proposed imputation, with θ_y and θ_x indicating the full set of parameters for the substantive model and for the marginal joint distribution of the covariates, respectively.

Because of the way the algorithm works, imputations which increase the likelihood of the substantive model are more likely to be accepted, and the sampler converges to the correct Bayesian posterior distribution (cf Appendix A).

Example 9.2 Improving medical records *(ctd)*

We return to the hospital records example and consider the appropriate imputation model. In line with the substantive model, this is multi-level, with patients at level 1 and clinicians at level 2. Ideally, we would have hospitals random at level 3, but our software does not accommodate this. As we have a fixed set of eight hospitals by design, it is reasonable to treat these as fixed effects for imputation.

Initially, we use a standard joint multi-level imputation model as described in Section 9.1.2. Because the data suggest that relations between variables may be different between the four hospitals randomised to receive the intervention (H1–H4) and those that did not (H5–H8), we impute separately in these two groups, always including a fixed effect of hospital. In addition, as we are interested in exploring the interaction between PAR use and whether or not a clinician undertakes CME, and PAR use is fully observed, within the randomised and control hospitals we further impute separately among those who do, and do not, use PAR. Thus, we split the data into four groups by hospital randomisation group and PAR use and impute separately in all four groups. Thus, for PAR users among H5–H8 (where CME was not on offer), the imputation model is

$$
\begin{aligned}
\text{completion}_{i,j,k} &= \beta^{(1)}_{1,0} + \sum_{l=2}^{4} \beta^{(1)}_{1,l} 1[k = 4 + l] + u^{(1)}_{1,j} + e^{(1)}_{1,i,j,k}, \\
\Pr(\text{female child}_{i,j,k}) &= \Pr\left\{ \beta^{(1)}_{2,0} + \sum_{l=2}^{4} \beta^{(1)}_{2,l} 1[k = 4 + l] + u^{(1)}_{2,j} + e^{(1)}_{2,i,j,k} > 0 \right\}, \\
\text{years experience}_{j,k} &= \beta^{(2)}_{1,0} + \sum_{l=2}^{4} \beta^{(2)}_{1,l} 1[k = 4 + l] + u^{(2)}_{1,j}, \\
\Pr(\text{female clinician}_{j,k}) &= \Pr\left\{ \beta^{(2)}_{2,0} + \sum_{l=2}^{4} \beta^{(2)}_{2,l} 1[k = 4 + l] + u^{(2)}_{2,j} > 0 \right\}, \\
(u^{(1)}_{1,j}, u^{(1)}_{2,j}, u^{(2)}_{1,j}, u^{(2)}_{2,j})^T &\sim N(\mathbf{0}, \mathbf{\Omega}_2),\ \mathbf{\Omega}_2 \text{ unconstrained except } \{\mathbf{\Omega}_2\}_{(4,4)} = 1, \\
\begin{pmatrix} e^{(1)}_{1,i,j,k} \\ e^{(1)}_{2,i,j,k} \end{pmatrix} &\sim N\left\{ \mathbf{0}, \begin{pmatrix} \sigma^2_{e,1} & \sigma_{e,1,2} \\ \sigma_{e,1,2} & 1 \end{pmatrix} \right\}.
\end{aligned}
\tag{9.11}
$$

We fitted each of the four models and imputed the missing values, using the `R` package jomo. Each imputation model was burned in for 5000 updates, and the model was updated 500 times between each of the 10 imputations. Examination of the chains showed the sampler had converged and had satisfactory mixing. The results were appended to give 10 imputed datasets.

Additionally, we imputed from a substantive model compatible imputation model, imputing compatibly with either analysis model (9.6) or (9.7). Using this approach, it is not necessary to split the data into four parts, as the imputation model is (by design) compatible with the interactions in the substantive model.

Table 9.4 shows the results. For all the analyses, PAR dramatically increases the percentage of completeness in the hospital admission record, and the randomised intervention adds an additional 10% to completeness on average. After imputation with any of the two methods, admission records from children admitted by a clinician who had participated in CME, but not used the PAR, have completion reduced by 5% ($p < 0.001$). Unsurprisingly, this is a small group of admissions (2.5% of those in H1–H4), yet still worth further investigation. Records from admissions by clinicians who took CME and used PAR show only a small and statistically non-significant increase in the completion of $(5.9 - 5.0) = 0.9\%$ over those who only used PAR. Turning to the variance components, the complete records analysis substantially underestimates both between clinician and between child variability in record completeness, with complete record estimates of variance components lying outside the corresponding 95% confidence intervals from the MI analysis. Residuals are slightly heavy tailed relative to the normal distribution, but this is insufficient to substantively affect these inferences.

The practically important difference between the complete records and MI analyses here is largely due to the additional information from the partially observed cases (typically where the clinician did not report their gender or years of experience). Unfortunately, there is very little information about the missing values of clinician's years of experience in the other variables. If available, auxiliary variables from the dataset could usefully be included to address this; since many clinicians report no experience, categorising this variable may also be appropriate. As usual, we make the assumption that MAR and sensitivity analysis are appropriate to explore the robustness of the inferences to plausible missing not at random (MNAR) mechanisms (see Chapter 12).

In conclusion, multi-level MI allows the imputation of missing variables at the child and clinician levels, respecting the multi-level structure. This confirms the substantive impact on the completion of paediatric admission procedures of PAR and the randomised intervention and reveals the CME (at least as provided) is unhelpful – at least in terms of improving the completeness of admissions records. □

9.2.4 Checking model convergence

As mentioned in Part I, when using joint modelling imputation, it is always important to check that the sampler has converged before starting to register imputations and that successive imputations are sufficiently apart to have low stochastic correlation. The simplest way to check this is by visual inspection of the MCMC chains for each parameter in the model alongside the corresponding auto-correlation plots. Additionally, it is advisable to estimate $\hat{R}$ for each parameter, which should be less than approximately 1.1 if the sampler has converged satisfactorily. The `R` package

Table 9.4 Results of fitting (9.6) and (9.7) to complete records and after multi-level multiple imputation.

Random-interc. model (1)	Complete records			Imputation model (9.11)			Substantive Model Compatible Multilevel MI		
Fixed-effect param:	Est.	SE	*p*-value	Est.	SE	*p*-value	Est.	SE	*p*-value
Intercept	26.3	2.30	<0.001	26.2	2.46	<0.001	26.6	2.30	<0.001
PAR use	50.2	0.43	<0.001	48.7	0.41	<0.001	48.7	0.41	<0.001
Female child	0.3	0.24	0.27	0.2	0.25	0.52	0.2	0.23	0.41
Female clinician	0.2	0.88	0.86	0.6	1.00	0.55	0.5	0.88	0.57
Years of experience	−0.3	0.08	<0.001	−0.4	0.20	0.064	−0.5	0.088	<0.001
Interventional hospital	10.0	3.10	0.016	11.2	3.25	0.001	11.0	3.15	<0.001
CME attendance	0.7	1.71	0.68	−5.1	1.58	0.001	−5.2	1.60	0.001
PAR × CME interaction	−0.5	1.37	0.74	5.9	1.17	<0.001	6.0	1.16	<0.001
Var. components:									
Hospital	17.09			19.03			17.80		
Clinician	41.06			50.23			48.00		
Child	88.95			100.15			100.36		
Random slope model (2)									
Fixed-effect param:	Est.	SE	*p*-value	Est.	SE	*p*-value	Est.	SE	*p*-value
Intercept	25.5	2.57	<0.001	25.5	2.68	<0.001	26.3	2.60	<0.001
PAR use	50.0	1.23	<0.001	48.9	1.10	<0.001	48.9	1.10	<0.001
Female child	0.2	0.22	0.37	0.2	0.22	0.42	0.2	0.21	0.47
Female clinician	0.3	1.05	0.77	0.5	1.09	0.63	0.1	1.10	0.89
Years of experience	−0.1	0.31	0.65	−0.4	0.27	0.16	−0.6	0.30	0.07
Years of exp squared	−0.011	0.013	0.39	−0.002	0.012	0.86	0.003	0.013	0.81
Interventional hospital	10.6	3.18	0.014	11.2	3.45	0.001	10.9	3.29	0.001
CME attendance	0.7	2.75	0.81	−3.1	2.35	0.19	−3.2	2.40	0.18
PAR × CME interaction	−0.5	2.84	0.86	4.0	2.51	0.11	4.1	2.53	0.11
Var. components:									
Hospital	17.12			21.11			19.01		
Clinician (int)	136.87			116.19			115.05		
Clinician (slope)	186.67			185.25			185.35		
Clinician (cov)	−125.56			−107.11			−107.20		
Child	73.66			82.25			82.24		

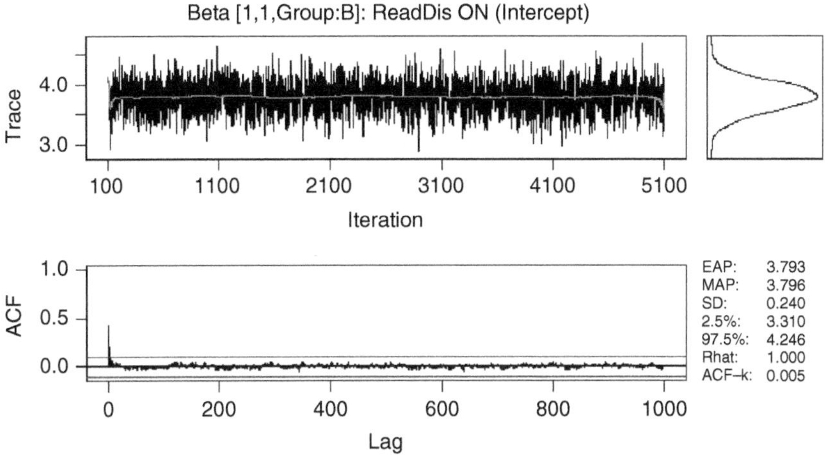

Figure 9.1 Example of trace plot and autocorrelation plot from R *package* `mitml`*.*

`mitml` (Grund *et al.*, 2019) includes functions to perform all the above checks and produce plots such as Figure 9.1.

9.3 Extensions

Here we introduce further extensions to the general algorithm introduced in Section 9.2. These include allowing for cross-classification, more than two levels and heteroscedasticity.

9.3.1 Cross-classification and three-level data

In principle, we can extend the multi-level model of Section 9.1 from two levels to as many as required. The Gibbs sampling algorithm in Section 9.2 extends directly to this setting; we need to include separate random effects and associated covariance matrices for each additional level and sample the associated parameters analogously to the level two random effects.

Cross-classified and associated multiple membership structures occur when observations are grouped by two separate hierarchies. For example, in an educational setting, children are grouped in classes within schools, but children are also grouped by residential neighbourhood, which is typically linked to social class and, hence, academic achievement. Such structures are considered in detail in Goldstein (2010, Chapter 12). When modelling such data, omitting the cross-classified structure can result in biased estimation of variance components because groups of units in the second (crossed) classification are treated as independent when they could be highly correlated. This in turn can lead to misleading inference.

It follows that when imputing such data, the model should allow for the cross-classified structure. Thus far, we have only considered hierarchical structure, and the full covariance matrix for the data has thus been block-diagonal. When modelling cross-classified data, we retain the block-diagonal structure for the first hierarchy, but the second hierarchy is captured through blocks of non-zero off-diagonal terms. It is computationally straightforward to update these terms one-at-a-time using Metropolis–Hastings steps. This proceeds in the way described, in the context of binary data, in Chapter 4.

9.3.2 Random level 1 covariance matrices

Yucel (2011) describes an extension to allow the level 1 covariance matrices to differ between level 2 units. An application where this may be useful is imputation for individual participant data meta-analysis. Here, the different entry criteria for the different studies may well result in different level 1 (within study) covariance matrices. However, we cannot impute each study separately, because – as discussed above – we need information from other studies to impute covariates that are not collected in specific studies. Another application arises in the context of multiple imputation with survey weights, discussed in Chapter 12.

In such situations, Yucel (2011) assumes that the level 1 precision (inverse covariance) matrices are drawn from a Wishart distribution. Thus, the common precision matrix $\mathbf{\Omega}_1$ in (9.8) is replaced by $\mathbf{\Omega}_{1,j}$, with marginal distribution

$$(\mathbf{\Omega}_{1,j})^{-1} \sim \mathrm{W}(a, A).$$

Here $a > p_1$ (the number of level 1 variables) is the degrees of freedom of the Wishart distribution, and A is the scale matrix.

In order to implement this, we need to extend the sampler described in Section 9.2. We first specify priors for $a \sim \chi^2_\eta$ and $A^{-1} \sim \mathrm{W}(\gamma, \Gamma)$. Here γ must be greater than the dimension of Γ, and the analyst needs to choose values of η, γ and Γ.

We first describe how to draw A, a and then describe how to draw $\mathbf{\Omega}_{1j}$. Other parameters are updated as described in Section 9.2, but now respecting the different level 1 covariance matrices, $\mathbf{\Omega}_{1j}$, for each of the level 1 units.

The inverse of A is drawn as follows:

$$A^{-1} \sim \mathrm{W}(\gamma + aJ, \Gamma^{\star}),$$

where J is the number of level 2 units, and $\Gamma^{\star} = (\Gamma^{-1} + \sum_j \mathbf{\Omega}_{1,j}^{-1})^{-1}$.

We update a using a Metropolis–Hastings step. First note that the conditional density of a is proportional to

$$f(a) = f_1(a)\left(\prod_{i=1}^{p_1} \Gamma\left(\frac{a+1-i}{2}\right)\right)^{-J} \left(\prod_{j=1}^{J} | \mathbf{\Omega}_{1,j}^{-1} |\right)^{-\frac{a+p_1+1}{2}}$$
$$\times |A_{-1} + \mathbf{\Omega}_{1,1}^{-1} + \cdots + \mathbf{\Omega}_{1,J}^{-1}|^{\frac{-aJ+\gamma}{2}} \left(\prod_{j=1}^{p_1} \Gamma\left(\frac{\gamma + aJ + 1 - j}{2}\right)\right)^{-1}, \tag{9.12}$$

where $f_1(a)$ is the prior distribution of a, i.e. χ^2_η.

We could use a symmetric Metropolis–Hastings sampler to update a. However, this will generally be awkward, as a has a skew distribution. Instead, Yucel (2011) proposes that since we must have $a > p_1$, we can write $u = \log(a + p_1)$, and then

$$f_U(u) = f(e^u - p_1)\left|\frac{\partial a}{\partial u}\right|,$$

where the function f on the right-hand side is given by (9.12). We then use a Metropolis–Hastings step to update u, where the proposal is a t_4 distribution centred at the mode of $f_U(u)$, with the same curvature (second derivative) at the mode. Denote the mode by u_m, calculated, say, using a numerical or Newton–Raphson search and denote the second derivative at the mode by

$$d(u_m) = \left.\frac{\partial^2}{\partial^2 u} f_U(u)\right|_{u=u_m}.$$

Then if we draw $T \sim t_4$, and set $U = \lambda T + u_m$, we have the proposal density

$$h(u) \propto \left[1 + \frac{(u - u_m)^2}{4\lambda^2}\right]^{-5/2}.$$

Since this has curvature $-5/(4\lambda^2)$ at the mode, to match the curvature of f_u, we choose

$$\lambda = \sqrt{-\frac{5}{4d(u_m)}}.$$

The Metropolis–Hastings sampler, currently at u, then accepts a proposed $u^\star$ with probability

$$\min\left\{1, \frac{f(u^\star)}{f(u)}\frac{h(u)}{h(u^\star)}\right\}.$$

Lastly, given draws of A, a, then for each j we draw

$$\boldsymbol{\Omega}_{1,j}^{-1} \sim \mathrm{W}(a + I, W_j^{-1}),$$

where $W_j = A^{-1} + \sum_{i=1}^{I} \boldsymbol{e}_{i,j}\boldsymbol{e}_{i,j}^T$ and

$$\boldsymbol{e}_{i,j} = \mathbf{Y}_{i,j}^{(1)} - (\boldsymbol{I}_{p_1} \otimes \mathbf{X}_{i,j}^{(1)})\boldsymbol{\beta}^{(1)} - (\boldsymbol{I}_{p_1} \otimes \mathbf{Z}_{i,j}^{(1)})\boldsymbol{u}_j^{(1)}.$$

Yucel successfully applies this to impute data from a crime victimisation survey, where level 2 units are city blocks.

Extending the imputation model in this way allows for different, cluster-specific, associations between outcomes of the imputation model. Hence, it is preferable to use this approach when the substantive model has missing data in both the outcome and a covariate with random slope. This issue was discussed by Quartagno and Carpenter (2016), and further explored by Enders *et al.* (2018) (among others). While an improvement over a homoscedastic imputation model in this setting, it is important to note that it still does not allow for full compatibility, for which the methods of Section 9.1.3 are necessary; the latter approach is therefore often preferable.

9.3.3 Model fit

Formal assessment of model fit is usually of secondary importance when constructing an imputation model, relative to selecting auxiliary variables and ensuring the structure in the model of interest is appropriately captured in the imputation model. This issue is discussed in Section 14.5.

Here we note that the deviance information criterion (DIC) (Spiegelhalter *et al.*, 2002) may provide useful additional information to choose between imputation models. In order to calculate the DIC, we need to calculate the log-likelihood at each cycle of the MCMC algorithm, say D_i, their average, $\overline{D}$, and also the log-likelihood at the final parameter estimates, say $D(\theta)$, where θ is usually obtained by averaging the post-convergence MCMC parameter chain. The DIC is then

$$\overline{D} + p_D, \text{ where } p_D = \{\overline{D} - D(\theta)\}.$$

Models with the smaller values of the DIC are then preferred. In applications with missing data, we have to be careful to calculate the log-likelihood for the observed data, rather than the log-likelihood for the observed and imputed data, and it may be useful to do this in stages, i.e. calculate the log-likelihood for the continuous variables given the categorical variables, and add the log-likelihood for the categorical variables (Goldstein *et al.*, 2009).

9.4 Other imputation methods

Thus far, in this chapter, we have focused on a single type of parametric multiple imputation based on the use of a joint imputation model for the partially observed variables which is fitted using MCMC. The main advantages of this method are that the extension to the multi-level settings is quite natural and that considerations around compatibility of imputation and analysis model are easier when the joint model is explicitly expressed.

On the other hand, it can be argued that JM imputation has drawbacks as well, particularly in terms of computational complexity Thus, in recent years, a number of alternative imputation methods - both of parametric and non-parametric nature - have been developed to handle missing multilevel data. In this section, we review and compare some of these methods, highlighting advantages and disadvantages of each.

9.4.1 One-step and two-step FCS

Full Conditional Specification remains one of, if not the, most used parametric imputation method with single-level data. Because of the complications introduced by the random effects, when imputing multi-level data FCS is less straightforward to apply. For example, Resche-Rigon and White (2018) showed that given a simple joint multi-level model, the conditional expectation of one predictor given the other depends on the cluster mean of that predictor and the size of the clusters. Hence, at least in theory, the cluster means should be included in the univariate imputation models, as well as the cluster level data, and the model should allow for heteroscedasticity.

But how can the FCS procedure be implemented with multi-level data exactly? In the last decade, various methods to perform multi-level FCS imputation have been developed. Among these, two in particular are available for imputation of a mix of different data types, and for both sporadically and systematically missing data, i.e. for both sporadic missingness within clusters and systematic missingness for certain variables in whole clusters.

The first method is FCS imputation based on generalised linear mixed-effects models (Jolani, 2018). This is perhaps the most natural extension of single-level FCS, where random effects are simply added to the standard univariate single-level models. The method was initially developed to handle systematically missing data only (Jolani *et al.*, 2015) and then extended to sporadically missing data (Jolani, 2018). In its current implementation in statistical software, it assumes homoscedasticity of level one variances. For this reason, it can only accommodate random-intercept substantive models. However, extending this to allow for heteroscedasticity is theoretically possible. With this method, the univariate imputation models are generalised mixed models and an approximate Bayesian step is used to draw the parameter values to be used for imputation after fitting the multi-level model. This extends a previous implementation (van Buuren, 2011) based on a full Gibbs sampler that was only able to handle partially observed continuous variables.

The second method is FCS based on a two-stage estimator. This is based on an idea similar to two-stage meta-analysis: first, a separate model within each cluster is fitted, and then the results are combined using multivariate random-effects meta-analysis models. This approach naturally allows for heteroscedasticity at level 1. Resche-Rigon and White (2018) compared two different methods of combining results from various clusters, and concluded that the method of moments was preferable, particularly because of its advantage in terms of computational speed over restricted maximum likelihood (REML).

9.4.2 Substantive model compatible imputation

In Section 9.1.3, we introduced the idea of substantive model compatible multilevel imputation based on the joint modelling framework. The same idea can be readily applied in the FCS framework, as described in Chapter 6. In the multilevel setting – as in the single level – the imputation step for the covariates could potentially be implemented via a rejection sampling step, instead of using Metropolis–Hastings. The advantage of the latter approach is that a new value is drawn at each step, although in some cases, the sampler might struggle to converge, failing to update certain imputed values.

Another possible option is to use the sequential modelling (SM) approach to imputation. This is a parametric method that sits roughly in between FCS and JM. Similarly to FCS, a set of univariate imputation models is specified, rather than the joint distribution. However, each model is not specified conditioning on all other variables as with FCS, but rather in a sequential way. Hence, a marginal model is proposed for the first covariate, followed by a model for a second covariate conditional on the first covariate only. Finally, a model for the outcome given all the covariates is assumed, and this can be made to match the substantive model. The main difference with respect to FCS imputation is that the SM approach defines the joint model at least in a factored way, while no joint model may correspond to the FCS univariate models. Similarly to SMC-JM, SMC-SM can be implemented in a relatively straightforward way with a full MCMC sampler. Hence, the most natural way of accepting the proposed imputations is via a Metropolis–Hastings step similar to that introduced in Section 9.2.

9.4.3 Non-parametric methods

While for single-level multiple imputation a multitude of non-parametric imputation methods have been developed, in addition to the classic parametric ones, for multi-level data non-parametric methods are less common. This may partly be due to the compatibility problems introduced by multi-level structures, or partly to the fact that the multi-level structure is most often defined in a fully parametric way, and hence, it is only natural to approach the problem of imputation in a similarly parametric way. Nevertheless, in recent years, a few imputation methods building on non-parametric ideas have been developed. For example, Vidotto *et al.* (2018) developed a Bayesian latent class imputation method for the imputation of categorical data, with latent classes both at levels 1 and 2, fitted with a Gibbs sampler. The advantage of the method is that it can theoretically handle complex interactions as well, although this comes at a cost in terms of simplicity in investigating congeniality of the imputation and analysis method. More recently, Husson *et al.* (2019) proposed a method based on multilevel singular value decomposition (SVD); this consists in decomposing the variability of the data into two components, one for each level, and in performing an SVD on both parts. At the moment, though, the method has only been developed to perform a single imputation, and hence, it is not clear how unbiased estimates of the variance of parameters estimates can be obtained.

9.4.4 Comparisons of different methods

A few papers have compared different methods of performing multilevel MI. Audigier *et al.* (2018) compared the two methods based on FCS imputation discussed above with a simple JM imputation (including a heteroscedastic model for the imputation of missing multi-level data), when the substantive model is a linear mixed model and data are both systematically and sporadically missing for a mix of continuous and binary variables. They concluded that all three methods perform better than simpler methods which do not properly account for the multilevel structure. Among the three, two-stage FCS was the most computationally efficient, when based on the method of moments, and the most robust to the number of clusters. JM was the most accurate with more than one binary partially observed variable and was recommended with a large number of clusters. One-stage FCS was recommended with small cluster sizes.

Similar results were obtained in Enders *et al.* (2018), while in an earlier paper, Mistler and Enders (2017) compared FCS and JM imputation, concluding that both are appropriate under a random intercept model, while FCS is preferable with random slopes and JM with analysis models that posit different within- and between-cluster associations. Grund *et al.* (2018) compared FCS and JM, similarly concluding that these work well in simple situations, but struggle to cope with more complex analysis models with random slopes and cross-level interactions. In order to overcome such problems, they suggested that substantive model compatible imputation might be needed.

Huque *et al.* (2020) compared different implementations of JM and FCS for both clustered and longitudinal data, obtaining similar results to Audigier *et al.* (2018) for clustered data; they also obtained good results with SMC-JM, which appropriately handles missing data in random covariates and non-linearities as well. For longitudinal data, they found the simpler implementations of JM and FCS to be unbiased and efficient with balanced data.

9.5 Individual participant data meta-analysis

An important application of multi-level imputation is individual participant meta-analysis, particularly when – as will usually be the case – not all contributing studies have followed the same protocol. For example, we may wish to estimate a risk model, but find that not all the contributing studies have collected the set of predictors we wish to include. Another issue that may arise alongside this is that studies may have recorded variables on different scales (e.g. continuous, ordinal). In addition to this, there will typically be missing data on variables that should have been recorded in a study, but for one reason or another were not.

The chief issue for applying multi-level MI using (9.8), and using the latent normal structure to handle discrete variables, is that there are usually a large number of variables relative to the number of studies. If there are p continuous variables, then the level two (study level) covariance matrix will have $p(p+1)/2$ parameters; unless the number of studies comfortably exceeds this, estimation is likely to be extremely imprecise, and may not be possible. In practice, there are therefore two options, which parallel those discussed in Section 14.8. We can either

1. stabilise the level 2 covariance matrix using a ridge-regression type approach, i.e. by adding a positive constant λ to the diagonal terms (variances) in the level 2 covariance matrix, or

2. restrict some of the level 2 covariance terms to zero, or restrict some of the partial correlation coefficients in the inverse level 2 covariance matrix to zero.

Given a (somewhat arbitrary) choice of ridge parameter λ, the first option is simpler computationally, especially if there are no categorical variables at level 2. In this case, the ridge-type approach still permits direct drawing of the level-two inverse covariance matrix from the Wishart distribution.

The second option is perhaps less arbitrary. However, since it involves constraining (typically to zero) level 2 covariances (and possibly variances) for which there is little information, we then have to update the covariance matrix element-wise, as discussed in Chapter 4.

One approach to decide which study-level variances/covariances should be set to zero is as follows. First, for each variable in turn fit a multi-level model with a component of variance at the patient- and study-level, and estimate the study-level residuals. Then calculate the sample covariances of the estimated study-level residuals. Variables for which the between study component of variance is very small, or inestimable, can be constrained to zero in the imputation model. Likewise, covariances which are practically unimportant can be constrained to zero in the imputation model.

In many examples, it may suffice to simply set all the level 2 covariance terms to zero. To understand the implication of this, consider an imputation model for individuals (level 1) within a study (level 2), who have data on systolic blood pressure (SBP) and diastolic blood pressure (DBP). The imputation model is

$$
\begin{aligned}
\mathrm{SBP}_{i,j} &= \beta_{0,1} + u_{0,1,j} + e_{1,i,j}, \\
\mathrm{DBP}_{i,j} &= \beta_{0,2} + u_{0,2,j} + e_{2,i,j}, \\
\begin{pmatrix} u_{0,1,j} \\ u_{0,2,j} \end{pmatrix} &\sim N\left[\begin{pmatrix} 0 \\ 0 \end{pmatrix}, \begin{pmatrix} \sigma^2_{u1} & \sigma_{u1,u2} \\ \sigma_{u1,u2} & \sigma^2_{u2} \end{pmatrix}\right], \\
\begin{pmatrix} e_{1,i,j} \\ e_{2,i,j} \end{pmatrix} &\sim N\left[\begin{pmatrix} 0 \\ 0 \end{pmatrix}, \begin{pmatrix} \sigma^2_{e1} & \sigma_{e1,e2} \\ \sigma_{e1,e2} & \sigma^2_{e2} \end{pmatrix}\right].
\end{aligned}
$$

Restricting $\sigma_{u1,u2} = 0$ does not formally affect the variance of SBP or DBP. The correlation of SBP and DBP from individual i in study j is

$$
\frac{\sigma_{e1,e2}}{\sqrt{(\sigma^2_{u1} + \sigma^2_{e1})(\sigma^2_{u2} + \sigma^2_{e2})}} \text{ instead of } \frac{\sigma_{u1,u2} + \sigma_{e1,e2}}{\sqrt{(\sigma^2_{u1} + \sigma^2_{e1})(\sigma^2_{u2} + \sigma^2_{e2})}},
$$

while for two different individuals in the same study, the correlation is

$$
0 \text{ instead of } \frac{\sigma_{u1,u2}}{\sqrt{(\sigma^2_{u1} + \sigma^2_{e1})(\sigma^2_{u2} + \sigma^2_{e2})}}.
$$

However, because $\sigma_{e1,e2}$, i.e. the within individual covariance, typically dominates $\sigma_{u1,u2}$, this is unlikely to cause serious bias in practice. Thus, under the multi-level imputation model even with constraints on the study-level covariance matrix, imputation takes account of the clustering within studies.

An alternative is to impute cross-sectionally, using a fixed effect for study. Such an imputation model does not take account of clustering within studies. In certain contexts, this may be non-trivial: for instance when different studies recruit patients with different illness severity, or otherwise different backgrounds. Further, for systematically missing variables within a study, we have to choose another study (with the variable observed) as the reference, to obtain a mean value about which to impute. Again, the appropriateness of this depends on the context of the various studies, but in general, it is advisable to avoid this, especially if we wish to do study-specific analyses and/or meaningful comparisons of summary statistics across studies. Nevertheless, in situations where the substantive model estimates a common effect of covariates adjusted for study, it may be that imputing using a fixed effect for study, and not formally taking account of the multi-level structure, is practically equivalent for estimating the coefficients of such covariates. This is because differences in the mean of covariates between studies will be accounted for in the coefficients for the study indicator variables in the substantive model.

9.5.1 Different measurement scales

We consider two scenarios: first, a measurement of the same underlying quantity is rounded in some studies but not in others. Second, closely related, yet different quantities are measured in different studies.

An example of the first is ejection fraction in patients with heart failure. Depending on how it is measured, this can be a percentage (between 0 and 100) but is quite often an ordinal score. If we wish to include the continuous variable in the model of interest, we can impute this for all participants, taking the ordinal values as bounds on the imputed values. For each patient, at each update of the imputation algorithm, the proposed imputed value is only accepted if consistent with the ordinal bounds. In the case of rejection, a new proposal is repeatedly drawn until one is accepted.

An example of the second is studies of lung function, which can be assessed, among other ways, using forced expiratory volume and forced vital capacity. Here the ideal is to have at least one study which has measured both and to include both variables in the imputation model. The desired measure can then be used in the model of interest.

Note that this issue is a particular example of measurement error, discussed in Chapter 11.

9.5.2 When to apply Rubin's rules

Another issue in this context is the choice of the appropriate point at which Rubin's rules are applied in the analysis. For example, suppose the goal of the analysis is estimation of a prognostic model. Then we can envisage two strategies:

Strategy 1: impute → meta-analysis → Rubin's rules.

This is appropriate when using a single multi-level imputation model across studies; we proceed as follows:

1. Fit the full imputation model, obtaining $k = 1, \dots, K$ imputations of all the constituent studies;
2. For imputation k,
   (a) fit the multi-level prognostic model to the data (with study as level 2);
3. Apply Rubin's rules to summarise the results of the $k = 1, \dots, K$ prognostic models.

Alternatively, we may use strategy 2: impute → fit the prognostic model to each imputation for each study→ apply Rubin's rules within studies → meta-analyse the results.

This is appropriate when imputing within studies; we proceed as follows:

1. Fit the full imputation model, obtaining $k = 1, \dots, K$ imputations of all the constituent studies *or* fit a separate imputation model within each study, again obtaining $k = 1, \dots, K$ imputations of all the constituent studies;
2. For study $j = 1, \dots, J$
   (a) fit the prognostic model to each of the $k = 1, \dots, K$ imputations for the study;
   (b) apply Rubin's rules to obtain parameter estimates and standard errors for that study;
3. Fit a meta-analysis to summarise the results across studies.

Strategy 1 is more consistent with the derivation of Rubin's rules, which are derived to summarise the posterior distribution of parameter estimates in models fitted to imputed data, and simulation studies by Burgess *et al.* (2013) have confirmed this.

If the model of interest is a survival model, and we are interested in assessing the improvement in prediction through adding additional variables, it is worth remembering that many of the commonly used measures depend implicitly on the underlying event rate; thus the same predictors will give different values of the predictive index with different underlying event rates. This is problematic with meta-analysis because usually different studies will have very different event rates. It is thus more meaningful to apply such measures to a multi-level predictive model for all studies, than to apply to individual studies and then attempt to summarise across studies.

9.5.3 Homoscedastic versus heteroscedastic imputation model

We have seen in this chapter that it is possible to fit a multi-level imputation model assuming either homoscedasticity, i.e. same covariance matrix for each level 2 unit, or heteroscedasticity, i.e. level 2-specific covariance matrices. Individual participant data meta-analyses are an application where it is often very common to deal with substantial heterogeneity between different clusters (i.e. studies). Hence, heteroscedastic models may be superior in this application. Quartagno and Carpenter (2016) investigated this, finding that, as expected, heteroscedastic models are superior in presence of heterogeneity, while they tend to be conservative in the absence of heterogeneity, without leading to substantial bias. Such heteroscedastic models can, if desired, in principle be combined with substantive model compatible imputation – this will be most useful in situations where the substantive model includes non-linearities and/or interactions and/or random slopes.

9.6 Software

Several software packages are available for performing multilevel MI. The following is not intended as an exhaustive list, and new packages continue to appear.

Joint modelling imputation is implemented in the `R` package `jomo` (Quartagno and Carpenter, 2023; Quartagno *et al.*, 2019). This allows for the imputation of a mix of continuous and categorical data at levels 1 and 2. Algorithms to perform both standard and substantive model compatible imputation are available, categorical data are handled with latent normal variables, and there is an option to allow for heteroscedastic imputation. A user-friendly interface is available in the package `mitml` (Grund *et al.*, 2019), which also provides a set of useful tools to inspect and analyse imputed multi-level data and an interface to the package `pan` (Zhao and Schafer, 2018). `pan` uses a very similar algorithm to jomo, but can only include level 1 continuous variables. In such restricted situations, it is much faster than all competing packages.

Some functions for multi-level FCS are included in the package `mice` (van Buuren and Groothuis-Oudshoorn, 2011), while `micemd` (Audigier and Resche-Rigon, 2019) provides the functions to perform two-stage FCS. There is currently no `R` package for performing substantive model compatible FCS imputation in multi-level settings, while two packages are available for substantive model compatible sequential modelling (SM) imputation, namely `mdmb` (Robitzsch and Luedtke, 2020) and `jointAI` (Erler *et al.*, 2021), though the latter is for a full Bayesian analysis combining analysis and imputation.

We are not aware of any functions for performing multi-level MI in Stata, but it is relatively simple to export data from Stata for imputation with `jomo` and then export the results back to Stata. In `SAS`, the `MMI_IMPUTE` macro implements multi-level JM with continuous data.

Finally, several standalone programmes allow for the imputation of multilevel data. `REALCOM-Impute` (Carpenter *et al.*, 2011a) uses a very similar algorithm to `jomo`, although it does not allow for random covariance matrices or substantive model compatible imputation. `MPlus` (Muthén and Muthén, 2011) similarly allows for the use of multi-level imputation through a latent normal model. Finally, `Blimp` (Keller and Enders, 2017) is a very flexible software package, allowing for both simple FCS multilevel imputation (Enders *et al.*, 2018) and substantive model compatible JM imputation (Hayes, 2019).

9.7 Discussion

In this chapter, we have considered imputation of multilevel data. We have proposed a general multi-level imputation model under the joint modelling framework, and illustrated some of the issues that may arise if the multi-level structure is ignored in imputation. We have illustrated the application of these methods to data with missing observations at level 2, and also considered the application to individual participant data meta-analysis, where some studies may not collect all of the variables we wish to include in the model of interest. We have seen the challenges of imputing when the substantive model includes random slopes and non-linearities, concluding that substantive model-compatible imputation can address both. Lastly, we have discussed extensions to more than two levels, cross-classified structures and random covariance matrices at level 1. As our applications illustrate, the class of multi-level imputation models described here allow congenial imputation for a range of models and data structures which are increasingly arising in applications, not least individual participant data meta-analysis.

Exercises

1. For this exercise, we use the 'class size' dataset. These data are derived from the class size study carried out by Peter Blatchford and colleagues at the Institute of Education (London) and kindly made available to us. The data contain simulated observations of standardised scores of pre-reception year maths and literacy scores and post-reception literacy scores. The data have a two-level hierarchical structure, with children clustered within schools. We consider two possible substantive models of interest:

    - A model for the `nmatpre` variable to investigate whether children from the same school have more similar pre-reception maths scores to each other than children from different schools. This is a linear model with a random school effect only, and no fixed effects, and is often called the random-intercept model.
    - A model to investigate if literature scores at the end of the year (`nlitpost`) are related to the literature and maths pre-reception scores (`nlitpre`, `nmatpre`). Since the observations are clustered within school, we again use a random-school intercept model.

    In this exercise, we explore the inferences from these models of interest, when we use different missing data handling strategies.

    (a) **Complete records analysis:** First, simply fit the two substantive models above to the partially observed data. Look at the results and interpret them. Under what missing data mechanisms these would be valid? Compare the random effect variance from the two models: would you expect these to be similar, and if so, why?

    (b) **Multiple imputation ignoring clustering:** Now impute the missing `nmatpre` values using an imputation model which completely ignores the clustering. Since data are missing in a single continuous variable, do you expect it would make a difference whether you choose to use single-level or multi-level imputation? Now, fit the substantive model and combine the estimates with Rubin's rules. Compare your parameter estimates with those from the complete records analysis. Are there any substantial differences? If so, can you explain them?

(c) **Including the cluster variable as a fixed effect:** Now repeat the same imputation routine, but this time including school as a fixed effect. Again, compare the estimates with those obtained from the previous missing data handling strategies. Are there any substantive differences? if so, can you explain them? When might using fixed effects for the cluster variable 'school' be a poor idea? In what circumstances might it be reasonable?

(d) **Homoscedastic multi-level multiple imputation:** Now impute using a multi-level imputation model under homoscedasticity, i.e. assuming the same variance applies to all schools. You can use the `R` package `jomo` to generate the imputations and, if you prefer working in Stata, you can save the data in `.dta` format using the `write.dta` function in the `foreign` package (cf also the `haven` package) and import the imputed data set in Stata using the `mi import` function. How do the parameter estimates compare with the complete records estimates and those based on a single-level imputation model? How do the standard errors compare with those from the complete records analyses?

(e) **Heteroscedastic multi-level multiple imputation:** Now impute using a similar imputation model, but in `jomo` set the option `meth='random'` to use a heteroscedastic model. How do the parameter estimates compare? What about the standard errors? Did you expect to see any substantial differences in this settings, and why? In what circumstances might this approach be more suitable?

(f) **Substantive model compatible imputation:** Finally, impute with substantive model compatible imputation, using the `jomo.lmer` function in `R`. Do you think this is different from the other multi-level imputation strategies for the first substantive model? What are the benefits of substantive model compatible imputation and do you think it was necessary here? What could be the disadvantage of such an approach? Can you create a single set of imputed data which is appropriate for both the substantive models considered here?

2. This exercise considers how to investigate the effect of a specific treatment on blood pressure. A number of studies have been published on this topic, and we wish to do an individual patient data meta-analysis to synthesize the results. Discuss what is, in your opinion, the best way to impute missing data for this meta-analysis under each of these scenarios in turn:

(a) All the studies are large randomised trials, all of which adjusted for the same two baseline variables. We do not anticipate much heterogeneity, as all trials targeted the same estimand, considered similar populations, in similar settings, and had very similar protocols. There are only few sporadically missing data in both confounders and in the outcome.

(b) All the studies are randomised trials, some larger and some smaller. Some trials are adjusted for two baseline variables, but some only for one because they did not collect data on the other. While the trials are similar, we expect that the slightly different settings in which they were conducted might lead to heterogeneous treatment effects. As well as the studies with systematically missing baseline variables, all the studies have sporadically missing data in all other variables.

(c) There is a mix of both randomised trials and observational studies. Some trials found that older people benefited less from the treatment, and observational studies always collected information on age. Our substantive model therefore includes an interaction between treatment and age. Given the nature of the studies, we anticipate there might be substantial heterogeneity.

(d) All studies are observational. Most studies adjusted for age and age squared, and so we aim to do the same. Not all studies collected and adjusted for the same baseline variables. Given the nature of the studies, we anticipate there might be substantial heterogeneity.

10

Sensitivity analysis: MI unleashed

Thus far we have applied MI under the assumption that data are MAR. In practice, we will often wish to explore whether our inferences are robust to this assumption. In order to do this, we typically need to impute data under a missing not at random (MNAR) mechanism, or approximate the results of so doing. This chapter explores both approaches. Unleashed from the restriction of MAR, MI provides a flexible, computationally straightforward route for inference under almost every conceivable MNAR assumption we may wish to explore.

While much of this book has been concerned with the details of choosing an imputation model, then imputing missing data under MAR, this should not detract from the practical importance of exploring the robustness of inference to the MAR assumption. This is because, as discussed at some length in Chapter 1, given a set of data, we cannot definitively identify the missingness mechanism. In order to draw conclusions from partially observed data, we therefore need to understand the extent to which the data support such conclusions under a range of plausible missingness mechanisms, which will generally include some MNAR mechanisms.

In applications, it is important for all those who have an interest in inference from a partially observed dataset to understand both the range of missingness mechanisms which support specific inferences, together with their plausibility in the context at hand (Carpenter *et al.*, 2013). In other words, it is necessary to be comfortable with the implications of the assumptions about missing data underpinning an analysis, if one is to be comfortable with decisions based on the resulting inferences. This is particularly so in the context of analysing randomised clinical trials, which has consequently provided much of the impetus for sensitivity analysis.

Multiple Imputation and its Application, Second Edition.
James R. Carpenter, Jonathan W. Bartlett, Tim P. Morris, Angela M. Wood, Matteo Quartagno and Michael G. Kenward.

This point informs the extended discussion of the role of sensitivity analysis in analysing trials in the ICH E9(R1) addendum on estimands ICH (2019). This draws on the recommendation 15 of the US National Research Council report entitled 'The prevention and treatment of missing data in clinical trials' (Panel on Handling Missing Data in Clinical Trials. Committee on National Statistics, Division of Behavioral and Social Sciences and Education. Washington, DC: The National Academies Press, 2010) which states 'Sensitivity analyses should be part of the primary reporting of findings from clinical trials. Examining sensitivity to the assumptions about the missing data mechanism should be a mandatory component of reporting'. However, the final recommendation, 18, notes '... There remain several important areas where progress is particularly needed, namely: (1) methods for sensitivity analysis and principled decision-making based on the results from sensitivity analysis....'

The plan for this chapter is as follows: In Section 10.1, we review the theory underlying the analysis of data when missing values are MNAR, in particular focusing on the contrast between the pattern mixture and selection model approaches. Then Section 10.2 reviews some of the issues that have to be considered in framing sensitivity analyses. Sections 10.3 and 10.4 outline the MI approach to pattern mixture modelling for cross sectional and longitudinal settings, illustrating with applications to clinical and social examples we have considered before. Reference-based sensitivity analysis – a particular form of pattern mixture modelling, where missing data are imputed by reference to particular groups of participants – is described in Section 10.5. An alternative, approximate, approach, which allows rapid exploration of local departures from MAR without re-imputing, is described in Section 10.6. We conclude with a discussion in Section 10.7.

10.1 Review of MNAR modelling

Suppose we have two variables, $\mathbf{Y}_1, \mathbf{Y}_2$, with $\mathbf{Y}_1$ partially observed, and $\mathbf{R}$ the vector of response indicators for $\mathbf{Y}_1$ ($R_i = 1$ if $Y_{i,1}$ is observed and 0 otherwise). Then, as described in Chapter 1, for each unit i, we have

$$f(Y_{i,1}, Y_{i,2}|R_i)f(R_i) = f(Y_{i,1}, Y_{i,2}, R_i) = f(R_i|Y_{i,1}, Y_{i,2})f(Y_{i,1}Y_{i,2}). \tag{10.1}$$

The central expression is the joint distribution of the data, comprising the variables and the selection indicator. On the right-hand side, this is written as the product of the density for selection given $Y_{i,1}, Y_{i,2}$ and a density for $Y_{i,1}, Y_{i,2}$. This is known in the literature as the *selection factorisation* or, more commonly, the *selection model* approach. A particular form of this relates $f(R_i|Y_{i,1}, Y_{i,2})$ and $f(Y_{i,1}Y_{i,2})$ through a shared parameter; for a review see Albert and Follman (2009), and an example of sensitivity analysis see Kenward and Rosenkranz (2011).

By contrast, on the left-hand side, we explicitly see a different distribution of $(Y_{i,1}, Y_{i,2})$ depending on whether $Y_{i,1}$ is observed. This is averaged over the probability that $Y_{i,1}$ is observed. In more realistic examples, there will be a number of *patterns* of missing observations, each potentially with a different joint distribution of partially observed and fully observed data, and the overall density as the average over these patterns, leading to the name *pattern mixture factorisation* or more commonly *pattern mixture model.*

The MAR assumption thus has two forms: the selection form,

$$f(R_i|Y_{i,1}, Y_{i,2}) = f(R_i|Y_{i,2}),$$

or the pattern mixture form

$$f(Y_{i,1}|, Y_{i,2}, R_i) = f(Y_{i,1}|Y_{i,2}).$$

In this simple case, it is obvious that the one implies the other; however, this holds true quite generally (e.g. Molenberghs *et al.*, 1998). This means that for sensitivity analysis, we can either focus on modelling the different patterns, or on modelling the selection process. In a complex analysis, we could do both, handling some aspects with a pattern mixture model and some aspects with a selection model.

If the focus is on pattern mixture modelling, then for each pattern, we need to specify the joint distribution of the partially and fully observed variables. In turn, this implies the conditional distribution of partially observed data given the fully observed data within each pattern. This can take any form commensurate with the data type (continuous/ordinal/categorical). However, the majority of these forms will be extremely implausible, given the scientific context and the observed data. We therefore advocate starting from the conditional distribution implied by MAR, and then changing this to reflect assumptions (which could be based on contextual knowledge or formally elicited expert belief, cf. Mason *et al.* (2017)) about the difference from the observed conditional distribution when the variable, or set of variables, is unobserved. Thus, a convenient starting point is writing

$$f(Y_{i,1}, Y_{i,2}|R_i) = f(Y_{i,1}|Y_{i,2}, R_i)f(Y_{i,2}|R_i),$$

keeping $f(Y_{i,2})$ (the marginal model for the fully observed variable) the same across patterns, and allowing $f(Y_{i,1}|Y_{i,2}, R_i)$ to differ with $R_i = 0,1$.

Under MAR, we estimate the distribution $f(Y_1|Y_2)$ from the observed data, typically using a regression model of some form. A simple example is linear regression:

$$Y_{i,1} = \beta_0 + \beta_1 Y_{i,2} + e_i, \quad e_i \overset{i.i.d.}{\sim} N(0, \sigma^2); \tag{10.2}$$

fitting this gives estimates $\hat{\beta}_0$, $\hat{\beta}_1$, and $\hat{\sigma}^2$.

Next, we need to specify $f(Y_1|Y_2, R = 0)$. A natural suggestion is

$$Y_{i,1} = (\beta_0 + \delta_0) + (\beta_1 + \delta_1)Y_{i,2} + e_i, \quad e_i \overset{i.i.d.}{\sim} N(0, (\sigma + \delta_2)^2). \tag{10.3}$$

Using this model, once we have specified the joint distribution of $\boldsymbol{\delta} = (\delta_0, \delta_1, \delta_2)^T$, say $f(\boldsymbol{\delta}; \boldsymbol{\eta})$, we have specified the distribution $f(Y_1|Y_2, R = 0)$. Since $f(R)$ is simply a Bernoulli distribution for the proportion of observed data, with say $\Pr(R_i = 1) = \alpha$, given a density $f(Y_2; \gamma)$, we therefore have the marginal likelihood (for $\boldsymbol{\beta}, \sigma, \gamma, \alpha, \boldsymbol{\eta}$)

of the observed data (i.e. integrating out the missing data and $\boldsymbol{\delta}$) as the product of terms:

$$L_i = \begin{cases} (2\pi\sigma^2)^{-\frac{1}{2}} \exp\left\{-\left(\frac{Y_{i1}-\beta_0-\beta_1 Y_{i,2}}{\sqrt{2}\sigma}\right)^2\right\} f(Y_{i,2};\gamma)\alpha & \text{if } R_i = 1, \\ \iint f(\boldsymbol{\delta})(2\pi(\sigma+\delta_2)^2)^{-\frac{1}{2}} \exp\left\{-\left(\frac{Y_{i,1}-(\beta_0+\delta_0)-(\beta_1+\delta_1)Y_{i,2}}{\sqrt{2}(\sigma+\delta_2)}\right)^2\right\} & \\ \quad \times f(Y_{i,2};\gamma)(1-\alpha)\, dY_{i,1}\, d\boldsymbol{\delta} & \text{if } R_i = 0. \end{cases} \tag{10.4}$$

Given $f(\boldsymbol{\delta};\boldsymbol{\eta})$, whose form and parameters cannot be estimated from the observed data (cf examples later in this chapter), inference for the parameters of interest is often conveniently obtained using MCMC. This has the attraction that, having specified $f(\boldsymbol{\delta};\boldsymbol{\eta})$ and priors for the other parameters, we can estimate any function of parameters or data from the MCMC draws from the posterior distribution. However, in principle, we could use (10.4) to obtain maximum likelihood estimates of $\boldsymbol{\beta}$, as a function of the parameters $\boldsymbol{\eta}$ of the distribution of $\boldsymbol{\delta}$.

Section 10.3 describes MI for pattern mixture modelling. Interesting examples of pattern mixture modelling include Little (1994), Molenberghs *et al.* (1998), Daniels and Hogan (2000), Thijs *et al.* (2002), Demirtas and Schafer (2003), Kenward *et al.* (2003).

Now consider the selection model approach. Assuming a linear-logistic model,

$$\text{logit}\{\Pr(R_i = 1 | Y_{i,1}, Y_{i,2})\} = \alpha_0 + \alpha_1 Y_{i,1} + \alpha_2 Y_{i,2}, \tag{10.5}$$

the likelihood of the data is the product of terms

$$L_i = \begin{cases} f(R_i|Y_{i,1}, Y_{i,2}) f(Y_{i,1}|Y_{i,2}) f(Y_{i,2}) & \text{if } R_i = 1, \\ \int f(R_i|Y_{i,1}, Y_{i,2}) f(Y_{i,1}|Y_{i,2}) f(Y_{i,2})\, dY_{i,1} & \text{if } R_i = 0. \end{cases} \tag{10.6}$$

The density $f(Y_{i,1}|Y_{i,2})$ is often a regression model such as (10.2); of course, the resulting parameter values and inferences differ in general to those from the subset of observed data.

Again, given the likelihood, we can estimate the parameters and draw inferences. We can often do this directly, using numerical integration (e.g. Diggle and Kenward, 1994, Verzilli and Carpenter, 2002) or using a Bayesian approach via MCMC (e.g., among many, Carpenter *et al.*, 2002).

Under the selection model approach, we can estimate the parameter α_1 in (10.5), and hence test for MNAR. However, such an approach is not advisable, because estimation rests on assumptions about the distribution of the missing data which are unverifiable from the observed data (e.g. Kenward, 1998). By contrast, in the pattern mixture approach, we clearly cannot estimate $f(\boldsymbol{\delta};\boldsymbol{\eta})$. The pattern mixture model's cleaner separation between what can, and cannot, be estimated is attractive in many contexts (cf. Daniels and Hogan, 2008). In practice, it is often sufficient to explore sensitivity to different fixed values of $\boldsymbol{\delta}$ in (10.4) or α_1 in (10.5).

Whichever approach is adopted, we reiterate that a useful sensitivity analysis must frame the assumptions in a way that is accessible to all those involved in the research, so they can in turn identify relevant, plausible departures from these assumptions to explore. In this respect, analysing data under MNAR models is qualitatively different from fitting a model to fully observed data, or examining diagnostics. Further, the correspondence between the pattern mixture and selection approaches mentioned above implies that if we adopt a pattern mixture approach for framing assumptions, the selection consequences should be plausible, and vice versa.

10.2 Framing sensitivity analysis: estimands

Analysis of partially observed data should consist of (i) a primary analysis, under a plausible primary missingness mechanism, and (ii) secondary analyses exploring the robustness of inference to departures from the primary missingness mechanism.

Framing both analyses requires careful consideration of the *estimand*. Simply speaking, the *estimand* is the quantity we wish to estimate and the population we wish to estimate it for. In the context of medical exposures or treatments, we may think of the estimand as a structured approach to defining the exposure or treatment effect. More formally, ICH (2019) defines the *estimand* as consisting of five attributes.

10.2.1 Definition of the estimand

In a trial, or observational study, an estimand is defined by

1. the population under study, from which the study participants are drawn;
2. the treatment or exposure regime;
3. the end point of interest (e.g. in an asthma study, lung function after 12 weeks follow-up);
4. the summary measure (e.g. mean), and
5. the *intercurrent events* and how they are to be handled.

For a more detailed discussion of estimands, see (among many) Cro *et al.* (2022), Clark *et al.* (2022).

While all aspects of the estimand are important in applications, here our focus is on the *intercurrent events*. An intercurrent event is an event that occurs after initiation of treatment (which is typically at baseline in a randomised trial), which affects either the existence or interpretation of the subsequent data. This often means that the data after the intercurrent event are (i) not necessarily directly relevant to the estimand of interest (e.g. because the patient has discontinued treatment), and (ii) often missing (e.g. because after treatment discontinuation the patient withdrew from follow-up). Note that the presence of missing data is not itself considered an intercurrent event but missing data are frequently caused by intercurrent events, such that they are closely related. The addendum uses the term *intercurrent event* rather than *post-randomisation event* because it seeks to include non-randomised (i.e. observational) studies.

To focus our discussion, we initially consider the clinical trials setting, where we have randomised treatment allocation and longitudinal follow-up. Examples of intercurrent events are (i) poor compliance with, or withdrawal from, the treatment; (ii) unblinding, either of treatment or evaluation, and (iii) study discontinuation, which leads to no further information on the patient being available.

10.2.2 Two common estimands

We now describe, in a highly simplified setting two estimands corresponding to using the *hypothetical* and *treatment policy* strategies for handling intercurrent events described by ICH (2019). Let Z denote randomised treatment ($Z = 1$ for active and $Z = 0$ for control treatment) and Y the outcome variable of interest. We assume that for each patient, the intercurrent event can occur during follow-up ($M = 1$) or not ($M = 0$). To define the two estimands, we use potential outcomes (see Section 13.1). We let $Y^{z,m}$ denote the potential outcome for a given patient were we to assign them to treatment level z ($z = 0,1$) and were we to intervene to set the intercurrent event to level m. The notion of intervening on an intercurrent event (such as patient discontinuation) may sometimes seem unnatural and reflects the fact that certain estimands may be ill-defined. For simplicity, we assume the summary measure of interest is the mean of Y.

If we take the *hypothetical* strategy to handle the intercurrent event, a possible estimand of interest is

$$E(Y^{1,0}) - E(Y^{0,0}).$$

This contrasts the mean outcome in the population if we assign active treatment and (somehow) prevent the intercurrent event from occurring, to the mean outcome if we assign control and similarly prevent the intercurrent event from occurring. In causal inference terminology, this is an example of a controlled direct effect. It isolates the direct effect of treatment on the outcome from the intercurrent event M. This estimand is likely to be of scientific interest in settings where the proportion of patients experiencing the intercurrent event differs materially between treatment groups.

For patients in the actual trial who did not experience the intercurrent event, we observe the outcome of interest $Y^{Z,0}$ under their randomised treatment Z. But for those who did experience the intercurrent event, we observe $Y^{Z,1}$ and the outcome of interest $Y^{Z,0}$ is counterfactual and missing. As such, estimation of this hypothetical estimand requires handling the missing counterfactual outcomes of interest. Within the analysis of clinical trials, estimation of such estimands has therefore tended to make use of missing data methods such direct likelihood and MI under MAR assumptions (Mallinckrodt *et al.*, 2020). The MAR assumption holds provided that all common causes of the intercurrent event M and the outcome Y are measured and conditioned on in the analysis (Olarte Parra *et al.*, 2022), but otherwise it may not. Therefore, a primary analysis for this hypothetical estimand might rely on an MAR assumption, with secondary MNAR analyses performed to assess the sensitivity of inferences to the MAR assumption. For further discussion of missing data approaches to causal inference problems, we refer the reader to Chapter 13.

If instead we take the *treatment policy* strategy to handle the intercurrent event, the estimand becomes

$$E(Y^{1,M}) - E(Y^{0,M}).$$

This estimand contrasts the mean outcome in the population were we to assign active treatment and let the intercurrent event M take its natural value (under active treatment) for each patient compared to assigning control treatment and again letting the intercurrent event M take its natural value. The estimand thus quantifies the effect of active versus control treatment, including any effects of the intercurrent event. In trials where the proportion of patients experiencing the intercurrent event differs between treatment groups, this estimand reflects not only the direct effect of treatment on the outcome but any indirect effect mediated via the intercurrent event.

For the treatment policy estimand, in contrast to the hypothetical estimand, there are no missing counterfactual outcomes. However, there may of course be missing actual outcomes, due to patients missing follow-up visits or being lost to follow-up. As such, there will generally still be missing data to accommodate in an analysis targeting the treatment policy estimand.

The hypothetical estimand defined above may often be useful in the earlier stages of drug development. In contrast, the treatment policy estimand may be of interest to regulatory agencies wishing to understand the cost/benefit return for a specific treatment policy. For example, in England, the National Institute for Health and Clinical Excellence (NICE, www.nice.org.uk/aboutnice/) provides national guidance on treating ill health, and typically needs answers to such questions. However, in this context, it is important to remember that the conditions in a clinical trial are often not reflective, in various respects, of real clinical practice, and so the treatment policy estimand targeted by the trial may differ from the treatment policy estimand that would be realised in clinical practice. Lastly, we note that treatment policy estimands have historically sometimes been referred to as 'Intention-to-treat' (ITT) effects. However, the latter term is sometimes used to refer to a set of patients and sometimes used to refer to an estimation method (e.g. Hollis and Campbell, 1999).

Whatever the estimand, we will generally wish to estimate the effect under a range of assumptions about missing values that are consistent with this estimand – i.e. often under both MAR and MNAR mechanisms. However, as we explore further in Section 10.4, the appropriate way to do this will typically vary with the estimand.

10.3 Pattern mixture modelling with MI

We motivate the discussion with an example, and then describe and illustrate a generic approach to pattern mixture modelling using MI, which – depending on the context – is relevant to a range of estimands.

Example 10.1 Peer review trial

Schroter *et al.* (2004) report a single blind randomised controlled trial among reviewers for a general medical journal. The aim was to investigate whether training improved the quality of peer review. The study compared two different types of training (face-to-face training or a self-taught package) with no training.

We restrict ourselves to the comparison between those randomised to the self-training package and no-training. Each participating reviewer was pre-randomised into their intervention group. Prior to any training, each was sent a baseline article to review (termed paper 1). If this was returned, then according to their randomised group, the reviewer was either (i) mailed a self-training package or (ii) received no further intervention.

Two to three months later, participants who had completed their first review were sent a further article to review (paper 2); if this was returned, a third paper was sent three months later (paper 3). The analysis excluded all participants who did not complete their first (i.e. baseline) review: this was not expected to cause bias since these participants were unaware of their randomised allocation.

Reviewers were sent manuscripts in a similar style to the standard British Medical Journal request for a review, but were told these articles were part of the study and were not paid. The three articles were based on three previously published papers, with original author names, titles, and location changed. In addition, nine major and five minor errors were introduced. The outcome is the quality of the review, as measured by the Review Quality Instrument. This validated instrument contains eight items scored from 1 to 5. Rating was done independently by two editors. The response in our analysis is the mean of the first seven items, averaged over the two editors. This ranges between 1 and 5, where a perfect review would score 5.

We restrict attention to the second review. For this, a complete records analysis showed a statistically significant difference at the 5% level in favour of the self-training package. Table 10.1 breaks down the results of the baseline review (paper 1) by whether reviewers responded to the request to review paper 2. It suggests that the missing paper 2 scores are not MCAR, and that they may be MNAR, even after accounting for baseline.

Table 10.1 Review quality index of paper 1 by whether or not paper 2 was reviewed.

		Group		
		Control	Postal	Face-to-face
Returned review of paper 2	n	162	120	158
	Mean	2.65	2.80	2.75
	SD	0.81	0.62	0.70
Did not return review of paper 2	n	11	46	25
	Mean	3.02	2.55	2.51
	SD	0.50	0.75	0.73

In this setting, we do not have information on the intercurrent events that may have occurred prior to the data being missing. For example, it could be that

(i) reviewers engaged with the material – but did not have time to complete the review, *or*

(ii) reviewers decided after the first review not to be further involved and disregarded the training material and subsequent review requests.

Suppose that we are interested in a treatment policy estimand. This estimand includes any effects of non-engagement with the training material. In the absence of further information about which of the two above intercurrent event types occurred, we will explore the robustness of conclusions for this estimand to (a) assuming all the intercurrent events are type (i) and (b) assuming all the intercurrent events are type (ii). Below, we explore how our conclusions about the benefit of offering reviewer training vary in these two cases. □

Consider variables $\mathbf{Y}_1, \dots, \mathbf{Y}_p$. For each unit, let $\mathbf{Y}_i^T = (Y_{i,1}, \dots, Y_{i,p})$ and $\mathbf{R}_i^T = (R_{i,1}, \dots, R_{i,p})$ be the vector of response indicators. Across all $i = 1, \dots, n$ units, suppose there are $M \ll n$ distinct response patterns, indexed by $\mathbf{R}_m$, $m \in (1, \dots, M)$. Each unit's missing and observed variables conform to one of these patterns, say $m(i)$, and one of the patterns corresponds to complete records on all p variables. Let $\mathbf{Y}_{\text{O},m(i)}, \mathbf{Y}_{\text{M},m(i)}$ be the observed and missing variables for unit i with response pattern $m(i)$.

For each unit with missingness pattern $m(i) = m$, let $\boldsymbol{\eta}_m$ denote the parameters of the joint distribution of the observed and missing data. From this we can derive the conditional distribution of the missing given the observed data, denoted by

$$f(\mathbf{Y}_{\text{M},m(i)} | \mathbf{Y}_{\text{O},m(i)}, \boldsymbol{\eta}_{m(i)}). \tag{10.7}$$

We have to estimate $\boldsymbol{\eta}_m$ before we can draw missing data from (10.7).

If data are MAR, then (10.7) does not depend on missingness pattern m; the parameters are common across patterns, $\boldsymbol{\eta}_m = \boldsymbol{\eta}$, $m \in (1, \dots, M)$, and we impute missing data from $f(\mathbf{Y}_{\text{M},i} | \mathbf{Y}_{\text{O},i}, \boldsymbol{\eta})$. However, if data are MNAR, the parameters will differ with missingness pattern m, and could further differ for different units within missingness pattern m.

Suppose that $\hat{\theta} = \hat{\theta}(\mathbf{Y}) = \hat{\theta}(\mathbf{Y}_\text{M}, \mathbf{Y}_\text{O})$ is of interest. For example, θ may be a regression coefficient. With no missing data, we would estimate this from $\mathbf{Y}$, using the appropriate generalised linear model. For each missingness pattern m, let $\mathbf{Y}_{\text{O},m}$ be the observed data from units i such that $m(i) = m$. Our approach is to define a form for (10.7), for each missingness pattern m, which reflects contextually relevant assumptions. Then we impute K 'complete' data sets by

MI1: Taking a draw from the Bayesian posterior distribution of $f(\boldsymbol{\eta}_m | \mathbf{Y}_{\text{O},m})$ and then

MI2: Imputing the missing data from (10.7) using the above draw of $\boldsymbol{\eta}_m$.

Both steps are repeated to create each imputed dataset. The parameter of interest is then estimated from each imputed data set in turn to give $\hat{\theta}_k$, with standard error $\hat{\sigma}_k$, $k = 1, \dots, K$. These are then combined using Rubin's rules to give a single multiple imputation estimate and associated standard error.

To implement MI1, we need to choose a model for the observed data. To implement MI2, we need to specify (10.7). Taking the former first, our approach is to estimate a common parameter vector $\boldsymbol{\eta}$ from all the observed data assuming MAR. We then use specific rules or information to derive, or draw, $\boldsymbol{\eta}_m$. This is of necessity-context specific. It could involve

1. explicitly specifying the distribution of $\boldsymbol{\eta}_m$ given $\boldsymbol{\eta}$, possibly using opinions elicited from experts, *or*

2. specifying how $\boldsymbol{\eta}_m$ is constructed from $\boldsymbol{\eta}$, for example in terms of rules across well-defined subsets of the data (such as treatment groups).

Consider now the pattern mixture model (10.2) and (10.3). In terms of the more general development here, $\boldsymbol{\eta}$, the parameters of the model for the observed data, are $(\beta_0, \beta_1, \sigma)$ and $\boldsymbol{\eta}_1$, the parameters of the model for the first (and only) missingness pattern, are $(\beta_0 + \delta_0, \beta_1 + \delta_1, \sigma + \delta_3)$. Thus, $\boldsymbol{\delta} = \boldsymbol{\eta}_1 - \boldsymbol{\eta}$.

The examples we consider below illustrate approaches 1 and 2 above. We take MAR as our starting point for sensitivity analysis. However, it is not necessary to do this in order to use MI for pattern mixture modelling, and the approach we describe can readily be adapted accordingly if desired.

Example 10.1 Peer review trial *(ctd)*

Focusing on the baseline adjusted comparison of the self-taught training package with no training, the model of interest is

$$Y_i = \beta_0 + \beta_1 X_{i,1} + \beta_2 X_{i,2} + e_i, \quad e_i \overset{i.i.d.}{\sim} N(0, \sigma^2), \tag{10.8}$$

where i indexes participant, $Y_i, X_{i,1}$ are the mean review quality index for paper 2 and paper 1, respectively, and $X_{i,2}$ is an indicator for the self-training group. Assuming all the missing data follow inter-current events of type (i) (see p. 253) that is reviewers engaged with the material but did not complete the review, we assume review 2 is MAR given baseline and intervention group. Under this assumption, we can obtain inference for β_2 from fitting (10.8) to the complete records. The estimates are shown in the first row of Table 10.2.

Multiple imputation analysis under MAR makes the same assumption: missing reviewer scores are imputed using information from participants who completed the second review and complied with the study protocol.

Now suppose all the intercurrent events are of type (ii): reviewers decided after the first review not to be involved. What would the effect in practice of implementing the self-taught training package if it was rolled out to all reviewers by the *British Medical Journal*? To answer this, White *et al.* (2007) devised a questionnaire which was completed by 2 investigators and 20 editors and other staff at the *British Medical*

Table 10.2 Peer review trial: inference for comparison of self-taught package with no training, under various assumptions. Parameter estimates are differences in mean review quality index, on a scale of 0–5.

Analysis	Est	SE	MI df	p-value	95% CI
Complete records, MAR	0.237	0.070	N/A	<0.001	(0.099, 0.376)
MAR, $K = 20$	0.245	0.073	302	<0.001	(0.102, 0.389)
MAR, $K = 10{,}000$	0.237	0.070	$\approx \infty$	<0.001	(0.099, 0.375)
MNAR, $\rho = 0$, $K = 20$	0.209	0.178	27	0.25	(−0.158, 0.575)
MNAR, $\rho = 0$, $K = 10{,}000$	0.193	0.151	$\approx \infty$	0.20	(−0.102, 0.488)
MNAR, $\rho = 0.5$, $K = 20$	0.205	0.167	27	0.23	(−0.141, 0.234)
MNAR, $\rho = 0.5$, $K = 10{,}000$	0.190	0.137	$\approx \infty$	0.17	(−0.089, 0.459)
MNAR, $\rho = 1$, $K = 20$	0.213	0.134	34	0.12	(−0.059, 0.486)
MNAR, $\rho = 1$, $K = 10{,}000$	0.190	0.123	$\approx \infty$	0.12	(−0.050, 0.431)

Journal. The questionnaire was designed to elicit the experts' prior belief about the difference between the average missing and average observed review quality index (RQI). White *et al.* (2007) show that it was reasonable to pool information from the experts. The resulting distribution is negatively skewed, with mean −0.21 and SD 0.46 (on the RQI scale). Suppose we denote by (δ_0, δ_1) draws from the distribution of the mean difference in review quality between observed and unobserved reviews, in, respectively, the control and self-training groups. We adopt a bivariate normal model approximation to the prior:

$$\begin{pmatrix} \delta_0 \\ \delta_1 \end{pmatrix} \sim N\left[\begin{pmatrix} -0.21 \\ -0.21 \end{pmatrix}, 0.46^2 \begin{pmatrix} 1 & \rho \\ \rho & 1 \end{pmatrix}\right]. \tag{10.9}$$

Unfortunately, it was not possible to elicit a prior on ρ from the experts; we therefore analyse the data with $\rho = 0, 0.5, 1$ below.

Given a draw (δ_0, δ_1) from this distribution, the model is

$$\begin{aligned} Y_i &= \beta_0 + \beta_1 X_{i,1} + \beta_2 X_{i,2} + e_i && \text{if } Y_i \text{ observed,} \\ Y_i &= (\beta_0 + \delta_0) + \beta_1 X_{i,1} + (\beta_2 + \delta_1 - \delta_0) X_{i,2} + e_i && \text{if } Y_i \text{ unobserved,} \\ e_i &\overset{i.i.d.}{\sim} N(0, \sigma^2). \end{aligned} \tag{10.10}$$

Thus conditional on baseline score, the mean review quality, relative to that estimated in the complete records, is changed by δ_0 in the control arm and δ_1 in the self-taught arm.

Following the general approach for estimating pattern mixture models via MI described above, we proceed as follows, noting that the imputation model under MAR and the substantive model are the same in this example:

1. Fit the imputation model (10.8) to the observed data and draw from the posterior distribution of the parameters $\boldsymbol{\eta} = (\beta_0, \beta_1, \beta_2, \sigma^2)$.

2. Draw (δ_0, δ_1) from (10.9)

3. Using the draws obtained in steps 1 and 2, impute the missing Y_i using (10.10).

Steps 1–3 are repeated to create K imputed datasets. Then we fit the model of interest (10.8) to each imputed dataset and apply Rubin's rules for inference.

The results are shown in Table 10.2. In line with theory, the results from MI under MAR agree with the complete records analysis, and this agreement is very close with $K = 10{,}000$ imputations (which in this example only take a matter of minutes). Imputing under MNAR, we see that the mean RQI in the self-training group is no longer statistically significantly different from the no training group. The standard error is largest when $\rho = 0$, and decreases as $\rho \to 1$. We also see that $K = 20$ imputations is enough to clearly show this conclusion, to practically relevant precision. Results with 10,000 imputations agree extremely closely with both a theoretical approximation and a full Bayesian analysis reported by White *et al.* (2007), even though the latter allow for uncertainty in estimating the proportion with missing data, which is conditioned on in the pattern mixture approach.

We conclude that, taking experts' prior belief into account, there is no evidence that self-training improves the quality of peer review. □

This approach can also be applied to directly to discrete outcomes. The attractions of interpretability and computational simplicity remain. For example, it could be applied in the setting of Magder (2003), who framed departures from MAR through the response probability ratio. It could equally be applied to estimation and inference with the 'Informative Missing Odds Ratio', proposed by Higgins *et al.* (2006). They framed departures from MAR through the ratio of the odds of response in patients whose data are observed to the odds of response in patients whose data are missing.

10.3.1 Missing covariates

We now consider sensitivity analysis for partially observed covariates in the substantive model. Exactly as above, we estimate the coefficients of the imputation model under MAR, but then modify them to reflect a departure from MAR before imputing the missing values. We illustrate with sensitivity analysis for the Youth Cohort Study.

Example 10.2 Youth Cohort Study

Consider again the youth cohort study (see, for example Chapter 5, p. 126). As shown there, the principle missing data pattern, in 11% of the records, is missing parental occupation but observed values for the other variables in our model of interest. The other, more complex patterns, account for <3% of the missing records between them. Since imputing with or without the latter records makes no difference to the resulting inference, we restrict to the 61,609 records with either complete records or only parental occupation missing.

As before, the substantive model is a linear regression of GCSE score on ethnic group, adjusted for sex, parental occupation, and cohort. Parental occupation

Table 10.3 Youth cohort study: model for the differences in GCSE points score (range 0–84) by ethnicity, adjusted for sex, parental occupation, and cohort. Analyses used 20 imputations.

Covariate	Estimates (standard errors) from:			
	Complete records	MAR	MNAR ($\delta_I = \delta_W = -2$)	MNAR ($\delta_I = 0, \delta_W = 1.8$)
Black	−5.39	−6.88	−6.92	−6.88
	(0.57)	(0.50)	(0.49)	(0.50)
Indian	3.83	3.25	3.22	3.22
	(0.44)	(0.41)	(0.41)	(0.41)
Pakistani	−1.79	−3.55	−3.59	−3.53
	(0.59)	(0.47)	(0.47)	(0.47)
Bangladeshi	0.69	−2.99	−4.93	−1.44
	(1.05)	(0.72)	(0.79)	(0.70)
Other Asian	5.79	4.90	4.89	4.86
	(0.69)	(0.63)	(0.62)	(0.63)
Other	0.37	−0.72	−0.71	−0.67
	(0.71)	(0.65)	(0.64)	(0.64)
Boys	−3.47	−3.37	−3.37	−3.36
	(0.13)	(0.13)	(0.13)	(0.13)
Intermediate	−7.46	−7.80	−7.73	−7.77
parental occupation	(0.15)	(0.16)	(0.17)	(0.16)
Working	−13.82	−14.33	−14.30	−14.37
parental occupation	(0.17)	(0.17)	(0.17)	(0.18)
1995 cohort	6.30	6.19	6.18	6.19
	(0.18)	(0.17)	(0.17)	(0.17)
1997 cohort	4.96	5.01	5.01	5.01
	0.18	(0.17)	(0.17)	(0.17)
1999 cohort	9.57	9.88	9.88	9.88
	0.19	(0.18)	(0.18)	(0.18)
Constant	4.81	4.11	4.07	4.10
	(0.15)	(0.15)	(0.15)	(0.15)

Table 10.4 Occupation of parents of students of Bangladeshi ethnicity, in complete records and under MAR, NMAR. Twenty imputations were used.

	Complete records	Imputation under		
		MAR	MNAR ($\delta_I = \delta_W = -2$)	MNAR ($\delta_I = 0, \delta_W = 1.8$)
Managerial	26 (12%)	48 (9%)	143 (26%)	34 (6%)
Intermediate	91 (41%)	215 (40%)	174 (32%)	126 (23%)
Working	104 (47%)	272 (51%)	221 (41%)	378 (70%)
Total	221	538	538	538

is a three-category variable, managerial, intermediate, and working. We use a multinomial logistic imputation model, with managerial as the reference category. Let $\pi_{iM}, \pi_{iI}, \pi_{iW}$ be the probability that pupil i's parental occupation is classed as managerial, intermediate, or working, respectively, where $\pi_{IM} + \pi_{iI} + \pi_{iW} = 1$. The imputation model is

$$\log(\pi_{iI}/\pi_{iM}) = \mathbf{X}_i\boldsymbol{\alpha}_I, \tag{10.11}$$

$$\log(\pi_{iW}/\pi_{iM}) = \mathbf{X}_i\boldsymbol{\alpha}_W, \tag{10.12}$$

where $\mathbf{X}_i$ is a $(n \times q)$ matrix with columns corresponding to the constant, pupil's GCSE score centred at 38 points, and indicators for boys, ethnicity (6 variables) and cohort (3 variables).

First, we assume the distribution of parental occupation is the same – given the other variables – whether it is observed or not. Under this MAR assumption, we estimate the parameters of (10.11), (10.12) from the complete records and create proper imputations as described in Chapter 5. The results of the complete records analysis and MAR imputation are shown in the left two columns of Table 10.3. Of particular interest are the coefficients for Pakistani and Bangladeshi ethnicity, which under MAR become substantially more negative and statistically significant. Focusing on Bangladeshi ethnicity, we explore the sensitivity of this result to the MAR assumption.

We consider two MNAR scenarios: for pupils of Bangladeshi ethnicity (i) missing parental occupations are predominantly 'managerial', and (ii) missing parental occupation scores are predominantly 'working'. In the former case we add to the Bangladeshi coefficients in (10.11), (10.12), respectively, $(\delta_I = -2, \delta_W - 2)$, and in the latter $(\delta_I = 0, \delta_W = 1.8)$. In the absence of prior information, in this example, we do not follow (10.9) but instead set $Var\ \boldsymbol{\delta} = 0$. The resulting imputed parental occupations are then, respectively, predominantly working, and predominantly managerial; when combined with the observed occupations we obtain the proportions shown in Table 10.4. The rightmost columns of Table 10.3 show the corresponding effect on the coefficient for Bangladeshi ethnicity in the model of inference: under both scenarios, inference is remarkably robust.

We conclude that on average pupils of Bangladeshi ethnic origin have significantly lower GCSE scores than the complete records analysis would suggest, and this result is robust to plausible MNAR mechanisms. □

10.3.2 Sensitivity with multiple variables: the NAR FCS procedure

In many applications, we will have more than one partially observed variable. To handle this situation, Leacy *et al.* (2017) proposed an extension to the full conditional specification algorithm for multiple imputation to include the missingness indicators, with practical implementation details given by Tompsett *et al.* (2018).

We outline the approach in the case of two partially observed variables, Y_1, Y_2 and fully observed variables $\mathbf{X}$; the extension to more complex settings is direct. As described in Section 3.3, full conditional specification imputation assuming MAR proceeds as follows:

Initialise For each variable, fill in all the missing values with starting values by drawing from observed values of the variable, or by using a monotone imputation procedure;

1. Return to the observed values of Y_1 and regress these on $Y_2, \mathbf{X}$, and properly impute the missing values of Y_1;
2. Return to the observed values of Y_2 and regress these on $Y_1, \mathbf{X}$, and properly impute the missing values in Y_2;

Steps 1 & 2 form a 'cycle'; we complete a number of cycles (a common default is 10) and then take the current values as an imputed dataset.

The extension to MNAR involves defining the two indicator variables for missing data in Y_1 and Y_2, say R_1 and R_2, and then including these in the procedure. Steps 1 & 2 therefore become

1. Return to the observed values of Y_1 and regress these on $Y_2, \mathbf{X}, R_1, R_2$ and properly impute the missing values of Y_1;
2. Return to the observed values of Y_2 and regress these on $Y_1, \mathbf{X}, R_1, R_2$ and properly impute the missing values in Y_2.

The difficulty is that there is no information to estimate the four additional coefficients of R_1, R_2. To address this, Tompsett *et al.* (2018) propose using the two coefficients, (i) δ_1, of R_1, in step 1 and (ii) δ_2, of R_2, in step 2, as sensitivity parameters. Their values can either be fixed, or their distribution can be elicited from experts. This gives sufficient information to estimate the conditional regression models in steps 1 and 2 (i.e. we do not need to additionally specify the coefficient of R_2 in step 1 and R_1 in step 2).

Once the values of δ_1 and δ_2 are chosen, each conditional imputation step is then performed in the same way as described above for pattern mixture sensitivity analysis for a single variable. Note that if δ_1 and δ_2 are set equal to zero we are imputing under MAR, but not strictly using the standard FCS algorithm because R_2 still remains in the imputation model for Y_1 and R_1 still remains in the imputation model for Y_2.

In applications, the challenge is to choose, or elicit information about, the distribution of (δ_1, δ_2). However, this is less straightforward than before, because now each of these represents a *conditional* difference (conditional on R_2 in step 1 and R_1 in step 2). This, and related issues, are discussed in more detail by Tompsett *et al.* (2018).

With multiple partially observed variables, the NAR-FCS procedure is theoretically a more appropriate approach than exploring sensitivity for each partially observed variable in turn (although this is often a useful first step). Further work is needed to understand the practical benefit of this joint procedure compared to simpler approaches.

10.3.3 Application to survival analysis

We now consider the pattern-mixture to sensitivity analysis for non-random censoring (i.e. non-random loss to follow-up) in survival analysis.

Example 10.3 Evaluation of antiretroviral treatment (ART) programmes in sub-Saharan Africa

HIV infection is a major cause of mortality and morbidity in sub-Saharan Africa, and between 2007 and 2010 the number of patients starting ART increased steeply (e.g. Boulle *et al.*, 2008), along with consequent interest in evaluating the efficacy of ART in this setting. However, during the same period, there has been increasing concern about loss to follow-up in these programmes (Brinkhof *et al.*, 2008), especially as those lost to follow-up may have substantially worse mortality than those who are followed up, which will bias the evaluation (Bartlett and Shao, 2009, Brinkhof *et al.*, 2009).

Accordingly, Brinkhof *et al.* (2010) decided to use a pattern mixture approach, estimated through multiple imputation, to explore the robustness of inferences about mortality to non-random censoring. □

To show how the pattern mixture approach can be applied to survival data, suppose that T is the random variable representing the time to event and C the random variable representing time to loss to follow-up (i.e. censoring). From each unit, or patient, we observe baseline covariates $\mathbf{X}_i$, and $Y_i = \min(T_i, C_i)$.

The Censoring at Random (CAR) assumption was introduced in Section 7.2, as the equivalent of the MAR assumption for survival data. Thus, CAR assumes T_i and C_i are conditionally independent given the covariates $\mathbf{X}_i$. Under CAR, valid estimates for coefficients $\boldsymbol{\beta}$ relating covariates to survival time are obtained from modelling the observed data, where censored units contribute $\Pr(T_i > C_i|\mathbf{X}_i, \boldsymbol{\beta})$ to the likelihood.

Similarly, the censoring not at random (CNAR) assumption is the MNAR assumption for survival data. Under CNAR, T_i and C_i are not independent, even given the covariates $\mathbf{X}_i$.

In order to obtain parameter estimates and inferences under CNAR, we adapt the strategy outlined on p. 253 to the survival setting; see also Jackson *et al.* (2014). Specifically, we obtain an estimate of the hazard assuming CAR, and then introduce a sensitivity parameter defining the ratio of the hazard of censored individuals to those that are not censored. Using the notation of Chapter 7, the hazard under CNAR is

$$h(t_i|C_i, \mathbf{X}_i) = \begin{cases} h_{\text{CAR}}(t_i|\mathbf{X}_i) & \text{if } t_i < C_i, \\ \exp(\delta) h_{\text{CAR}}(t_i|\mathbf{X}_i) & \text{if } t_i \geq C_i. \end{cases} \tag{10.13}$$

If $\delta = 0$, then given $\mathbf{X}_i$, the hazard is the same, irrespective of censoring; in other words CAR holds. Otherwise, the hazards are different. The parameter δ is once again the sensitivity parameter, but this time it is the log-hazard ratio of censored to uncensored. As usual, the data at hand give no information on the value of δ. However, information on this may be elicited from experts or other data sources; alternatively, we may re-analyse the data with δ successively further from 0 and then assess the plausibility of the value of δ at which our conclusions change substantively.

For now, we assume that we have a prior distribution for the log hazard-ratio

$$\delta \sim N(\mu_\delta, \sigma_\delta^2), \tag{10.14}$$

although in seeking prior information it will usually be better to work on the hazard-ratio scale itself. We also assume a parametric model for survival. Then, given (10.14) and (10.13), we can apply the approach described on p. 335 directly, giving the following algorithm:

1. Assuming CAR, fit the survival model to the data, obtaining parameter estimates $\hat{\boldsymbol{\beta}}$ relating the log-hazard to the covariates, with associated estimated covariance matrix $\hat{\boldsymbol{\Sigma}}$, typically obtained from the observed information (Kenward and Molenberghs, 1998).
2. Draw δ^* from (10.14) and $\boldsymbol{\beta}^* \sim N(\hat{\boldsymbol{\beta}}, \hat{\boldsymbol{\Sigma}})$.
3. With these values, for each censored unit i impute the time to event from the hazard $\exp(\delta^*)h_{\text{CAR}}(t|\boldsymbol{\beta}^*, \mathbf{X}_i)$. If a unit's imputed time is less than the censoring time we draw again, until it is greater than the censoring time. The observed and imputed event times together make the imputed dataset under CNAR.

Repeating steps 2 and 3, we can generate K imputed data sets, to each of which we fit the substantive model. This could be a parametric or semi-parametric survival model; at its simplest it could be the Kaplan–Meier estimate of survival at a specific time. This gives K point estimates and their standard errors, which can be combined for final inference by applying Rubin's rules on an appropriate scale. For example, for an estimate of the probability of surviving past time t, $\hat{S}(t)$, appropriate choices would be the probit, logit, or complementary log–log scale. We would transform the estimate from each imputed data set, apply Rubin's rules, and then back transform the point estimate and confidence interval.

In practice, in order to draw the survival times, we will often want to calculate the cumulative distribution function of the survival time, $F(t; \mathbf{X}, \boldsymbol{\beta}^*, \delta^*)$, corresponding to the hazard $\exp(\delta^*)h_{\text{CAR}}(t|\mathbf{X}, \boldsymbol{\beta}^*)$. Once we have done this, then since

$$F(T; \mathbf{X}, \boldsymbol{\beta}^*, \delta^*) \sim U[0,1]$$

we can draw a survival time for censored unit i by drawing u_i from the uniform distribution on $[F(C_i), 1]$ and then calculating

$$T_i^* = F^{-1}(u_i; \mathbf{X}_i, \boldsymbol{\beta}^*, \delta^*).$$

This approach is convenient under a parametric survival model. If we adopt a Cox proportional-hazards model, then generating proper imputations is harder, as uncertainty in estimating both the coefficients of the relative hazard as well as the baseline hazard needs to be taken into account. We do not view this as a major limitation, since within the rich families of parametric survival models, it is likely that an appropriate choice can be found for imputation. Of course, the Cox proportional hazards model can be fitted to the imputed data. If there are concerns about inconsistencies between the imputation model and model of interest, a natural first check is to impute the censored data assuming CAR (i.e. $\delta = 0$), fit the substantive model to each imputed dataset and combine the results using Rubin's rules. Just as in Table 10.2 rows 1–3, the resulting inferences should be very close to those from the observed data.

Again, exactly as in application to the peer review trial, it may well be appropriate to have different means and variances for δ in different treatment or other groups. In that case, values for the correlation between these also need to be selected. In trials, it is also possible to envisage piecing post-censoring hazards together by drawing on other trial arms, much as in the longitudinal trials discussion in Section 10.4 – see Atkinson *et al.* (2019,2021), and references therein, for examples.

Example 10.3 Evaluation of ART programmes in sub-Saharan Africa *(ctd)*

Brinkhof *et al.* (2010) apply the approach set out above to explore the robustness of inference about mortality of patients receiving ART in studies conducted in sub-Saharan Africa to CNAR. Their estimand of interest was survival 1-year following initiation of ART, estimated using the Kaplan–Meier method. They chose a Weibull model for imputation. Under this model, (10.13) becomes

$$h(t|\mathbf{X}, \boldsymbol{\beta}, C) = \begin{cases} \exp(\mathbf{X}^T\boldsymbol{\beta})\gamma t^{\gamma-1} & \text{if } t < C, \\ \exp(\delta)\exp(\mathbf{X}^T\boldsymbol{\beta})\gamma t^{\gamma-1} & \text{if } t \geq C, \end{cases} \tag{10.15}$$

where $t > 0, \gamma > 0$, δ is unrestricted and the $p \times 1$ vector $\mathbf{X}$ includes the intercept. As discussed below, they explore sensitivity for fixed values of δ; they do not sample it as in (10.14).

To implement the algorithm described above, the Weibull model is first fitted to the observed data in the usual way. Then, using the observed information, to create each imputed dataset we draw from the distribution of the parameters, $\boldsymbol{\beta}^*, \gamma^*$, then with these parameter draws, sample survival times for censored observations from $S(t|t > C, \mathbf{X}_i, \boldsymbol{\beta}^*, \gamma^*, \delta)$. Under the Weibull distribution, this is

$$S(t|t > C, \mathbf{X}_i, \boldsymbol{\beta}^*, \gamma^*, \delta) = \frac{S(t|\mathbf{X}_i, \boldsymbol{\beta}^*, \gamma^*, \delta)}{S(C|\mathbf{X}_i, \boldsymbol{\beta}^*, \gamma^*, \delta)} = \exp\{-e^{\delta}(t^{\gamma^*} - C^{\gamma^*})\exp(\mathbf{X}_i^T\boldsymbol{\beta}^*)\}.$$

We can draw from this distribution as described above, since the cumulative distribution function $F = 1 - S$. The results for two of the five studies analysed by Brinkhof *et al.* (2010) are shown in Table 10.5. The estimated 1-year survival probabilities from each imputed dataset, $\hat{S}(1)_k$, $k = 1, \dots, K$, were transformed using the complementary log–log link, $Z_k = \log[-\log\{\hat{S}(1_k)\}]$ to be approximately normally distributed. Rubin's rules were applied to the transformed values to obtain point estimates and confidence intervals, which were then back transformed to the original scale.

The estimated 1-year survival in the observed data, and after CAR imputation ($\delta = 0, K = 10$ imputations) agrees closely. This is what theory predicts: imputation of censored survival times under CAR should give the same results as the observed data CAR analysis.

Table 10.5 Illustration of sensitivity analysis for increased mortality among patients lost to follow-up.

Study	$\exp(\delta_{\text{study}})$	One year mortality			Relative increase
		In observed data	Under (10.15) $\delta = 0$	Under (10.15) $\delta = \delta_{\text{study}}$	
Lighthouse	6	10.9% (9.6–12.4%)	10.8% (9.4–12.3%)	16.9% (15.0–19.1%)	56%
AMPATH	12	5.7% (4.9–6.5%)	5.9% (5.1–6.9%)	10.2% (8.9–11.6%)	73%

Source: Adapted from Brinkhof *et al.* (2010).

For the sensitivity analyses, Brinkhof *et al.* (2010) used meta-regression of other studies available to them to estimate plausible values of δ for the Lighthouse and AMPATH studies. For each study, the sensitivity parameter δ was then fixed at the estimated value rather than drawn from a distribution as in (10.14). The results show a substantial, practically important, relative increase in mortality in these studies if the hazard ratio relating those lost to follow-up to those remaining in follow-up is consistent with that estimated in the meta-regression.

We conclude this example by noting that while, given δ, the point estimates in Table 10.5 could be approximated analytically, MI also provides estimates of the standard errors, and resulting confidence intervals. The ability to do this when δ has a prior distribution, and this distribution is allowed to differ by treatment arm or other subgroups, makes MI a very attractive method for estimation and inference. □

10.4 Pattern mixture approach with longitudinal data via MI

We now extend this approach to longitudinal data, focusing particularly on longitudinal data arising from clinical trials, although the same ideas will typically be applicable to longitudinal data arising in other settings.

Suppose we intend to observe a response at baseline, and p follow-up times, $Y_{i,0}, Y_{i,1}, \dots, Y_{i,p}$. For a given estimand, an *intercurrent event relevant to the estimand* (hereafter *intercurrent event*) is a post-randomisation event such that post-intercurrent event data (if available) cannot be directly used for inference about the estimand. Here we assume that post-intercurrent event data are missing. When available, relevant post-intercurrent event data can naturally be incorporated within this framework to inform the analysis.

While the precise definition of an estimand and associated intercurrent events will be trial-specific (e.g. Clark *et al.*, 2022), for pragmatic, treatment policy estimands, we typically regard the first instance of the following as relevant intercurrent events:

- unblinding, for example of treatment allocation, and
- unknown events resulting in loss to follow-up (after which no data are available in any case);

whereas the following intercurrent events would typically not be relevant under the treatment policy estimand, so outcome data collected after these events is still included in the analysis:

- moving to partial compliance with treatment, and
- withdrawal from treatment (e.g. following an adverse event).

For hypothetical estimands, where – for example – we wish to estimate the treatment effect in the hypothetical scenario all patients complied with the protocol, we typically regard the first instance of any of these as relevant intercurrent events:

- unblinding;
- moving to partial compliance with treatment;
- withdrawal from treatment, and
- loss to follow-up.

We emphasise 'typically'; in applications, intercurrent events need to be carefully defined in the protocol.

Having pre-specified the estimands and associated intercurrent events, we are left with a dataset in which (i) each patient has longitudinal follow-up data until either they have an intercurrent event, or reach the scheduled end of the study, and (ii) the nature of each intercurrent event is available. The approach we describe here is that, for each intercurrent event (or – more likely – group of similar intercurrent events occurring for similar reasons) we build an appropriate post-intercurrent event distribution taking account of (i) the patient's pre-intercurrent event observations; (ii) pre-intercurrent event data from other patients in the trial; (iii) the nature of the intercurrent event, and (iv) the reason for the intercurrent event.

We stress that we do not advocate building the post-intercurrent event distribution after unblinding. Instead, for a given estimand, and associated pre-specified primary outcome measure, we advocate pre-specifying (i) a *primary* and (ii) *one or more secondary* post-intercurrent event distributions. The former gives the primary answer to the question; the latter provide sensitivity analyses.

10.4.1 Change in slope post-deviation

Suppose that in the post-intercurrent event, patients have a different, usually poorer response than predicted under MAR. For example in an asthma trial, FEV_1 might

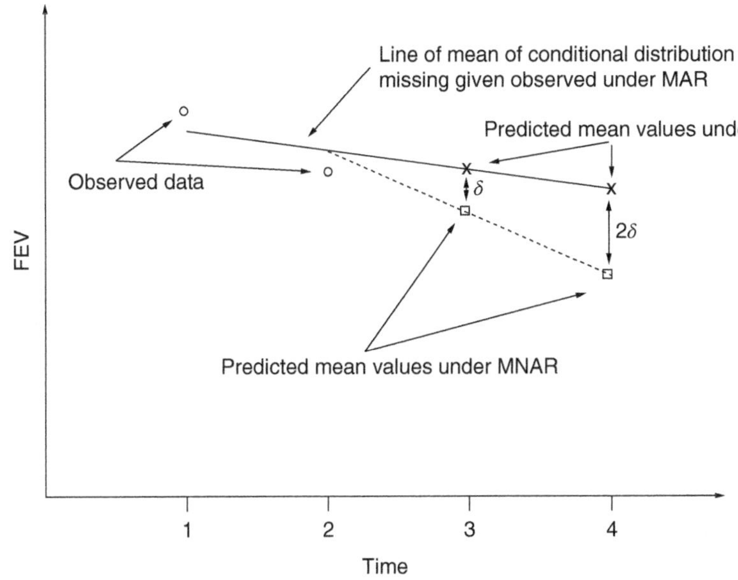

Figure 10.1 Schematic illustration of increasing the rate of decline by δ post-intercurrent event.

improve more slowly (or decline more quickly) after the intercurrent event which results in missing data. If the change in rate of decline post-intercurrent event in arm a is denoted δ_a, then the MAR conditional mean for the first scheduled post-intercurrent event observation is reduced by δ_a, the second by $2\delta_a$, and so on. This is schematically illustrated in Figure 10.1.

As in Example 10.1, if possible we can elicit from experts a prior distribution for the joint distribution of δ_a, for a indexing the different treatment groups. If, for example we assume this is a multivariate normal, we require the mean and variance of δ_a in the intervention arm a, which is assumed to be normally distributed, and $\text{Cor}(\delta_a, \delta_{a'})$, for all treatment groups a and a'. In practice, White *et al.* (2007) show the widest confidence intervals occur when the correlation is zero (assuming it is not negative), and often useful information can be obtained by assuming the distribution of δ_a is the same across arms.

Computationally, we follow the approach described on p. 253. First, separately within each treatment arm, we use the pre-intercurrent event data to generate K imputations under MAR. Then, if we have two intervention arms, for each imputation, $k = 1, \dots, K$, we sample

$$\begin{pmatrix} \delta_{1,k} \\ \delta_{2,k} \end{pmatrix} \sim N\left[\begin{pmatrix} \mu_{\delta_1} \\ \mu_{\delta_2} \end{pmatrix}, \begin{pmatrix} \sigma_1^2 & \rho\sigma_1\sigma_2 \\ \rho\sigma_1\sigma_2 & \sigma_2^2 \end{pmatrix}\right].$$

For each patient, in each intervention arm $a = 1,2$, for imputation k, we then increase the first MAR imputed observation by $\delta_{a,k}$, the second by $2\delta_{a,k}$, and so on. We then analyse the resulting datasets and combine the estimates using Rubin's rules. If the time between observations is not constant, we may want to change the multipliers of δ from $1,2,3,\ldots$, to maintain a linear change. We can handle interim missing observations by decreasing them by δ_a, or simply leaving them with their MAR imputed values. The latter is consistent with a different mechanism driving interim missing data and the intercurrent event.

As discussed above, the confidence intervals are going to be narrower, the greater the correlation between the δ's for different treatment arms. In practice, information on this correlation is unlikely to be available, so as the correlation is unlikely to be negative, a conservative approach is to set $\rho = 0$. Likewise, often, in the absence of prior information, we may set $\delta_1 = \delta_2$. Depending on the context, one approach may then be to increase δ until the treatment effect is no longer clinically relevant (often referred to as a tipping-point analysis).

Example 10.4 Asthma study

We now illustrate this approach using the asthma study (see p. 25). As before, we compare the placebo and lowest active dose arms. Our substantive model is the regression of 12 week FEV_1 on treatment, adjusted for baseline. This is essentially the primary analysis of the original study. We focus on the hypothetical estimand, asking what would be the treatment effect if patients in both were able (or made) to endure remaining in the study under the protocol, despite worsening asthma. In this study patients are followed up systematically until they have an intercurrent event. The intercurrent events are typically discontinuing or unblinding treatment for a variety of reasons. Only limited post-intercurrent event data are available, and we disregard these for our analyses.

The first row of Table 10.6 shows the analysis of the 108/180 patients who completed the 12-week follow-up. Treatment increases lung function by a clinically relevant 0.25 l on average, and this estimate is significant at the 5% level. This analysis addresses the hypothetical estimand of the effect of treatment if taken as specified in the protocol. The MAR assumption is a reasonable primary assumption for this

Table 10.6 Asthma study: estimates of the treatment effect in the hypothetical case that all patients remain on treatment, assuming MAR, and MNAR with increasing post-intercurrent event increments, δ. MI analyses used $K = 1000$ imputations.

Analysis	Treatment estimate (l)	Standard error	p-value
Complete records, hypothetical	0.247	0.100	0.0155
MI, hypothetical, randomised arm MAR	0.335	0.107	0.0017
MI, hypothetical, $\mu_\delta = 0.1, \sigma_\delta = 0$	0.361	0.108	0.0008
MI, hypothetical, $\mu_\delta = 0.1, \sigma_\delta = 0.1$	0.362	0.156	0.0207
MI, hypothetical, $\mu_\delta = 0.2, \sigma_\delta = 0.0$	0.388	0.110	0.0004
MI, hypothetical, $\mu_\delta = 0.2, \sigma_\delta = 0.1$	0.392	0.158	0.0132

estimand, since the distribution of the missing data given baseline and treatment is estimated from patients who complied – i.e. whose data are observed. A more plausible assumption is that data are MAR given baseline, treatment, and intermediate measurements. Under this assumption, and imputing separately in the treatment arms, the 12-week effect increases to 0.36 l, with a much reduced p-value. Following Figure 10.1, the third analysis (which assumes MNAR) decreases the MAR conditional mean by 0.1 l each post-intercurrent event follow-up visit. In other words, in (10.4.1) $\mu_{\delta_{\text{active}}} = \mu_{\delta_{\text{placebo}}} = \mu_\delta = 0.1$ and $\sigma_{\text{active}} = \sigma_{\text{placebo}} = 0$.

Since 53/90 in the placebo, but only 19/90 in the lowest active arm, have intercurrent events before 12 weeks, the consequence is to increase the treatment effect. The precision is unchanged from the randomised arm MAR analysis because $\sigma_{\text{active}} = \sigma_{\text{placebo}} = 0$; with a relatively large $\sigma_{\text{active}} = \sigma_{\text{placebo}} = 0.1$, and $\rho = 1$, it is increased but the effect remains significant. Analysis with $\mu_{\delta_{\text{active}}} = \mu_{\delta_{\text{placebo}}} = 0.2$, retaining $\sigma_{\text{active}} = \sigma_{\text{placebo}} = 0.1$, $\rho = 1$, yields similar results. We conclude that, under the MNAR mechanism represented by this particular model for sensitivity analysis, inference for the hypothetical treatment effect estimand inference is robust to the MNAR mechanisms considered. □

10.5 Reference based imputation

Thus far, our pattern mixture sensitivity analyses have all relied on specification of the prior distribution of the sensitivity parameter vector, $\boldsymbol{\delta}$. Carpenter *et al.* (2013) propose an alternative approach in the context of randomised clinical trials, which is to piece together the post-intercurrent event distribution by making qualitative, not quantitative, reference to other arms. This is in the spirit of an approach to sensitivity analysis proposed by Little and Yau (1996); see also Carpenter and Kenward (2009), who provide an early implementation of this approach using sequential regression imputation. Its theoretical and empirical behaviour has been explored by Cro *et al.* (2019), and is illustrated in a tutorial by Cro *et al.* (2020).

Here, while the generic algorithm remains that described on p. 253, we specify how the joint distribution of post-intercurrent event data in the treatment arms is constructed *by reference to other treatment arms*, as follows:

1. Separately for each treatment arm, take all patients' relevant pre-intercurrent event data and – assuming MAR – fit a multivariate normal distribution with unstructured mean (i.e. a separate mean for each of the $1 + p$ baseline plus post-randomisation observation times) and unstructured variance-covariance matrix (i.e. a $(1 + p) \times (1 + p)$ covariance matrix), as described in Chapter 3.
2. Separately for each treatment arm, draw a mean vector and variance-covariance matrix from the posterior distribution.
3. For each patient who has a relevant intercurrent event before the end of the study, use the draws from step 2 to build the joint distribution of their pre- and

post-intercurrent event outcome data. Suggested options for constructing this are given below.

4. For each patient who has a relevant intercurrent event before the end, use their joint distribution in step 3 to construct their conditional distribution of post-intercurrent event given pre-intercurrent event outcome data. Sample their post-intercurrent event data from this conditional distribution, to create a 'completed' dataset.
5. Repeat steps 2–4 K times, resulting in K imputed datasets.
6. Fit the substantive model to each imputed dataset, and combine the resulting parameter estimates and standard errors using Rubin's rules (Rubin, 1987) for final inference.

As usual, we use MCMC to sample from the appropriate Bayesian posterior in step 2, updating the chain sufficiently between successive draws to ensure they are effectively independent.

10.5.1 Constructing joint distributions of pre- and post-intercurrent event data

We now give some examples of methods for constructing the joint distribution of each patient's pre- and post-intercurrent event outcome data in step 3. Each option represents a difference in the post-intercurrent event outcome distribution. Many others are possible, but these are sufficient to explain our approach and illustrate its flexibility. Our experience is they are likely to prove appropriate in many settings.

Randomised-arm MAR: The joint distribution of the patient's pre- and post-intercurrent event outcome data is multivariate normal with mean and covariance matrix from their randomised treatment arm.

Jump to reference: Post-intercurrent event, the patient ceases their randomised treatment, and their mean response distribution is now that of a 'reference' group of patients (typically, but not necessarily, control patients). Such a change may be seen as extreme, and choosing the reference group to be the control group might be used as a worst-case scenario in terms of reducing any treatment effect since patients on active who discontinue their randomised treatment will lose the effect of their period on treatment.

In the implementation presented here, post-intercurrent event data in the reference arm are imputed under randomised-arm MAR, but in applications other assumptions may be more appropriate.

Last mean carried forward: Post-intercurrent event, it is assumed that the patient is expected, on average, to neither get worse nor better. So the mean of their distribution stays constant at the value of the mean for their randomised treatment arm at their last pre-intercurrent event measurement. The variance-covariance matrix remains that for their randomised treatment arm.

Thus a patient who is well above the mean for their arm at the last pre-intercurrent event measurement (giving a large positive pre-intercurrent event residual) will tend to progress back across later visits to within random variation of the mean value for their arm at their pre-intercurrent measurement visit. The speed and extent of that progression will depend on the strength of the correlation between successive measurements.

Copy increments in reference: After a patient's intercurrent event, their mean increments copy those from the reference group (typically, but not necessarily, control patients). Post-intercurrent event data in the reference arm are imputed under randomised-arm MAR. If the reference is chosen to be the control arm, the patient's mean profile following their intercurrent event tracks that of the mean profile in the control arm, but starting from the benefit already obtained. This is what we might hope for in an Alzheimer's study where treatment halts disease progression. After stopping therapy, the disease continues to progress again.

Copy reference: Here, for the purpose of imputing the missing response data, a patient's whole distribution, both pre- and post-intercurrent event, is assumed to be the same as the reference (typically, but not necessarily, control) group. Post-intercurrent event data in the reference arm are imputed under randomised-arm MAR.

Perhaps surprisingly, this may often have a less extreme impact than 'jump to reference' above. This is because if a patient on active treatment is well above the reference mean, then this relatively large positive residual will feed through into subsequent draws from the conditional distribution of post-deviation data, to a degree determined by the correlation in the reference arm. Thus, the patient's profile will decay back towards the mean for control at later visits relatively slowly.

Note that 'last mean carried forward' and 'copy increments in reference' have an important feature in common. For an active and a reference patient whose intercurrent events occur at the same time, the difference between their two post-intercurrent event means is maintained at a constant value up to the end of the trial. In the former case, the individual group mean profiles are held constant over time, in the latter, they are allowed to vary across time. In this sense, they both represent ways of implementing in a principled modelling framework, the assumptions that might be implied by 'last observation carried forward' (LOCF) type methods.

10.5.2 Technical details

We now describe how step 3 works under 'jump to reference'. This leads to a brief presentation of the approach for the other options. Suppose there are two arms, active and reference.

In step 2, denote the current draw from the posterior for the $1 + p$ reference arm means and variance-covariance matrix by $\mu_{r,0}, \dots, \mu_{r,p}$, and $\boldsymbol{\Sigma}_r$. Use the subscript a

for the corresponding draws from the other arm in question (which will depend on the arm chosen as reference for the analysis at hand).

Under 'jump to reference', suppose patient i is not randomised to the reference arm and their last observation, prior to the intercurrent event, is at time d_i, $d_i \in (1, \dots, p-1)$. The joint distribution of their pre- and post-intercurrent event outcomes is multivariate normal with mean

$$\boldsymbol{\mu}_i^* = (\mu_{a,0}, \dots, \mu_{a,d_i}, \mu_{r,d_i+1}, \dots, \mu_{r,p})^T;$$

that is post-intercurrent event they 'jump to reference'.

We construct the new covariance matrix for these observations as follows. Denote the covariance matrices from the reference arm (without relevant intercurrent events) and the other arm in question (without relevant intercurrent events), partitioned at time d_i according to the pre- and post-intercurrent measurements, by

$$\text{Reference } \boldsymbol{\Sigma}_r = \begin{bmatrix} \mathbf{R}_{11} & \mathbf{R}_{12} \\ \mathbf{R}_{21} & \mathbf{R}_{22} \end{bmatrix} \text{ and other arm: } \boldsymbol{\Sigma}_a = \begin{bmatrix} \boldsymbol{A}_{11} & \boldsymbol{A}_{12} \\ \boldsymbol{A}_{21} & \boldsymbol{A}_{22} \end{bmatrix}.$$

We want the new covariance matrix, $\boldsymbol{\Sigma}$ say, to match that from the active arm for the pre-intercurrent event measurements, and the reference arm for the *conditional* components for the post-intercurrent event given the pre-intercurrent event measurements. This also guarantees positive definiteness of the new matrix, since $\boldsymbol{\Sigma}_r$ and $\boldsymbol{\Sigma}_a$ are positive definite. That is, we want

$$\boldsymbol{\Sigma} = \begin{bmatrix} \boldsymbol{\Sigma}_{11} & \boldsymbol{\Sigma}_{12} \\ \boldsymbol{\Sigma}_{21} & \boldsymbol{\Sigma}_{22} \end{bmatrix},$$

subject to the constraints

$$\begin{aligned} \boldsymbol{\Sigma}_{11} &= \boldsymbol{A}_{11}, \\ \boldsymbol{\Sigma}_{21}\boldsymbol{\Sigma}_{11}^{-1} &= \mathbf{R}_{21}\mathbf{R}_{11}^{-1}, \\ \boldsymbol{\Sigma}_{22} - \boldsymbol{\Sigma}_{21}\boldsymbol{\Sigma}_{11}^{-1}\boldsymbol{\Sigma}_{12} &= \mathbf{R}_{22} - \mathbf{R}_{21}\mathbf{R}_{11}^{-1}\mathbf{R}_{12}. \end{aligned}$$

The solution is

$$\begin{aligned} \boldsymbol{\Sigma}_{11} &= \boldsymbol{A}_{11}, \\ \boldsymbol{\Sigma}_{21} &= \mathbf{R}_{21}\mathbf{R}_{11}^{-1}\boldsymbol{A}_{11}, \\ \boldsymbol{\Sigma}_{22} &= \mathbf{R}_{22} - \mathbf{R}_{21}\mathbf{R}_{11}^{-1}(\mathbf{R}_{11} - \boldsymbol{A}_{11})\mathbf{R}_{11}^{-1}\mathbf{R}_{12}. \end{aligned}$$

Under 'jump to reference', we have now specified the joint distribution for a patient's pre- and post-intercurrent event outcomes, when inter-current event is at time d_i. This is what we require for step 4.

For 'copy increments in reference', we use the same $\boldsymbol{\Sigma}$ as for 'jump to reference' but now

$$\begin{aligned} \boldsymbol{\mu}_i = \{&\mu_{a,0}, \dots, \mu_{a,d_i-1}, \mu_{a,d_i}, \mu_{a,d_i} + (\mu_{r,d_i+1} - \mu_{r,d_i}), \\ &\mu_{a,d_i} + (\mu_{r,d_i+2} - \mu_{r,d_i}), \dots\}^T. \end{aligned}$$

For 'last mean carried forward', $\boldsymbol{\Sigma}$ equals the covariance matrix from the randomisation arm. The important change is the way we put together $\boldsymbol{\mu}$. Thus, for patient i in arm a under 'last mean carried forward',

$$\boldsymbol{\mu}_i = (\mu_{a,0}, \dots, \mu_{a,d_i-1}, \mu_{a,d_i}, \mu_{a,d_i}, \dots)^T; \quad \boldsymbol{\Sigma} = \boldsymbol{\Sigma}_a.$$

Finally for 'copy reference', the mean and covariance both come from the reference (typically, but not necessarily, control) arm, irrespective of inter-current event time.

10.5.3 Software

SAS macros, help files and examples implementing this (and a range of related) approaches can be downloaded from the 'DIA' tab of https://missingdata.lshtm.ac.uk. In Stata, the approach is implemented in the '`mimix`' macro (Cro *et al.*, 2016). In `R`, the approach is implemented in the '`rbmi`' package (Gower-Page *et al.*, 2022) and the '`RefbasedMI`' available from https://github.com/UCL/RefbasedMI. The approach has been successfully applied to cost-effectiveness data, with associated Stata software (Leurent *et al.*, 2018, Leurent and Cro, 2022).

Example 10.4 Asthma study *(ctd)*

We return to the asthma study, and again focus on the placebo and lowest active dose arms, with the same definition of an intercurrent event as before. For each imputation analysis, the substantive model is the ANCOVA regression of 12-week lung function on baseline and treatment.

The first row of Table 10.7 (analysis HY1) shows the complete records analysis (cf Table 10.6) by ANCOVA using the week 12 data, using the 108 patients with data at 12 weeks. It follows from the definition of the intercurrent event that the MAR assumption implies that, conditional on treatment and baseline, the distribution of unobserved and observed 12-week responses is the same. As the latter is estimated from on-treatment, protocol adhering patients, this analysis addresses the hypothetical question of the treatment effect if all patients were somehow made to comply fully with the protocol. However, there are only 37 out of 90 patients with 12-week data in the placebo arm, compared with 71 out of 90 in the active.

Analysis HY2 includes all observed pre-intercurrent event data in a saturated repeated measurements (SRM) model. This fits a separate mean for each treatment and time, with a full baseline-time interaction and common unstructured covariance matrix. Analysis HY3 further allows a separate, unstructured covariance matrix in each arm. The results show inference from the primary analysis (HY1: 0.247 litres), $p = 0.0155$), which addresses the hypothetical (on-treatment) estimand, is robust to the different assumptions made by HY2, HY3; indeed HY3 gives both the largest and most significant treatment estimate (0.346 l, $p = 0.0013$).

Analysis HY4, randomised MAR using MI makes a very similar MAR assumption as HY3. In line with theory, the result from the SRM model with separate variance-covariance matrices agrees closely with that from using multiple imputation because the data are well modelled by the normal distribution. The only difference in the underlying imputation model for HY4

Table 10.7 Estimated 12-week treatment effect on FEV_1 (litres), from ANCOVA, mixed models, multiple imputation, and sensitivity analyses. All multiple imputation analyses used 1000 imputations, with a 'burn-in' of 1000 updates and 500 updates between imputations.

	Analysis estimate (litres)	Treatment	Std. Err.	DF (model)	*t*-statistic	*p*-value
Hypothetical						
HY1	ANCOVA (completers), joint variance	0.247	0.101	105	2.46	0.0155
HY2	Mixed model, joint covariance matrix	0.283	0.094	131	3.02	0.0030
HY3	Mixed model, separate covariance matrices	0.346	0.104	72.8	3.34	0.0013
HY4	Randomised-arm MAR MI	0.334	0.107	130.6	3.13	0.0022
Treatment policy						
TP1	Last mean carried forward option	0.296	0.102	141.6	2.90	0.0043
TP2	Jump to reference (active)	0.141	0.119	102.7	1.18	0.2390
TP3	Jump to reference (placebo)	0.264	0.108	135.5	2.46	0.0153
TP4	Copy reference (active)	0.252	0.087	139.4	2.88	0.0046
TP5	Copy reference (placebo)	0.295	0.105	146.5	2.82	0.0055
TP6	Copy incr. in reference (active)	0.295	0.103	139.7	2.87	0.0048
TP7	Copy incr. reference (placebo)	0.323	0.104	139.6	3.12	0.0022

from the SRM model HY3 is that the multiple imputation approach implicitly allows a full three-way interaction of baseline with treatment and time, whereas the SRM model has the same regression coefficients for baseline × time in the two arms. Apart from this, they are structurally equivalent.

We now consider the treatment policy estimand and explore the implications of different assumptions about post-intercurrent event behaviour in TP1–TP7 in Table 10.7. Each of these assumes a different joint distribution for pre- and post-intercurrent event data.

Analysis TP1 corresponds to the underlying mean response remaining static after intervention stops (this is applied to both active and reference, i.e. placebo arms). This would address the treatment policy question when after an intercurrent event active arm patients took no further relevant medication and their condition was stable. If, allowing for the personal covariates such as baseline, they have a positive residual at their final pre-intercurrent event visit, we expect that post-intercurrent event their residuals will decrease (but continue to randomly vary), so on average they will get closer to their own conditional mean.

In the asthma setting, this flat mean profile post-intercurrent event may be plausible for a week or two after the intercurrent event in the active treatment arm. In these data, the downward trend in the placebo arm (Table 1.3) suggests that LMCF is likely to yield higher estimates of the latter placebo means than analyses addressing the hypothetical estimand, while estimates for the active arm will change in the other direction. This leads to a smaller treatment estimate (0.296 *l*), but not as low as that for HY1.

We now apply the 'jump to reference' (HY2, HY3), 'copy reference' (HY4, HY5) and 'copy increments in reference' (HY6, HY7) options. We discuss the implications for the interpretation of choice of the 'reference' arm under these two approaches (in this example it could either be the placebo, or the lowest active dose arm).

Suppose we wish to address the question corresponding to the assumption that, post-intercurrent event, (i) patients on placebo obtain a treatment equivalent to the active, and (ii) the active treatment patients continue on treatment and adhere to the protocol, so that their post-intercurrent event data can be imputed assuming randomised-arm MAR. In this case, we specify the *active arm* as 'reference'. The early part of the study suggests that 2 and 3 weeks are needed for a treatment to take effect. Further, the patients have chronic asthma, so it is likely that they will seek an active treatment on discontinuation from the placebo treatment. For the treatment policy estimand, this assumption is thus arguably more plausible than considering placebo as 'reference'. Nevertheless, for discussion we also present results where the placebo is 'reference'; that is where post-intercurrent event (i) patients on the active treatment switch to a placebo equivalent, and (ii) the placebo treatment patients continue on placebo adhering to the protocol, and their post-intercurrent data can be imputed assuming randomised-arm MAR. This latter assumption might be appropriate where no alternative treatment is generally available.

Analysis TP2 estimates the treatment effect under 'jump to reference' when the 'reference' is the active arm. Of all the treatment policy analyses, this is the most extreme in terms of effect on the treatment difference, since the means prior to

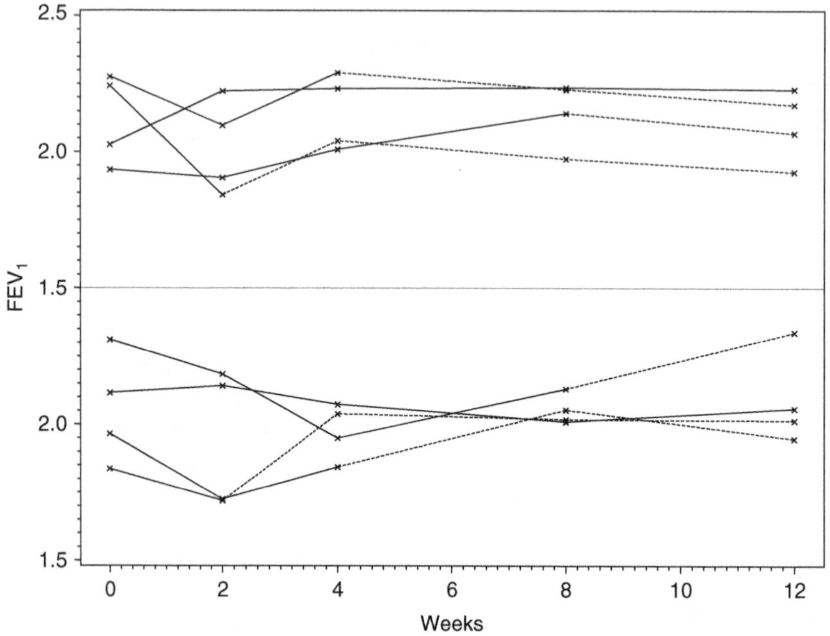

Figure 10.2 Mean FEV_1 (litres) against time for the four different intercurrent event patterns. Solid lines join observed means (before inter-current event) and dotted lines join the means of the imputed data for that pattern. Top panel: lowest active dose, imputed under randomised-arm MAR; bottom panel: placebo arm imputed under 'jump to reference' (where 'reference' is lowest active dose).

intercurrent event follow the patients randomised arm and then abruptly switch to that of the specified 'reference' arm. The effect of this is shown in Figure 10.2; we find plots like this very useful tools for conveying the implications of assumptions. This big change in placebo patients' post-intercurrent event means results in a substantially reduced treatment estimate (0.141 l, $p = 0.24$). We conclude that, if post-intercurrent event medication has comparable effect to the lowest active dose, patients from both arms will have comparable lung function at the end of the study. This analysis mimics what we might expect for a *retrieved dropout analysis* (Committee for Medicinal Products for Human Use, 2010) where placebo patients are allowed to switch to active treatment.

Analysis TP3 corresponds to the less-plausible reverse option where after withdrawal the active patients now 'jump to reference' and the reference is the placebo. Since far fewer patients have intercurrent events in the active arm, the change from the hypothetical MAR analysis is much smaller: the treatment difference remains significant (0.264 l, $p = 0.015$).

We now consider two further sets of assumptions for addressing the treatment policy estimand: 'copy reference' and 'copy increments in reference'. The former replaces both pre-intercurrent event and post-intercurrent event means with those of the specified 'reference', when constructing the joint distribution of pre- and post-intercurrent event data in step 3 of the algorithm at the start of Section 10.4.1. The latter, 'copy increments in reference', has the randomised profile prior to intercurrent event, but then the incremental changes in mean FEV_1 from visit-to-visit track those in the 'reference' arm.

When the active arm is specified as the 'reference', 'copy reference' (TP4), and 'copy increments in reference' (TP6) give 12-week treatment estimates of 0.252 *l* and 0.295 *l* respectively. In this case, 'copy reference' has a larger treatment effect than 'jump to reference' because under 'copy reference', pre-intercurrent event placebo patients have relatively larger residuals (differenced from the mean for the active arm), which implies that after the intercurrent event they track to the active means more slowly; with 'jump to reference' pre-intercurrent event placebo patients have smaller residuals (differenced from the mean for the placebo arm), so post-intercurrent event, they track to the active means more rapidly.

When placebo is specified as the 'reference', 'copy reference' (DF5) and 'copy increments in reference' (DF7) give much smaller changes from the randomised-arm MAR estimate, for the same reason as 'jump to reference' (DF7), discussed above.

In summary, the primary analysis addressing the (hypothetical) treated-as-per-protocol estimand assuming MAR is consistent with a significant beneficial effect of treatment relative to placebo. Addressing the treatment policy estimand with a conservative assumption about the effect of post-intercurrent event (withdrawal) switching to active ('copy reference' or 'copy increments in reference') continues to show a significant improvement at the 5% level. However, if instead, we use 'jump to reference' ('reference' is active treatment), then the treatment benefit is reduced by over 50% relative to randomised-arm MAR, and is no longer statistically significant. If the many placebo patients who discontinue early switch to the active treatment, this is to be expected. □

Before moving on, we note that the copy reference and jump to reference sensitivity analysis can be re-framed in terms of the proportion of treatment benefit retained, which has the attraction of giving a single sensitivity parameter to work with (White *et al.*, 2019). The approach has also been extended to survival data (Atkinson *et al.*, 2019, 2021).

10.5.4 Information anchoring

While the discussion thus far has focused on how the mean of the imputation distribution (conditional predictive distribution) of the missing data given the observed can be changed to reflect departures from MAR, it is also important to keep in mind the variance of the imputation distribution, as this directly relates to whether the sensitivity analysis increases, holds constant, or decreases the information about a parameter of interest – such as a treatment or exposure effect, relative to that in the primary analysis. This is explored in detail by Cro *et al.* (2019).

Example 10.5 Information in sensitivity analysis

Suppose a study intends to take measurements on n patients $Y_1, \ldots, Y_n$, from a population with known variance σ^2, and the estimator is the mean. If no data are missing, then the variance of the mean is σ^2/n.

Now suppose that n_d observations are missing. Our estimator is the mean for both our primary and sensitivity analysis. Our primary analysis will assume data are missing completely at random, and the sensitivity analysis will assume that the missing values are from patients with the same mean, but a different variance, σ_m^2. Since the distribution of the missing data are assumed different from the observed, this corresponds to a particular MNAR assumption.

Under our primary analysis assumption, we can obtain valid inference by an observed data likelihood analysis. Here this corresponds to calculating the mean of the $n - n_d$ observed values. Alternatively, we can use multiple imputation for the missing values. In both cases, the variance of the estimator is the same: $\sigma^2/(n - n_d)$.

Under our sensitivity analysis, the MNAR *observed* data likelihood estimator and variance remain the same, since those with missing data are assumed to have the same mean as those observed. The fact that we now assume the missing values have a different variance makes no difference to our inference for μ.

Alternatively, we can multiply impute the missing data under our assumption, and suppose again our full data estimator is the sample mean. Now, however, the variance will be approximately $\{(n - n_d)\sigma^2 + n_d\sigma_m^2\}/n^2$. Further, the information (recall this is 1/variance) about the mean from the sensitivity analysis depends on σ_m^2. Since σ_m^2 is not estimable, this information is under the control of the analyst.

This is illustrated by Figure 10.3, which shows how the information (1/variance), based on Rubin's variance estimator about the mean varies with σ_m^2, when $n = 100$,

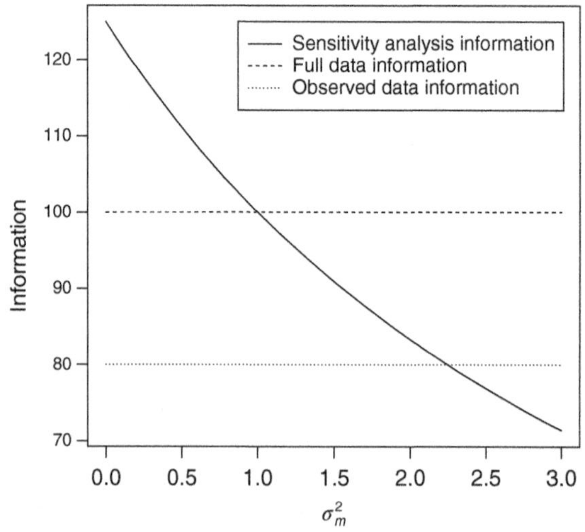

Figure 10.3 Information about the sample mean varies with σ_m^2 (recall information is 1/variance).

$n_d = 20$ and $\sigma^2 = 1$. When $\sigma_m^2 < \sigma^2$, the information about the mean in the sensitivity analysis is greater than from the intended 100 observations; when $1 \leq \sigma_m^2 \leq 2.25$ then the information is greater than in the $(n - n_d)$ observations we were able to obtain, and when $\sigma_m^2 > 2.25$, the information is less than in the observed data $(n - n_d)$ observations we were able to obtain.

The discrepancy between the variance/information from the observed data likelihood analysis and MI is due to uncongeniality. The full data analysis model applied to the imputed datasets is the simple sample mean. This is however not congenial with the imputation model; a congenial full data analysis model would weight the means from those with Y observed and missing according to the relative size of σ^2 and σ_m^2. Indeed, one can see that in this simple example, as $K \to \infty$, the MI estimator converges to the observed data mean of Y, and consequently, the true frequentist variance of the MI estimator (with $K = \infty$) is $\sigma^2/(n - n_d)$. □

Definition of information anchoring

We have seen in the simple example above how a sensitivity analysis can change, or apparently change, the statistical information about a treatment estimate. We now define *information-anchored* sensitivity analyses, which hold the proportion of information lost due to missing data constant across the primary and sensitivity analyses.

Suppose that a clinical trial intends to collect data from $2n$ patients, denoted $\mathbf{Y}$, in order to estimate a treatment effect θ. However, a number of patients do not give complete data. Denote the observed data by $\mathbf{Y}_{\text{obs}}$, and missing data by $\mathbf{Y}_{\text{miss}}$. Consistent with the ICH-E9 (R1) addendum (ICH, 2019), we make a *primary* set of assumptions, under which we perform the primary analysis. We then make a *sensitivity* set of assumptions, under which we perform the sensitivity analysis. Both primary and sensitivity assumptions (i) specify the distribution $f(\mathbf{Y}_{\text{miss}}|\mathbf{Y}_{\text{obs}})$, (ii) could be true, yet (iii) cannot be verified from $\mathbf{Y}_{\text{obs}}$.

Let $\hat{\theta}_{\text{obs, primary}}$ be the estimate of θ under the primary analysis assumption. Further, suppose we were able to observe a realisation of $\mathbf{Y}_{\text{miss}}$ under the primary assumption. Putting these data together with $\mathbf{Y}_{\text{obs}}$ gives us a complete set of observed data, which actually follows the primary assumption: we denote this by $\mathbf{Y}_{\text{primary}}$, and the corresponding estimate of θ by $\hat{\theta}_{\text{full, primary}}$. We denote the observed information about θ by $I(\hat{\theta}_{\text{obs, primary}})$ and $I(\hat{\theta}_{\text{full, primary}})$, respectively. Then,

$$\frac{I(\hat{\theta}_{\text{obs, primary}})}{I(\hat{\theta}_{\text{full, primary}})} < 1,$$

reflecting the loss of information about θ due to missing data.

Defining corresponding quantities under the sensitivity assumptions for the chosen sensitivity analysis procedure we have,

$$\frac{I(\hat{\theta}_{\text{obs, sensitivity}})}{I(\hat{\theta}_{\text{full, sensitivity}})} < 1,$$

again reflecting the loss of information about θ due to missing data – but now under the sensitivity assumptions.

Comparing these leads us to the following definitions:

$$\begin{aligned}
&\frac{I(\hat{\theta}_{\text{obs, primary}})}{I(\hat{\theta}_{\text{full, primary}})} > \frac{I(\hat{\theta}_{\text{obs, sensitivity}})}{I(\hat{\theta}_{\text{full, sensitivity}})} : \text{Information-}\textit{negative}\text{ sensitivity analysis,}\\
&\frac{I(\hat{\theta}_{\text{obs, primary}})}{I(\hat{\theta}_{\text{full, primary}})} = \frac{I(\hat{\theta}_{\text{obs, sensitivity}})}{I(\hat{\theta}_{\text{full, sensitivity}})} : \text{Information-}\textit{anchored}\text{ sensitivity analysis,}\\
&\frac{I(\hat{\theta}_{\text{obs, primary}})}{I(\hat{\theta}_{\text{full, primary}})} < \frac{I(\hat{\theta}_{\text{obs, sensitivity}})}{I(\hat{\theta}_{\text{full, sensitivity}})} : \text{Information-}\textit{positive}\text{ sensitivity analysis.}
\end{aligned} \tag{10.16}$$

When analysing a clinical trial, an information-positive sensitivity analysis is hard to justify, because it implies that the more data are missing, the more information there is about the treatment effect under the sensitivity analysis. Conversely, while information-negative sensitivity analyses provide an incentive for minimising missing data, there is no natural consensus about the appropriate loss of information. Therefore, we argue that information-anchored sensitivity analyses are the natural starting point. They provide a level playing field between regulators and industry, allowing the focus to be on the average response to treatment among the unobserved patients.

The definitions above are quite general, applying directly to all the estimands and sensitivity analyses considered in this chapter.

Which sensitivity analyses are information anchored?

Cro *et al.* (2019) show that MI with Rubin's variance estimator is information anchored for the $\boldsymbol{\delta}$-method sensitivity analysis approach, when fixed values of $\boldsymbol{\delta}$ are used. If a prior distribution for $\boldsymbol{\delta}$ is specified, this results in an information negative analysis – because uncertainty about $\boldsymbol{\delta}$ increases the uncertainty about the treatment effect.

The reference-based MI approach can be information positive, when information is judged by repeated sampling variance of the observed data likelihood information. This means that as the amount of missing data increases, uncertainty about the treatment effect can decrease (Seaman *et al.*, 2014). Fortunately, Cro *et al.* (2019) show however that if one uses Rubin's variance estimator, inferences remain approximately information anchored. The discrepancy between the observed data likelihood based information and information judged by Rubin's variance estimator is, as in Example 10.5, due to uncongeniality between the imputation and analysis models. For further discussion of this subtle issue, we refer the reader to Cro *et al.* (2019) and Bartlett (2021).

10.6 Approximating a selection model by importance weighting

Thus far we have explored sensitivity analysis using a pattern mixture approach. In particular, having chosen a model for the observed data, we specified models for the various patterns of missing data relative to this. Missing data were then imputed from these models, then the model of interest fitted to each of the imputed datasets and the results combined using Rubin's rules.

While this approach involved no approximations, it did require that data be explicitly imputed under the MNAR model, and then the model of interest fitted to this imputed data. Assuming that imputation had previously been performed under MAR, this approach therefore entails imputing a new set of data under each MNAR mechanism considered.

By contrast, here we describe an approximate approach, initially proposed by Carpenter *et al.* (2007) and improved upon by Beesley and Taylor (2021), for exploring the sensitivity of conclusions to MNAR mechanisms without the need for imputing under the MNAR mechanism.

The idea is simple: impute under MAR as usual and then up-weight imputed values that are more likely under the MNAR mechanism we are considering, and hence approximate the parameter estimate under this MNAR mechanism. Both approaches calculate the same weight for each imputed observation, but while Carpenter *et al.* (2007) proposed combining these to re-weight the parameter estimates from fitting the substantive model to each imputed dataset, Beesley and Taylor (2021) propose stacking the imputed data with the weights alongside, then fitting a single weighted regression to obtain the MNAR parameter estimate.

Both approaches use the idea of importance sampling. Suppose we draw

$$Z_1, \dots, Z_K \overset{i.i.d.}{\sim} g,$$

for some distribution g, but wish to estimate the expectation of some function, $h(Z)$ when Z is drawn from the distribution f. Provided the support of f is contained in that of g, and f/g is bounded, if we calculate $w_k = f(Z_k)/g(Z_k)$,

$$E_f[h(Z)] \approx \frac{\sum_{k=1}^{K} w_k h(Z_k)}{\sum_{k=1}^{K} w_k}, \tag{10.17}$$

with the approximation tending to equality as $K \to \infty$.

Essentially, we apply this result to MI, identifying g with the imputation distribution under MAR, f with the imputation distribution under MNAR, k indexing imputations, and Z_k with the kth imputation of the missing values under MAR.

To explore how this works, consider a very simple setting of two variables, partially observed $\mathbf{Y}_1$ and fully observed $\mathbf{Y}_2$. Write the estimator of the parameter of interest as $\hat{\theta} = \hat{\theta}(\mathbf{Y}_1, \mathbf{Y}_2)$.

Suppose $Y_{i,1}$ is missing. As usual, denote the missingness indicator by R_i, so that $R_i = 0$. Suppose, we have drawn K imputations of $Y^*_{i,1,k}$ under MAR, i.e. from the conditional predictive distribution

$$f(Y_{i,1} | Y_{i,2}, R_i = 1). \tag{10.18}$$

However, we wish to impute under MNAR, i.e. draw from

$$f(Y_{i,1} | Y_{i,2}, R_i = 0). \tag{10.19}$$

In the first part of this chapter, we took a pattern mixture approach and defined (10.19) by reference to (10.18) via sensitivity parameters. Here we consider a selection model, that is we define the relationship implicitly through the logistic regression of R_i on $Y_{i,1}, Y_{i,2}$:

$$\text{logit } \Pr(R_i = 1 | Y_{i,1}, Y_{i,2}) = \alpha_0 + \alpha_1 Y_{i,1} + \alpha_2 Y_{i,2}. \tag{10.20}$$

In this case, for imputed value $Y^*_{i,1,k}$, the weight is the ratio

$$\begin{aligned} \frac{f(Y^*_{i,1,k} | Y_{i,2}, R_i = 0)}{f(Y^*_{i,1,k} | Y_{i,2}, R_i = 1)} &= \frac{f(Y^*_{i,1,k}, Y_{i,2}, R_i = 0) f(Y_{i,2}, R_i = 1)}{f(Y^*_{i,1,k}, Y_{i,2}, R_i = 1) f(Y_{i,2}, R_i = 0)}, \\ &= \frac{f(R_i = 0 | Y^*_{i,1,k}, Y_{i,2}) f(Y_{i,2}, R_i = 1)}{f(R_i = 1 | Y^*_{i,1,k}, Y_{i,2}) f(Y_{i,2}, R_i = 0)}. \end{aligned} \tag{10.21}$$

Now consider $f(R_i = 0 | Y^*_{i,1,k}, Y_{i,2})$. Under model (10.20), this is $\{1 + \exp(\alpha_0 + \alpha_1 Y^*_{i,1,k} + \alpha_2 Y_{i,2})\}^{-1}$, and $f(R = 1 | Y^*_{i,1,k}, Y_{i,2}) = 1 - f(R_i = 0 | Y^*_{i,1,k}, Y_{i,2})$. So (10.21) is

$$\exp\{-(\alpha_0 + \alpha_1 Y^*_{i,1,k} + \alpha_2 Y_{i,2})\} \frac{f(Y_{i,2}, R_i = 1)}{f(Y_{i,2}, R_i = 0)}.$$

Therefore, the non-normalised weight for imputation k is

$$\tilde{w}_{i,k} = \exp(-\alpha_1 Y^*_{i,1,k}) \left\{ \exp[-(\alpha_0 + \alpha_2 Y_{i,2})] \frac{f(Y_{i,2}, R_i = 1)}{f(Y_{i,2}, R_i = 0)} \right\}. \tag{10.22}$$

Because the terms between the braces { } are common to all weights $\tilde{w}_{i,k}$, the normalised weights

$$w_{i,k} = \frac{\tilde{w}_{i,k}}{\sum_{k=1}^{K} \tilde{w}_{i,k}} \tag{10.23}$$

are proportional to $\exp(-\alpha_1 Y^*_{i,1,k})$. In other words, we do not need estimates of α_0, α_2 to estimate the weights; all we need are the imputed values under MAR, $\{Y^*_{i,1,k}\}_{k=1}^{K}$ and α_1. As with pattern mixture modelling, we do not estimate α_1 (cf Kenward, 1998). Instead, we explore the sensitivity of the results as α_1 varies from 0, which corresponds to MAR.

In fact, in the linear predictor, $\alpha_0 + \alpha_1 Y_{i,1} + \alpha_2 Y_{i,2}$, we can have any function of the observed data: it will cancel out of the weights. This means that, in contrast to full joint modelling approaches, our inference is robust to possible mis-specification of the relationship between the probability of observing $Y_{i,1}$ and the observed part of the data *provided* the relationship of the missingness process on the unseen data is correctly specified.

10.6.1 Weighting the imputations

Carpenter *et al.* (2007) proposed using (10.21) to weight the parameter estimate from each imputed dataset. Because conditional on the observed data and imputation-specific parameter draws, the imputed values are independent, the weight w_k for imputation k is given by

$$\tilde{w}_k = \exp\left(-\alpha_1 \sum_{i=1}^{n_{\text{miss}}} Y^*_{i,1,k}\right), \quad w_k = \frac{\tilde{w}_k}{\sum_{k=1}^{K} \tilde{w}_k}. \tag{10.24}$$

where we have re-ordered the data vector so that units $i = 1, \ldots, n_{\text{miss}}$ have missing $Y_{i,1}$ and units $i = (n_{\text{miss}} + 1), \ldots, n$ have observed $Y_{i,1}$.

Having done this, let $\hat{\theta}_k$ denote the estimate of θ obtained from the kth imputed dataset under MAR, and $\hat{\sigma}^2_k$ the corresponding variance. To obtain an estimate of θ when data are MNAR the analyst first chooses a plausible value of α_1 for the selection model

$$\text{logit}\{\Pr(R_{i,1} = 1 | Y_{i,1}, Y_{i,2})\} = \alpha_1 Y_{i,1} + g(Y_{i,2}). \tag{10.25}$$

Then, under the MNAR model implied by the analyst's choice of α_1 in (10.25), with weights w_k given by (10.24), the estimate of θ and its variance are

$$\hat{\theta}_{\text{MNAR}} = \sum_{k=1}^{K} w_k \hat{\theta}_k, \tag{10.26}$$

with variance

$$\hat{V}_{\text{MNAR}} \approx \hat{V}_W + (1 + 1/K)\hat{V}_B, \tag{10.27}$$

where now

$$\hat{V}_W = \sum_{k=1}^{K} w_m \hat{\sigma}^2_m, \quad \hat{V}_B = \sum_{k=1}^{K} w_m (\hat{\theta}_k - \hat{\theta}_{\text{MNAR}})^2. \tag{10.28}$$

Reliability of the approximation

The accuracy of the approximation justifying $\hat{\theta}_{\text{MNAR}}$ and $\hat{V}_{\text{MNAR}}$ improves as the number of imputations, K increases, provided the two importance sampling conditions hold

I1: The support of the MNAR distribution of the parameter estimates is contained within the support of the MAR distribution of the parameter estimates, and

I2: The ratio of the MNAR distribution to the MAR distribution is bounded.

This has a number of practical implications.

First, for the full generality of MNAR models, I1 cannot hold. Thus, the method is suitable for exploring local departures from MNAR. Second, even locally, it may be that the ratio of the distributions is unbounded. For example, if the MAR imputation distribution is $N(1,1)$ and the MNAR imputation distribution is $N(0.5, 1)$, this occurs in the left tail.

More subtly, the justification for the weights relies on (10.21), which has the true MAR distribution, in our notation $f(Y_{i,1} | Y_{i,2}, R_i = 1)$, in the denominator. In practice, of course, this is estimated from the observed data. If the dataset is very small, or there are many missing data, this estimate will be noisy, and in particular the proper imputation distribution often has a considerably heavier tail than $f(Y_{i,1} | Y_{i,2}, R_i = 1)$. As Smuk (2015) shows, this causes re-weighted estimates to overshoot the true MNAR value, because the imputed data drawn from the heavy tail of the imputation distribution gets disproportionately up-weighted. These two issues are the cause of the residual bias reported by Hayati Rezvan *et al.* (2015).

Smuk (2015) proposes and evaluates a solution, namely multiplying the weight for each imputed dataset by the ratio of the improper to proper imputation density. This was applied in Carpenter *et al.* (2011b). However, while this correction substantially improves the performance of the method, the additional calculations entailed mean the essential simplicity is lost, and the limitation of condition [I1] above still applies.

10.6.2 Stacking the imputations and applying the weights

These limitations led Beesley and Taylor (2021) to propose using weights again derived from $-\alpha_1 Y^*_{i,1,k}$, but now applied to the stacked imputed data. Specifically, under model (10.25), we have that the weight for $Y^*_{1,i,k}$ is

$$w_{i,k} = \frac{\exp(-\alpha_1 Y^*_{i,1,k})}{\sum_{k=1}^{K} \exp(-\alpha_1 Y^*_{i,1,k})}. \tag{10.29}$$

In other words, we now normalise the weights across imputed values for the same individual, rather than across imputations – i.e. apply the importance sampling argument at the individual, rather than the imputation, level. Continuing with the two variable example from Section 10.6.1, this gives the following algorithm:

Algorithm for re-weighting sensitivity analysis

1. Impute the missing $Y_{i,1}$ under MAR in the usual way, giving K imputations $\{Y^*_{i,1,k}\}_{k=1}^{K}$ for each of the n_{miss} missing values.

2. Form the expanded $(n \times 3)$ data as

$$\mathbf{Y}_{\text{expanded,k}} = \begin{pmatrix} Y^*_{i,1,k} & Y_{i,2} & w_{1,k} \\ \vdots & \vdots & \vdots \\ Y^*_{n_{\text{miss}},1,k} & Y_{n_{\text{miss}},2} & w_{n_{\text{miss}},k} \\ Y_{n_{\text{miss}}+1,1} & Y_{n_{\text{miss}}+1,2} & 1/K \\ \vdots & \vdots & \vdots \\ Y_{n,1} & Y_{n,2} & 1/K \end{pmatrix}, \tag{10.30}$$

where fully observed records are each given weight $1/K$.

3. Stack the $\mathbf{Y}_{\text{expanded},k}$, $k = 1, \ldots, K$, giving an $(nK \times 3)$ data matrix $\mathbf{Y}_{\text{stacked}}$.
4. Use weighted linear regression, with weights $w_{i,k}$, fit the substantive model using the stacked data $\mathbf{Y}_{\text{stacked}}$. Let y_i^k denote the $(n \times K)$ values of the dependent (i.e. outcome) variable in this substantive model, $\hat{y}_i^k$ the fitted values and $\hat{\theta}_{\text{MNAR}}$ the parameter estimate.

   Using the fitted values from this weighted regression, calculate the weighted estimate of the residual variance,

$$\hat{\sigma}^2 = \sum_{k=1}^{K} \sum_{i=1}^{n} w_{i,k}(y_i^k - \hat{y}_i^k)^2.$$

   Let $\mathbf{X}$ be the $(n \times p)$ design matrix for the substantive model, with $p = 2$ in our underlying setup with one covariate. For the coefficient of interest, estimate the 'within' imputation component of variance, σ_W^2, as the corresponding diagonal element of

$$(\mathbf{X}^T\mathbf{X})^{-1}\hat{\sigma}^2.$$

5. Use the jack-knife to estimate the between imputation variance, as follows:

   (a) Define $\hat{\theta}_{\text{MNAR},(k)}$ to be the estimate of θ obtained from $\mathbf{Y}_{\text{stacked}}$ *after omitting imputed data set k*. Note, before calculating $\hat{\theta}_{\text{MNAR},(k)}$, the weights must be re-normalised for the imputed values, and those for the observed values be set to $1/(K-1)$.

   (b) Calculate the jack-knife estimate of variance as

$$\hat{\sigma}_{\text{jack}}^2 = \frac{K-1}{K} \sum_{k=1}^{K} (\hat{\theta}_{\text{MNAR},(k)} - \overline{\theta})^2, \quad \text{where} \quad \overline{\theta} = \frac{1}{K} \sum_{k=1}^{K} \hat{\theta}_{\text{MNAR},(k)}.$$

   (c) Beesley and Taylor (2021) propose that because $\hat{\sigma}_{\text{jack}}^2$ is approximately $(1/K)$ of the usual between imputation variance – being an estimate of the variance of $\overline{\theta}$, not the variance of $\hat{\theta}^k$ across the imputation distribution – we set

$$\hat{\sigma}_B^2 = K(1 + 1/K)\hat{\sigma}_{\text{jack}}^2 = (K+1)\hat{\sigma}_{\text{jack}}^2.$$

   The variance of $\hat{\theta}_{\text{MNAR}}$ is then estimated by

$$\hat{\sigma}_{\text{MNAR}}^2 = \hat{\sigma}_W^2 + \hat{\sigma}_B^2.$$

While this algorithm has been presented with the underlying two variable example in mind (where the outcome variable in the substantive model is partially observed and the covariate fully observed), the algorithm can be applied when the outcome is fully observed and the missing values to which the sensitivity analysis are applied are in the covariate.

Note that criteria (I1) and (I2) above still need to hold for this approach to work, but they are now applied at the individual, rather than the imputation, level. This turns out to be a key advantage, because the estimates $\hat{\theta}_{\text{MNAR}}$ can now lie outside the range of the K MAR imputation parameter estimates. However, it is good practice to check that the weights for a small number of individuals are not dominating.

Beesley and Taylor (2021) evaluate two alternative approaches to calculating the variance of $\hat{\theta}_{\text{MNAR}}$, using the bootstrap and Louis' formula. In their simulation study, the jack-knife approach performs at least as well as the other methods, is computationally less burdensome than the bootstrap, and avoids the need for the score equations of the substantive model in Louis' formula.

Thus far we have considered only the simple example of two variables, Y_1 and Y_2. However, as Beesley and Taylor (2021) point out, we can use the same approach if Y_2 now represents a set of variables, some of which may be missing (and imputed), but which can all be assumed to be MAR. We are simply assuming that only Y_1 is MNAR, or – more likely in practice – that we are principally concerned with exploring the sensitivity of inference for θ to Y_1 being MNAR. They further discuss alternative selection models to (10.25), but once we move away from the logistic link, functions of the observed values no longer cancel out of the weights.

Lastly, we note that while the approach can be applied to longitudinal data, we then generally have more than one sensitivity parameter. For example, let $Y_{i,1}, Y_{i,2}, Y_{i,3}$ be three longitudinal measurements on subject i. Let $R_i = 1$ if $Y_{i,3}$ is observed. A general model for this is

$$\text{logit}\{\Pr(R_i = 1 | Y_{i,1}, Y_{i,2}, Y_{i,3})\} = \alpha_0 + \alpha_1 Y_{i,1} + \alpha_2 Y_{i,2} + \alpha_3 Y_{i,3}.$$

If some subjects have $Y_{i,2}$, and/or $Y_{i,3}$ missing, then we need to specify both sensitivity parameters α_2, α_3, since no parameter in the selection model involving missing data cancels out when we normalise the weights. One possible approach to this would be to specify say α_3, and use an EM type approach to estimate other parameters; however, given that typically there is relatively little information on these in the data, both a large number of imputations and a large number of observations are likely to be needed.

Example 10.6 Simulation study: sample mean

We now extend the simulation study of Carpenter *et al.* (2007) to include the approach proposed by Beesley and Taylor (2021). Draw 100 pairs of observations $(Y_{1,1}, Y_{1,2}), \ldots, (Y_{100,1}, Y_{100,2})$ from

$$N\left\{\begin{pmatrix}0\\0\end{pmatrix}, \begin{pmatrix}1 & 0.5\\0.5 & 1\end{pmatrix}\right\},$$

and for each pair calculate

$$p = \frac{e^{Y_1+Y_2}}{1 + e^{Y_1+Y_2}}, \tag{10.31}$$

draw u from a uniform distribution on [0,1], and set Y_2 missing if $u > p$. This is equivalent to selecting observations using

$$\text{logit } \Pr(\text{observe } Y_{i,2} | Y_{i,1}, Y_{i,2}) = \alpha_0 + \alpha_1 Y_{i,1} + \alpha_2 Y_{i,2},$$

with $\alpha_0 = 0$, $\alpha_1 = \alpha_2 = 1$. We then estimate $E(Y_2)$ (true value 0) using:

1. the average of the observed Y_2's, which assumes observations are missing completely at random;
2. K multiply imputed data sets, generated assuming observations are missing at random;
3. by re-weighting the imputations drawn in 2, using (10.24), and
4. using Beesley & Taylor's proposal.

In 3 & 4 we re-weight using the true value of $\alpha_2 = 1$, as we wish to see how close the estimated mean is to the true value of zero.

We performed 1000 such simulations, with various values of K, and averaged the resulting estimates of $E(Y_2)$. Table 10.8 summarises the results. The first row gives the average of the 1000 estimates of $E(Y_2)$ from the observed part of each simulated dataset (i.e. the complete records). As this does not depend on the number of imputations, this is only shown in the second column. As the selection model (10.31) means we tend to observe larger values of Y_2, this estimate is biased upwards from the true value of 0.

Multiple imputation under MAR reduces the MCAR estimate by about 34%; although the precise estimates of $E(Y_2)$ vary slightly with different choices of K, this is beyond the precision shown. As the underlying MAR model is wrong, no matter how large K the estimate will never converge to 0.

Re-weighting the MI estimates obtained under MAR is a simple calculation, hence, fast computationally. It removes substantially more of the bias than MI under MAR. As the number of imputations increases, steadily more of the bias is removed. This makes sense and is a direct consequence of the fact that the approximation in (10.17) improves as the number of imputations increases.

Table 10.8 Results of simulation study. Estimated standard errors of the estimates over 1000 replications are all around 0.005.

	No. imputations, M:				
	5	10	50	100	1000
Method 1: average observed data (assumes MCAR)	0.5				
Method 2: MI under MAR	0.33	0.33	0.33	0.33	0.33
Method 3: re-weighting MAR imputations (Carpenter)	0.20	0.16	0.1	0.06	−0.01
Method 4: re-weighting MAR imputed values (Beesley)	0.07	0.04	−0.03	−0.03	−0.03

The results show that Beesley's proposal converges to zero quite rapidly, although it tends to slightly underestimate the true value of zero. It is possible that, as discussed on p. 282 this over-shoot is because the MAR imputation distribution has heavier tails than the true distribution. The original proposal of Carpenter *et al* converges more slowly, but is at increased risk of markedly overshooting if the number of imputations is increased (c.f. discussion in Hayati Rezvan *et al.*, 2015).

Clearly, $K = 1000$ imputations is more than would be used in many applications. However, the results suggest that even with, as here, typically 50% of the observations missing, useful results can be obtained with Beesley's method with $K = 10$. □

Example 10.7 Simulation study *(ctd)*

To complete the picture, we summarise some further simulation results from Beesley and Taylor (2021). Let $n = 100$, draw $X_i \overset{i.i.d.}{\sim} N(0,1)$ and $Y_i \overset{i.i.d.}{\sim}$ Bernoulli$(\exp(\beta X_i)/(1 + \exp(\beta X_i)))$, with $\beta = 0.5$. We make about 50% of the Y values missing under the model $\text{logit}(Y_i\text{observed}|X_i, Y_i) = \alpha Y_i + X_i$, with $\alpha = 0.5$.

We evaluate the bias in estimates of β using complete records, and methods (3) and (4) from the previous simulation study. The results are shown in Figure 10.4.

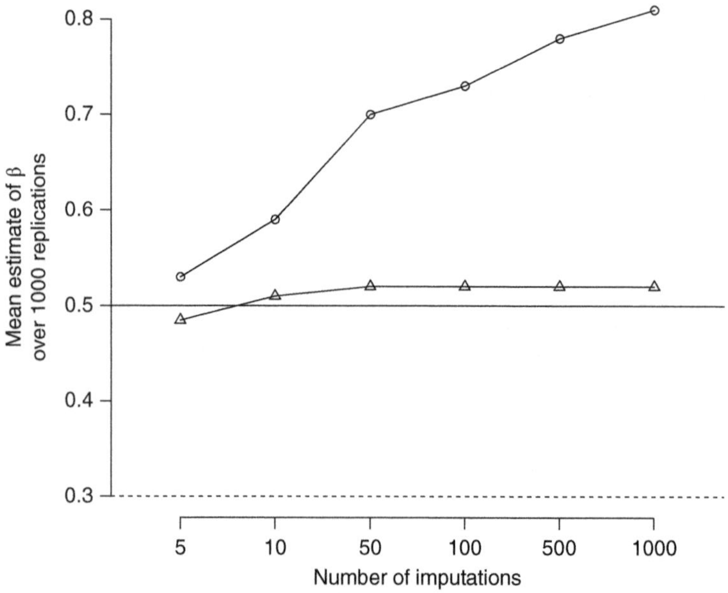

Figure 10.4 Simulation results for sensitivity analysis by re-weighting in logistic regression (details in the text). Key: — true MNAR value; – – estimate assuming MAR; –△– re-weighting individual imputed values; -o- re-weighting imputed parameter estimates. Source: Adapted from Beesley and Taylor (2021).

Here we see how the original proposal can lead to unsatisfactory over-correction, while re-weighting the imputed values, as proposed by Beesley and Taylor (2021), performs well. □

Example 10.8 Peer review trial *(ctd)*

We now perform a second sensitivity analyses for these data by imputing under MAR and re-weighting to explore sensitivity to MNAR. Specifically, we investigate the sensitivity of the results to the possibility that the RQI from paper 2, Y_i, is MNAR. Let $R_i = 1$ if the Y_i is observed and 0 otherwise. We use the following selection model

$$\text{logit } \Pr\{(R_i = 1|X_{i,1}, X_{i,2}, Y_i)\} = \alpha_0 + \alpha_1 X_{i,1} + \alpha_2 X_{i,2} + \alpha_3 Y_i, \tag{10.32}$$

where $X_{i,1}$ is the review of the baseline paper and $X_{i,2}$ is an indicator for the self-training group. If $\alpha_3 = 0$, then Y is MAR. As α_3 increases from 0 the probability of Y being observed increases with Y (i.e. increases with the review quality). If $\alpha_3 = 0$, we can fit this model using logistic regression. This gives the results shown in the left column of Table 10.9. Overall, the probability of withdrawing decreases as baseline review quality increases and is much higher in the self-training arm.

The estimate $\hat{\alpha}_1 = 0.21$ suggests that each point rise in the baseline average RQI increases the odds of response by 1.23. In light of this we carry out sensitivity analyses with $\alpha_3 = 0.3$ and $\alpha_3 = 0.5$ in (10.32). These correspond, on the odds-scale, to roughly 10% and 35% stronger adjusted association between the chance of seeing the second review and its quality.

We obtain estimates of the effect of the self-training intervention versus control using `winBUGS` by fitting models (10.8) and (10.32) jointly. We also obtain estimates and standard errors by re-weighting the imputed values obtained under MAR using Beesley & Taylor's proposal (10.29). We do this using $K = 50, 150, 250$, and 1000 imputations. The results presented below are based on analyses including the face-to-face training group, with corresponding indicator variables added to (10.8), (10.32).

Table 10.10 shows the results. As expected, the estimated effect of the self-training intervention is reduced, but it remains significant at the 5% level. The `winBUGS` estimates (point estimates and standard errors) agree well with the estimates obtained by re-weighting using Beesley and Taylor's proposal, and good results are obtained with $K = 50$ imputations.

Table 10.9 Parameter estimates (log odds ratios) for logistic regression for probability of paper 2 being reviewed, model (10.32), with $\alpha_3 = 0$.

	Parameter		
	α_0	α_1	α_2
Estimate	2.14	0.21	−1.75
Std.Err.	(0.64)	(0.22)	(0.35)

Table 10.10 Peer review trial: estimated effects of the self-training intervention versus the control, obtained from `winBUGS` analysis and re-weighting K imputed values using Beesley and Taylor (2021)'s proposal. All models adjusted for baseline review quality index. Uncertainty in parameter estimates from `winBUGS` due to Monte Carlo estimation is less than ± 0.001.

Method	Estimated effect of self-training intervention versus control	Standard error
Missing at random		
Regression	0.236	0.070
Multiple imputation, $M = 1000$	0.237	0.070
Regression using `winBUGS`	0.236	0.070
Missing not at random, $\alpha_3 = 0.3$		
`winBUGS`	0.215	0.071
Weighting, $K = 50$	0.212	0.071
Weighting, $K = 150$	0.206	0.072
Weighting, $K = 250$	0.205	0.071
Weighting, $K = 1000$	0.207	0.070
Missing not at random, $\alpha_3 = 0.5$		
`winBUGS`	0.202	0.071
Weighting, $K = 50$	0.193	0.071
Weighting, $K = 150$	0.187	0.072
Weighting, $K = 250$	0.186	0.071
Weighting, $K = 1000$	0.189	0.071

In conclusion, this analysis, by re-weighting after MAR imputation, confirms the results for the self-training arm are sensitive to poorer reviewers not returning the second paper and hence withdrawing. Specifically, if the adjusted log odds of returning the second paper increases by 0.5 (OR 1.65) for every point increase in the RQI, the confidence interval for the self-training intervention comes close to the null value. Analysis using `winBUGS` and weighting give similar conclusions. However, the latter is far quicker, even taking into account the time taken to draw the MAR imputations, and requires relatively little specialist programming. In comparing the results of this analysis with those presented in Table 10.2, the principle difference is in the standard errors. The reason for this is that in the selection modelling we have fixed the sensitivity parameter α_3 at certain values, where as in the pattern mixture modelling, the corresponding sensitivity parameter, δ, had a prior distribution. □

In applications, it is important to check whether all the weights are concentrated on a relatively small number of imputed values (across the stacked dataset); in such cases importance of sampling estimates are less reliable. Usually simply checking the overall range of the weights is sufficient. In the previous example, for $\alpha = 0.5$ and $K = 1000$ they range from 0.0003 to 0.0031.

Further developments

Carpenter *et al.* (2011b) apply this approach to publication bias in meta-analysis, and Héraud-Bousquet *et al.* (2012) apply the method to sensitivity analysis for missing covariates. Promising results were found in both cases; however, if readers wish to apply the method we recommend re-weighting the individual-level imputed values using the improved approach of Beesley and Taylor (2021), rather than the original proposal of Carpenter *et al.* (2007).

10.7 Discussion

In this chapter, we have described a comprehensive approach to sensitivity analysis with inference via multiple imputation. In the first part of the chapter, we considered the pattern-mixture approach; in the latter half the selection approach. In both cases, MI provides a practical computational approach to estimation and inference. In passing, we saw how MNAR inference could proceed by direct likelihood modelling (albeit with numerical integration). There is also an extensive literature on sensitivity analysis using inverse probability weighting (e.g. Scharfstein *et al.*, 1999), but this is not our focus here.

In collaborations, we have found that the pattern-mixture approach is most readily understood by non-statistically trained experts. One reason is that distributions estimated from the complete records, together with imputed values under MAR, can be graphed as a starting point for discussion about MNAR distributions. By contrast, discussions about the selection sensitivity parameter are less natural, as it is the adjusted log-odds ratio relating the chance of observing a variable to its underlying (possibly unseen) value. However, the imputation-based approach has the advantage that it is straightforward after using a pattern mixture approach to explore the selection implications, and vice versa. For example, having created imputed datasets using the pattern mixture approach under MNAR, we can fit selection models to the imputed data, combine the results using Rubin's rules, and check with experts they are contextually plausible. Going in the reverse direction, Carpenter *et al.* (2011b) illustrate calculating weighted averages of the imputed data to graph the difference in mean between the observed and imputed data as selection increases.

A feature of our proposed reference-based pattern mixture approach for longitudinal data is the avoidance of explicit specification of sensitivity parameters by specifying instead patterns of profiles. This seems most natural in the clinical trials setting, where we have data in active and control arms and the appropriate approach to imputation depends on the estimand at hand. As we argued above, in this setting, post-intercurrent event distributions can be accessibly framed with reference to the various imputation arms.

In conclusion, as Rubin stressed in his original book (Rubin, 1987, Ch. 6), the analysis of partially observed data involves untestable assumptions, and MI provides a practical framework for sensitivity analysis. The MAR assumption is a natural starting point, with its implication that conditional distributions of partially observed given fully observed data do not differ by missingness pattern. Moving to

MNAR mechanisms, we have illustrated the flexibility, and hence broad utility, of an imputation-based approach.

Exercises

1. This exercise repeats some of the analyses of the peer review study discussed in this chapter. The variables in Table 10.11 are available in `reviewer_sensitivity.dta`.

Focusing on the control and self-taught arms, use the data to answer the following questions.

(a) Describe the data: How many reviewers are there in each arm? How does the number returning a review of paper 2 vary by baseline and randomised arm? Obtain the results shown in Table 10.1 and satisfy yourself that the data suggest a disproportionate number of poor reviewers in the self-taught group failed to review paper 2.

(b) Use linear regression to obtain an estimate of the intervention effect assuming missing outcome data are MAR. What do you conclude?

(c) Use MI to impute the missing outcome data assuming MAR, using a common imputation model across randomised arms and $K = 50$ imputations. Are the assumptions of this analysis the same as part (b)? How do the results compare?

(d) Use the imputed data from part (c) to carry out a simple pattern mixture sensitivity analysis using the prior given in (10.9) with $\rho = 0$, as follows:

For imputation $k = 1, \ldots, K$:

(i) draw a value, $(\delta_{\text{control}}, \delta_{\text{self}})$ from (10.9);

(ii) add δ_{control} to the imputed values only in the control arm, and

(iii) add δ_{self} to the imputed responses only for the self-taught arm;

Fit the substantive model to each imputed dataset and combine the results using Rubin's rules.

Interpret your results.

Table 10.11 Description of variables in the `reviewer_sensitivity.dta` dataset.

Variable	Description
`id`	Reviewer identifier
`inter`	Intervention group: 0 – no training; 1 – self-taught; 2 – face-to-face
`base`	mean review quality index for paper 1 (baseline)
`resp`	mean review quality index for paper 2 (response)

(e) Repeat (d) with $\rho = 0.3$, $\rho = 0.6$ and $\rho = 1$: what do you conclude?

(f) Now repeat (d) but fixing $\delta_{\text{cont}} = \delta_{\text{self}} = 0.21$ (i.e. setting the variance matrix in (10.9) to zero. What do you conclude

(g) Which of the analyses (e) and (f) is information anchored?

2. Consider a clinical trial with two arms, a binary baseline and outcome, and missing outcome values in both arms. Devise a multiple imputation algorithm for sensitivity analysis using the 'informative missing odds ratio (p. 256, cf Higgins *et al.*, 2006)).

3. Repeat the simulation study described in Example 10.6.

4. Use the algorithm for sensitivity analysis by re-weighting on p. 282 to reproduce the results in Table 10.10, with $K = 50$ imputations and outcomes MNAR with $\alpha = 0.3$, and then $\alpha = 0.5$ Why is this analysis approximately information anchored?

5. This exercise explores reference-based sensitivity analysis for the asthma study data (Section 10.4.1). To do this exercise you will need to use either the `mimix` package in Stata, or the `RefBasedMI` package in `R`, or the SAS 5-macros package. Further details from https://missingdata.lshtm.ac.uk.

The data are available in `asthma_sensitivity.dta`, which contains the following variables: `id`–patient identifier; `time`–time of clinic visit (since randomisation) in weeks; `treat`–randomised treatment arm; `base`–baseline FEV_1 (litres), and `fev`–FEV_1 (litres) recorded at clinic visit.

(a) Use the data to reproduce Table 10.12.

(b) We see that dropout is much higher in the placebo arm (60%) than in the lowest active arm (22%).

What do you think is the likely reason for this? Does the information in Table 10.12 support your reasoning?

(c) We begin with the 'on treatment' estimand, exploring the treatment effect we would obtain under the (hypothetical) assumption that patients continued on treatment after their intercurrent event. The substantive model is the regression of 12-week FEV_1 on baseline and treatment.

To do this, separately in each treatment group, assume MAR and use all the FEV_1 data to impute the missing values at 12 weeks. Create $K = 50$ imputations. Fit the substantive model to each imputed dataset and combine the results using Rubin's rules. What do you conclude about the treatment effect? How do the results compare with a regression of the observed 12-week data on baseline and treatment?

(d) Now consider what the results might look like if, post-intercurrent event, the benefit (or deficit) that patients had obtained during treatment was maintained.

Explore this using the 'Last Mean Carried Forward' assumption. This says that, post-intercurrent event, the mean at each visit for the patient is held

Table 10.12 Summary results for the asthma study: the outcome is FEV_1 (litres) measured at baseline, 2, 4, 8, and 12 weeks after randomisation.

	Mean FEV_1 (litres) measured at week					Number	Percent
Dropout pattern	0	2	4	8	12		
Placebo arm							
1	2.11	2.14	2.07	2.01	2.06	37	40
2	2.31	2.18	1.95	2.13	—	15	16
3	1.96	1.73	1.84	—	—	22	24
4	1.84	1.72	—	—	—	16	17
All patients (mean)	2.11	1.97	1.98	2.04	2.06	90	100
All patients (std.)	0.57	0.67	0.56	0.58	0.55		
Lowest active arm							
1	2.03	2.22	2.23	2.24	2.23	71	78
2	1.93	1.91	2.01	2.14	—	8	9
3	2.28	2.10	2.29	—	—	8	9
4	2.24	1.84	—	—	—	3	3
All patients (mean)	2.03	2.17	2.22	2.23	2.23	90	100
All patients (std.)	0.65	0.75	0.80	0.85	0.81		

at the mean of their treatment group at the time of their intercurrent event. Perform this analysis, again using $K = 50$ imputations, and compare with the results from part (b). Do they seem plausible? Is the treatment policy estimand addressed by the LMCF assumption sensible in this trial?

(e) Jump to reference (placebo)

Now suppose that post-dropout, patients in the active arm switch to the placebo treatment. When imputing their missing values, post-intercurrent event means are therefore those from the placebo treatment.

By contrast, for patients in the placebo arm, post-intercurrent event they are imputed assuming MAR – i.e. that their statistical behaviour is 'like' those who remain in the placebo arm.

In order to do this, you will have to tell the software that treatment group 2 (the placebo) is the 'reference' group.

Perform the analysis and compare the results with those above. Are they in line with your expectations? How plausible is this assumption for these data?

(f) Jump to reference (active)

Last, suppose that in the placebo group, patients who have an intercurrent event switch to the active treatment (or equivalent). Conversely, in the active group, patients who have an intercurrent event continue with a similar treatment.

To assess this, again use the 'Jump to Reference' assumption, but this time making the reference treatment the active. Simply instruct the software to change the 'reference' group from placebo to active.

Carry out the analysis and note your results. Can you explain why they are markedly different from having the placebo group as the 'reference'? Is this assumption plausible for these data?

(g) Summarise your conclusions from your analyses of these data in a form suitable for a medical journal.

6. Use the data `ycs_sensitivity.dta` (recall the description of the variables in this dataset in Example 1.2). Reproduce the sensitivity analysis shown in Table 10.3 with $\delta_I = \delta_W = -2$.

11

Multiple imputation for measurement error and misclassification

In this chapter, we consider the use of multiple imputation (MI) for handling measurement error and misclassification in variables. In Section 11.1, we give an overview of the consequences of measurement error for statistical analyses and outline how tackling them can be viewed as a particular type of missing data problem. In Section 11.2, we consider the case where validation data are available, meaning that the true value of the covariate(s) is available in at least a subset of the dataset. In Section 11.3, we then turn to the replication setting, where we do not observe the true covariate on any individuals, but have replicate error-prone or misclassified measurements available. In Section 11.4, we consider a setup where information about the measurement process is provided via some external information and describe a modified version of Rubin's rules suitable for this setting. We conclude in Section 11.5 with a discussion, considering some particular practical issues which arise when applying MI to handle measurement error and misclassification.

11.1 Introduction

In a given statistical analysis, some of the variables we have available might be error-prone versions of what would be considered the 'true' values of the variables of interest. For example, if we are interested in the effects of blood pressure on some later outcome, we may have a single measurement W of blood pressure from each participant. Blood pressure measurements on a given individual change over time,

Multiple Imputation and its Application, Second Edition.
James R. Carpenter, Jonathan W. Bartlett, Tim P. Morris, Angela M. Wood, Matteo Quartagno and Michael G. Kenward.

both because of technical measurement error and also because the underlying true blood pressure varies over time. In such cases, our interest may lie in the effects of shifts in individual's underlying 'true' blood pressure X, perhaps defined as the average over a baseline period of time. The single blood pressure measurement W is then an error-prone measure of this 'true' blood pressure value.

We suppose that interest lies in fitting a substantive model for an outcome Y with covariates X and Z. If the substantive model is fitted using an error-prone or misclassified version W in place of X, the resulting estimates are typically biased (Carroll *et al.*, 2006). The effects of, and methods for handling, measurement error or misclassification, require some level of modelling assumptions regarding the measurement error or misclassification process. In the case of continuous X, the simplest assumption is that of classical measurement error:

$$W = X + U,$$

where $E(U|X) = 0$. If a regression model for an outcome Y is fitted using W and other variables Z as covariates, the coefficient corresponding to W is generally diluted towards the null relative to the value that would be obtained had the true value X been used (Keogh *et al.* (2020), Section 3.1.2). Moreover, the coefficients of the other covariates Z are also biased whenever they are correlated with X. When X represents an exposure of interest, these results mean that classical measurement error leads to estimates of exposure effect which are smaller than they should be. When X represents a confounder to be adjusted for, estimates of the effects of the exposure(s) will not be fully adjusted for confounding. In the extreme scenario of very large measurement error, it is clear that adjusting for W will hardly adjust for the confounding effects of X at all.

Because of the adverse effects on inferences caused by measurement error and misclassification, a wide range of statistical methods have been developed to adjust for their effects (Grace *et al.*, 2021). These include maximum likelihood-based methods, Bayesian methods, semi-parametric methods, and others such as simulation extrapolation. Whichever approach is used, one has to either (i) make assumptions about certain parameters in the measurement error or misclassification model (e.g. concerning $\text{Var}(U)$ in the classical error model) based on estimates from prior studies, or (ii) use data internal to the study at hand to estimate such parameters. In the latter case, we can distinguish between studies with *validation* data and studies with *replication* data. In the case of a study with validation data, while every individual has W recorded, a subset of individuals additionally has the true value X measured. In the case of continuous X in a study having replication data, every individual has an error-prone measurement $W_1 = X + U_1$ available, and in addition, a subset has a second independent replicate measurement $W_2 = X + U_2$ (assuming classical error).

Measurement error and misclassification can be viewed as a particular type of missing data problem. In a regular missing data problem, a variable is either observed or not for a particular individual or unit. In the case of a variable measured with error or possible misclassification, we have partial information about the variable's true value but do not know its value exactly. Moreover, if only replication data are available, the error-free version of the variable is missing for all individuals. Indeed, measurement error, misclassification, and missing data are all examples of the more general notion of 'coarsened data' (Heitjan and Rubin, 1991), in which the data we observe are some coarsened version of the data we would wish to have measured.

Given the view of measurement error and misclassification as a special kind of missing data problem, in this chapter, we consider how multiple imputation methods can be applied to adjust for measurement error and misclassification in covariates.

11.2 Multiple imputation with validation data

In this section, we consider how MI can be used to impute the missing values of the true variable of interest X when internal validation data are available, meaning that X is observed for some individuals but missing for others, while an error-prone or misclassified version W is available for all. In this setting, the subset of individuals with X observed is almost always selected at random in practice, such that we know that the missing X values are missing completely at random (MCAR) by design. The structure here is then identical to that in a standard missing data problem. Thus, the outstanding task is to ensure that X is imputed from a suitable model. Having created multiple imputations of X, the substantive model can be fitted and estimates pooled using Rubin's rules in the usual way.

In the case of internal validation data being available, the missing values of X can (at least for certain types of substantive model) be imputed using standard MI software, specifying a suitable imputation model for $f(X|W,Y,Z)$. Following our earlier developments, what constitutes a suitable imputation model depends on the form of the substantive model and the measurement error or misclassification model assumptions we make.

To impute X, we need to specify a model for $f(X|W,Y,Z)$. The substantive model is a model for $f(Y|X,Z)$, without W, and so W plays the role of an auxiliary variable here. One route to specifying the imputation model is via the factorisation

$$\begin{aligned} f(X|W,Y,Z) &\propto f(Y,W,X,Z) \\ &\propto f(Y|W,X,Z)f(W|X,Z)f(X|Z). \end{aligned} \tag{11.1}$$

This factorisation is natural because it is composed of an extended (due to the inclusion of W as a covariate) outcome model $f(Y|W,X,Z)$, a measurement error model $f(W|X,Z)$, and a true covariate model $f(X|Z)$. Note that no model is needed for the error-free covariate(s) Z. Suppose for $f(Y|W,X,Z)$ we assume that

$$Y = \alpha_0 + \alpha_X X + \alpha_Z Z + \alpha_W W + \epsilon_Y \tag{11.2}$$

with $\epsilon_Y \sim N(0,\sigma_Y^2)$, independent of X, Z, and W.

Often, we are willing to make the so-called *non-differential* error assumption. One way of expressing this assumption is that $Y \perp\!\!\!\perp W|X,Z$. This assumption is often plausible if the measurement error or misclassification errors are simply random noise, unrelated to the outcome. The non-differential error assumption implies $\alpha_W = 0$, whereas including the $\alpha_W W$ term allows for the possibility of *differential error*. Note however that even in this case, we still assume that our substantive model of interest for Y only contains X and Z as covariates.

We now consider separately the cases where X is continuous and measured with error by W, then when X is binary and is measured by a misclassified version W.

11.2.1 Measurement error

For the measurement model $f(W|X,Z)$, consider first the case that X is a continuous variable and suppose we assume

$$W = \delta_0 + \delta_X X + \delta_Z Z + \epsilon_W \tag{11.3}$$

with $\epsilon_W \sim N(0, \sigma_W^2)$, independent of X and Z. Unlike the classical error model mentioned earlier, this non-classical measurement model allows for the possibility that the error-prone measurements are biased, and that Z may affect W conditional on X. Lastly, suppose we assume $f(X|Z)$ is given by

$$X = \gamma_0 + \gamma_Z Z + \epsilon_X \tag{11.4}$$

with $\epsilon_X \sim N(0, \sigma_X^2)$, independent of Z. The joint model thus defined implies that (Y, W, X) is tri-variate normal given Z, with each variable's mean a linear function of Z. From the properties of the multivariate normal distribution, the conditional distribution $f(X|W, Y, Z)$ required for imputation of X is also normal with mean a linear function of W, Y, and Z. As such, standard normal regression MI software can be used to impute the missing values of X.

Recall that although the outcome model specified in equation (11.2) allows for the possibility that W is informative for Y conditional on X and Z, we assume that the substantive model of interest does not include W as a covariate. Under the joint model we have described, since (Y, W, X) is tri-variate normal given Z, it follows that $f(Y|X,Z)$ is also normal. As such, imputing X using a normal imputation model given W, Y, and Z is compatible with a linear regression substantive model for Y which has X and Z but not W as covariates.

11.2.2 Misclassification

Now, consider the case where X is binary and W is a misclassified version. In the place of the normal models given by equations (11.3) and (11.4), we might now assume for $P(W = 1|X,Z)$ that

$$P(W = 1|X,Z) = \delta_0 + \delta_X X, \tag{11.5}$$

where we have assumed that Z is not informative for W conditional on X. For $P(X = 1|Z)$, now that X is binary we could, for example choose to assume that

$$\text{logit}P(X = 1|Z) = \gamma_0 + \gamma_Z Z. \tag{11.6}$$

Then following equation (11.1), one can show (Exercise 1) that $P(X = 1|W, Y, Z)$ follows a logistic regression model with main effects of W, Y, and Z. As such, standard MI software can be used to impute X using the latter model, and this is compatible with the linear regression outcome model given in equation (11.2). This logistic regression imputation model is also implied from an alternative joint model specification that assumes that $X|W, Z$ is a logistic regression with main effects of W and Z.

We note that with W and X binary, if $f(Y|W, X, Z)$ is described by the linear model in equation (11.2), $f(Y|X, Z)$ is no longer a normal distribution with constant variance unless $\alpha_W = 0$. Nonetheless, one can show (Exercise 2) using equation (11.5) that $E(Y|X, Z)$ is still linear in X and Z. In this case, we would expect MI to give consistent estimates of the substantive model parameters, but a robust sandwich variance estimator may be needed to give a consistent within-imputation variance estimate.

Example 11.1 Simulation study with validation data

Cole *et al.* (2006) explored the performance of this approach in a simulation study but with the outcome a censored time to event variable. Specifically, they simulated a true binary exposure X with $X \sim$ Bernoulli(0.4). Event times were simulated from a Weibull distribution with shape parameter 2 and with hazard ratio equal to 2.25. Censoring times were simulated from a Weibull distribution with shape 2 and scale exp(−1.85), which resulted in 80% of event times being censored. The error-free exposure X was observed in 15% or 25% of the 600 observations in each simulated dataset, while every individual had a misclassified version W available. The substantive model was a Cox proportional-hazards regression of survival time on X. For MI the imputation model used was

$$\text{logit } \Pr(X = 1) = \beta_0 + \beta_1 W + \beta_2 D + \beta_3 \log(T), \tag{11.7}$$

where T and D denote the event or censoring time variable and D is the event indicator. They compared the following methods to estimate the exposure hazard ratio:

(a) use W, the exposure measure subject to misclassification;

(b) use X, but only the subset of data where X is observed;

(c) use MI as described above;

(d) use regression calibration for the measurement error: the naive estimate from (a) is divided by the coefficient of W estimated from a linear model for X with W as covariate (Spiegelman *et al.*, 2000); and

(e) analyse the 'full' data on X (known, because this was a simulation study and used as the benchmark).

The relationship between W and X is defined by the sensitivity and specificity of W as a surrogate for error-free X. Eight scenarios were considered with sensitivity 0.7, 0.9, specificity 0.7, 0.9, and validation study 15% and 25% of the study size. Across all eight scenarios (a) was badly biased, with poor coverage. Method (e) was unbiased as expected, with greatest power and confidence interval coverage close to 95%. Methods (b)–(d) also had relatively small bias. In six of the eight scenarios considered, regression calibration, (d), was slightly more powerful than (c) and substantially more powerful than (b). In the remaining two (sensitivity = specificity = 0.7, proportion in validation study 15%, 25%) MI, (c), was more powerful than (b) which was more powerful than (d). Confidence interval coverage was close to the nominal 95% level for (b) but fractionally higher for (c) and (d), with a suggestion that it was higher for MI than regression calibration.

The results confirmed that MI is a valid and practical alternative to regression calibration for measurement error, although as White (2006) points out, we might have expected MI to perform better, because unlike regression calibration, it uses the true value when it is available. One possible reason was that as described by Cole *et al.* (2006), their MI approach did not exploit the non-differential error assumption, which in this case was correct. Moreover, we note that the imputation model (11.7) is mis-specified given the way the data were generated. Following Section 7.1.1 and the results of White and Royston (2009), we should include the baseline cumulative hazard function as a covariate rather than $\log(T)$. In the simulations conducted by Cole *et al.* (2006), the Weibull shape parameter was 2, such that $H_0(t) \propto t^2$, indicating that including T^2 as the covariate in the imputation model rather than $\log(T)$ would be preferable. □

11.2.3 Imputing assuming error is non-differential

If one is willing to assume that measurement error or misclassification is non-differential, the assumption ought to be used in the imputation process to increase statistical efficiency. In the joint model defined by equations (11.2), (11.3), and (11.4), the non-differential error assumption, that Y is independent of W conditional on X and Z, is encoded by setting $\alpha_W = 0$ in (11.2). This restriction implies certain constraints between the parameters of $f(X|W, Y, Z)$, but standard MI software cannot utilize this constraint, and thus cannot exploit the efficiency gain from making the non-differential error assumption. The assumption can however be exploited by using substantive model compatible MI software (Section 6.4). To do so, W must be used as a covariate in the model for X but excluded from the model specified for Y. This is, for example possible (Exercise 11.3) using the R or Stata packages `smcfcs` (Bartlett, 2019; Bartlett and Morris, 2015).

In some cases, we may wish to go further and assume that the measurement error is classical, such that $\delta_0 = 0$, $\delta_X = 1$, and $\delta_Z = 0$ in equation (11.3). As before, these additional restrictions imply further constraints between the parameters in the model for $f(X|W, Y, Z)$. At the time of writing neither standard MI software nor substantive model-compatible MI implementations are capable of utilising these in the validation data setting.

11.2.4 Non-linear outcome models

Our developments so far have focused on the case where Y is continuous and is modelled by a normal regression model (equation (11.2)). Following the developments in

Chapter 6, in general a directly specified imputation model for $f(X|W,Y,Z)$ will not be compatible with the desired substantive model for the outcome, but exceptions exist. For example, suppose the outcome Y is binary and that X and Z are jointly normal conditional on Y. Then this implies that Y follows a logistic regression given X and Z (Freedman *et al.*, 2004). If one then assumes that W is conditionally normal given X and Z, as per equation (11.3), and that the measurement error is non-differential, we can once again use a normal regression imputation model for $f(X|W,Y,Z)$.

More generally, given the increasing availability of substantive model-compatible approaches to MI, we would advocate their use in the case of imputation of mismeasured covariates when validation data are available, since these ensure the imputation distribution is substantive model compatible by design, and moreover, can exploit the non-differential error assumption when desired.

A further strength of the substantive model-compatible MI approach (and naturally a full Bayesian analysis; see Section 9.5 of Carroll *et al.* (2006)) in this context is the ease with which it can accommodate more complex relationships between the outcome Y and covariates X and Z, for example including interactions or non-linear effects. In the case of non-linear relationships between the outcome Y and X, classical measurement error generally leads to the association seeming more linear than it ought to be (Keogh *et al.*, 2012). In such settings, substantive model-compatible MI can be used to impute X allowing for the possibility of non-linear effects on the outcome (Gray, 2018).

Example 11.2 Simulation study with validation data revisited

We now revisit the simulation study of Cole *et al.* (2006) to explore the potential benefits of including the censored event time variable based on the results of White and Royston (2009) and the potential gain of imputing using an approach which exploits the non-differential error assumption. In addition to regression calibration and full conditional specification (FCS) using log(T) as a covariate (plus the event indicator D), as performed by Cole *et al.* (2006), we additionally show the results for FCS using T^2 as covariate, using the results of White and Royston (2009) and the fact that the Weibull shape parameter in the simulation study was 2. Lastly, we show the results obtained using SMC-FCS in R, which exploits the non-differential error assumption by including W as a covariate for imputing X but not including W as a covariate in the substantive model.

Table 11.1 shows estimates of the bias and empirical standard error for the different methods, with $K = 40$ imputations used for the MI methods. For bias, we see that for some scenarios regression calibration shows a small bias. In contrast all MI methods are (up to Monte Carlo error) unbiased. Interestingly, using log(T) as a covariate in the imputation model for X, which following the results of White and Royston (2009) ought to be biased, shows little bias. A potential explanation is that since W is such a good predictor of X here, incorporating the outcome variables in the imputation model in exactly the correct form is not critical. In terms of empirical standard error, the MI approaches are uniformly less variable than regression calibration, with a larger advantage when the sensitivity and specificity

Table 11.1 Results of the simulation study with misclassified binary exposure.

Sensitivity, specificity	% in validation substudy	Regression calibration	Multiple imputation using …		
			FCS log(T)	FCS T^2	SMC FCS
		Bias			
0.7, 0.7	15	0.034	−0.001	0.009	0.009
	25	0.023	−0.018	−0.002	−0.002
0.7, 0.9	15	−0.021	−0.003	0.003	0.003
	25	−0.013	−0.011	0.000	0.002
0.9, 0.7	15	0.055	0.002	0.009	0.010
	25	0.036	−0.015	−0.002	0.007
0.9, 0.9	15	0.003	−0.001	0.004	0.005
	25	0.007	−0.005	0.002	0.007
		Empirical SE			
0.7, 0.7	15	0.470	0.193	0.196	0.195
	25	0.469	0.206	0.210	0.210
0.7, 0.9	15	0.282	0.189	0.191	0.190
	25	0.288	0.200	0.204	0.204
0.9, 0.7	15	0.321	0.189	0.191	0.191
	25	0.326	0.201	0.204	0.203
0.9, 0.9	15	0.226	0.188	0.189	0.188
	25	0.235	0.196	0.198	0.197

Bias and empirical standard errors of the estimated log hazard ratio from 2000 repetitions are shown. The true log ratio is $\log(2.25) = 0.811$. Note the Monte Carlo SE of bias can be computed by dividing empirical SE by $\sqrt{2000}$.

are lower. This is likely to be due to the fact, as noted previously, that MI uses X in the model for Y when available, whereas RC does not. Somewhat surprisingly, the SMC-FCS empirical SEs were no smaller than those from FCS, despite the fact SMC-FCS exploits the non-differential error assumption. Again, this could be due to the fact that W is such a good proxy (auxiliary variable) for X. □

11.3 Multiple imputation with replication data

In this section, we consider MI when internal replication data are available. Here X is not directly observed on any individuals. Rather each has an error-prone or misclassified measurement W_1, and a subset has an additional error-prone measurement W_2. Since X is missing for all individuals, unlike in the case of validation data, standard MI software cannot be used to impute X with replication data. Nevertheless, the steps required to impute remain the same – we specify an imputation model, take draws from the posterior distribution of its model parameters, and draw random imputations from the model conditional on these parameter values.

Compared to the models used in the case of validation data (Section 11.2), the only part of the joint model that requires changing is the measurement model. Whereas in the validation case, we specified a model for $f(W|X,Z)$, in the replication case, we specify a model for $f(W_1, W_2|X,Z)$. In the following, we again consider separately the cases of continuous X measured with error by W and binary X whose misclassified version is W.

11.3.1 Measurement error

With X continuous, the simplest model for $f(W_1, W_2|X,Z)$ is that W_1 and W_2 follow a normal classical error model and are conditionally independent given X and Z. That is, $W_1 = X + U_1$ and $W_2 = X + U_2$, with U_1 and U_2 mean zero normals, independent of X and Z and of each other. These assumptions allow σ_U^2 to be estimated despite never observing X, since

$$\begin{aligned}\text{Var}(W_1 - W_2) &= \text{Var}((X + U_1) - (X + U_2))\\ &= \text{Var}(U_1 + U_2)\\ &= 2\sigma_U^2.\end{aligned}$$

For individuals in the subset who had W_2 measured, we must impute from $f(X|W_1, W_2, Y, Z)$; for those without W_2 measured, we must impute from $f(X|W_1, Y, Z)$. Suppose we adopt the normal model for $f(Y|W,X,Z)$ given in equation (11.2), assuming non-differential error so that $\alpha_W = 0$, and that we assume the normal model for $f(X|Z)$ as given in equation (11.4). Then from the properties of the multivariate normal distribution, both $f(X|W_1, W_2, Y, Z)$ and $f(X|W_1, Y, Z)$ are normal linear models. Since X is never observed, we cannot directly fit these models. In fact, the implied conditional model for $f(W_1, W_2|Y,Z)$ is a linear mixed model with W_1 and W_2 as the dependent variables, fixed effects of Y and Z, and a random individual intercept (Bartlett *et al.*, 2009). If this model is fitted using a Bayesian approach, one could obtain the draws from the posterior distribution of the model parameters, and hence, generate multiple imputations from the corresponding conditional normal distributions. This approach can also be used when Y is binary, under the assumption that $f(X|Y,Z)$ is normal.

As in the case of missing covariates considered in Chapter 6, the difficulty of directly specifying imputation models for covariates is that if the substantive model for Y is non-linear or contains non-linear functions of X, ensuring X is imputed from a model compatible with the substantive model requires problem-specific derivations and implementations. Thus, the substantive model-compatible approaches described in Section 6.4 are in principle attractive. Unfortunately, most substantive model compatible imputation implementations thus far do not have functionality for a covariate X which is wholly missing but measured with error by replicates W_1, W_2. One exception is the `smcfcs` package in R (Bartlett, 2019), which can impute X when error-prone replicates are available, under an assumption that these follow the normal classical error model.

Example 11.3 NHANES III analysis with covariate measurement error and missing covariates

Bartlett and Keogh (2018) performed illustrative analyses of data from the Third National Health and Nutrition Examination Survey (NHANES III) survey, in which there was a combination of covariate measurement error and missing data to handle in the analysis. NHANES III was a survey conducted in the United States between 1988 and 1994 in 33,994 individuals aged two months and older. Bartlett and Keogh (2018) considered a model relating known risk factors for cardiovascular disease measured at the original survey to subsequent hazard of death due to cardiovascular disease. They analysed the data from those aged 60 years and above at the time of the original survey and used a Weibull substantive model model for hazard for death due to cardiovascular disease, with age, sex, smoking status, diabetes status, and systolic blood pressure at the time of the survey as covariates. Here we consider instead a Cox proportional hazards model for the cause-specific hazard of death due to cardiovascular disease:

$$h_i(t) = h_0(t)e^{\beta_1 \text{sbp}_i + \beta_2 \text{male}_i + \beta_3 \text{age}_i + \beta_4 \text{smoker}_i + \beta_5 \text{diabetes}_i},$$

where $\beta_1, \dots, \beta_5$ are log hazard ratios, and t is time since the original survey for each individual. For systolic blood pressure, Bartlett and Keogh (2018) assumed the first systolic blood pressure measurement taken at the original survey, sbp_{i1}, to be an error-prone measurement of each individual's underlying true systolic blood pressure sbp_i, subject to normal classical error. An approximate 5% subset of individuals was selected in the survey to participate in a second examination, during which systolic blood pressure was again measured. This second exam took place on average 17.5 days after the first exam. Bartlett and Keogh (2018) assumed this second measurement of systolic blood pressure, sbp_{i2}, to be an independent error-prone measurement of each individual's underlying systolic blood pressure, sbp_i.

Table 11.2 shows the distributions of the baseline variables and, for each, how many values were missing. Due to the large proportions of missingness in the smoker and SBP_1 (sbp_{i1}) variables, a complete records analysis here will be quite inefficient statistically. Based on mortality information up to 2011, of the 6526 individuals, 1472

Table 11.2 Distribution of, and missing values in, baseline variables from illustrative analysis of data from NHANES III.

Variable	Mean (SD) or No. (%)	No. (%) missing
SBP_1^a	142.0 (24.1)	1488 (22.8%)
SBP_2^a	137.4 (21.1)	6125 (93.9%)
Male	3076 (47.1%)	0 (0%)
Age (years)	72.9 (8.4)	0 (0%)
Smoker	981 (28.5%)	3088 (47.3%)
Diabetes	1019 (15.6%)	7 (0.1%)

[a]SBP – systolic blood pressure in mm Hg.

(22.6%) had died due to cardiovascular disease, 931 (14.3%) had died due to cancer, and 2714 (41.6%) had died due to other causes.

Bartlett and Keogh (2018) compared regression calibration with a fully Bayesian approach. One could contemplate using MI to impute the missing covariates, and then performing regression calibration on each imputed dataset. The difficulty with this approach is that there is no software to calculate analytical standard errors for regression calibration estimators, which would be needed for the within-imputation variance calculation. Consequently, for regression calibration they performed it on the complete records and used bootstrapping to obtain confidence intervals.

Keogh and Bartlett (2021) extended the same analysis, using SMC-FCS to generate multiple imputations, accommodating the covariate measurement error in systolic blood pressure and the missingness in covariates. However, both Bartlett and Keogh (2018) and Keogh and Bartlett (2021) handled missing data (either via a full Bayesian or MI approach) assuming a substantive model for the cause-specific hazard for death due to cardiovascular disease, treating failures from other causes as censoring. While doing this is entirely correct for the purposes of fitting models for the cause-specific hazard for death due to cardiovascular disease when covariates are fully observed, it is not generally valid when missing values in covariates are being imputed. Specifically, Bartlett and Taylor (2016) showed that if the covariate(s) being imputed is related to the cause-specific hazards of other causes, to obtain valid inferences, the imputation process must additionally specify models for these other cause-specific hazards and impute compatibly with the set of cause-specific hazard models.

We therefore re-analyse the data here using four methods:

(a) Complete records analysis naïve Cox model, ignoring covariate measurement error; the Cox model was fitted to the complete records, using the error-prone sbp_{i1} in place of the unobserved true systolic blood pressure sbp_i.

(b) Complete records regression calibration; a linear mixed model was fitted to the repeat measures of systolic blood pressure, with the other substantive model covariates as fixed effects and random individual intercepts. The Cox model was then fitted, using the conditional mean of sbp_i from the mixed model in place of the unobserved sbp_i value. Percentile-based bootstrap confidence intervals (10,000 bootstraps).

(c) SMC-FCS survival; imputing missing values in smoker_i and diabetes_i using logistic regression models and sbp_i assuming normal classical error model. Imputation performed compatibly with a Cox model for the cause-specific hazard of death due to cardiovascular disease, treating deaths from other causes as censoring. $K = 100$ imputations generated using `smcfcs` in R, with 100 iterations per imputation.

(d) SMC-FCS competing risks; same as (c), except that imputation was performed compatibly with separate Cox models for each of the three (cardiovascular, cancer, and other causes) cause-specific hazard functions, entering the same covariates into all three models.

Table 11.3 Log hazard ratio estimates and 95% confidence intervals for the NHANES III data.

Covariate	CRA naïve complete	CRA RC	SMC-FCS survival	SMC-FCS competing
SBP[a]	0.088	0.118	0.138	0.126
	(0.016, 0.159)	(0.014, 0.222)	(0.062, 0.214)	(0.053, 0.198)
Male	0.49	0.5	0.47	0.47
	(0.31, 0.68)	(0.32, 0.69)	(0.37, 0.58)	(0.37, 0.57)
Age[b]	0.92	0.91	1.04	1.05
	(0.8, 1.04)	(0.79, 1.03)	(0.97, 1.12)	(0.98, 1.13)
Smoker	0.28	0.28	0.26	0.3
	(0.08, 0.47)	(0.08, 0.47)	(0.09, 0.44)	(0.14, 0.45)
Diabetes	0.52	0.52	0.7	0.7
	(0.3, 0.74)	(0.29, 0.74)	(0.56, 0.83)	(0.57, 0.83)

CRA naïve – complete records analysis ignoring covariate measurement error, CRA RC – complete records regression calibration, SMC-FCS survival – substantive model compatible MI assuming survival outcome, SMC-FCS competing – substantive model compatible MI assuming competing risks outcome.

[a] Systolic blood pressure per 20 mmHg.

[b] Age per 10 years.

Table 11.3 shows the results from the four methods. Going from the naive complete records analysis to the complete records analysis using regression calibration, we see as expected that the log hazard ratio corresponding to systolic blood pressure increases in magnitude, due to the correction for covariate measurement error. These analyses are based on the $n = 2667$ complete records.

The two SMC-FCS analyses are based on all $n = 6526$ individuals, and so as expected, the confidence intervals are narrower than for the two complete records analyses. We also see some material changes in coefficients between the complete records regression calibration analysis and the SMC-FCS results, with the MI based analyses suggesting larger effects of age and diabetes.

Comparing the SMC-FCS survival with SMC-FCS competing risks, we see that the estimates are mostly very close, although the coefficient for true systolic blood pressure is somewhat smaller for SMC-FCS competing risks, whereas the coefficient for smoker is somewhat larger. Some changes are to be expected through accommodating the outcome as competing risks, since additional analyses (results not shown) suggested that smoking (but not systolic blood pressure) is associated with increased cause-specific hazard of death due to cancer, and smoking and increased systolic blood pressure are associated with increased cause-specific hazard of death due to other causes. □

We earlier wrote that the steps involved in an MI algorithm are essentially the same in the case of replication data as with validation data. One aspect in which it is different concerns the use of prior distributions on the parameters in models. In many implementations of MI for missing data, the implementation is based on an assumption of improper flat priors for the model parameters. For example, the MI procedure for a single normally distributed variable subject to missingness is constructed based on an improper uniform prior for the mean parameter. Note that by improper here we mean a function which is not a valid probability density, as opposed to the meaning of proper and improper in the context of Rubin's 'proper imputation'. In general, there is no guarantee that the use of improper priors will lead to proper posteriors. In the present case of covariate measurement error with replication data, use of a default improper prior for the variances in the conditional models may lead to an improper posterior (Gustafson, 2003). Moreover, an MCMC sampler constructed based on such improper priors will run without apparent problems, despite the non-existence of the posterior it purportedly targets (Hobert and Casella, 1996). To ameliorate this, the implementation in `smcfcs` in R follows the suggestion of Gustafson (2003) by using vague proper inverse-gamma priors for the measurement error variance parameter σ_U^2 and the parameter for the conditional variance of X given Z.

We have described an implementation based on the simplest normal classical error model, but extensions in different directions are possible. For example Freedman *et al.* (2008) considered a setup where the measurement W_1 available for all individuals is subject to non-classical error, and in a subset two additional measurements, W_2 and W_3 are obtained, which are subject to classical error.

11.3.2 Misclassification

Now suppose again that X is binary and W_1 and W_2 are misclassified versions of X, with W_2 measured on a subset of individuals. Analogous to the measurement error case, suppose we assume that W_1 and W_2 are conditionally independent given X, and that their misclassification probabilities are the same, i.e. $P(W_1 = 1|X = 1) = P(W_2 = 1|X = 1)$ and $P(W_1 = 0|X = 0) = P(W_2 = 0|X = 0)$. Even under these strong assumptions, the misclassification probabilities cannot be estimated (see Exercise 4).

In the case when X is binary, in many applications, W_1 and W_2 will be obtained using different methods, such that their misclassification mechanisms likely differ. In turn this means that an assumption that the misclassification probabilities for W_1 and W_2 are the same will often not be plausible. Analogous to the continuous case, we might assume that the W_1 and W_2 are conditionally independent given the underlying X, but allow them to have distinct misclassification probability parameters. In the case of a case-control study with binary Y, Hui and Walter (1980) showed that likelihood inference is in fact feasible, allowing W_1 and W_2 to have different misclassification probability parameters. It follows that Bayesian inference (Gustafson, 2003) and hence MI inference is also possible in principle. Thus far however to our knowledge no MI approach for this setting has been explored, which we conjecture is primarily due to the fact that, with X entirely missing, standard MI software cannot be applied.

11.4 External information on the measurement process

Sometimes information about the measurement error or misclassification process is only available from data external to the study at hand. Suppose an external study had previously been conducted, which collected data $D_{\text{ext}} = \{(Y_i, X_i, W_i), i = 1, \dots, n_{\text{ext}}\}$. Suppose further that those analysing the external data D_{ext} have released estimates of the parameters θ in a model for $f(X|W,Y)$, but not the data themselves. In our study, we have data $D_{\text{int}} = \{(Y_i, W_i), i = 1, \dots, n_{\text{int}}\}$, with the error-prone W_i recorded but not the error-free version X_i. If we are willing to assume that the conditional distribution needed for imputation of X can be transported from the external study to ours, how should we perform MI?

A natural approach would be to use the parameter estimates from the external study to generate K draws θ^k, $k = 1, \dots, K$ from the posterior distribution of the parameters θ indexing our model for $f(X|W,Y)$. This could be achieved approximately if we were willing to assume that (on some scale) the posterior is approximately multivariate normal and provided that in addition to the estimates of the parameters, we had access to their estimated variance covariance matrix. For imputation k, we can generate the kth imputed dataset by drawing from $f(X|W, Y, \theta^k)$. We then analyse our imputed datasets and combine estimates and variances using Rubin's rules.

Unfortunately, Reiter (2008) showed that the preceding approach does not lead to valid variance estimates. Specifically, he demonstrated that Rubin's variance estimator is biased upwards, as a result of the fact that the analysis or substantive model is not exploiting records used in the fitting of the imputation model. This can be seen as an example of uncongeniality, where the imputation model assumes that $f(X|W,Y)$ is the same across both studies (subsets), whereas the substantive model fitted only to the internal study data can be cast as part of a larger substantive model which fits two distinct models to the two studies' datasets. Since this is an example where the imputation model can be viewed as making stronger assumptions than the substantive model, the upward bias in Rubin's variance estimator is in line with the results of Xie and Meng (2017) described in Section 2.8.3.

To overcome this, Reiter (2008) proposed a nested two-stage imputation process and an alternative variance estimator which allows for the fact that the records used to fit the imputation model are not being used when fitting the substantive model. In the proposed two-stage imputation process, for each $k = 1, \dots, K_1$, we draw $\theta^{(k)} \sim f(\theta|D_{\text{ext}})$, i.e. a draw from the posterior distribution of θ indexing $f(X|W,Y)$ given the data from the external study. Next, for each $k = 1, \dots, K_1$, we generate K_2 imputations of X in our study data. That is, for each $i = 1, \dots, n_{\text{int}}$, we generate K_2 draws from $f(X|W_i, Y_i, \theta^{(k)})$.

The result is a set of $K_1 K_2$ nested imputations of the internal study data. Let $\hat{\beta}_{k,l}$ denote the estimate of the parameter of interest from the lth imputation generated using $\theta^{(k)}$ and $\hat{V}_{k,l}$ the corresponding variance estimate. Let $\hat{\beta}_k = \frac{1}{K_2} \sum_{l=1}^{K_2} \hat{\beta}_{k,l}$ denote the average of the point estimates across the K_2 imputations generated using $\theta^{(k)}$. The overall point estimate is then $\hat{\beta}_{K_1K_2} = \frac{1}{K_1}\sum_{k=1}^{K_1}\hat{\beta}_k$, i.e. the average of $\hat{\beta}_k$ across the K_1 parameter draws, which is equivalent to the average of all K_1K_2 point estimates. The variance of $\hat{\beta}_{K_1K_2}$ can be estimated by

$$\hat{W} - \hat{B}_{K_2} + (1 + 1/K_1)\hat{B}_{K_1} - \hat{B}_{K_2}/K_2,$$

where

$$\hat{B}_{K_2} = \frac{1}{K_1}\sum_{k=1}^{K_1}\frac{1}{K_2-1}\sum_{l=1}^{K_2}(\hat{\beta}_{k,l} - \hat{\beta}_k)^2,$$

$$\hat{B}_{K_1} = \frac{1}{K_1-1}\sum_{k=1}^{K_1}(\hat{\beta}_k - \hat{\beta}_{K_1K_2})^2,$$

$$\hat{W} = \frac{1}{K_1K_2}\sum_{k=1}^{K_1}\sum_{l=1}^{K_2}\hat{V}_{k,l}.$$

It is possible for this variance estimator to be negative, in which case Reiter (2008) proposes using $(1 + 1/K_1)\hat{B}_{K_1}$ as the variance estimate. We refer the interested reader to Reiter (2008) for a derivation of the variance estimator and details on the degrees of freedom calculation for confidence interval construction and hypothesis tests. A simulation study by Reiter (2008) indicated generally good performance of the proposed approach.

We have introduced this two-stage MI approach as a potentially useful approach when information about the measurement or misclassification process is only available from an external study whose data will not be used in the analysis. However, as noted by Reiter (2008), the above approach is in fact much more general. For example it could be used when we want to impute values for a variable in one dataset in which that variable was never recorded. If we have another dataset which does have the variable(s) of interest, and there exist a common set of variables which both datasets contain, the approach is potentially applicable. Of course, its validity rests critically on the (untestable) assumption that the imputation model fitted to what we have called the external dataset can be transported for use in the internal dataset.

11.5 Discussion

Multiple imputation is a potentially attractive solution to handling covariate measurement error and misclassification, particularly in settings (e.g. Example 11.3) where there is a combination of missing data in the usual sense and additionally measurement error or misclassification. Due to the relationship between MI and likelihood-based methods, if the MI implementation exploits the assumptions the analyst wishes to make (e.g. the non-differential error assumption), an MI analysis is expected to be efficient.

There are however a number of practical issues to be wary of when using MI to handle covariate measurement error or misclassification. One is that the fraction of missing information is inevitably high, particularly in the replication data case, where X is missing for all individuals. This suggests that in general a larger number of imputations (see Section 14.6) will be required to reduce Monte Carlo error to an acceptable level compared to the setting of MI for missing data. A further consequence of the large fraction of missing information is that convergence will typically take more iterations than in the regular missing data setting if the imputation model fitting is based on an MCMC type approach (Bartlett, 2019).

A further potential issue is that the normality assumptions underpinning the justification of Rubin's rules (see Section 2.4) may not hold particularly well in the case of measurement error or misclassification (Bartlett and Keogh, 2018). In particular, estimators adjusting for classical measurement error can often have quite skewed sampling distributions, such that the frequentist properties of normal-based inferences based on Rubin's rules may be poor. This is particularly likely when estimates of the measurement error model are imprecise. In such settings, a fully Bayesian approach may be preferable, since the full posterior distribution of the substantive model parameters can be obtained (or approximated based on samples), and mildly informative priors can be used to stabilise inferences (Bartlett and Keogh, 2018). Moreover, the Bayesian approach may be attractive when only external estimates of error or misclassification parameters are available.

There are naturally a number of important areas within measurement error and misclassification that we have not covered here. One is the possibility of error or misclassification in the outcome variable Y (see Section 5.4 of Shaw *et al.* (2020)). This is often neglected in practice. One reason may be because at least in some settings, error in the outcome does not cause bias in parameter estimates. For example, if the substantive model is a linear regression model and if the outcome Y is subject to independent measurement error, this simply becomes part of the residual error in the model and does not cause bias in parameter estimates. For further coverage of such topics, the interested reader is referred to Carroll *et al.* (2006), Keogh *et al.* (2020), Shaw *et al.* (2020), and Grace *et al.* (2021).

Exercises

1. Suppose that $f(Y|W, X, Z)$ is given by

$$Y = \alpha_0 + \alpha_X X + \alpha_Z Z + \alpha_W W + \epsilon_Y, \tag{11.8}$$

with $\epsilon_Y \sim N(0, \sigma_Y^2)$, independent of X, Z, and W. Suppose that W and X are binary, with

$$P(W = 1|X, Z) = \delta_0 + \delta_X X. \tag{11.9}$$

Lastly, suppose that

$$\text{logit}P(X = 1|Z) = \gamma_0 + \gamma_Z Z.$$

Show that these model assumptions imply that $P(X|W, Y, Z)$ is a logistic regression with main effects of W, Y, and Z.

2. Suppose that X is binary and that W is a misclassified version. Show that if $f(Y|W,X,Z)$ is as given by equation (11.8) and $P(W = 1|X,Z)$ is as given by equation (11.9), then $E(Y|X,Z)$ is a linear function of X and Z.

3. Simulate a dataset with n =10,000, where $X \sim N(0,1)$, $W = X + U$ with $U \sim N(0,1)$, and $Y = X + \epsilon$ with $\epsilon \sim N(0,1)$. Delete a random 90% of the observations of X.

   (a) Fit the linear model for Y with W (naive analysis) and examine the coefficient of W. Is it as you would expect?

   (b) Use multiple imputation with $K = 50$ imputations to impute the missing values of X using a normal linear regression model with W and Y as covariate and compare your estimates to those obtained from the naive analysis.

   (c) Use substantive model-compatible MI (e.g. `smcfcs` in R or Stata) to impute X, specifying that the substantive/outcome model contains X but not W. To get the software to use W in the covariate model for X, you will need to use the `predictorMatrix` argument in R or the `eq` option in Stata. Compare the estimate and standard error you obtain with those obtained from the previous MI analysis.

   (d) Simulate a new dataset using the same setup, except with $n = 200$. Use substantive model compatible MI again to impute X and estimate the fraction of missing information for the coefficient of X in the substantive model for Y. Based on this, what do you conclude regarding how many imputations would be needed to reduce Monte Carlo error to an acceptable amount (see Section 14.6)?

   (e) Using the same dataset simulated in part 3d, re-run `smcfcs` with one imputation and 100 iterations. Plot the saved values of the substantive model coefficients from the 100 iterations to examine how many iterations might be needed to achieve convergence.

4. Show that with binary X and two independent (conditional on X) misclassified versions W_1 and W_2, the misclassification probabilities and $P(X = 1)$ are not identifiable from data on (W_1, W_2) if one assumes that $P(W_1 = 1|X = 1) = P(W_2 = 1| X = 1)$ and $P(W_1 = 0|X = 0) = P(W_2 = 0|X = 0)$. Hint: consider the distribution of $W_1 + W_2$.

5. In this exercise, we will explore the performance of Reiter's modified combination rules when we use external data (Section 11.4) to fit the imputation model but do not use these data when fitting the substantive model.

   (a) Write code which simulates $X \sim N(0,1)$, $W|X \sim N(X, 1)$ and $Y|X \sim N(X, 1)$ for a dataset of a given size.

(b) Use your code to simulate an 'external' dataset of size 100, and a separate 'internal' dataset of size 200, with the latter not including the simulated X values. Both datasets have the same data-generating mechanism defined in part (a).

(c) Write code to fit a normal linear regression model for $X|W, Y$, and apply it to the external dataset.

(d) Add code to simulate $K_1 = 10$ sets of parameter values from the posterior distribution of the linear regression model, following the algorithm given in Section 3.1.

(e) Add code which, for each $k = 1, \ldots, K_1$, generates $K_2 = 5$ imputations of X for the internal dataset, based on the kth posterior draw.

(f) To each of the $K_1 \times K_2$ imputations of the internal data, fit the normal linear model for $Y|X$, and save the estimated coefficient of X and its estimated variance.

(g) Calculate the average of the K_1K_2 estimates and implement Reiter's modified variance estimator as described in Section 11.4.

(h) Wrap all your code into a loop in order to run 1000 simulations, saving the overall point estimate and Reiter's variance estimate from each simulation. Compare the empirical variance of the point estimates to the mean of Reiter's variance estimates.

12

Multiple imputation with weights

Throughout this book, we have been focusing on multiple imputation (MI) in the context of conventional model-based statistical analysis, and we have used the Bayesian paradigm that sits at core of the technique to provide a broad justification for its use. In this chapter, we instead consider settings that are common in survey sampling (the original setting where Rubin proposed MI; Rubin, 1987) in which account must be taken of the sampling scheme, typically through appropriate weighting. Comprehensive references for the use of model-based analyses in this setting are Särndal *et al.* (1992), Särndal *et al.* (2003). The main problem with the justification of MI in the sample survey setting is the absence of methods for the construction of proper imputation schemes. Thus, we cannot, in general, make recourse to the direct Bayesian arguments set out in Chapter 2. Hence, exploration of the behaviour of MI schemes in the sample survey literature is usually based on direct assessment of the behaviour of the statistics involved, and it is much harder to provide very general results. It has been known for a long time (e.g. Fay (1992,1993), Kott (1995)) that a naive application of the MI variance formula in non-trivial survey settings will produce a biased estimator because the sets of multiply imputed datasets do not follow from the actual sampling mechanism. Kim *et al.* (2006) provide an exposition of the problem and derive some quite general results for the special case of estimators that are linear functions of the data. Much of Section 12.2 is based on their development. Then, in Section 12.3, we discuss how to include weights in MI, before introducing a general approach which exploits multi-level MI in Section 12.4. Estimation in domains is discussed in Section 12.5.1, further issues in Section 12.5.2 and we conclude with a discussion in Section 12.6. We begin, though, by considering a special setting where these problems can be avoided.

Multiple Imputation and its Application, Second Edition.
James R. Carpenter, Jonathan W. Bartlett, Tim P. Morris, Angela M. Wood, Matteo Quartagno and Michael G. Kenward.

12.1 Using model-based predictions in strata

Consider a setting in which we are able to link the goal of our analysis, typically involving weights derived from the sampling scheme, directly to the model-based approach used in the rest of this book. The connection is made through model-based *prediction* in a survey setting, see for example Royall (1992), Särndal *et al.* (1992). Suppose that the data are grouped or clustered, and we have a substantive model with parameter vector $\boldsymbol{\beta}_j$ in the jth of N clusters. Our goal is to estimate a weighted combination of some prediction $g(\boldsymbol{\beta}_j)$:

$$\theta = \sum_{j=1}^{N} w_j g(\boldsymbol{\beta}_j), \tag{12.1}$$

for known weights w_j, $j = 1, \ldots, N$. It is important that we allow the substantive model parameters to differ in some way across clusters; otherwise, the weighting is irrelevant as far as bias (and hence consistency) of the estimator is concerned, although it may of course have a bearing on precision. A simple example is estimating a weighted average of the cluster means (of a variable), in which case $g(\boldsymbol{\beta}_j) = \beta_j$ is the mean for the jth cluster:

$$\theta = \sum_{j=1}^{N} w_j \beta_j.$$

If sampling is completely random within clusters, and missing data are missing at random (MAR), then we can apply the conventional MI procedure *separately* within each cluster to produce a set of MI estimators $\widehat{\boldsymbol{\beta}}_{MI,j}$ and corresponding MI variance estimators $\widehat{\mathbf{V}}_{MI,j}$, $j = 1, \ldots, N$. A consistent estimator of θ is then given by

$$\widehat{\theta} = \sum_{j=1}^{N} w_j g(\widehat{\boldsymbol{\beta}}_{MI,j}),$$

and a consistent estimator of the variance of this can obtained from Rubin's variance estimators, $\widehat{\mathbf{V}}_{MI,j}$, in the usual way. This is particularly simple when $g(\boldsymbol{\beta}_j) = \boldsymbol{\beta}_j$, for then

$$\widehat{\theta} = \sum_{j=1}^{N} w_i \widehat{\boldsymbol{\beta}}_{MI,j},$$

with variance estimator

$$\sum_{j=1}^{N} w_i^2 \widehat{\mathbf{V}}_{MI,j}.$$

This gives valid inference because we are using valid MI procedures within each cluster.

Unfortunately, the applicability of this approach is limited. The data structure may be more complex than simple clustering and, even with a single set of clusters, these need to be of sufficient size to support MI within each cluster. There are many situations, for example when the weights are inverse response probabilities, when the weights may be unique to each unit. Clearly, this approach cannot then be applied, unless we form groups defined by suitably similar weights. Although this is ad hoc, it may nevertheless work acceptably.

If we eschew this approach, we might consider instead applying MI to the whole dataset. However, the survey structure will, in general, cause problems for Rubin's MI variance formula. It may also cause some bias in point estimates. This is because MI must now be applied across the whole weighted data, rather than separately within each cluster. Specifically, if the sampling structure of the imputations does not match that of the data, then the Rubin's variance formula will be biased. We explore this next, and consider how this bias can be minimised (and sometimes avoided). This motivates our multi-level imputation approach, which we discuss in Section 12.4.

12.2 Bias in the MI variance estimator

Kim *et al.* (2006) derive quite general conditions for approximate unbiasedness of the MI variance estimator, which we give shortly. They confine their development to linear estimators of the form

$$\hat{\theta}_C = \mathbf{a}_O{}^T\mathbf{Y}_O + \mathbf{a}_M{}^T\mathbf{Y}_M, \tag{12.2}$$

where 'C' indicates the estimate from the complete (or completed by imputation) data, and both of coefficient vectors $\mathbf{a}_O$ ($n_O \times 1$) and $\mathbf{a}_\mathrm{M}$ ($n_M \times 1$) have no missing values. The elements of $\mathbf{a}$ are assumed to contain weights and other relevant quantities from the survey design, as well as covariate values. For example (exercise 1), the estimator of any linear function $\mathbf{c}^T\boldsymbol{\beta}$ of the linear regression parameter $\boldsymbol{\beta}$ can be expressed in this form. Unfortunately, this theory does not cover the case of missing values in both $\mathbf{Y}$ and $\mathbf{a}$, although the insights it gives are helpful for developing strategies that reduce the bias in applying Rubin's MI variance formula.

Recall that, in the scalar setting, the conventional MI variance estimator of $\hat{\theta}_{MI}$ is

$$\widehat{V_{MI}} = \widehat{W} + (1 + 1/K)\widehat{B}$$

for $\widehat{W}$ the average of the within-imputation set variance estimators, and $\widehat{B}$ the between-imputation variance

$$\widehat{B} = \frac{1}{K-1}\sum_{k=1}^{K}(\hat{\theta}_k - \hat{\theta}_{MI})^2.$$

We are interested in the bias in $\widehat{V_{MI}}$ (i.e. the difference between the MI variance estimate and the long-run frequentest variance of $\widehat{\theta}_{MI}$) when survey weights are introduced. Let the estimator (which now includes weights) when there are no missing data be $\widehat{\theta}_C$. The MI estimator can be written as follows:

$$\widehat{\theta}_{MI} = \widehat{\theta}_C + (\widehat{\theta}_{MI,\infty} - \widehat{\theta}_C) + (\widehat{\theta}_{MI} - \widehat{\theta}_{MI,\infty}) \tag{12.3}$$

where $\widehat{\theta}_{MI,\infty}$ is the limiting form of the MI estimator as the number of imputations increases:

$$\widehat{\theta}_{MI,\infty} = \lim_{K\to\infty} \widehat{\theta}_{MI}.$$

Given a set of assumptions that will be satisfied in typical survey settings, Kim *et al.* (2006) show that the three components on the right of (12.3) need to be uncorrelated for Rubin's variance estimator to be approximately unbiased. One implication of this is that

$$\text{Var}(\widehat{\theta}_{MI,\infty}) \simeq \text{Var}(\widehat{\theta}_C) + \text{Var}(\widehat{\theta}_{MI,\infty} - \widehat{\theta}_C) \tag{12.4}$$

which is another way of expressing the self-efficiency requirement of Meng (1994), discussed in Section 2.8.3. Kim *et al.* (2006) also show that this is equivalent to the requirement that the average covariance of $\widehat{\theta}_C$ and the difference $(\widehat{\theta}_k - \widehat{\theta}_C)$ be zero when the expectation is taken over the entire sampling process, for $\widehat{\theta}_k$ the estimator from the kth imputed data set. From (12.4) we can see that, if this holds approximately, then

$$\text{E}(\widehat{B}) \simeq \text{Var}(\widehat{\theta}_{MI,\infty} - \widehat{\theta}_C).$$

For the congenial examples considered in Chapter 2, with completely random sampling, it is easy to see that this will be true exactly, at least when the expectation of the imputed values consists of linear functions of the observed data, that is,

$$\text{E}(\mathbf{Y}^*_{M,k} \mid \mathbf{Y}_O) = \mathbf{H}\mathbf{Y}_O, \tag{12.5}$$

for some fixed $n_M \times n_O$ matrix $\mathbf{H}$.

As a simple example of this, consider the linear regression imputation model whose properties were explored in Section 2.7. We have

$$\widehat{\beta}_{MI} = \widehat{\beta}_O + (\mathbf{X}^T\mathbf{X})^{-1}{\mathbf{X}_M}^T(\mathbf{X}_M\overline{\boldsymbol{b}}_{.} + \overline{\boldsymbol{e}}_{.}),$$

from which

$$\widehat{\beta}_{MI,\infty} = ({\mathbf{X}_O}^T\mathbf{X}_O)^{-1}{\mathbf{X}_O}^T\mathbf{Y}_O$$

and

$$\widehat{\beta}_C = (\mathbf{X}^T\mathbf{X})^{-1}{\mathbf{X}_O}^T\mathbf{Y}_O + (\mathbf{X}^T\mathbf{X})^{-1}{\mathbf{X}_M}^T\mathbf{Y}_\text{M}.$$

The difference of these is

$$\widehat{\beta}_{MI,\infty} - \widehat{\beta}_C = \{({\mathbf{X}_O}^T\mathbf{X}_O)^{-1} - (\mathbf{X}^T\mathbf{X})^{-1}\}{\mathbf{X}_O}^T\mathbf{Y}_O - (\mathbf{X}^T\mathbf{X})^{-1}{\mathbf{X}_M}^T\mathbf{Y}_\text{M}$$

and so

$$\begin{aligned}\mathrm{Var}(\widehat{\beta}_{MI,\infty} - \widehat{\beta}_C) &= \sigma^2\{(\mathbf{X}_O{}^T\mathbf{X}_O)^{-1} - (\mathbf{X}^T\mathbf{X})^{-1}\}\mathbf{X}_O{}^T\mathbf{X}_O \\ &\quad \{(\mathbf{X}_O{}^T\mathbf{X}_O)^{-1} - (\mathbf{X}^T\mathbf{X})^{-1}\} \\ &\quad + \sigma^2(\mathbf{X}^T\mathbf{X})^{-1}\mathbf{X}_M{}^T\mathbf{X}_M(\mathbf{X}^T\mathbf{X})^{-1} \\ &= \sigma^2\{(\mathbf{X}_O{}^T\mathbf{X}_O)^{-1} - (\mathbf{X}^T\mathbf{X})^{-1}\}.\end{aligned}$$

which, as shown in Section 2.7, is equal to $\mathrm{E}(\widehat{\mathbf{B}})$.

However, when survey weights enter the definition of $\widehat{\theta}_C$, the conventional MI variance estimator will typically be biased. Kim *et al.* (2006) show that this bias can be expressed as a function of the covariance between $\hat{\boldsymbol{\theta}}_C$ and $\hat{\boldsymbol{\theta}}_{MI,\infty}$,

$$\mathrm{E}(\widehat{\mathbf{V}}_{MI}) - \mathrm{Var}(\widehat{\boldsymbol{\theta}}_{MI}) \simeq -2\mathrm{E}\{\mathrm{Cov}(\widehat{\boldsymbol{\theta}}_k - \hat{\boldsymbol{\theta}}_C, \hat{\boldsymbol{\theta}}_C)\}.$$

In the particular case in which the observations Y_i are independent with common variance σ^2, this expression takes a particularly simple form:

$$\mathrm{Cov}(\widehat{\boldsymbol{\theta}}_k - \hat{\boldsymbol{\theta}}_C, \hat{\boldsymbol{\theta}}_C) = \sigma^2\mathbf{a}_\mathrm{M}{}^T(\mathbf{H}\mathbf{a}_\mathrm{O} - \mathbf{a}_\mathrm{M}),$$

where $\mathbf{H}$ is defined in (12.5), giving the bias

$$\mathrm{Bias} = \mathrm{E}(\widehat{\mathbf{V}}_{MI}) - \mathrm{Var}(\hat{\boldsymbol{\theta}}_{MI}) = 2\sigma^2\mathbf{a}_M{}^T(\mathbf{a}_M - \mathbf{H}\mathbf{a}_O). \tag{12.6}$$

As an illustration, consider again the situation in which the imputation model is a linear regression, this time with simple inverse probability weighting, with weights the elements of $\mathbf{w}_O$ and $\mathbf{w}_M$ for the observed and missing data, respectively. That is the substantive and imputation models are both based on the same linear regression model

$$\mathbf{Y} \sim N(\mathbf{X}\boldsymbol{\theta}, \sigma^2\mathbf{I}), \tag{12.7}$$

but because of the sampling design, we need to use the weighted least squares estimator

$$\hat{\theta} = (\mathbf{X}^T\mathbf{W}\mathbf{X})^{-1}\mathbf{X}^T\mathbf{W}\mathbf{Y}, \tag{12.8}$$

for $\mathbf{W}$ the diagonal matrix of weights w_i. In the notation we have used earlier, the bias in the MI variance estimator (12.6) for this setup can be written as

$$\mathrm{Bias} = 2\sigma^2\left[\mathbf{w}_M{}^T\mathbf{w}_M - \mathrm{tr}\left\{\mathbf{w}_O{}^T\mathbf{X}_O(\mathbf{X}_O{}^T\mathbf{X}_O)^{-1}\mathbf{X}_M{}^T\mathbf{w}_M\right\}\right]. \tag{12.9}$$

A practically important consequence follows from this expression: if the weights are included in the space spanned by the variables in the regression model, that is, if we can write

$$\mathbf{w}_O = \mathbf{X}_O\mathbf{d} \quad \text{and} \quad \mathbf{w}_M = \mathbf{X}_M\mathbf{d},$$

for some fixed $(1 \times p)$ vector $\mathbf{d}$, then

$$\begin{aligned}\mathrm{Bias} &= 2\sigma^2\left[\mathbf{d}^T\mathbf{X}_M{}^T\mathbf{X}_M\mathbf{d} - \mathrm{tr}\left\{\mathbf{d}^T\mathbf{X}_O{}^T\mathbf{X}_O(\mathbf{X}_O{}^T\mathbf{X}_O)^{-1}\mathbf{X}_M{}^T\mathbf{X}_M\mathbf{d}\right\}\right] \\ &= 2\sigma^2\left[\mathbf{d}^T\mathbf{X}_M{}^T\mathbf{X}_M\mathbf{d} - \mathbf{d}^T\mathbf{X}_M{}^T\mathbf{X}_M\mathbf{d}\right] = 0.\end{aligned} \tag{12.10}$$

This suggests a practical approach for correcting for the bias in Rubin's variance estimator when using weights at least with linear regression: introduce these into the linear predictor. We now consider the implications of this in more detail for the special case of simple weighted estimation schemes.

12.3 MI with weights

Seaman *et al.* (2012a) develop the results of Kim *et al.* (2006) for the general regression setting, and much of this section follows their development. We first consider the conditions for the multiple imputation estimator, $\widehat{\theta}_{MI}$ to be consistent, and then consider the closely related conditions for the multiple imputation estimator of variance, $\widehat{\mathbf{V}}_{MI}$, to be consistent.

12.3.1 Conditions for the consistency of $\widehat{\theta}_{MI}$

We begin by moving from the direct expression of the estimator given in (12.2) to its representation as a solution of set of estimating equations. In this subsection only, we let $\mathbf{Y}_i$ be the multivariate data collected on individual i, which we may think of as comprising the dependent and independent variables in some regression model of interest. We suppose that in the absence of weights (i.e. for a sampling scheme that does not require weights), the required estimator of $\boldsymbol{\theta}$ from the substantive model is the solution of the unbiased estimating equation

$$\sum_{i=1}^{n} \mathbf{U}(\widehat{\theta}; \mathbf{Y}_i) = \mathbf{0}.$$

Then, because of the sampling scheme, we need to include design weights w_i, $i = 1, \dots, n$. In the absence of missing data, we would estimate $\boldsymbol{\theta}$ by solving

$$\sum_{i=1}^{n} w_i \mathbf{U}(\widehat{\theta}; \mathbf{Y}_i) = \mathbf{0}.$$

Now suppose that for units (typically individuals) $i \in \mathcal{M}$ one or more component variables are missing and denote by $\mathbf{Y}^*_{i,k}$ the kth the imputed value for unit i. Seaman *et al.* (2012a) give conditions under which multiple imputation will give consistent parameter estimators under a general pattern of MAR missingness. These are

1. The design weights are correct.
2. Given the variables used to calculate the weights, the probability of an individual i being included in the sample does not depend on their data $\mathbf{Y}_i$.
3. Within the sample observations, $i = 1, \dots, n$, data are missing at random given the weights and observed data.
4. The imputation model includes the weights and is correctly specified.

Then if $\hat{\theta}_k$ is the estimate obtained by using the kth set of imputed data to solve

$$\sum_{i \in \mathcal{O}} w_i \mathbf{U}(\hat{\theta}; \mathbf{Y}_i) + \sum_{i \in \mathcal{M}} w_i \mathbf{U}(\hat{\theta}; \mathbf{Y}^*_{i,k}) = \mathbf{0},$$

we have, as usual, that the MI estimator is

$$\hat{\theta}_{MI} = \frac{1}{K} \sum_{k=1}^{K} \hat{\theta}_k \tag{12.11}$$

and it is consistent for θ when $K = \infty$.

In the context of design weights, condition 2 above will hold if the data have been collected according to the design. Conditions 3 and 4 are sufficient to ensure the imputed data comes from the correct distribution, taking into account the weights and the missingness mechanism.

For condition 4 to hold, the minimum we will have to do is include the weights in our imputation model as an additional variable. However, to correctly specify the imputation the model we may also need to include interactions between the variables making up multivariate $\mathbf{Y}$ and the weights. Since a number of these variables may have missing values, this in turn means we may need to handle interactions between the weights and partially observed variables in our imputation model. Thus, we may need to apply one of the approaches discussed in Chapter 6. In many settings though, including relevant interactions between the weights and the fully observed variables will be sufficient. Including all, or too many, interactions in the imputation model risks losing efficiency or inducing imputation model fitting problems. In Section 12.4, we discuss a random effects approach implemented in `jomo` which shows promise for minimising these issues.

In many settings, we may wish to use estimated weights. For example we may wish to weight for unit non-response and impute for item non-response (the motivation for Seaman *et al.*, 2012a). Provided our weight model is correct, (12.11) is again consistent. Further, if desired we can combine design weights with estimated weights (e.g. estimated unit non-response weights).

While the condition requiring $K = \infty$, i.e. an infinite number of imputations, is required to formally establish consistency, in practice it does not appear that more imputations are needed in this than in other settings.

We conclude by reiterating that the result in this subsection applies whatever the pattern of missingness in the covariates and response comprising the substantive model, and for any probability model or link function that gave rise to the score equations.

12.3.2 Conditions for the consistency of $\hat{\mathbf{V}}_{MI}$

For MI to be of practical use, we also need to be able to use Rubin's variance formula with confidence. Unfortunately, at present this is only formally justified in the special case of a partially observed outcome (dependent) variable in the substantive model, and fully observed covariates. Encouragingly, though simulation results (e.g. Seaman *et al.*, 2012a) show good performance when covariates also have missing values.

To set out the result, we consider a linear regression of partially observed Y_i on p explanatory variables $\mathbf{X}_i$, where we have q auxiliary variables $\mathbf{Z}_i$. As usual we stack the data from the individuals, giving the $(n \times 1)$ vector $\mathbf{Y}$, the $(n \times p)$ matrix $\mathbf{X}$ and the $(n \times q)$ matrix $\mathbf{Z}$. Additionally, let the $(n \times n)$ weight matrix $\mathbf{W}$ have diagonal entry the ith weight w_i and zeros elsewhere.

Suppose that the substantive model and accompanying weighted estimator, follow (12.7) and (12.8). If data were complete, we assume the 'sandwich' variance estimator for the variance of $\hat{\theta}$ would be used:

$$\hat{\mathbf{V}} = (\mathbf{X}^T\mathbf{W}\mathbf{X})^{-1}\{\mathbf{X}^T\mathbf{W}(\mathbf{Y} - \mathbf{X}\hat{\theta})(\mathbf{Y} - \mathbf{X}\hat{\theta})^T\mathbf{W}\mathbf{X}\}(\mathbf{X}^T\mathbf{W}\mathbf{X})^{-1}. \tag{12.12}$$

Now consider the auxiliary variables, $\mathbf{Z}$, and form the extended $[(2p + 2q) \times n]$ covariate matrix $\mathbf{X}_{\text{ext}} = (\mathbf{X}, \mathbf{W}\mathbf{X}, \mathbf{Z}, \mathbf{W}\mathbf{Z})$. Seaman *et al.* (2012a) show that if

1. conditions (1)–(4) from Subsection 12.3.1 hold, and
2. the imputation model for missing Y_i is

$$\mathbf{Y} \sim N(\mathbf{X}_{\text{ext}}\boldsymbol{\beta}, \sigma^2\mathbf{I}), \tag{12.13}$$

   and

3. for each imputed dataset, $\mathbf{Y}_k^*$ we use the weighted estimator

$$\hat{\theta}_k = (\mathbf{X}^T\mathbf{W}\mathbf{X})^{-1}\mathbf{X}^T\mathbf{W}\mathbf{Y}_k^*$$

   and variance estimator

$$\mathbf{V}_k^* = (\mathbf{X}^T\mathbf{W}\mathbf{X})^{-1}\{\mathbf{X}^T\mathbf{W}(\mathbf{Y}_k^* - \mathbf{X}\hat{\theta}_k)(\mathbf{Y}_k^* - \mathbf{X}\hat{\theta}_k)^T\mathbf{W}\mathbf{X}\}(\mathbf{X}^T\mathbf{W}\mathbf{X})^{-1}$$

   then if we apply Rubin's rules in the usual way:

$$\hat{\theta}_{MI} = \frac{1}{K}\sum_{k=1}^{K}\hat{\theta}_k,$$

$$\hat{\mathbf{V}}_{MI} = \frac{1}{K}\sum_{k=1}^{K}\mathbf{V}_k^* + \frac{K+1}{K(K-1)}\sum_{k=1}^{K}(\hat{\theta}_k - \hat{\theta}_{MI})(\hat{\theta}_k - \hat{\theta}_{MI})^T.$$

we have

1. $\hat{\boldsymbol{\theta}}_{MI}$ is consistent for $\boldsymbol{\theta}$ (as in Subsection 12.3.1);
2. $\hat{\mathbf{V}}_{MI}$ is asymptotically unbiased for $\text{Var}(\hat{\boldsymbol{\theta}}_{MI})$ as $n \to \infty$; and
3. at $K = \infty$, $\hat{\mathbf{V}}_{MI}$ is consistent for $\text{Var}(\hat{\boldsymbol{\theta}}_{MI})$.

If we omit $\mathbf{W}\mathbf{Z}, \mathbf{W}\mathbf{Z}$ from (12.13), imputing in the standard way with just the covariates $\mathbf{X}$ and the auxiliary variables $\mathbf{Z}$, then consistency (3) no longer holds and our MI variances will typically be too large.

We note that this result only holds for linear regression, where the response has missing observations. With missing covariates, there will be an asymptotic upward bias in the variance; Seaman *et al.* (2012a) use Theorems 1 and 2 of Robins and Wang (2000) to derive this for their simulation study, and find it is $< 4\%$ for all parameters, and $< 1\%$ for the majority.

Up to now, we have assumed the weights are known. If they are estimated, then strictly we need to replace (12.12) with a sandwich variance estimator that accounts for uncertainty in the weights (Robins *et al.*, 1994); otherwise the variance will be biased upwards.

Seaman *et al.* (2012a) further explore the performance of this approach when the model of interest is logistic, with missing response or missing covariate. In the latter case, there is a small, but practically negligible, upward bias in the variance estimate.

In summary, these results show that we can use multiple imputation for weighted estimators; at a minimum, we need to include the weights in the imputation model. Ideally, we should also include the interactions of weights with all the variables, though in many applications, failure to do this will not incur a substantial penalty in terms of over estimation of the imputation estimate's variance by the MI variance estimator.

12.4 A multi-level approach

We have seen above that, with design weights, estimated weights, or a combination of the two, for Rubin's variance formula to be valid, the weights (and potentially a full interaction with the other variables) must be included in the imputation model. Further, the imputation model must be correctly specified. However, in general, correct specification of the imputation model may also involve including non-linear effects of the weights, or the inverse weights.

In general, then, the consequence is likely to be a complex imputation model. Even if it is not formally over-specified, the resulting imputations are likely to be noisy.

We have already noted that the bias in Rubin's MI variance formula, given by (12.10), vanishes if the weights are included in the space of the variates spanned in the regression model, i.e. if we write $\mathbf{w}_o = \mathbf{X}_o\mathbf{d}$ and $\mathbf{w}_m = \mathbf{X}_m\mathbf{d}$, for some value of $\mathbf{d}$.

Specifically, suppose that we have p covariates for each unit, of which the first is the intercept, and the second the weight. Then if the $p \times 1$ vector $\mathbf{d} = (0, 1, 0, \dots, 0)^T$, this criterion is satisfied. However, while this is sufficient for valid variance estimation using Rubin's rules for a mean, as noted above, it is insufficient when we have covariates (including variables identifying groups, sometimes termed domains) in our data; then we need to include both the covariates and their interactions with the weights.

As an alternative, now suppose that we group the weights, without loss of generality into $g = 1, \dots, G$ groups. We include an additional G dummy variables as the leftmost covariates in $\mathbf{X}$. These index which of the groups unit i's weight belongs to. Also, let $\mathbf{d} = (\overline{w}_1, \overline{w}_2, \dots, \overline{w}_G, 0, \dots, 0)^T$, where $\overline{w}_g$ is the mean weight for group g. Now the criteria for the bias in the variance vanishing (12.10) is approximately satisfied. Further, the approximation will improve if we choose our weight groups so the weight SD within the groups is small. This is often possible to do in applications because the weights are calculated (often by the data provider) from a set of categorical predictors.

While approximately satisfying the criterion for Rubin's variance formula to work, this approach also has the advantage that it does not require the relationship between the weights and the dependent variable to be linear; it is unstructured across the groups. However, in general fitting a large number of fixed parameters is not desirable.

Instead, we propose letting the G weight groups define a second level in the data, and including random intercepts. This still approximately satisfies the criterion, but now we can pool information across weight groups where appropriate.

This is not sufficient in general, though, because ideally (as discussed in Section 12.3) we should allow for an interaction between the weights and the other variables in the imputation model. We can do this by allowing the covariance matrix of the (level-1) variables to vary across the (level-2) weight-strata. This links back to the stratum-specific imputation approached of Section 12.1. The key difference is that – rather than introduce a lot of parameters – we now give the covariance matrix a random distribution across strata.

For example, suppose that the substantive model is a weighted linear regression of $y_{i,j}$ on $x_{1,i,j}, x_{2,i,j}$, where $i = 1, \dots, n_j$ indexes units in strata $j = 1, \dots, J$, with weight w_j.[1] Suppose data are MAR. Let the weight strata define level 2, so that our joint imputation model is

$$\begin{pmatrix} y_{i,j} \\ x_{1,i,j} \\ x_{2,i,j} \end{pmatrix} \sim N\left(\begin{pmatrix} \theta_{0,0,j} + u_{0,j} \\ \theta_{1,0,j} + u_{1,j} \\ \theta_{2,0,j} + u_{2,j} \end{pmatrix}, \mathbf{\Omega}_j\right)$$
$$\begin{pmatrix} u_{0,j} \\ u_{1,j} \\ u_{2,j} \end{pmatrix} \sim N\left(\begin{pmatrix} 0 \\ 0 \\ 0 \end{pmatrix}, \mathbf{\Psi}\right) \tag{12.14}$$
$$\Omega_j \sim W^{-1}(a, A^{-1}),$$

where W^{-1} denotes the inverse Wishart distribution. Notice this includes the random intercepts for each variable, and that the level 1 covariance matrix varies across weight strata j, so allowing the association of y, x_1, x_2 to vary across strata. This model was proposed in different context by Yucel (2011) and developed for individual patient data meta-analysis by Quartagno and Carpenter (2016) and has been introduced in Section 9.3.2.

Compared with including the weights as a linear term in the imputation model, together with their interaction with the other variables, model (12.14) has the advantage that the relationship across the weight strata is not required to be linear; it is driven by the data, and information is pooled across strata as appropriate. Further,

[1] For consistency with standard multi-level modelling notation, the weight groups are here indexed by j rather than g.

while in general it only approximately satisfies the criteria for Rubin's variance formula to hold, in many applications, the difference between the empirical and Rubin's MI variance is small, or negligible, so this may well be satisfactory.

Note that if the weight is common in each group G, then as the number of observations in each strata gets large this approach tends to the natural, and often optimal, approach of imputing separately in each strata. However, if the proportion of missing in some strata is high, the multi-level approach may be able to improve on this.

12.4.1 Evaluation of the multi-level multiple imputation approach for handling survey weights

We now evaluate this approach in a simulation study, comparing it with imputing separately in each strata, ignoring the weights in the imputation, and including them in various ways. Further simulation results (including for logistic regression) are given by Quartagno *et al.* (2020).

Data-generating mechanism

Imagine we aim to collect data on three variables, Y, X_1, and X_2; our total sample size is 400 individuals, but the sampling scheme is stratified in 10 strata, each with 40 individuals and a corresponding known weight. We generate data from the following model:

$$\begin{aligned}
\begin{pmatrix} x_{1,i,j} \\ x_{2,i,j} \end{pmatrix} &\sim N\left(\begin{pmatrix} 0 \\ 0 \end{pmatrix}, \begin{pmatrix} 0.5 & 0.2 \\ 0.2 & 0.5 \end{pmatrix}\right) \\
e_{i,j} &\sim N(0,1) \\
\boldsymbol{\beta}_0 &= (1,2,3,4,5,6,7,8,9,10) \\
\boldsymbol{\beta}_1 &= 0.2\boldsymbol{\beta}_0 \\
\boldsymbol{\beta}_2 &= 0.5\boldsymbol{\beta}_0 \\
y_{i,j} &= \beta_{0,j} + \beta_{1,j}x_{1,i,j} + \beta_{2,j}x_{2,i,j} + e_{i,j},
\end{aligned} \qquad (12.15)$$

where j indexes different weight strata.

After generating data from (12.15), the substantive model is a weighted linear regression:

$$Y_{i,j} = \alpha_0 + \alpha_1 X_{1,i,j} + \alpha_2 X_{2,i,j} + \epsilon_{i,j}, \qquad (12.16)$$

with weights

$$w = \left(\frac{1}{0.1}, \frac{1}{0.2}, \dots, \frac{1}{1}\right) = (10, 5, \dots, 1). \qquad (12.17)$$

The population values of $\boldsymbol{\alpha}$ (estimated numerically) are $(\alpha_0, \alpha_1, \alpha_2) = (3.414, 0.685, 1.707)$.

This relatively extreme choice is chosen to distinguish the behaviour of the various methods; in real applications, weights (and fixed effect parameters $\boldsymbol{\beta}$) would typically be more similar. We fit the substantive model on the full data (FD) and, after introducing missing values, we compare the results of simple complete records (CRs) analysis, i.e. excluding all the units with any item missing, with those of inference after imputing missing data with the following imputation models.

Multiple imputation with no weights (MI-noW)

This, the simplest imputation model, consists of a multivariate normal model for the three partially observed variables and does not use the weights:

$$\begin{pmatrix} y_{i,j} \\ x_{1,i,j} \\ x_{2,i,j} \end{pmatrix} \sim N(\boldsymbol{\theta}, \boldsymbol{\Omega}). \tag{12.18}$$

As this approach ignores the weights, we do not expect it to give good results.

Multiple imputation with weights (MI-W)

The next approach is to use an imputation model where weights are included as additional variables. We do this by including them as an additional covariate in the multivariate normal model, assuming a linear relation between weights and all the three variables:

$$\begin{pmatrix} y_{i,j} \\ x_{1,i,j} \\ x_{2,i,j} \end{pmatrix} \sim N\left(\begin{pmatrix} \theta_{0,0,j} + \theta_{0,1,j} w_j \\ \theta_{1,0,j} + \theta_{1,1,j} w_j \\ \theta_{2,0,j} + \theta_{2,1,j} w_j \end{pmatrix}, \boldsymbol{\Omega}\right). \tag{12.19}$$

By including the weights as a linear term in the imputation model, this approach takes the first step to satisfying the criteria set out in Section 12.2 equation 12.10.

Multiple imputation with weights and interactions (MI-xW)

As explained earlier, we expect better performance from an imputation model which includes not only the weights but also all the interactions between weights and covariates. This can be done easily when missing data are confined to the outcome variable, but not when data are missing in all variables. In this case, we need to rely on the methods for substantive model compatible imputation (see Chapter 6). Here we use the multilevel substantive model compatible approach described in Section 9.1.3. Following this approach, we partition the joint distribution of the three variables between a joint distribution for the covariates and a conditional distribution for the outcome given the covariates:

$$\begin{gathered} \begin{pmatrix} x_{1,i,j} \\ x_{2,i,j} \end{pmatrix} \sim N\left(\begin{pmatrix} \theta_{1,0,j} + \theta_{1,1,j} w_j \\ \theta_{2,0,j} + \theta_{2,1,j} w_j \end{pmatrix}, \boldsymbol{\Omega}\right) \\ y_{i,j} | x_{1,i,j}, x_{2,i,j} = \beta_0 + \beta_1 x_{1,i,j} + \beta_2 x_{2,i,j} + \beta_3 w_j + \beta_4 w_j x_{1,i,j} + \beta_5 w_j x_{2,i,j} + \epsilon_{i,j} \\ \epsilon_{i,j} \sim N(0, \sigma^2). \end{gathered} \tag{12.20}$$

Missing data in Y are imputed from the conditional model given the covariates, while missing data in the covariates are imputed compatibly with the model for Y, by means of a Metropolis–Hastings step within the Gibbs sampler. The model specified for Y in the imputation model is usually the same as the substantive model of interest, but in this case, because the substantive model is a weighted marginal model (12.16), we instead impute compatibly with a simple linear regression model with interactions.

While this approach should give better results than both (12.18) and (12.19), two possible limitations are (i) with an increasing number of covariates, the conditional model for Y becomes extremely complicated, and we might struggle to estimate its parameters, especially with small strata, and (ii) the weights are assumed linearly related to the outcome.

Note that while the simulation study implemented (12.18), (12.19), and (12.20) using joint model imputation, similar results would be obtained with full conditional specification (or substantive model-compatible full conditional specification for (12.20)).

Multiple imputation by stratum (MI-S)

Another possibility is to impute separately in each of the ten weight strata:

$$\begin{pmatrix} y_{i,j} \\ x_{1,i,j} \\ x_{2,i,j} \end{pmatrix} \sim N(\boldsymbol{\theta}_j, \boldsymbol{\Omega}_j), \qquad j = 1, \dots, 10. \tag{12.21}$$

This method is theoretically valid, but with small strata, we may struggle to estimate the parameters of some of the strata-specific imputation models.

Homoscedastic multi-level multiple imputation (MLMI-Hom)

Here we use a multi-level imputation model, with weight strata defining the second level, in order to have the advantage of shrinkage for small strata, without forcing a linear relationship with the weights. The simplest joint multi-level imputation model has a common covariance matrix, $\boldsymbol{\Omega}$ across the ten weight strata:

$$\begin{pmatrix} y_{i,j} \\ x_{1,i,j} \\ x_{2,i,j} \end{pmatrix} \sim N\left(\begin{pmatrix} \theta_{0,0,j} + u_{0,j} \\ \theta_{1,0,j} + u_{1,j} \\ \theta_{2,0,j} + u_{2,j} \end{pmatrix}, \boldsymbol{\Omega} \right)$$

$$\begin{pmatrix} u_{0,j} \\ u_{1,j} \\ u_{2,j} \end{pmatrix} \sim N\left(\begin{pmatrix} 0 \\ 0 \\ 0 \end{pmatrix}, \boldsymbol{\Psi} \right). \tag{12.22}$$

The limitation of this approach is that (because the covariance matrix $\boldsymbol{\Omega}$ is common across the strata) it assumes a common linear relationship between the variables across the strata.

Heteroscedastic multilevel multiple imputation (MLMI-Het)

Our next approach is to use model (12.14); recall this is

$$\begin{pmatrix} y_{i,j} \\ x_{1,i,j} \\ x_{2,i,j} \end{pmatrix} \sim N\left(\begin{pmatrix} \theta_{0,0,j} + u_{0,j} \\ \theta_{1,0,j} + u_{1,j} \\ \theta_{2,0,j} + u_{2,j} \end{pmatrix}, \boldsymbol{\Omega}_j\right)$$

$$\begin{pmatrix} u_{0,j} \\ u_{1,j} \\ u_{2,j} \end{pmatrix} \sim N\left(\begin{pmatrix} 0 \\ 0 \\ 0 \end{pmatrix}, \boldsymbol{\Psi}\right)$$

$$\Omega_j \sim W^{-1}(a, A^{-1}).$$

We assume an inverse-Wishart distribution for the stratum-specific covariance matrices because using this conjugate distribution for the covariance matrix of multivariate normally distributed data simplifies the calculations substantially.

As discussed in Section 12.4, theory suggests this approach should be able to allow a non-linear relationship between weights and the variables, as well approximately satisfying the criteria needed for Rubin's rules to hold.

Substantive model compatible multilevel MI (MLMI-SMC)

Our final approach extends (12.20) by adding level 2 strata defined by the weight groups:

$$\begin{pmatrix} x_{1,i,j} \\ x_{2,i,j} \end{pmatrix} \sim N\left(\begin{pmatrix} \theta_{1,0,j} + u_{1,j} \\ \theta_{2,0,j} + u_{2,j} \end{pmatrix}, \boldsymbol{\Omega}\right)$$

$$\begin{pmatrix} u_{1,j} \\ u_{2,j} \end{pmatrix} \sim N\left(\begin{pmatrix} 0 \\ 0 \end{pmatrix}, \boldsymbol{\Psi}\right)$$

$$y_{i,j} | x_{1,i,j}, x_{2,i,j} = \beta_0 + v_{0,j} + (\beta_1 + v_{1,j})x_{1,i,j} + (\beta_2 + v_{2,j})x_{2,i,j} + \epsilon_{i,j}$$

$$\epsilon_{i,j} \sim N(0, \sigma^2)$$

$$\begin{pmatrix} v_{0,j} \\ v_{1,j} \\ v_{2,j} \end{pmatrix} \sim N\left(\begin{pmatrix} 0 \\ 0 \\ 0 \end{pmatrix}, \boldsymbol{\Psi}_Y\right). \tag{12.23}$$

Examining this imputation model, we see it allows a different linear relationship between $y_{i,j}$ and the $x_{1,i,j}$, $x_{2,i,j}$ across weight strata, but it imposes a common covariance matrix, Ω; given the data generation model (12.15) this is actually a better choice here and may improve the results.

12.4.2 Results

Table 12.1 presents the results of using these approaches when data are missing in all three variables, in proportion to the weights:

$$p_{\text{miss},j} = \frac{2w_j}{\sum_{j=1}^{10} w_s} \tag{12.24}$$

Table 12.1 Simulation results: mean, empirical SE, multiple imputation SE, and coverage level for the three fixed-effect parameters of the substantive weighted regression model, α_0, α_1, and α_2 (see (12.16)).

	α_0				α_1				α_2			
	Mean	Emp. SE	MI SE	Cov.	Mean	Emp. SE	MI SE	Cov.	Mean	Emp. SE	MI SE	Cov.
True value	3.414				0.685				1.707			
Full data	3.428	0.097	0.096	0.946	0.682	0.278	0.276	0.942	1.723	0.292	0.283	0.939
Complete records	5.343	0.177	0.199	0.000	1.077	0.372	0.355	0.775	2.676	0.405	0.372	0.302
MI-noW	5.182	0.133	0.272	0.000	1.204	0.341	0.448	0.846	2.775	0.341	0.432	0.285
MI-W	2.435	0.247	0.316	0.070	1.102	0.580	0.619	0.907	1.899	0.653	0.726	0.961
MI-xW	2.142	0.478	0.509	0.281	0.100	0.763	0.801	0.926	0.771	0.667	0.923	0.939
MI-S	3.476	0.155	0.182	0.974	0.796	0.353	0.422	0.961	1.461	0.420	0.501	0.958
MLMI-Hom	3.567	0.283	0.248	0.859	1.187	0.335	0.355	0.729	2.650	0.397	0.394	0.353
MLMI-Het	3.527	0.175	0.191	0.928	0.781	0.450	0.445	0.924	1.656	0.483	0.482	0.942
MLMI-SMC	3.535	0.157	0.193	0.959	0.717	0.354	0.393	0.958	1.783	0.393	0.432	0.941

Data are generated from (12.15) and missingness (in all three variables) is directly proportional to weights, following (12.24).

with j indexing weight strata. We generated 1000 simulated datasets. Each imputation method used `jomo` with $K = 20$ imputations, a burn-in of 500 updates and 500 further updates between each imputed dataset.

For each method, we report the bias, the square root of the empirical variance of the parameter estimates across the 1000 replications (empirical standard error) and the square root of the average of Rubin's variance estimates across the 1000 replications (MI SE), and the coverage. Ideally, a method should have small bias, similar empirical and imputation standard errors, and hence good coverage.

We see that in this, relatively demanding setting, that the best results are obtained with 'MLMI-Het' or 'MLMI-SMC' – that is (12.14) and (12.22), respectively. Possibly MLMI-Het has closer agreement between the empirical and MI variance, but MLMI-SMC lower bias. These results, together the theory and additional results reported by Quartagno *et al.* (2020), support the use of one of these multi-level approaches in applications.

Quartagno *et al.* (2020) further explore the setting of a logistic substantive model. In this setting, (12.22) performs slightly better than (12.14).

Example 12.1 Millennium Cohort Study

To illustrate this approach, we consider an analysis of the Millennium Cohort Study dataset (Plewis, 2007). This was a multi-disciplinary research project following the lives of around 19,000 children born in the United Kingdom in 2000/2001. We focus on the second wave (children around three years of age), where some items are missing, particularly in the family income and hearing problems variables (around 12% missing).

The substantive model is the weighted regression of the Bracken school readiness score on three explanatory variables: logarithm of family income, whether the child has hearing problems (1 = yes; 0 = no), and the number of siblings. Sampling weights used were described by Plewis (2007).

We analysed the CRs and then we multiply imputed data (i) omitting the weights (MI-noW); (ii) including the weight interactions (MI-xW); separately in each weight stratum (MI-S) and using the multi-level approach (12.14). We used `jomo` with a burn in of 500 updates and imputed $K = 20$ datasets, updating the sampler 500 times between each imputation. As there are only nine distinct weight values, we use these to define the strata for MI-S and the second level for the multi-level imputation method. Table 12.2 summarises the results, in terms of parameter estimates and associated standard errors.

Results after MI are slightly different than with CRs, suggesting the missingness mechanism involves the outcome; looking at the standard error estimates, MI-xW and MI-S, though theoretically correct, lead to slightly larger estimates, because they are less efficient than MLMI-Het. Estimates of standard errors from MLMI-Het are smaller than CR, suggesting that some information has been recovered. However, it is important not to over-interpret this because if the missingness mechanism involved the outcome, CR would be invalid, so that comparing standard error estimates would become unimportant. □

Table 12.2 Analysis of millennium cohort study: parameter estimates and associated standard error estimates for the four fixed-effect parameters of the substantive model.

Coefficient of	Constant		Log (family income)		Hearing problems		No. siblings	
	Mean	SE	Mean	SE	Mean	SE	Mean	SE
CR	−0.683	0.051	0.292	0.013	0.101	0.033	−0.198	0.011
MI-noW	−0.749	0.047	0.313	0.012	0.090	0.030	−0.208	0.009
MI-xW	−0.744	0.049	0.311	0.011	0.089	0.032	−0.208	0.009
MI-S	−0.703	0.083	0.309	0.021	0.074	0.049	−0.206	0.016
MLMI-Het	−0.772	0.046	0.320	0.011	0.090	0.031	−0.206	0.009

Full details in the text.

12.5 Further topics

12.5.1 Estimation in domains

On occasion, analysts are interested in estimating summary statistics, or relationships between variables, in a specific subset or domain of the data. Perhaps this is most common in the analysis of survey data, where, for example economic data are summarised within social and ethnic groups.

In terms of handling missing data by MI, summarising variables within domains not recognised within the imputation model does not result in a biased estimate within those domains, if the imputation model is correctly specified. However, as the discussion in Section 12.2 shows, if the domain indicator and its interaction with the weights is not included in the imputation model, the corresponding MI variance estimate will, generally, be too large.

If the imputer is the analyst, this problem can readily be avoided, for example by using the multi-level approach discussed above. If the imputer and analyst are separate (e.g. when data are imputed for public use), then ideally the imputation model would be published. If it is not published, or if the published imputation model does not include the domain indicator and its interaction with the weights, then the correspondence between this issue and congeniality Meng (1994) (see the discussion in Section 2.8.3) suggests that the MI variance is still usually smaller than the complete records analysis variance, and that the resulting MI confidence intervals (though they may over-cover) and inferences are therefore preferable.

12.5.2 Two-stage analysis

Valid imputation in conjunction with estimated weights unlocks the possibility of a two-stage approach, which was the motivation of Seaman *et al.* (2012a). Under this approach, handling missing data can be broken down into two parts. A natural (but not the only) way to do this is by unit non-response and item non-response. Unit non-response can be handled by weighting, and then item non-response through multiple imputation which takes appropriate account of the weights.

The usefulness of dissecting the problem this way is that weighting and/or imputation models are simplified, and thus more likely to be correctly specified. Nevertheless, using MI in both stages will likely be more efficient, and this will thus be attractive for the final analysis. Exploring robustness by using weighting for the first stage is however an attractive, relatively straightforward, diagnostic. Practically relevant differences between the two point estimates suggest further investigation into the structure of the data, particularly possible interactions, is warranted.

12.5.3 Missing values in the weight model

Another issue that frequently arises, particularly if weights are estimated, is that some variables involved in the derivation are partially observed and the corresponding weights are missing. In this setting, using substantive model compatible multiple imputation offers a potential way forward (albeit one that has not yet been explored in the literature). We simply include weight in the imputation model as an additional covariate, whose missing values can be imputed compatible with the substantive model. Once missing weights have been imputed, each unit will either have an observed, or average imputed, weight. These can then be used to form weight strata so that the multi-level approach described above can be applied. Alternatively, if relatively few weights are missing, it may be preferable to substitute a 'best guess' of the missing weight, using, for example the calibration procedure proposed by Carpenter and Plewis (2011), and then apply the multi-level approach.

12.6 Discussion

In this chapter, we have explored some of the issues raised by design weights, and estimated weights, in the context of MI. In both settings, if our imputation model excludes the weights, but we fit a weighted substantive model to each imputed dataset and apply Rubin's rules for inference, in general our point estimates will not be consistent and our standard errors (usually upwardly) biased.

Kim *et al.* (2006) cite the issues raised by MI and domain estimation – particularly the need to include in the imputation model both the domain indicator and potentially its interactions with the other variables – as sufficient reason to conclude that MI 'is not generally recommended for public use data'. However, in the light of the more recent developments reported in this chapter, we find this conclusion unduly negative.

The extent to which including the weights is a practically relevant issue in any specific analysis is hard to predict. If there is little difference in the CRs analysis when design weights are included/omitted, concerns about specifying the imputation model to appropriately include the design weights are secondary. This will often be the case when the substantive model is a regression model because the covariates and auxiliary variables needed to make the missing at random assumption plausible are often good working surrogates for the variables that define the weights.

In settings where it is important to include the weights in the imputation model, we propose either the 'MI-xW' approach (using substantive model compatible multiple imputation) or, preferably, one of the multi-level approaches 'MLMI-het' or 'MLMI-SMC'.

Exercises

1. For linear regression of a $(n \times 1)$ vector $\mathbf{Y}$ on a $(n \times p)$ covariate matrix $\mathbf{X}$, satisfy yourself that the least squares estimate of the regression parameters, $\hat{\beta} = (\mathbf{X}^T\mathbf{X})^{-1}\mathbf{X}^T\mathbf{Y}$ can be written as

$$\hat{\beta} = \left(\sum_{i=1}^{n} \mathbf{x}_i^T \mathbf{x}_i\right)^{-1} \sum_{i=1}^{n} (\mathbf{x}_i^T y_i),$$

where $\mathbf{x}_i$ is the ith row of $\mathbf{X}$, $i = 1, \dots, n$.
Now suppose we have missing values in $\mathbf{Y}$ only, that we partition $\mathbf{Y}$ into observed and missing parts $\mathbf{Y}_O$ and $\mathbf{Y}_M$.
Show that $\hat{\beta}$, and any linear transformation of $\hat{\beta}$, can be written in the form of (12.2).

2. This exercise uses simulated data with four strata, each of which has a different 'design' weight, and compares complete records analysis with MI excluding weights, stratum-specific MI, MI including the weights, and multilevel MI using `jomo`.
The data are available in `svyweight.dta` and were simulated as follows:

- Let $i = 1, \dots, 40$ index the observations in each stratum, and $j = 1, 2, 3, 4$ index the strata so that there are 160 observations in total.
- Draw $X_{i,j} \overset{i.i.d.}{\sim} N(\mu = 0, \sigma^2 = 2)$.
- Let $\beta_0 = 0$ and $\beta_j = j$. Draw $Y_{i,j} = \beta_0 + \beta_j X_{i,j} + \epsilon_{i,j}$, $\quad \epsilon_{i,j} \overset{i.i.d.}{\sim} N(\mu = 0, \sigma^2 = 1)$.
- Set the sampling weights for the four strata to be $w_{i,1} = 2, w_{i,2} = 1.6, w_{i,3} = 1.3$, and $w_{i,4} = 1$.
- Let the substantive model be the weighted linear regression

$$Y_{ij} = \alpha_0 + \alpha_1 X_{ij} + \epsilon_{i,j}. \tag{12.25}$$

The variables available in `svyweight.dta` are `Y`, `X`, `wt`, `XobsMCAR`, and `XobsMAR`, where the last two are partially observed versions of `X`, with missing values generated as described below.

For regression with survey data, users of `R` should use the `svyglm` command from the `survey` library. Users of Stata should use and the `svy:` prefix (having `svyset` their data).

(a) Calculate the expected values of $(\hat{\alpha}_0, \hat{\alpha}_1)$. Fit the weighted substantive model (12.25) to the 160 simulated observations and check that the 95% confidence intervals include your expected values.

(b) The variable `XobsMCAR` has about 25% of the values of $X_{i,j}$ missing completely at random.

Using `Y`, `XobsMCAR`, and the weights `wt`, perform the following analyses to estimate α_0, α_1 in the substantive model (12.25):

(i) complete records analysis;

(ii) standard multiple imputation (K=20 imputations), ignoring the weights;

(iii) stratum-specific multiple imputation, i.e. (a) imputing separately in each stratum (ignoring the weights), then (b) appending the kth imputed dataset for each stratum to form the kth imputed dataset ($k = 1, \dots, 20$), and (c) fitting the weighted substantive model (12.25) to each imputed dataset and combining the results using Rubin's rules;

(iv) standard MI but now including the weight variable and its interaction with fully observed Y in the imputation model; and

(v) multi-level multiple imputation (using the `jomo` package in `R`). As only X has missing values, it is natural to condition on Y, so the multi-level imputation model is

$$X_{i,j} = \gamma_0 + u_{0,j} + (\gamma_1 + u_{1,j})Y_{i,j} + \epsilon_{i,j},$$

$$\begin{pmatrix} u_{0,j} \\ u_{1,j} \end{pmatrix} \overset{i.i.d.}{\sim} N(\mathbf{0}, \mathbf{\Omega})$$

$$\epsilon_{i,j} \overset{i.i.d.}{\sim} N(0, \sigma_j^2), \quad \sigma_j^2 \overset{i.i.d.}{\sim} \sigma^2 / \chi_a^2, \tag{12.26}$$

$i = 1, \dots, 160$; $j = 1, \dots, 4$. Create $K = 20$ imputations and burn in the model for 1000 updates before the first imputation and between subsequent imputations.

(vi) Compare the results of your analyses: what do you conclude?

(c) The variable `XobsMAR` has values that are missing at random, following the mechanism:

$$\Pr(X_{i,j} \text{ is observed}) = 1/(1 + \exp(Y_{i,j})).$$

Repeat (b) using the variable `XobsMAR`, and discuss your results.

3. Multiple imputation for the Youth Cohort Study, including the survey weights. Consider again the Youth Cohort study (see pages 128 and 256). Our previous analyses showed (i) that the missingness mechanism depends on the response and ethnic group so that under MAR, the complete records analysis gives biased estimation of the coefficients for ethnic group, which is corrected by MI and (ii) that this correction is robust to plausible MNAR mechanisms.

We now complete the analysis by including the survey weights, supplied with each cohort of the data, in the imputation model. The data are available in the file `ycs_ch12.dta`. This contains the subset of 61,609 records which are either complete (n =54,872) or have only parental occupational group is missing.

The weights were derived to adjust for student non-response (i.e. missingness at the unit level). Ideally, the variables used to derive these weights would be available and included in the imputation model. However, this is not the case, and neither is there any documentation about how the weights were calculated.

Therefore, we wish to compare a number of analyses:

(a) an unweighted complete records analysis;

(b) a weighted complete records analysis;

(c) standard MI, but including the weight as a covariate; and

(d) multi-level MI, (12.14) with the weights defining level-2 units.

Across the 61,609 records, the weights supplied with the data range between 0.2 and 3.6, with mean 1.0.

Carry out the four analysis above, and discuss the results.

For the multi-level approach, form level-2 strata from students with identical weights, regardless of cohort. This assumes that the weights can be interpreted similarly across cohorts, which seems reasonable (because non-response adjustment is likely to be similar over waves). It gives over 850 weight strata, with a minimum of 10 observations in each. The multi-level imputation model should have the three category variable *parental occupation* as the dependent (Y) variable, and the other variables as covariates, with random intercepts and random level-1 covariance matrices across strata.

4. (hard) By referring to Kim *et al.* (2006), show that for linear estimators of the form (12.2), the three components on the right of (12.3) need to be uncorrelated for Rubin's variance estimator to be approximately unbiased. Use this result to deduce (12.4).

5. (hard) Referring to Kim *et al.* (2006), build on the results of the previous question to show that when survey weights enter the definition of $\hat{\theta}_C$, the bias in Rubin's MI variance estimator is given by (12.9).

13

Multiple imputation for causal inference

In this chapter, we consider ways in which MI can be used to tackle problems in causal inference. As we describe below, the basic problem in causal inference can be viewed as a missing data problem (Westreich *et al.*, 2015; Ding and Li, 2018), so it is not surprising that missing data techniques, and MI in particular, can potentially be useful. We begin in Section 13.1 by considering how MI can be used to estimate the causal effect of a treatment or exposure which is assigned at one point in time, first in the randomised trial setting and then in observational studies. Propensity scores are an increasingly popular approach to estimating causal effects in observational studies. In Section 13.2, we consider how MI should be carried out when a propensity score analysis is to be performed on the imputed datasets. In Section 13.3, we describe how the principal stratification approach can be implemented using MI. When the no unmeasured confounders assumption is in doubt, an approach sometimes adopted for causal effect estimation is based on so-called instrumental variables (IVs) – in Section 13.4, we consider how MI can be used to perform an IV analysis. Having seen throughout the chapter, the close connections between missing data and causal inference, we conclude in Section 13.5 by noting some of the differences between them.

13.1 Multiple imputation for causal inference in point exposure studies

The so-called 'modern' approach to causal inference is often based on the notion of potential outcomes or counterfactuals (Hernán and Robins, 2020). For a given individual, let Y^0 denote the outcome they would experience if they were assigned to

Multiple Imputation and its Application, Second Edition.
James R. Carpenter, Jonathan W. Bartlett, Tim P. Morris, Angela M. Wood, Matteo Quartagno and Michael G. Kenward.

a control treatment (or not exposed to some agent) and Y^1 the outcome they would experience if assigned to receive active treatment (or some exposure). The causal effect of active treatment compared to control at the individual level is then some contrast of these potential outcomes, such as the difference $Y^1 - Y^0$.

Letting Z denote the individual's assigned treatment or exposure, the observed outcome Y is then linked to the potential outcomes *via*

$$Y = (1 - Z)Y^0 + ZY^1,$$

if we make the so-called *counterfactual consistency* assumption (not to be confused with the usual statistical meaning of consistency) that states that $Y = Y^0$ if $Z = 0$ and $Y = Y^1$ if $Z = 1$. This basic causal inference problem can be viewed as a missing data problem since for every individual one of the potential outcomes is observed but the other is missing (Tsiatis, 2006; Westreich *et al.*, 2015). Table 13.1 shows data for this simple setup from a fictitious study. For those who received control treatment ($Z = 0$), Y^0 is observed, but Y^1 is missing, while for those who received active treatment ($Z = 1$), Y^1 is observed, but Y^0 is missing.

Since we never jointly observe Y^0 and Y^1, we should not expect to be able to estimate individual-level causal effects, except if we make strong untestable assumptions, such as that these individual-level effects are the same for all individuals. A less ambitious but more realistic goal is to estimate population level or marginal causal effects.

For example, we might be interested in the average causal effect $E(Y^1) - E(Y^0)$. This measures how the mean outcome in the population changes if we give everyone the active treatment versus giving everyone the control treatment. Since

$$E(Y^1) - E(Y^0) = E(Y^1 - Y^0),$$

the average treatment effect is also the mean of the individual-level effects. This is, however, not true in general. For example, the marginal risk ratio $\frac{E(Y^1)}{E(Y^0)}$ is not the average of individual-level ratio effects Y^1/Y^0. Indeed, the latter is not even well defined for individuals with $Y^0 = 0$.

Table 13.1 Data from a fictitious study with Z indicating treatment, Y observed outcome, Y^0 potential outcome under control treatment, Y^1 potential outcome under active treatment.

Z	Y	Y^0	Y^1
0	3.4	3.4	–
1	4.2	–	4.2
1	6.7	–	6.7
0	2.4	2.4	–
0	7.2	7.2	–

13.1.1 Randomised trials

Consider now a randomised trial in which the outcome Y is fully observed. In this setting, the missing values of Y^0 and Y^1 are known to be missing completely at random by design. In this case, we know that a complete records analysis, which here corresponds to analysing Y^0 in those allocated to control and analysing Y^1 in those allocated to active, is unbiased. Taking a missing data perspective, we could attempt to multiply impute the missing values in Y^0 and Y^1.

Since we never jointly observe Y^0 and Y^1, there is no information in the data about their so-called cross-world dependence. However, we could impute Y^0 from a marginal model for $f(Y^0)$ and similarly for $f(Y^1)$. However, we know from earlier developments that in the absence of auxiliary variables, there is no advantage from a precision perspective of doing so. If we have baseline variables X which are predictive of outcome, these can be viewed as auxiliary variables from an MI perspective – they could be used to reduce the uncertainty about the missing values of Y^0 and Y^1 but are not used in the substantive model, at least not in the simplest analysis that calculates the difference between the mean of Y^1 and the mean of Y^0. There is a rich literature on statistical methods for covariate adjustment in randomised trials, with the objective of increasing precision and statistical power (Morris *et al.*, 2022), but this literature has thus far to the best of our knowledge not viewed the problem from a missing data perspective.

13.1.2 Observational studies

In observational studies, treatment or exposure is not assigned completely at random. To make progress, the standard approach is to measure confounding variables X thought to influence the treatment assignment and also the outcome Y. We then may be willing to assume that treatment is assigned at random conditional on X, which typically would be referred to as an assumption of no unmeasured confounding. One version of this assumption is that

$$Z \perp\!\!\!\perp Y^0|X \text{ and } Z \perp\!\!\!\perp Y^1|X. \tag{13.1}$$

In words this says that among individuals with the same values of the confounders X, treatment assignment is unrelated to the potential outcome Y^0, and also unrelated to the potential outcome Y^1. Viewing Z as the missingness pattern indicator, we can see that assumption (13.1) is equivalent in the missing data perspective to Y^0 being missing at random (MAR) given X, and Y^1 being MAR given X (Tsiatis, 2006; Westreich *et al.*, 2015). As such, we can contemplate using MI to provide valid inferences.

Westreich *et al.* (2015) proposed using MI for causal inference in this setting. Specifically, they proposed that the missing values in Y^0 be multiply imputed from an appropriate imputation model for $f(Y^0|X)$ and similarly the missing values in Y^1 be imputed from an appropriate imputation model for $f(Y^1|X)$. For analysing the resulting imputed datasets, they suggested a marginal analysis which estimates, for example the marginal mean of Y^0 and the marginal mean of Y^1, and then contrasts these, for example by their difference. For variance estimation, they suggested that Rubin's rules cannot be used because each individual contributes to both the treated (exposed) and untreated (unexposed) calculations, and instead proposed that bootstrapping be used. In fact, it may well be reasonable to use Rubin's variance estimator (Exercise 1). To see this, note that marginal to X, Y^0, and Y^1 will be correlated in the imputed datasets due to the fact that each has been imputed using X. This leads to dependence between the means $\overline{Y^0}$ and $\overline{Y^1}$ within each imputation. Provided however the variance of $\overline{Y^1} - \overline{Y^0}$ can be estimated accounting for their dependence, we would expect Rubin's variance estimator to be unbiased.

The more common approach to estimating marginal effects of treatment (exposure) in observational studies where the outcome (as opposed to the treatment assignment) is modelled is to use the G-formula (sometimes known as G-computation) (Hernán and Robins, 2020; Westreich *et al.*, 2015). The G-formula involves fitting models for the potential outcomes, simulating the potential outcomes for *all* individuals and analysing the resulting fully simulated datasets. Although this approach, where after having fitted the models we discard the observed data, may seem strange, it is important to remember that the simulated datasets are derived from the fitted models, and these are in turn derived from the observed data. Since an MI approach here uses observed potential outcomes at the analysis stage, we might expect inferences from MI to be more precise than from G-formula. In fact, it has been shown that, at least in certain settings, the point estimates from the two approaches are (up to Monte Carlo error) identical (Olarte Parra *et al.*, 2022).

We now demonstrate this equivalence in the point exposure setting where linear outcome models are used. Suppose we have data (Z_i, X_i, Y_i) for $i = 1, \dots, n$. Consider estimation of $E(Y^1)$ using the G-formula approach. This involves first fitting a model for $f(Y|X, Z)$ or alternatively, since we are targeting $E(Y^1)$, it suffices to fit a model $f(Y|X, Z = 1)$. Suppose for simplicity we assume a normal linear regression model for this:

$$Y|X, Z = 1 \sim N(\beta_0 + \beta_1 X, \sigma^2).$$

Let $\hat{\beta}_0$ and $\hat{\beta}_1$ denote the ordinary least squares (and also the maximum likelihood estimate (MLE)) estimates of β_0 and β_1. In general, with time-varying treatment and confounding, implementations of G-formula simulate potential outcomes sequentially over time. In the present simpler point exposure/treatment setting, it is equivalent and more efficient to simply take the predicted mean of the potential outcomes. Thus, the G-formula estimator of $E(Y^1)$ is

$$\frac{1}{n}\sum_{i=1}^{n} \hat{\beta}_0 + \hat{\beta}_1 X_i. \tag{13.2}$$

G-formula is predicting the outcome under treatment for each patient, given their confounder value X_i.

Now consider the MI approach described by Westreich *et al.* (2015). This involves fitting a model for $f(Y^1|X)$, which under counterfactual consistency and the no unmeasured confounding assumption is equal to $f(Y|X, Z = 1)$. Suppose we fit the same normal linear regression model for this as we used in G-formula, and let $\hat{\sigma}^2$ denote the MLE of the residual variance σ^2. Suppose now that we multiply impute Y^1 from the model, using the MLEs of the model parameters, rather than posterior draws as normally we would do in 'proper' MI. We do this because it makes the following argument easier, and at the end, we will consider what would change if we were to use conventional 'proper' MI. Thus, for each individual with missing Y_i^1, i.e. those with $Z_i = 0$, we generate $k = 1, \dots, K$ imputations

$$Y_i^{1(k)} = \hat{\beta}_0 + \hat{\beta}_1 X_i + \epsilon_i^{(k)},$$

where $\epsilon_i^{(k)} \sim N(0, \hat{\sigma}^2)$. In the resulting imputed datasets, we can then calculate the sample mean of Y^1 (consisting of observed and imputed), and average these across the K imputations in Rubin's rules. This is of course equivalent to simply averaging Y^1 across imputed datasets and individuals, so we obtain that our MI point estimator of $E(Y^1)$, which we denote $\hat{\mu}_1^{MI}$, is equal to

$$\hat{\mu}_1^{MI} = \frac{1}{nK} \sum_{k=1}^{K} \sum_{i=1}^{n} Z_i Y_i + (1 - Z_i) Y_i^{1(k)}.$$

We can rewrite $\hat{\mu}_1^{MI}$

$$\begin{aligned}
\hat{\mu}_1^{MI} &= \frac{1}{n} \sum_{i=1}^{n} \left[Z_i Y_i + \frac{1}{K} \sum_{k=1}^{K} (1 - Z_i)(\hat{\beta}_0 + \hat{\beta}_1 X_i + \epsilon_i^{(k)}) \right] \\
&= \frac{1}{n} \sum_{i=1}^{n} \left[Z_i Y_i + (1 - Z_i)(\hat{\beta}_0 + \hat{\beta}_1 X_i) \right] + \frac{1}{nK} \sum_{k=1}^{K} \sum_{i=1}^{n} (1 - Z_i) \epsilon_i^{(k)}.
\end{aligned}$$

As the number of imputations K gets larger, the final term in the preceding expression goes to zero. Thus, for large K, we have that

$$\hat{\mu}_1^{MI} \approx \frac{1}{n} \sum_{i=1}^{n} Z_i Y_i + (1 - Z_i)(\hat{\beta}_0 + \hat{\beta}_1 X_i). \tag{13.3}$$

Comparing the G-formula estimator (equation (13.2)) with the MI estimator (equation (13.3)), they do not appear the same, since the G-formula uses predicted outcomes for individuals with $Z = 1$, whereas MI uses the observed outcomes. However, we now exploit the fact that for generalised linear models with canonical link, including the normal linear model, the mean of the predictions in the sample used to fit the model equals the sample mean of the outcomes. As such, we have that

$$\sum_{i=1}^{n} Z_i (\hat{\beta}_0 + \hat{\beta}_1 X_i) = \sum_{i=1}^{n} Z_i Y_i,$$

recalling that we fit the model only to those with $Z = 1$. Consequently, we can rewrite $\hat{\mu}_1^{MI}$ as

$$\begin{aligned}
\hat{\mu}_1^{MI} &\approx \frac{1}{n} \sum_{i=1}^{n} Z_i (\hat{\beta}_0 + \hat{\beta}_1 X_i) + (1 - Z_i) \left(\hat{\beta}_0 + \hat{\beta}_1 X_i \right) \\
&= \frac{1}{n} \sum_{i=1}^{n} \hat{\beta}_0 + \hat{\beta}_1 X_i,
\end{aligned}$$

such that the G-formula and MI estimators are, as $K \to \infty$, identical. Recall that our derivation was based on generating each imputed dataset using the MLEs of the imputation model parameters, whereas in order for Rubin's rules to provide valid inferences, we must impute each dataset using a draw from their posterior distribution given the observed data. However, with a large number of imputations K and large sample sizes n, this difference has negligible impact on the point estimate (von Hippel and Bartlett, 2021). In fact, for the normal model considered here, with large K adding posterior draws has no impact on the point estimate, even for small n, since the posterior draws of β_0 and β_1 are from a (bivariate) normal centred at the MLE (see Section 3.1). Thus for all intents and purposes, we can view the G-formula and MI estimators of $E(Y^1)$ here (and obviously analogously also for $E(Y^0)$) as being equivalent.

The fact that G-formula and MI are essentially equivalent, at least in certain important cases such as the one shown above, suggests the choice of which method to adopt should be driven by other considerations, such as software availability. An attractive feature of the MI route is that, as in the case of measurement error and/or misclassification (Chapter 11), MI can potentially handle both missingness of potential (counterfactual) outcomes and 'regular' missingness in variables intended to be collected.

13.2 Multiple imputation and propensity scores

In the preceding section, we discussed methods which can provide unbiased estimates of treatment or exposure effects in observational studies which are based on modelling how outcomes depend on the treatment and the confounders. An alternative approach to confounder adjustment is based on modelling the treatment assignment process using so-called *propensity scores*. We begin this section by first providing a brief introduction to methods for confounder adjustment based on propensity scores.

13.2.1 Propensity scores for confounder adjustment

To estimate the average causal effect, we need to estimate $E(Y^1)$ and $E(Y^0)$. To estimate $E(Y^1)$, we could naïvely use the sample mean of Y in those assigned to treatment:

$$\frac{\sum_{i=1}^n Z_i Y_i}{\sum_{i=1}^n Z_i} = \frac{\sum_{i=1}^n Z_i Y_i^1}{\sum_{i=1}^n Z_i}.$$

Viewing this as a complete records analysis, with Z playing the role of the observation/missingness indicator, we know from Chapter 1 that it will be unbiased only if $Z \perp\!\!\!\perp Y^1$. Recall that the assumption of no unmeasured confounders (at least the version we use in this chapter) is that

$$Z \perp\!\!\!\perp Y^0 | X \text{ and } Z \perp\!\!\!\perp Y^1 | X.$$

Under this assumption, while $Z \perp\!\!\!\perp Y^1 | X$, it will not generally be the case that $Z \perp\!\!\!\perp Y^1$, such that the complete records mean of Y^1 will be biased.

Inverse probability of missingness/treatment weighting (IPW) modifies the complete records mean by weighting observations according to the probability that their Y^1 value was observed, or equivalently, the probability that they were treated (Hernán and Robins, 2020). To define the IPW estimator of $E(Y^1)$, we must first define the *propensity score*, which is the probability that an individual receives the treatment (exposure) given their value of the confounders:

$$\pi(X) = P(Z = 1|X).$$

The IPW estimator of $E(Y^1)$ is then given by

$$\frac{\sum_{i=1}^{n} \frac{Z_i Y_i^1}{\pi(X_i)}}{\sum_{i=1}^{n} \frac{Z_i}{\pi(X_i)}} = \frac{\frac{1}{n}\sum_{i=1}^{n} \frac{Z_i Y_i^1}{\pi(X_i)}}{\frac{1}{n}\sum_{i=1}^{n} \frac{Z_i}{\pi(X_i)}}. \tag{13.4}$$

To see why this estimator is consistent for $E(Y^1)$, we note that, by the law of large numbers, the numerator, which is the sample mean of $\frac{ZY^1}{\pi(X)}$, is a consistent estimator of $E\left\{\frac{ZY^1}{\pi(X)}\right\}$ (Tsiatis, 2006). We then have that

$$\begin{aligned}
E\left\{\frac{ZY^1}{\pi(X)}\right\} &= E\left[E\left\{\frac{ZY^1}{\pi(X)}|Y^1, X\right\}\right] \\
&= E\left[\frac{Y^1}{\pi(X)}E\{Z|Y^1, X\}\right], \text{ then using } Z \perp\!\!\!\perp Y^1|X \\
&= E\left[\frac{Y^1}{\pi(X)}P(Z = 1|X)\right], \text{ then using } P(Z = 1|X) = \pi(X) \\
&= E[Y^1],
\end{aligned}$$

where in the third line, we use the no unmeasured confounding assumption expressed in equation (13.1) and in the fourth line, the fact that $P(Z = 1|X) = \pi(X)$. A similar argument shows the denominator of equation (13.4) is consistent for 1, and consequently, the IPW estimator is a consistent estimator of $E(Y^1)$. A similar argument shows that

$$\sum_{i=1}^{n} \frac{(1 - Z_i)Y_i^0}{1 - \pi(X_i)} \bigg/ \sum_{i=1}^{n} \frac{1 - Z_i}{1 - \pi(X_i)}$$

is a consistent estimator of $E(Y^0)$.

In practice in observational studies, we do not know how the confounders X influence treatment assignment. To make progress, we can postulate a parametric model for $P(Z = 1|X) = \pi(X, \psi)$, such as a logistic regression model. We can estimate ψ, for example by maximum likelihood and replace $\pi(X)$ in the foregoing expressions by $\pi(X, \hat{\psi})$. Inferences for the IPW estimators which account for the fact that ψ is estimated can be obtained using sandwich methods (Lunceford and Davidian, 2004). In fact, somewhat surprisingly, it turns out that if one ignores the uncertainty in $\hat{\psi}$ when estimating the variance, one obtains conservative inferences.

An alternative approach for confounder adjustment using propensity scores is to match, not weight, treated to untreated individuals using the propensity score. Typically, this involves finding, for each treated individual, an untreated individual with equal or close value of the propensity score (Rosenbaum and Rubin, 1983). It can be shown that conditional on the propensity score, treated and untreated individuals have the same distribution of the confounders X. As such, after matching, we can simply compare the outcomes in the treated to the outcomes in the untreated:

$$\frac{1}{\sum_{i=1}^{n} Z_i} \sum_{i:Z_i=1} Y_i - Y_{i(u)},$$

where $i(u)$ denotes the index of the untreated individual matched to the treated individual i. Because we have matched untreated individuals to the treated, the resulting estimator is targeting the so-called average treatment effect in the treated: $E(Y^1 - Y^0|Z = 1)$. An alternative matching estimator can be constructed which targets the average treatment effect $E(Y^1 - Y^0)$ (Abadie and Imbens, 2016).

Lastly, we note that there are yet further alternative approaches for using the propensity score to adjust for confounding, including stratification by the propensity score and regression modelling adjusting for the propensity score as a covariate (Vansteelandt and Daniel, 2014).

13.2.2 Multiple imputation of confounders

In practice some of the confounders in X may be missing for some individuals, and indeed, there could also be missing values in the exposure Z. This complicates the process of fitting the propensity score model. Suppose we wish to use MI to impute the missing values in X. It is not immediately clear however, how this should be done in conjunction with the propensity score modelling.

Qu and Lipkovich (2009) proposed using MI to impute missing values in the confounders X, using an imputation model which conditions on the observed confounders, treatment Z, and outcome Y. Their approach then involved applying the IPW propensity score method within each imputed dataset. That is, within each imputation, they fitted the propensity score model, calculated each individual's propensity score value, and then calculated the IPW estimator. The estimated causal effects were then averaged across imputations. Simulation results suggested this approach gave unbiased estimates under missing completely at random (MCAR) or MAR missingness in the confounders. Qu and Lipkovich (2009) also proposed a modified version where the missingness pattern was added as a covariate in the logistic regression propensity score model fitted to each imputed dataset, motivated by the idea that this modification may reduce bias under missing not at random (MNAR) mechanisms. While simulations suggested that this modification may reduce bias somewhat under MNAR, estimates remained materially biased in general.

Seaman and White (2014) subsequently investigated the two MI approaches proposed by Qu and Lipkovich (2009). They proved that when values in X are MCAR or MAR and the imputation model is correctly specified, the MI approach provides consistent point estimates. Moreover, simulation evidence suggested that Rubin's variance estimator performs well when the sandwich variance estimator described by Lunceford and Davidian (2004) is used for the within-imputation variance. For the approach proposed by Qu and Lipkovich (2009), where the missingness indicator(s) are included in the propensity score model, Seaman and White (2014) showed that it can be biased under MAR if missingness in a confounder depends on the outcome Y. Under MNAR, in accordance with the motivation given by Qu and Lipkovich (2009), including the missingness indicator(s) in the propensity score model can reduce bias relative to not doing so.

Mitra and Reiter (2016) investigated two MI approaches in the context of matching by the propensity score. In both, the missing values in X are first multiply imputed using treatment Z but not the outcome Y, with the latter omitted on the intuitively reasonable basis that the propensity score does not involve the outcome. The propensity score model is then fitted separately to each imputed dataset, and each individual's propensity score is estimated, using their confounder values (some of which will have been imputed). In the 'within' approach, treated and untreated individuals are matched within each imputed dataset, the difference in mean outcomes is estimated within each imputation, and the treatment effect estimates across imputations are averaged. In the 'across' approach, for each individual, their propensity score values are averaged across the imputed datasets, and then the matching estimator is calculated using these averaged propensity score values.

Simulation studies performed by Mitra and Reiter (2016) revealed that both approaches can give biased estimates. Subsequent simulation investigations by Leyrat *et al.* (2019) using IPW by the propensity score suggested these biases were likely due to the omission of the outcome Y in the imputation models. To see why, consider matching by the propensity score as investigated by Mitra and Reiter (2016), and suppose there is just one continuous confounder X. In this case, matching on the propensity score is equivalent to matching on the single confounder X. Suppose that the single confounder X is missing in almost all individuals completely at random, but that our study is very large. Further, suppose we then impute the missing X values using only their treatment variable Z. This means that X in the treated individuals will have the correct distribution, and similarly, it will have the correct distribution for untreated individuals. However, when we then match a treated individual with imputed X value x_1 to an untreated individual with imputed X value close to x_1, in truth their missing X values may be completely different – we have not really matched on the confounder at all. As such, we would not expect matching on the imputed X to have removed the confounding effects of X. While this scenario is extreme and unusual, it demonstrates why imputation of missing confounders omitting the outcome does not lead to valid inferences.

Thus, if we multiply impute missing values in confounders, we must impute conditional on the observed confounders, treatment Z, *and* outcome Y. Leyrat *et al.* (2019) showed that if one does this, within each of the imputed datasets, the no unmeasured confounders assumption (equation (13.1)) holds. That is, if we let $X = (X_{\text{obs}}, X_{\text{miss}})$, and let $X_{\text{miss}}^{(k)}$ denote the kth imputation of X_{miss}, then

$$Z \perp\!\!\!\perp Y^0 | X_{\text{obs}}, X_m^{(k)} \quad \text{and} \quad Z \perp\!\!\!\perp Y^1 | X_{\text{obs}}, X_{\text{miss}}^{(k)}.$$

As a result, IPW by the propensity score after imputation results in consistent estimators of $E(Y^1)$ and $E(Y^0)$.

Leyrat *et al.* (2019) also considered two 'across'-type approaches. One, as proposed by Mitra and Reiter (2016), termed 'MIps' by Leyrat *et al.* (2019), involves estimating the propensity score model in each imputed dataset, calculating each individual's propensity score in each imputation, and then averaging these at the individual level across imputations. The second, termed 'MIpar', calculates a propensity score for each individual using the average of the logistic regression coefficient estimates across the imputed datasets and setting the individual's confounders equal to their average across the imputed datasets. Leyrat *et al.* (2019) argued why both of these approaches lead to a propensity score that does not satisfy the so-called *balancing property* that, conditional on the resulting propensity score, the confounder distribution is the same in the treated as in the untreated individuals. As such, they argued and demonstrated *via* simulation studies that the 'MIps' and 'MIpar' approaches are not consistent estimators of the (average) causal effect of treatment.

When propensity score matching is used, while all individuals are used to fit the propensity score model, only the matched subset are used to estimate the causal effect. This means that when MI is used to impute missing values prior to use of propensity score matching, while the imputation models are fitted using the observed data from all individuals, the causal effect is estimated only using a subset of these. As described in Section 11.4, fitting the substantive model to a subset of the records used to fit the imputation model generally leads to uncongeniality, such that Rubin's variance estimator may be biased. Ségalas *et al.* (2023) demonstrated that this is indeed the case when MI is used to handle missing data in a propensity score matching analysis, with Rubin's rules confidence intervals having coverage above the nominal level. Moreover, they demonstrated that the modified procedure proposed by Reiter (2008) (described in Section 11.4) results in confidence interval coverage closer to the nominal level.

In conclusion, when using MI in conjunction with propensity scores methods, one should impute missing confounders conditional on both observed confounders, treatment Z, and the outcome Y. The propensity score model should be fitted in each imputation and the causal effect estimated within each imputation using the propensity score in the desired way (e.g. weighting, stratifying, matching). For weighting or stratification by the propensity score, Rubin's rules should be used, whereas with propensity score matching the modification proposed by Reiter (2008) is recommended.

13.2.3 Imputation model specification

Having concluded that if we are to use propensity scores to adjust for confounding, we should impute missing confounder values from an imputation model that conditions on the observed confounders, treatment Z, *and* outcome Y, we now consider *how* the imputation model should be specified. Throughout most of this book, we have considered that after imputation, a parametric or semi-parametric substantive model for the outcome is to be fitted, which models how the outcome Y depends on covariates. In a propensity score analysis, the substantive model essentially consists of a non-parametric marginal model for $f(Y^0)$ and a non-parametric model for $f(Y^1)$. In order to estimate the means of these marginal distributions, we specify a parametric model for $P(Z = 1|X)$, which does not involve the outcome. When imputing missing values in X, it is sensible to impute from a model that does not conflict with the assumptions encoded in the propensity score model. That is, we would like to impute from a model for X such that both it and the propensity score model can be correctly specified. To this end, we might factorise $f(X|Z, Y)$ as

$$f(X|Z, Y) \propto f(X)P(Z|X)f(Y|X, Z), \tag{13.5}$$

where $P(Z|X)$ corresponds to the propensity score model. This shows that to specify an imputation model that is compatible with the propensity score model and conditions on Y, we must also specify a model for $f(Y|X, Z)$. This is somewhat unfortunate, given that one of the reasons one might have chosen to use a propensity score approach rather than an outcome modelling approach is that the propensity score approach does not require specification of a model for the outcome given treatment and confounders. Since in the analysis of the imputed datasets we do not fit a model for $f(Y|X, Z)$, a sensible approach may be to specify $f(Y|X, Z)$ when constructing the imputation model to be as flexible as we think is reasonable and necessary. Unfortunately, at the time of writing, standard MI software is not capable of imputing missing values in X using the model given by equation (13.5). As such, a sensible practical alternative approach when the treatment (exposure) variable Z is fully observed may be to impute separately in the $Z = 0$ and $Z = 1$ groups.

Eiset and Frydenberg (2022) investigated how to impute missing confounder values in a propensity score analysis of a study investigating post-traumatic stress disorder in Syrian refugees. With the aim of imputing missing covariates compatibly with the propensity score model, they used `smcfcs` in R to impute missing values, specifying the chosen propensity score model as the substantive model. The post-traumatic stress disorder outcome variable (Y) was conditioned on in the 'covariate models' but omitted from the substantive model since this was specified as per the chosen propensity score model (a model for $P(Z = 1|X)$). While the resulting imputation model is then compatible with the specified propensity score model, it would not be expected to lead to unbiased results, since by omitting the outcome Y from the substantive model argument passed to `smcfcs`, one is (inadvertently and incorrectly) specifying that $Z \perp\!\!\!\perp Y|X$.

13.3 Principal stratification *via* multiple imputation

Principal stratification (Frangakis and Rubin, 2002) involves defining exposure or treatment effects in subsets (strata) of the population defined by post-baseline variables. Some clinical examples where principal stratification may be useful include

- comparing the effects of treatments on an outcome Y measured at time $\tau > 0$ among the principal strata of individuals who would survive to time τ under assignment to either treatment (missingness or truncation due to death);
- comparing the effects of treatments on outcome within the principal strata of individuals who would adhere to their assigned treatment regardless of which treatment they are assigned to (non-adherence);
- in clinical trials where a rescue treatment may be given if needed, comparing effects of randomised treatments on outcome among those patients who would not require rescue treatment under assignment to either treatment.

For further clinical trial examples of principal stratification, we refer readers to Bornkamp *et al.* (2021) and Lipkovich *et al.* (2022).

13.3.1 Principal strata effects

Suppose in a randomised trial in patients with HIV we are interested in the treatment effects on CD4 (Y), a measure of immune system response, at one year after randomisation. Unfortunately, some patients will have died (indicated by $D = 0$) by this time point, such that their CD4 values are missing. In fact, it is arguably more appropriate to say such values are undefined – once the patient has died, there is no meaningful CD4 value after death. As such, approaches based on imputing the 'missing' CD4 values are generally not advisable. In the terminology of the ICH E9(R1) addendum on estimands (ICH, 2019), the occurrence of death is an 'inter-current event' (see Section 10.2.1).

A naïve approach to estimating the effect of treatment Z on outcome Y in such a trial is to compare the outcomes Y between randomised treatment groups Z among those who survived to 1 year on their treatment ($D = 1$). Unfortunately, the estimand targeted by such an analysis does not have a valid causal interpretation, since the subset of patients surviving on control treatment will generally differ from the subset of patients surviving on active treatment in respect of baseline variables which affect outcome.

In the principal stratification approach to solving this problem, we consider the potential outcomes of the death by one year variable, under control and active treatments, which we denote D^0 and D^1 (= 0 if dead and = 1 if alive). Since the CD4 values are undefined if a patient dies, we compare the CD4 count distribution between treatment groups among the principal stratum of patients who would survive to one year under both treatments, i.e. those with $D^0 = D^1 = 1$. For those randomised to control, we observe D^0, while for those randomised to active, we observe D^1. If a patient died in the trial, we know they did not belong to the principal stratum of 'always-survivors'. If they survived on their assigned treatment, we need to know whether or not they would have died on the treatment they did not receive to determine if they belong to the always-survivor stratum. Thus estimation of principal strata effects can be viewed as a missing data problem – if we can impute the potential outcome D^0 or D^1, whichever is unobserved for each patient, then the analysis is straightforward.

13.3.2 Estimation

Estimation of principal strata effects requires untestable assumptions of one form or another to be made. One of the earliest proposals for estimation of a principal stratum effect, by Rubin (1998), was based on multiply imputing the missing potential outcome D^{1-Z} using baseline covariates X. This approach was expanded on by Mallinckrodt *et al.* (2019) (Section 24.6) and consists of the following:

1. Fit a logistic regression model for $P(D = 1|Z, X)$:

$$\text{logit}(P(D = 1|Z = z, X = x)) = \alpha_0 + \alpha_1 z + \alpha_2^T x$$

with parameter vector $\boldsymbol{\alpha} = (\alpha_0, \alpha_1, \alpha_2)$.

2. For $k = 1, \dots, K$:

   (a) Generate a posterior draw $\boldsymbol{\alpha}^* = (\alpha_0^*, \alpha_1^*, \alpha_2^*)$ from its posterior distribution.

   (b) For each patient with $Z = 0$, impute the missing D^1 potential outcome from $D^{1(k)*} \sim \text{Bern}(\text{expit}(\alpha_0^* + \alpha_1^* + \alpha_2^{T*}X))$. For each patient with $Z = 1$, impute D^0 from $D^{0(k)*} \sim \text{Bern}(\text{expit}(\alpha_0^* + \alpha_2^{*T}X))$.

   (c) Estimate difference in mean of Y between those with $Z = 1$, $D^{0*} = 1$ and $D^1 = 1$ and those with $Z = 0$, $D^0 = 1$ and $D^{1*} = 1$:

$$\hat{\beta}_k = \frac{\frac{1}{n}\sum_{i=1}^n Y_i Z_i D_i^{0(k)*} D_i^1}{\frac{1}{n}\sum_{i=1}^n Z_i D_i^{0(k)*} D_i^1} - \frac{\frac{1}{n}\sum_{i=1}^n Y_i (1 - Z_i) D_i^0 D_i^{1(k)*}}{\frac{1}{n}\sum_{i=1}^n (1 - Z_i) D_i^0 D_i^{1(k)*}}. \tag{13.6}$$

3. Pool point estimates $\hat{\beta}_k$ and corresponding within-imputation variances using Rubin's rules.

In step 1, an alternative to fitting a single model for $P(D = 1|Z, X)$ would be to fit separate models in each randomised treatment group.

It can be shown (Exercise 3) that the preceding algorithm will give consistent estimates of the principal strata effect $E(Y^1 - Y^0|D^0 = D^1 = 1)$ under the assumptions given by Hayden *et al.* (2005), who took a weighting rather than imputation approach. Specifically, sufficient assumptions are that

$$D^0 \perp\!\!\!\perp D^1 | X \tag{13.7}$$

and

$$D^0 \perp\!\!\!\perp Y^1 | X, D^1 = 1 \quad \text{and} \quad D^1 \perp\!\!\!\perp Y^0 | X, D^0 = 1. \tag{13.8}$$

The first assumption states that the survival outcomes D^0 and D^1 are independent conditional on the baseline covariates X. This is a so-called cross-world assumption, since it specifies independence of potential outcomes that cannot be simultaneously observed or realised in a single world. As such, it cannot be assessed from the observed data. If one does not measure any variables X, such that we require $D^0 \perp\!\!\!\perp D^1$, the assumption seems highly implausible, due to the almost certain existence of factors which influence mortality irrespective of which treatment is received. As such, we should include in X all variables that we think influence D.

The second assumption states that survival on control treatment, D^0, is independent of the outcome under active treatment Y^1, among those with the same covariates X and who survive under active treatment ($D^1 = 1$) (and also that $D^1 \perp\!\!\!\perp Y^0 | X, D^0 = 1$). This is another cross-world assumption, and hence cannot be verified or refuted from the observed data. One can readily imagine scenarios where it might not hold. Suppose the active treatment is highly efficacious at preventing death and improving outcomes. Then among those who survive on active treatment ($D^1 = 1$), one would imagine the outcome Y^1 could be predictive of survival on control D^0 – those who survive but have poor outcomes on active treatment may well be more likely to die under control treatment than those who survive on active and have good outcomes. Thus again to make the assumption more tenable we should measure and adjust for variables X which may influence both death D and the outcome Y. Ideally, sensitivity of inferences to such assumptions should be assessed – Wang *et al.* (2022) describe an approach to this based on MI.

13.4 Multiple imputation for IV analysis

Although in randomised clinical trials patients are assigned to receive one of the treatments being compared, in many trials, for a variety of reasons, some patients may not receive the treatment assigned to them. This is sometimes referred to as non-adherence or non-compliance.

In the presence of treatment non-adherence, an intention to treat analysis which compares outcomes between randomised groups, ignoring adherence, validly estimates the effect of treatment assignment on outcomes. It does not however estimate the effect of actually receiving one treatment versus the other, due to the non-adherence. That this is the case can be seen from a contrived and extreme example: suppose no patients assigned to the active treatment take it, instead receiving the control treatment (e.g. usual care), and all the patients assigned to control receive the control treatment. Then it is clear that the intention to treat analysis is not estimating the effect of taking the active treatment compared to the control, since no patients took the active treatment.

In this section, we consider the instrumental variable (*IV*) approach to estimating the effects of receiving or taking active treatment versus control. We first review the idea of the complier (adherer) average causal effect (CACE) and the IV approach to its estimation. Next, we explore the use of MI to performing an IV analysis.

13.4.1 Instrumental variable analysis for non-adherence

Let Z denote the binary variable indicating an individual's randomised treatment, with $Z = 1$ indicating active treatment and $Z = 0$ indicating control treatment. Let Y denote the outcome variable. We let D denote the binary variable indicating whether the patient receives active treatment ($D = 1$) or control treatment ($D = 0$). Further, let

D^z denote the treatment received when Z is set to level z, and $Y^{z,d}$ denote the potential outcome with treatment assigned to level z and actual treatment received set to level d.

A CACE of possible interest is

$$E(Y^{1,D^1} - Y^{0,D^0} | D^0 = 0, D^1 = 1) = E(Y^{1,1} - Y^{0,0} | D^0 = 0, D^1 = 1),$$

that is the effect of assigning active *versus* control treatment on outcome among those who would adhere with their assigned treatment whichever they are assigned to. This effect is an example of a principal stratum effect (Section 13.3.1).

The naïve approach to estimating the CACE is to compare outcomes according to treatment received (D):

$$E(Y|D = 1) - E(Y|D = 0).$$

This in general is not an unbiased estimator of the CACE because of the presence of unmeasured confounders – variables U that influence both which treatment the individual receives (D) and the outcome Y.

Thus in order to estimate the CACE, further assumptions must be made. The IV approach uses the random treatment assignment Z as an instrument. What this means can be encoded graphically in the causal directed acyclic graph (DAG) in Figure 13.1. The DAG shows the unmeasured confounders U that affect D and Y. It also encodes the key exclusion restriction assumption that the effect of treatment assignment Z on outcome Y is mediated wholly *via* the treatment receipt variable D.

Following Hernán and Robins (2020), the IV assumptions can be formulated in terms of potential outcomes as follows:

$$Z \perp\!\!\!\perp D, \text{relevance},$$

$$Y^{z,d} = Y^{z',d} = Y^d, \text{exclusion restriction},$$

$$Z \perp\!\!\!\perp Y^{z,d}, \text{marginal exchangeability}.$$

These can be shown to hold under the DAG in Figure 13.1. In a randomised trial, the relevance assumption ought to always hold – we should expect more active treatment to be taken in the $Z = 1$ group compared to the $Z = 0$ group. The exclusion restriction may be plausible, if we think that the treatment assignment process has no effect other than *via* its effect on which treatment the individual actually takes. Lastly, in a randomised trial, the marginal exchangeability assumption holds because Z is randomly assigned.

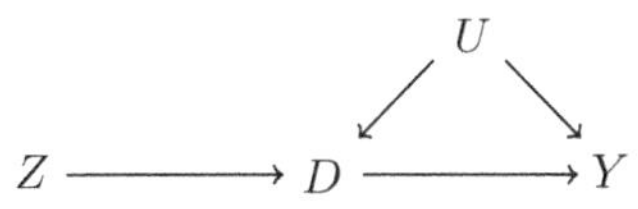

Figure 13.1 Directed acyclic graph depicting Z as an instrumental variable for the effect of treatment D on outcome Y. U represents unmeasured confounders of the effect of D on Y.

The so-called *IV estimand* is defined as

$$\frac{E(Y|Z=1)-E(Y|Z=0)}{E(D|Z=1)-E(D|Z=0)}. \tag{13.9}$$

Under certain effect homogeneity assumptions, the IV estimand equals the average causal effect of D on Y in the whole population (Hernán and Robins, 2020). These assumptions are however often implausible and, hence, difficult to justify. Instead, we may be willing to assume the following so-called monotonicity assumption, that $D^1 \geq D^0$. The monotonicity assumption means that there are no so-called *defiers*, those with $D^0 = 1$ and $D^1 = 0$. Monotonicity is often a reasonable assumption in randomised trials. Furthermore, if it is impossible for patients assigned to control treatment to receive active treatment, monotonicity holds (there are no defiers or so-called *always takers* in this case).

Under the monotonicity or no-defiers assumption, the IV estimand is equal to the CACE. Intuitively, it can be seen that this is true as follows (Hernán and Robins, 2020). With Z randomly assigned, the numerator of the IV estimand is the average effect of Z on Y. This is a weighted average of the effects of Z on Y in the adherers ($D^0 = 0$, and $D^1 = 1$), the always takers ($D^0 = 1$ and $D^1 = 1$), and the never-takers ($D^0 = 0$ and $D^1 = 0$), with the weights corresponding to the proportions of the different adherence types in the population. The average effect of Z on Y in the always-takers and never-takers is however zero because of the exclusion restriction: in these two subsets, Z has no effect on D, and the exclusion restriction says that any effects of Z on Y are mediated *via* D. Thus, the numerator of the IV estimand is equal to the effect of Z on Y in the adherers multiplied by the proportion of adherers in the population:

$$E(Y^{z=1} - Y^{z=0}|D^0 = 0, D^1 = 1)P(D^0 = 0, D^1 = 1).$$

Next, note that the proportion of always-takers $P(D^0 = 1, D^1 = 1) = P(D^0 = 1)$, since $D^0 = 1 \Rightarrow D^1 = 1$ by the monotonicity assumption. The proportion of always-takers $P(D^0 = 1)$ can then be estimated by $E(D|Z = 0)$. Similarly, the proportion of never-takers $P(D^0 = 0, D^1 = 0) = P(D^1 = 0)$ which can be estimated by $1 - E(D|Z = 1)$. The proportion of adherers is then

$$1 - \{E(D|Z = 0) + 1 - E(D|Z = 1)\} = \mathrm{E}(D|Z = 1) - \mathrm{E}(D|Z = 0).$$

Hence, the IV estimand (equation (13.9)) is equal to the CACE.

13.4.2 Instrumental variable analysis *via* multiple imputation

The standard IV estimator replaces the expectations involved in the formula for the IV estimand (equation (13.9)) with their sample counterparts:

$$\frac{\hat{E}(Y|Z=1)-\hat{E}(Y|Z=0)}{\hat{E}(D|Z=1)-\hat{E}(D|Z=0)}.$$

The resulting estimator is consistent for the CACE under the previously stated assumptions.

The CACE compares the *mean* outcome under the two treatments among the always-adherers. Imbens and Rubin (1997) showed that in fact the outcome *distributions* under control and active for the adherers can be identified from the observed data. Through doing this, they showed that the standard IV estimator is implicitly based on estimates of the densities of the two potential outcome distributions, with no guarantee that these are non-negative. Motivated by this finding, they proposed some alternative estimators of CACE which correspond to valid (i.e. non-negative) estimates of the adherer potential outcome densities. One is a fully parametric normal model, where the outcome is assumed to be normal with distinct mean parameters in the (i) never-takers, (ii) always-takers, and (iii) adherers (one mean under control, one mean under active treatment). In a small simulation study, they found that this parametric estimator of CACE could be considerably less variable and biased than the standard IV estimator. This occurred in their simulation setup because they had a small (10%) adherer stratum. As such, the denominator of the IV estimator could sometimes be close to zero, resulting in a very large CACE estimate. In such cases, the IV assumptions together imply the ITT (treatment policy) effect cannot be large, since the only stratum with a possible non-zero effect of treatment assignment is the adherers. This suggests that the ITT effect targeted by the numerator of the IV estimator ought to be small also, but the IV estimator does not exploit this.

Little and Yau (1998) developed the parametric approach further. They considered the special case where, in addition to no defiers, there are also assumed to be no always-takers. This setup could be appropriate in trials where it is impossible for those assigned to control treatment to receive active treatment. Again using a normal model, there are now three distinct mean parameters, and the model can be expressed as

$$Y = \beta_0 + \beta_C C + \beta_{CZ} CZ + \epsilon, \tag{13.10}$$

where $C = 1$ if the individual is a adherer and $C = 0$ if they a never-taker. The interaction coefficient β_{CZ} then corresponds to the CACE. Note the absence of a main effect of Z in the model, which is implied by the exclusion restriction assumption. We then have a model for the binary adherence status variable C which is simply a Bernoulli. Under this model, the adherence status variable is partially observed – for individuals assigned to active treatment ($Z = 1$), we can ascertain from their treatment received variable D whether they are adherers or never-takers. But in those assigned to control ($Z = 0$), who all have $D = 0$, we cannot tell which are adherers and which are never-takers. The problem can thus be cast as a missing data problem with C being partially observed. As such Imbens and Rubin (1997) and Little and Yau (1998) proposed using the EM algorithm for estimation (Dempster *et al.*, 1977).

The preceding model can be readily extended to incorporate baseline covariates X which may affect the outcome and/or the adherence membership variable C in order to improve precision. Specifically, the outcome model could now be extended to

$$Y = \beta_0 + \beta_C C + \beta_{CZ} CZ + \beta_X X + \beta_{CX} CX + \beta_{CZX} CXZ + \epsilon. \tag{13.11}$$

This model allows the effect of treatment (active versus control) to differ according to the level of the covariate X. The coefficient β_{CZ} now represents the effect of active treatment (relative to control) among adherers with $X = 0$. The probability of being an adherer can then be modelled using a suitable (e.g. logistic) regression conditional on X.

A drawback to fitting such models by maximum likelihood (through the EM algorithm) or by Bayesian methods is the need to use specialist software. More recently, DiazOrdaz and Carpenter (2019) proposed an MI approach to impute the partially observed adherence variable C. A difficulty with applying standard MI software to the problem is to ensure that C is imputed compatibly with the outcome model (e.g. equation (13.10) or (13.11)), particularly because of the presence of the CZ interaction term. Due to the presence of this interaction term, DiazOrdaz and Carpenter (2019) proposed using a substantive model compatible (SMC) imputation approach (Section 6.4). Here we specify that $f(C|X,Z) = f(C|X)$ is a logistic regression model and that the substantive model for the outcome Y is as per equation (13.11) or a possibly simpler version which omits the CX and CXZ interactions.

Simulation studies reported by DiazOrdaz and Carpenter (2019) showed good performance of SMC full conditional specification (FCS) compared to a two-stage least-squares IV estimator, which can be viewed as an extension accommodating baseline covariates of the simple IV ratio estimator discussed above. They investigated settings with either a continuous or binary outcome Y. In the latter case, the two-stage least-squares IV estimator targets the difference in risk between active treatment and control among adherers. Instead, we may be interested in estimating alternative effect measures, such as an odds ratio, either conditional on X or marginal to X (Daniel *et al.*, 2021). The MI approach makes estimation of such measures straightforward – we can impute C, exploiting baseline covariates X for improved efficiency but, if desired, omit X when fitting the outcome model to the imputed datasets.

In principle, a SMC MI approach can also be used for the case where there are always-takers (but still no defiers) (DiazOrdaz and Carpenter (2019)). In this case, the adherence class variable can take three values. The difficulty is that, while we can identify some individuals who are always-takers from the observed data (those with $Z = 0$ and $D = 1$) and some who are never-takers (those with $Z = 1$ and $D = 0$), we cannot definitively identify any adherers: those with $Z = 0$ and $D = 0$ could be never-takers or adherers, and those with $Z = 1$ and $D = 1$ could be always-takers or adherers. As such, the partially observed version of the adherence class variable only takes two, rather than three values. Because of this, most SMC MI software (such as SMC-FCS in R and Stata) will not be able to impute C correctly, since there are no observed values of C corresponding to the adherer class.

13.5 Discussion

We have seen that a variety of important causal inference problems can be cast as missing data problems. On the surface, assumptions that appear distinct – not least because of their different names, such as missing at random and no unmeasured confounding or conditional exchangeability – are seen to be closely related.

Methods developed from one area may potentially be fruitfully applied to the other, while in some situations, as seen in Section 13.1, methods that appear at first sight distinct may in fact in some cases turn out to be identical.

Despite the close connections between causal inference and missing data, there are important differences (Ding and Li, 2018). In particular, whereas the fundamental goal in causal inference is the comparison of potential outcomes under two versions of treatment or exposure, missing data methods have as their objective reliable inference on a statistical parameter relating to the distribution of the full or complete data. The latter parameters(s) may in some settings have causal interpretations, but there are of course many research endeavours where the parameter of interest does not have a direct causal interpretation. A further difference is that the missingness patterns that occur when viewing causal inference from a missing data perspective (Table 13.1) tend to be simple and highly structured. In contrast, 'regular' missing data in studies can appear in multiple variables in complex patterns. Moreover, in the basic causal inference problem (Section 13.1), we never jointly observe Y^0 and Y^1, and thus cannot hope to estimate their joint distribution. In contrast, in missing data problems, under an assumption such as MAR, we would generally be able to estimate the joint distribution of the variables under study.

Many of the causal inference ideas outlined in this chapter, such as estimation of IV and CACE estimands, were described for simple randomised trials. An advantage of viewing these as a missing data problem and constructing MI estimators is that this may open the door to using them in settings, both experimental and observational, where in addition to missing potential outcomes, we also have missing data in the usual sense. As was demonstrated in Chapter 11 in the case of simultaneously handling covariate measurement error and missing data, the estimation task is simplified by being able to use MI for both.

Exercises

1. **Multiple imputation for causal inference in a randomised trial**
   In this question, we explore the properties of MI for causal inference in a randomised trial, following the developments in Section 13.1.1.

   (a) Simulate data for a trial with $n = 100$ patients, with a value $Y^0 \sim N(\mu_0, \sigma^2)$ and a value $Y^1 \sim N(\mu_1, \sigma^2)$ for each patient, choosing your own values for the true parameters. Generate a random treatment assignment variable Z. Generate $Y = ZY^1 + (1 - Z)Y^0$ and calculate the difference in the sample mean of Y between treatment groups $Z = 1$ and $Z = 0$.

   (b) Create the observable versions of Y^0 and Y^1 based on the patient's assigned treatment Z. Then write your own code to create multiple imputations of the missing values in Y^0 using a normal imputation model with no covariates (i.e. only an intercept), utilising the known value of σ^2. Impute the missing values in Y^1 similarly. Use $K = 1{,}000$ imputations for each, calculate the difference between the mean of Y^0 and Y^1 in each imputed dataset, and average these across the K imputations. Compare your answer to that obtained from the difference in sample means in part (a).

(c) Give an analytical argument that as $K \to \infty$, the MI estimator of the difference in means of Y^0 and Y^1 converges in probability to the difference in observed sample means.

(d) Apply Rubin's rules to the estimates from the $K = 1000$ imputed datasets, where for the within-imputation variance assume that the two sample means are independent, and assuming that σ^2 is known. Compare it with the estimated variance from the difference in observed sample means from part (a), with the latter also calculated using the known value of σ^2.

(e) Based on what you observe in the last part, derive an analytical result relating Rubin's variance estimator to the variance of the difference in observed sample means.

2. **Imputation with propensity scores**

(a) For a dataset of size n =10,000, assign 2000 to be treated ($Z = 1$), and 8000 to be untreated ($Z = 0$). Simulate a confounder $X|Z \sim N(0.5Z, 1)$. Simulate the outcome $Y|X, Z \sim N(X + Z, 1)$.

(b) Show analytically the true values of the average treatment effect (ATE) $E(Y^1 - Y^0)$ and the average treatment effect in the treated (ATT) $E(Y^1 - Y^0| Z = 1)$ based on the data generating mechanism and by assuming causal consistency and conditional exchangeability.

(c) Use the data to estimate the ATT by matching on X and compare your estimate to the value you derived for the ATT derived analytically.

(d) Now imagine that X is missing for all individuals, but someone has told you the true conditional distribution for $X|Z$, i.e. that $X|Z \sim N(0.5Z, 1)$. Use this to generate a single imputed X value for each individual in the data. Then re-estimate the ATT by matching on the now wholly imputed X. Examine the mean outcomes in the treated and matched untreated individuals, and explain any differences.

(e) Use your knowledge of the true data generating mechanism to derive the conditional distribution of $X|Z, Y$. From this, generate a new single imputation of X for each individual. Then again match on the resulting X and compare the means of the treated and matched untreated individuals to the values you should expect.

3. **Imputation for principal stratification – theory**

In this question, we show that MI using the algorithm described in Section 13.3.2 yields consistent estimates of the always-survivor principal stratum effect under the assumptions in equations (13.7) and (13.8). We assume that the logistic regression imputation model(s) for D^0 and D^1 are correctly specified, so that as $n \to \infty$, D^{1*} is a draw from $f(D^1|X)$ and D^{0*} is a draw from $f(D^0|X)$.

(a) Show that the mean outcome under active treatment in the always-survivor principal stratum

$$E(Y^1|D^0 = D^1 = 1)$$

can be expressed as

$$\frac{E(Y^1 D^0 D^1)}{E(D^0 D^1)}. \tag{13.12}$$

(b) Argue why the denominator of the preceding expression can be expressed as

$$E[E(D^0|X)E(D^1|X)].$$

(c) Show that for the estimator given by equation (13.6) which is applied to each imputed dataset, the denominator of the first term consistently estimates

$$(1/2)E[E(D^0|X)E(D^1|X)].$$

(d) Show that the numerator of equation (13.12) can be expressed as

$$E[D^1 E(Y^1|X, D^1 = 1)E(D^0|X)].$$

(e) Show that in the estimator given by equation (13.6), the numerator of the first term consistently estimates

$$(1/2)E[D^1 E(Y^1|X, D^1 = 1)E(D^0|X)].$$

(f) Conclude your argument for why the MI approach yields a consistent estimator of the always-survivor principal stratum effect under the assumptions of equations (13.7) and (13.8).

4. Imputation for principal stratification – simulation

(a) For a dataset of size $n = 500$, simulate a baseline variable $X \sim N(0,1)$. Simulate the survival potential outcomes D^0 and D^1 for each individual independently from

$$P(D^0 = 1|X) = \text{expit}(X),$$
$$P(D^1 = 1|X) = \text{expit}(-1 + X),$$

where $\text{expit}(x) = \frac{\exp(x)}{1+\exp(x)}$.
Simulate potential outcomes Y^0 and Y^1 from

$$Y^0|X \sim N(X, 1),$$
$$Y^1|X \sim N(1 + 0.5X, 1).$$

(b) Calculate a 'full data' estimate of the always-survivor principal stratum effect $E(Y^1 - Y^0|D^0 = D^1 = 1)$ using the potential outcomes Y^0, Y^1, D^0, D^1.

(c) Generate a random treatment assignment variable Z with 250 individuals assigned to the control treatment and 250 assigned to the active treatment. Generate the observable versions of Y and D according to which treatment each individual is assigned to.

(d) Based on the observable data, calculate a naïve estimate of the principal stratum effect by comparing mean outcomes in the $Z = 1$ and $Z = 0$ among those with $D = 1$.

(e) Put your code in a loop to repeat the simulation process 1000 times. Perform a two-sample paired t-test on the resulting 'full data' and naïve estimates of the effect and confirm that the naïve estimator is biased.

(f) Create the partially observed versions of D^0 and D^1 using Z and D. Add code to implement the MI algorithm described in Section 13.3.2, using the variable X to impute the missing values in D^0 and D^1. Re-run your simulation and examine whether the MI estimator is biased relative to the full data estimator. Are the results as you expect?

(g) Re-run your simulation study after modifying the imputation step so that D^0 and D^1 are imputed using a logistic regression model with only an intercept parameter, i.e. without using X. How do the full data, naïve, and MI estimators now compare?

14

Using multiple imputation in practice

This book is titled *Multiple Imputation and Its Application* and Part III has focused on details of its application to specific problems. This chapter offers some more general advice on using multiple imputation. We begin in Section 14.1 with a general strategy for using multiple imputation in practice. No applied strategy will be perfect or universal, but having a clear strategy is nonetheless worthwhile: in any particular application, you may wish to modify or diverge from it, but it is useful to consider what you are diverting from, what (if anything) to do instead, and why.

Even when you have decided that multiple imputation is appropriate, it is possible that collaborators and/or reviewers will disagree. In Section 14.2, we present and respond to some common objections to multiple imputation that have arisen in our work. Some objections are well founded, some are not; for many it depends on the context.

It is very common to read methods sections along the lines of, 'All analyses used multiple imputation (10 imputations using the MICE method), assuming data were missing at random,' with a possible reference to software. Such a description leaves many important aspects and choices of what was done unspecified. Section 14.3 offers some suggestions for reporting analysis involving multiple imputation. The remainder of the chapter addresses a range of practical issues that have repeatedly arisen in workshops we have run.

14.1 A general approach

This section describes 10 steps we regard as always or usually relevant when applying multiple imputation. We focus attention on the missing data setting rather

Multiple Imputation and its Application, Second Edition.
James R. Carpenter, Jonathan W. Bartlett, Tim P. Morris, Angela M. Wood, Matteo Quartagno and Michael G. Kenward.

than the measurement error or causal inference settings described in Chapters 11 and 13. We further assume that data have already been collected. Of course, at an earlier stage in the study, strategies to minimise missing data should be taken (e.g. Panel on Handling Missing Data in Clinical Trials. Committee on National Statistics, Division of Behavioral and Social Sciences and Education. Washington, DC: The National Academies Press, 2010; Hussain *et al.*, 2022). The points covered here also relate to practical issues that arise in applying the 'Treatment and Reporting of Missing Data in Observational Studies' (TARMOS) framework (Lee *et al.*, 2021); see also Carpenter and Smuk (2021).

In randomised clinical trials, and increasingly elsewhere, analyses are pre-specified before seeing the outcome data. In this case, we advise constructing one or more plausible datasets to represent the anticipated data and inform the statistical analysis plan. Whether or not a formal statistical analysis plan is required prior to seeing the data, it is worth writing down the statistical analysis procedures (specifically the primary substantive model) that would be undertaken in the ideal case with no missing data. The MI paradigm allows this to remain unchanged, despite the missing data. This provides an anchor for analysis and differentiates decisions that inform the choice of the substantive model from those taken to address issues raised by the missing data.

14.1.1 Explore the proportions and patterns of missing data

Explore which variables have the most missing values and discuss this with the research team. Are there any (i) surprises? (ii) patterns that are particularly common? How many in/complete records are there? UpSet plots (Figure 14.1) are a useful visualisation tool (Tierney *et al.*, 2021; Tierney and Cook, 2018).

14.1.2 Consider plausible missing data mechanisms

This task can be difficult because, as we have emphasised, assumptions about missingness cannot be definitely verified without seeing the missing data. The difficulty can sometimes be addressed using information beyond the data at hand. For example, discussions with those involved in 'on-the-ground' data collection are often revealing. A data collection process that allows recording of reasons for missing data is also helpful. For example, missing outcomes on a study participant may be viewed differently depending on whether they moved abroad, died during the study, or withdrew from the treatment following adverse effects. Consideration of missing data mechanisms may ultimately lead the analysis away from using multiple imputation (cf. discussion of complete records analysis in Chapter 1).

14.1.3 Consider whether missing at random is plausible

When using multiple imputation, missing at random (MAR) is a desirable assumption because it the most general missingness mechanism under which we can recover the lost information without injecting information external to the observed data.

This means that the assumption almost represents a conflict of interest for analysts: by assuming missing at random, we can make our task slightly easier. It is important to consider whether conditioning on the observed data makes MAR plausible. Considering what might be the causal relationships between the variables involved may help in this regard, and expressing this through graphical models can be useful (Daniel *et al.*, 2011; Moreno-Betancur *et al.*, 2018; Hughes *et al.*, 2019).

14.1.4 Choose the variables for the imputation model

These should include all the variables in the substantive model (including the outcome when imputing covariates), together with any auxiliary variables identified. To help select auxiliary variables, recall:

(a) A useful auxiliary variable must sometimes be observed when the incomplete variable/s are not. Otherwise, it does not contain any information about the missing values and need not be included in the imputation model. This point is frequently overlooked when missingness patterns are inspected.

(b) An auxiliary variable predictive of both missingness and of the incomplete variable should be included in the imputation model to reduce the bias of a complete records analysis.

(c) Variables that are highly correlated with an incomplete variable but that do not predict missingness will not affect bias but will improve efficiency.

(d) Variables that predict missingness but are uncorrelated with the incomplete variable will not add information and should be omitted from the imputation model (Spratt *et al.*, 2010) – though often you may not know this *a priori*. If this is counter-intuitive, consider that including such a variable in the imputation model does not change (in expectation) the distribution from which imputations are drawn, meaning that omitting it did not introduce bias.

14.1.5 Choose an appropriate imputation strategy and model/s

The general strategy may be to base imputation on a joint model or full conditional specification (FCS). The specific imputation model/s to be used can then be chosen. This should reflect the data types, any interactions, and non-linear structure, and multilevel structure if relevant. Choices should reflect details of the methods described in Parts II and III.

14.1.6 Set and record the seed of the pseudo-random number generator

This is to ensure the results are reproducible. Multiple imputation is inherently simulation-based and in practice uses pseudo-random number generation. To reproduce the results exactly, an analysis must at least set the same random-number seed. It will also typically be necessary to have the data sorted in the same order and the variables in the same order in the database. Slightly more detail is required for others to reproduce a multiple imputation analysis: the *method of random number generation*, the *stream* used by the random number generator (in Stata, for example each possible input seed can be specified in any of 32,000 streams for certain methods of random number generation), the *version number* of the software, and the *operating system* on which the analysis was run.

14.1.7 Fit the imputation model

Create a small number of imputed datasets (say three). Check that the imputations appear plausible, fit the substantive model to the imputed datasets, and combine the results using Rubin's rules, as summarised on page 71. Consider diagnostics for the imputation models, such as convergence diagnostics when using joint-model imputation. Also consider whether any diagnostics are needed for the substantive model and whether these should be done on the combined substantive model or separately for each imputed dataset; see Section 14.5. For the latter choice, consideration is needed as to how problems will be handled if they occur in some imputed datasets but not others. The fraction of missing information can sometimes help to diagnose issues: we have seen examples where a variable with around 10% missing data has fraction of missing information(FMI) close to 1, which highlighted problems with the imputation model.

14.1.8 Iterate and revise the imputation model if necessary

There are many things that can go wrong once an imputation model has been specified. This is frequently the realisation that something intended was omitted, such as an important variable or a structure. Issues such as *separation* (sometimes called *perfect prediction*) in the imputation model are not uncommon, particularly with categorical data and good auxiliary variables. In one sense, it is advantageous if the observed data perfectly predict the missing values, but makes it difficult to draw from the posterior. This then needs to be dealt with by changing the features of the imputation model or by augmenting the observed data as advocated by White *et al.* (2010); see the discussion in Chapter 4, Section 4.6.

14.1.9 Estimate monte carlo error

Multiple imputation is inherently simulation-based and thus subject to Monte Carlo error (Section 14.6, Koehler *et al.*, 2009, White *et al.*, 2011). This may lead to the decision to increase the number of imputations. For scalar parameter estimates, Monte Carlo error is readily estimated as $\sqrt{\hat{B}/K}$ and can be estimated for other statistics using a jack-knife procedure (White *et al.*, 2011; Efron, 1992). If the estimated Monte Carlo error is unacceptably high for statistics of key substantive interest, then the number of imputations should be increased and Monte Carlo error re-estimated. See Section 14.6 for how to choose K.

14.1.10 Sensitivity analysis

Explore the sensitivity of inferences to departure from the primary missing data assumption (typically MAR), as discussed in Chapter 10. Unless the missing data mechanism is known with certainty, or conclusions are irrefutable, it is useful to explore the sensitivity of the results (though the context of Chapter 8 may sometimes be an exception). Sensitivity analysis does just this, holding the estimand fixed. If, for example a specific missing not at random (MNAR) assumption was made for the primary analysis, it is worth also knowing what the result would be under MAR or alternative plausible MNAR assumptions. MI is a particularly flexible and practical tool for sensitivity analysis, as described in Chapter 10.

14.2 Objections to multiple imputation

There are many objections to multiple imputation. Some are well founded; others are not. For a given objection, its legitimacy frequently depends on context. We discuss the objections we have encountered; hopefully, this will help readers understand and deal with them in their own work.

Multiple imputation must not be used because you could end up with several different results from your statistical analysis.
This objection typically arises for one of two reasons. The first is simply that some people assume multiple imputation returns K sets of results and do not know about Rubin's combination rules, a misunderstanding which can be easily put right. The second is an objection that multiple imputation is inherently simulation-based. For the researcher using multiple imputation, there is a responsibility to use a sufficient number of imputations to minimise Monte Carlo error (see Section 14.6) and reassure critics that they would not have seen results with the same MI procedure but a different random number seed differ by an amount that materially affects the inferences. □

Multiple imputation assumes missing at random and this assumption may be wrong.
It is true that default implementations of multiple imputation require data to be missing at random (as readers will know by now, there are further conditions for its validity). However, multiple imputation is flexible and sensitivity parameters can be included in imputation models to reflect departures from missing at random (see Chapter 10). The fact that the assumption about the missingness mechanism may be wrong is a fair criticism, but it is a criticism that can be levelled at *any* analysis with incomplete data.

Therefore, the appropriate response to this objection prompts is *compared to what?* The alternative of no missing data is not an option. Instead, the analyst must do the best they can in the presence of incomplete data, or do no analysis – in some cases, the wisest decision. □

Outcome variables should not be imputed.
It is sometimes true that imputing outcome variables is a pointless exercise. However, if the imputation model is appropriately specified, the worst that can happen is that it induces some (generally negligible) additional Monte Carlo error (cf. p. 481). To avoid this Monte Carlo error, von Hippel (2007) suggests deleting imputed outcomes before fitting the substantive model to each imputed dataset. We do not believe that this is worth the effort in most applications; moreover, retaining the imputed outcome data is preferable when the imputation model includes information and/or structure, not in the substantive model (e.g. auxiliary variables, sensitivity parameters, non-linear relationships). In such cases deleting the imputed outcomes will likely cause problems (Sullivan *et al.*, 2015). □

Covariates should not be imputed
Multiple imputation is particularly attractive when covariates are incomplete and data are missing at random. Chapters 3–6 focused on such settings.

However, as discussed in Section 1.6.2, if the probability of a complete record depends only on the values of covariates, complete records analysis is valid. Moreover, if it depends on the values of covariates which themselves have missing values, data are MNAR, and so strictly MI will be biased – though in some applications, the gain in precision will mean the mean square error of parameter estimates is smaller. This is particularly the case when the probability of a complete record depends on both outcome and covariates so that a complete records analysis is biased. In fact, as the simulation study in Bartlett *et al.* (2014) illustrates, you have to work quite hard to get significant bias with a MNAR mechanism in this setting.

A subtly different setting is when missingness depends on the value of other covariates only when these covariates are observed; then multiple imputation assuming MAR is valid, but complete records should be unbiased.

Because, in most applications, the outcome will be measured after the incomplete covariate, it seems that if covariates are MAR involving the outcome, then this must imply a causal effect backwards in time. However, this is not the case because association is not causation. The most common explanation is that there exists a common, unmeasured cause of missingness and outcome. Less plausibly, missingness could be a cause of Y: for example, the presence or the absence of data could affect some subsequent decision that could be a cause of Y. □

Multiple imputation requires a model for incomplete covariates.
With complete data, most regression analyses model some function of the outcome distribution conditional on covariates. As the covariates are observed, fitting the regression model does not require a covariate model.

However, beyond complete records, all methods for handling missing covariates require an assumption about their missingness mechanism; likelihood-based methods (including MI and Bayesian approaches) additionally require a model for their distribution.

Specifically, for regression, we have already noted that complete records analysis is valid if the probability of a complete record is conditionally independent of the dependent variable given (partially observed) covariates. By contrast, for valid inference from inverse probability weighting, data must be missing at random and the weights must correctly model this mechanism. Neither method, though, requires model for the distribution of covariates.

However, this objection does not invalidate MI, but in fact makes it more attractive – because it allows MI to bring back into the analysis of the substantive model (and hence our inferences) all the observed data on each individual (or unit), regardless of whether it is complete, as well as including information in auxiliary variables. In non-standard settings, contextually important misspecification of the imputation model can be avoided by using the approaches described in the earlier part of this book.

An accessible discussion of the pros and cons of MI versus complete records and inverse probability weighting is given by Little *et al.* (2022). □

Multiple imputation should only be used when the power of complete records analysis is low.
We do not agree with this above argument in general. We advocate first considering the missing data assumptions, then using a method that will give valid inference under those assumptions, and then performing sensitivity analysis. When multiple imputation and complete records analysis are both valid, multiple imputation will typically be more powerful and allow the inclusion of auxiliary variables. See the discussion of the objection that *Outcome variables should not be imputed.* □

Multiple imputation uses simulation, so one person would get different results from another.
This is true, but rather an odd objection. It implies we should not use multiple imputation simply because it uses simulation. Yet simulation-based methods are widely used; for example bootstrapping and Markov chain Monte Carlo methods. Further, we can quantify random error due to simulation as Monte Carlo error and control it by increasing the number of imputations (Section 14.6). □

Multiple imputation can only be used when data are missing at random.
While, by default, multiple imputation software assumes data are missing at random, Chapter 10 shows how to apply it when data are missing not at random. This requires additional information that does not come from the observed data, and so typically requires more care than multiple imputation assuming MAR. □

Multiple imputation under missing not at random is not appropriate because sensitivity parameters are not informed by the data; it is just making it up!
Suppose we have a single quantitative variable to impute. The imputation model assumes missing not at random by imputing under MAR and adding a fixed value δ to each imputed value. Arguably, this sensitivity δ is not informed by the observed data and so is 'made up'. However, now consider the case of missing at random. This

can be viewed as fixing $\delta = 0$, which is as 'made up' as any other value of δ. This goes back to the point that the missing data mechanism is unknown because we cannot compare the missing values with the observed. The question then is whether we are willing to proceed with any (ideally a range) assumptions or not.

We emphasise that, while δ cannot be known, it can be informed by knowledge external to the data at hand. This may be through those responsible for collecting data, such as research nurses who follow up patients in a longitudinal study, or based on external data (Pham *et al.*, 2018), or based on carefully elicited expert opinion (Mason *et al.*, 2017). □

Rubin's variance formula may be too conservative or too liberal.
This issue is carefully explored in Section 2.8.3, see also p. 97. In summary, this is unlikely to be a materially relevant concern, especially if the methods described in this book are appropriately applied. Should concerns persist, bootstrapping (Bartlett and Hughes, 2020) could be considered. □

Multiple imputation should only be used with a small/large percentage of missing values.
Sometimes we are asked: 'at what percentage of missingness does MI become inappropriate?', suggesting that when the percentage is large, use of MI is inadvisable. As often is the case in statistics, there is no simple answer to such a question.

First, when addressing any scientific question, the concern is not the proportion of missing values *per se*, but the impact of the missing values in terms of loss of information relevant to the question – and the increased ambiguity about the answer. However, this depends on the question: when crossing a road, all data about the condition of the on-coming traffic's rear lights is missing – but this represents no loss of information. At the other extreme, when estimating incidence or prevalence of a rare disease, a few missing disease classifications can greatly impact the estimates. Further, the extent of the missing information depends on the assumption about the missingness mechanism.

Second, the validity of an MI analysis does not depend on the proportion of missing values, but rather on the veracity of the missingness and modelling assumptions made. Nevertheless, inferences will generally be more susceptible to violations of these assumptions the larger the amount of missingness, such that we might be more wary about imputing when the percentage missing is very large (Section 7.4.4) – or more inclined to carefully check our modelling and missing data assumptions and perform sensitivity analysis. Having said this, in a setting where we have a strongly predictive auxiliary variable, although the percentage missing may be high, we may be able to recover a large amount of the missing information *via* imputation.

Other times critics argue 'the percentage missing is so small, there is no point in using MI'. It is true that in general with a small percentage missing, inferences will often be similar from a complete records analysis and an MI analysis. However, it is difficult to be sure of this without actually performing both and checking. Moreover, there are (admittedly fairly uncommon) situations where with even a small percentage missing, a complete records analysis can be badly biased and an MI analysis may be unbiased. □

Having said all this, we must acknowledge that – at least in the medical research world – MI has to some extent become a victim of its own success. It is frequently requested by co-authors or demanded by reviewers when unnecessary, or even inappropriate. One example is in randomised clinical trials with missing outcome values. When the statistical analysis plan and protocol specify an 'intention-to-treat' (ITT) analysis, it is not uncommon to see multiple imputation of outcomes justified as 'preserving ITT' (see White *et al.* (2012); examples of this can be readily found in the literature). However, while multiple imputation directly respects the requirement to 'analyse all randomised individuals', when only outcomes are missing this does not mean inferences will differ from a correspondingly specified likelihood analysis of all the observed data (modulo Monte-Carlo error) – cf. Section 1.6.1, and the discussion and examples in Carpenter and Kenward (2008), ch. 4. To recap, in regression analysis with longitudinal partially observed outcomes and fully observed covariate data, MI and a likelihood-based analysis of the observed data will agree when:

1. a fully efficient, likelihood-based analysis is used for all the observed data;
2. MI is implemented assuming missing at random, and
3. the parameter of interest in the substantive model is either directly estimated by the likelihood analysis of the observed data or is a function of parameters of this analysis.

14.3 Reporting of analyses with incomplete data

For most applied analyses with incomplete data, the missing data are a nuisance that complicate the analysis (with the missing indicator method, Section 8.8.2 a possible exception). This frequently leads to published research including only a terse description of how missing data were handled, such as 'missing data were multiply imputed 10 times using the MICE method'. Unless buttressed by details in the supplementary material, this is inadequate, because the reported analysis is not reproducible.

In particular, choices about how missing data are handled have implications for bias (in particular) and results will depend in part on untestable assumptions. Therefore, ensuring that assumptions are clearly described facilitates critical appraisal and understanding of analysis as a whole.

In a review of handling of missing covariate data, Carroll *et al.* (2020) found a common practice was to exclude people with incomplete data from the study through the 'eligibility' criteria (106 of 148 articles). This makes it difficult for readers to determine the true extent of missing data, since the 'total' sample size typically reported is *after* this step. Such pre-filtering may or may not be well intended, but it is clear that it does not facilitate understanding or appraisal. It effectively tells readers 'There is no missing data problem to deal with now that all patients with missing data have been eliminated' (Çay *et al.*, 2021).

What is needed for reporting is rather difficult to say for any specific case. However, the goal is clear: readers should be able to find sufficient detail (across the primary report and supplementary material) that, if they were given the data, they could reproduce the analysis. Useful suggestions are given by Sterne *et al.* (2009). A natural structure is reporting the decisions made for each of the subheadings in Section 14.1 along with their rationale.

14.4 Presenting incomplete baseline data

Most analysis reports begin with a data summary. The idea is to give readers an understanding of the makeup of the dataset and provide context for the subsequent analyses. Indeed, beginning with descriptive results is a common theme in reporting guidelines relating to ætiological and prognostic research.

We advised in Section 14.1 that imputed data be checked before fitting the substantive model. The aim is to identify obvious unexplained issues with the imputation model. For example a contextually substantial discrepancy between observed and imputed values should be explainable either due to MAR or through an imputation method that deliberately causes this (e.g. as part of sensitivity analysis). However, we emphasised in Chapter 1 that the purpose of multiple imputation is not to recover the missing values, and so checking the imputations is only an informal procedure for flagging possible issues.

Before describing the observed data, it is good practice to summarise the proportions and patterns of missing data. That is, it is useful to know the amount of missingness in each variable and the frequency of certain combinations of missing values. For example, if an oncology study includes several tumour measurements, then these may always be missing together. In particular, *UpSet plots* provide a clear visualisation of missing data frequencies according to missing data pattern. An example is given in Figure 14.1 using the fictional 'heart attack data' from Stata's `mi` help files (StataCorp, 2021b) and created using the R package `naniar` Tierney *et al.* (2021), Tierney and Cook (2018). Each vertical bar depicts the frequency (not percentage) of a given missing data pattern ('intersection'), with the particular pattern visualised by the black dots below the bar. When black dots are connected vertically, this indicates a pattern in which two or more variables are missing at the same time. The horizontal bars to the left of the variable names give the frequency (not %) of missing data for that variable.

In trials with missing outcome data, the question arises as to how to summarise the data beyond describing missingness. A typical 'table 1' contains summaries of baseline data for each randomised arm, and sometimes overall as well. The purpose is to reassure readers about randomisation; it should demonstrate that the groups were exchangeable at baseline. With incomplete outcome data, we have to decide whether to present baseline summary data for all randomised individuals or only those whose outcome was observed. Both may be informative: it is quite possible for 'table 1' to appear reassuring among those randomised but concerning when we restrict to individuals with observed outcomes. Such imbalance implies that data are not MCAR, but may be consistent with outcomes missing at random due to an interaction between

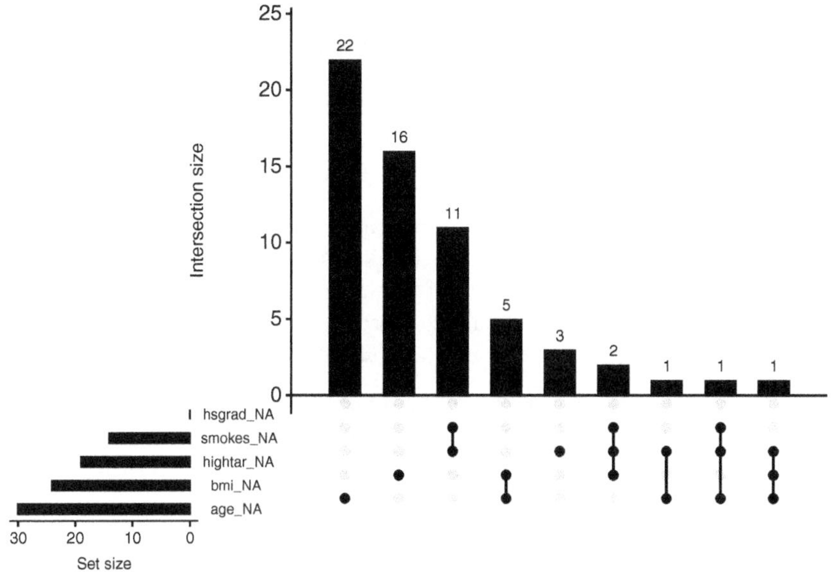

Figure 14.1 An UpSet *plot for the fictional 'heart attack data'; details in the text.*

randomised arm and/or covariates and/or intermediate outcomes. Variables predictive of the missing outcomes should be adjusted for in the substantive model and/or included as an auxiliary variables in any imputation model. Similar considerations apply to observational studies, except for the expectation that distributions of baseline variables are the same across exposure groups.

When either outcomes or baseline covariates are to be imputed, the interpretation of descriptive summaries may differ among the available records (all data available for that variable), complete records, and imputed data. Among the available records and the complete records, we have a description of only a subset of the data that will contribute to the substantive model. We argue that summarising the available records on each variable is always appropriate, as described by what has been observed. Alongside this, it may be appropriate to summarise the observed and imputed data, especially if either (i) they differ materially, or (ii) the primary analysis uses multiple imputation.

14.5 Model diagnostics

Fitting a substantive model to complete data is ideally followed by a series of model diagnostics to evaluate the model assumptions and to identify any influential observations. The multiple imputation procedure presents specific challenges for such assessments (Marshall *et al.*, 2009; Vergouwe *et al.*, 2010; White *et al.*, 2011; Wood *et al.*, 2015). We recommend model diagnostics, say $\hat{Q}_k$, be calculated separately for each imputed dataset (or for the substantive model fitted to each imputed dataset). Then they should be checked and extreme values investigated – as would be done in the complete-data setting. While reporting space will typically limit a detailed description, checking of diagnostics should be mentioned.

In many cases, it may be useful to summarise the $\hat{Q}_k$ across the datasets. Care needs to be taken to use the appropriate form of Rubin's rules. Specifically:

(a) Diagnostics that take the form of parameter estimates (e.g. a time interaction parameter to test for non-proportionality in a Cox model) should be combined using the usual standard of Rubin's rules. As usual, estimators with a non-normal distribution should be appropriately transformed before combining (e.g. Fisher's z-transformation for correlations).

(b) Diagnostics that take the form of p-values may be combined using combination rules for p-values (p. 73); alternatively, the logistic transform of the p-values may be combined using Rubin's rules – it is not clear which is the best approach.

(c) Diagnostics that take the form of a likelihood ratio test may be combined using a version of Rubin's rules for likelihood ratio statistics (Subsection 2.5.4).

The literature suggests that the inferential properties of the versions of Rubin's rules for p-values and likelihood ratio tests are less good than for parameter estimates, and in particular may lack power. Therefore, if there is a choice, (a) should be used. Nevertheless, a non-significant combined diagnostic test across imputations, combined with exploration of any imputed datasets in which $\hat{Q}_k$ are extreme, provides useful reassurance that there are not major violations of the assumptions.

14.6 How many imputations?

When considering how to choose the number of imputations, the first key point is that a small number of imputations gives statistically *valid* inference, but could be inefficient compared with using a larger number. For example, under congenial MI, using Rubin's rules with $K = 5$ or $K = 500$ imputations will produce confidence intervals with the correct frequentist coverage but the former will be wider (on average) than the latter. The ability to get valid inference with a small number of imputations was a key advantage of MI when computational power was limited and remains an attraction when analysing very large datasets.

The difference between the confidence interval widths in the previous paragraph is due to simulation error, termed *Monte Carlo* error. As we increase K, we reduce the Monte Carlo error.

To illustrate Monte Carlo error, we use the fictional 'heart attack data' from Stata's `mi` help files (StataCorp, 2021a). Using the imputation model and substantive model described in the Stata help files for `mi impute chained` and `mi estimate`, $K =$ 10 imputations were generated, twice over, using two different random number seeds.

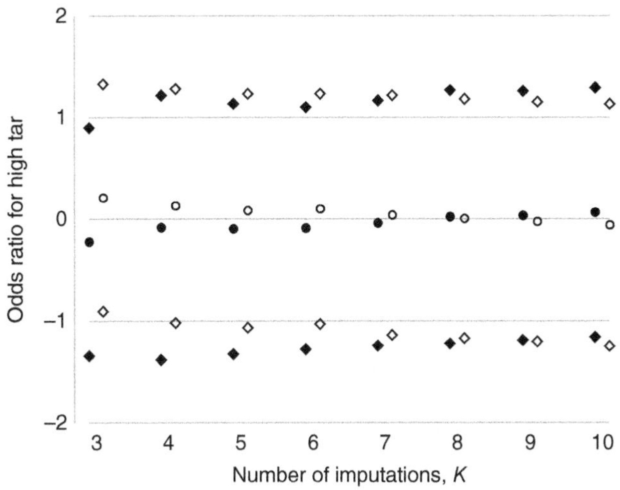

Figure 14.2 Illustration of Monte Carlo error in estimating the odds ratio and 95% confidence limits for 'high tar' smoking. The substantive model was fitted in turn to the first $K = 3, 4, \ldots, 10$ imputations, for two separate sets of 10 imputations. Key: solid symbols from the first set of 10 imputations, open symbols from the second; ∘, • – point estimates; ◇, ■ – 95% confidence limits.

Figure 14.2 displays the estimated odds ratio and 95% confidence interval for high-tar smoking on heart attack as a result of fitting the substantive model. We see that the estimated statistics move around as each new imputation is added, but that this is less pronounced as k increases. This is Monte Carlo error: the statistics oscillate around, and converge towards, their limiting values as $K \to \infty$. However, as the figure shows, after 10 imputations, there are still discrepancies in the odds ratios and confidence limits between the two sets of imputations.

Figure 14.2 helps clarify our aim in choosing K: we require a sufficient number of imputations that, were another analyst, starting with a different random number seed, to repeat the analysis, the discrepancy in their results would be suitably small. What is deemed 'suitably small' will depend on the user and the context. A pharmaceutical company using MI to analyse a clinical trial will want to ensure that the p-value corresponding to the treatment effect is estimated with very little noise if it is around the infamous 0.05 level. In contrast, in an analysis of a very large electronic health records database, where uncertainty (conditional on modelling assumptions) of estimates may be very small, this will be less of a concern.

Suppose, for some statistic $\hat{S}$ estimated by multiple imputation (e.g. parameter, standard error, or p-value), we have a corresponding estimate of the Monte-Carlo standard error, $\hat{\sigma}_{MC,S}$. Assuming the estimator of Monte Carlo error is consistent, repeating the MI analysis (using a different random number seed) and calculating $\hat{S} \pm 1.96\hat{\sigma}_{MC,S}$ would trap the infinite-K value of S 95% of the time. This may help guide the choice of K. For example, if we want to report an estimate reproducible to 1 decimal place, we need to choose K such that – at least – $1.96\hat{\sigma}_{MC,q} < 0.5$, i.e. $\hat{\sigma}_{MC,q} < 0.026$.

Towards this end, there have been various proposals for how to choose the number of imputations required; see Bodner (2008), White *et al.* (2011), and von Hippel (2020). The rule-of-thumb proposed by Bodner (2008) and explained by White *et al.* (2011) is simple and attractive: the number of imputations should be greater than or equal to the per cent of incomplete records. The justification is that, for a given statistic, the percentage of incomplete records is (typically) a conservative estimate of the fraction of missing information $\gamma \in (0,1)$ and, if a value of K is chosen such that $\gamma/K \leq 0.01$, we obtain Monte Carlo standard errors that are 'suitably low' for various statistics of interest (White *et al.*, 2011). Note that γ will vary from statistic to statistic: in applications we might, therefore, wish to use the largest value of γ across the range of statistics of interest.

Unfortunately, von Hippel (2020) pointed out that this 'linear' rule is incorrect because, for standard errors, the required value of K is a quadratic function of the fraction of missing information, $\gamma \in (0,1)$. To control the Monte Carlo SE for standard errors,

$$K = 1 + 0.5\left(\frac{\hat{\gamma}E[\widehat{\text{SE}}]}{\sqrt{\text{Var}[\widehat{\text{SE}}]}}\right)^2. \tag{14.1}$$

Since $\hat{\gamma}, E[\widehat{\text{SE}}], \text{Var}[\widehat{\text{SE}}]$ have to be estimated, von Hippel (2020) proposed the following two-step strategy:

1. Draw a small number of initial imputations to obtain estimates of $\hat{\gamma}, E[\widehat{\text{SE}}]$ and $\text{Var}[\widehat{\text{SE}}]$.
2. Plug these estimates in to equation (14.1) to determine the number of additional imputations required to control Monte Carlo SE.

Note that the fraction of missing information may itself be estimated with appreciable uncertainty. When γ is underestimated, this procedure will underestimate the number of imputations required; when it is overestimated, the procedure will produce more imputations than required. Therefore, as well as using the obvious estimate $\hat{\gamma}$, von Hippel (2020) suggested as a conservative strategy plugging the upper 95% confidence limit for $\hat{\gamma}$.

14.6.1 Using the jack-knife estimate of the Monte-Carlo standard error

In deciding on the required number of imputations, we regard obtaining a suitably small Monte Carlo error for key statistics of interest as the correct aim, because this allows the analyst to choose K such that their published results are accurate to the number of decimal places reported.

The key attractions of the proposal by Bodner (2008) are that it involves one stage and tends to be conservative. However, given that von Hippel (2020) showed it is not correct for standard errors, and proposed a two-stage procedure, we propose the following two-stage algorithm as the most direct approach to achieve the above aim:

1. Decide which statistics S (e.g. point estimates, p-values, CI limits) produced by fitting the substantive model are of central interest;
2. Produce a small initial number of imputations, say $K_{\text{init}} = 10$, fit the substantive model and use the jack-knife[1] to estimate $\widehat{\text{MCSE}}_{K_{\text{init}}}(\hat{S})$;
3. If $\widehat{\text{MCSE}}_{K_{\text{init}}}(\hat{S})$ is larger than desired, estimate the required number of imputations K_{req} by noting that $\text{MCSE}(\hat{S})$ is locally approximately proportional to $\sqrt{K^{-1}}$, so that if our target Monte Carlo standard error is $\text{MCSE}_{\text{target}}$,

$$\text{MCSE}_{\text{target}}(\hat{S}) \approx \frac{\sqrt{K_{\text{init}}}\widehat{\text{MCSE}}_{K_{\text{init}}}(\hat{S})}{\sqrt{K}}$$

suggesting that we should carry out a further

$$K_{\text{req}} = K - K_{\text{init}} = K_{\text{init}}\left(\frac{\widehat{\text{MCSE}}_{K_{\text{init}}}(\hat{S})}{\text{MCSE}_{\text{target}}(\hat{S})}\right)^2 - K_{\text{init}}$$

imputations;
4. Produce a further K_{req} imputations and re-estimate $\text{MCSE}(\hat{S})$, using all the $(K_{\text{init}} + K_{\text{req}})$ imputed datasets;
5. Repeat steps 3 and 4 as necessary until $\text{MCSE}_{\text{target}}(\hat{S})$ is achieved.

We emphasise this proposal has yet to be comprehensively evaluated relative to the two previous proposals; the final exercise in this chapter explores this further.

14.7 Multiple imputation for each substantive model, project, or dataset?

While this book has generally discussed *a* (singular) substantive model, most research projects or datasets will involve more than one. The question then arises as to how to approach multiple imputation. Consider the following three broad strategies:

1. Multiple imputation for each substantive model;
2. Multiple imputation for a specific project, such as a research paper;
3. Multiple imputation for a dataset.

[1] Available in Stata as option `mcerror` to the `mi estimate:` command (StataCorp, 2021b), with a beta version available for R available (Gasparini, 2022).

The first option will, perhaps, ensure the best answer to each question. Each substantive model can have its tailored imputation model and, in each case, we can produce a sufficient number of imputations for our conclusions to be reproducible (Section 14.6). This strategy may be too time-consuming in some settings. Further, when preparing descriptive tables (see Section 14.4), the analyst needs to decide, preferably *a priori*, which imputation model is most appropriate to use. This is because different imputation models will likely give rise to slightly different summaries – while these differences should be inconsequential, it is easy to envisage them causing readers to be confused or even suspicious.

The second option may be attractive if we intend to perform multiple analyses of a partially observed dataset using multiple imputation and do not wish to specify a different imputation model for each one – say to avoid introducing additional Monte Carlo error. However, it requires considerable care to choose the imputation model: we need to ensure it is sufficiently inclusive to support all the planned analyses. This requires a consideration of different outcome variables and covariates, different models, different linear predictors, and so on. For example, in the context of using substantive model-compatible imputation, Bartlett *et al.* (2015b) suggested that imputation of missing covariates could be performed compatible with a rich (flexible) outcome model, with the idea that a range of different nested substantive models can then be fitted to the resulting set of imputed datasets.

If we wish to do sensitivity analyses and avoid any further imputation, the weighting approach described in Section 10.6 is natural. For continuous data, pattern mixture 'δ-method' sensitivity analyses (Section 10.3) do not require further imputation, but further imputation is required for categorical data (Subsection 10.3.1).

In the survey setting – for which multiple imputation was originally conceived – Rubin envisaged the third option, with multiply imputed datasets being created by an 'imputer' to be released to multiple 'analysts' (Rubin, 1987). This may be reasonable for fairly simple datasets with a small number of possible substantive model's. However, for datasets and/or substantive model's with any level of complexity, this places an unbearable burden on the imputer, who has to try to anticipate all possible analyses and impute in a way that accommodates them.

In practice, analysts who need to use such externally imputed datasets need to be provided with information about how the imputations were constructed. In light of this information, it is then the analyst's responsibility to judge whether it is sensible to fit their particular substantive model(s) to the imputed datasets.

14.8 Large datasets

Large datasets raise various issues for multiple imputation. These could be large cross-sectional datasets, but they could also be longitudinal with regular, or irregular observation times. We considered multi-level, or hierarchical, imputation models in Chapter 9. Here our focus is addressing issues raised by imputing a large number of variables simultaneously, rather than those specifically raised by hierarchical/ multi-level structure.

We first consider these issues in the context of joint modelling, and then in the context of FCS.

14.8.1 Large datasets and joint modelling

Consider joint multivariate normal modelling first, so that either all the variables are continuous, or they are being treated as continuous for the purpose of imputation. The key difficulty which is likely to arise is an ill-conditioned covariance matrix, whose determinant is close to zero. This can arise when:

1. two or more variables are highly correlated; and/or
2. the number of variables is 'large' relative to the number of observations.

The first cause can be dealt with relatively easily; after removing any variables that are structurally dependent on others, we can calculate the sample correlation matrix of the data, taking care to use all available data to estimate each pairwise correlation, and remove variables that have a correlation of above 0.9, say. For the general treatment of such problems see Hansen (1998).

The second potential problem is that there are p means and $p(p+1)/2$ variance/covariance parameters with the p-variate normal, and issues of both statistical precision and numerical stability arise in its estimation. As far as precision is concerned, a good rule of thumb is that the unstructured covariance matrix will perform well compared with more parsimoniously parameterised alternatives provided $n > 10p$ (see Section 5.6 of Molenberghs and Kenward, 2007). If there are concerns about the numerical stability of the covariance matrix estimator, then it is helpful to monitor the convergence to identify potential ill-conditioning. When there are such problems, there are two broad approaches which can be taken:

1. increase the diagonal terms; and/or
2. set some off-diagonal terms of the inverse to zero.

Approach 1 has a long history and is known as ridge regression (Hoerl and Kennard, 1970), and see Schafer (1997) p. 155–156 for a discussion in the MI context. For the imputation of quantitative data, recall from p. 110 that the update step for the precision matrix $\mathbf{\Omega}^{-1}$ with prior $\text{W}(\nu, \mathbf{S}_P)$ is

$$f(\mathbf{\Omega}^{-1}|\boldsymbol{\beta}, \mathbf{Y}) \sim \text{W}\left[n+\nu, \left\{\mathbf{S}_P^{-1} + \sum_{i=1}^{n}(\mathbf{Y}_i - \boldsymbol{\beta})(\mathbf{Y}_i - \boldsymbol{\beta})^T\right\}^{-1}\right].$$

Under ridge regression, for a chosen scalar $\lambda > 0$, this becomes

$$f(\boldsymbol{\Omega}^{-1}|\boldsymbol{\beta}, \mathbf{Y}) \sim \mathrm{W}\left[n + \nu, \left\{ \mathbf{S}_P^{-1} + \sum_{i=1}^{n} (\mathbf{Y}_i - \boldsymbol{\beta})(\mathbf{Y}_i - \boldsymbol{\beta})^T + \lambda \boldsymbol{I}_p \right\}^{-1}\right], \tag{14.2}$$

where $\boldsymbol{I}_p$ is the p-dimensional identity matrix. An alternative proposal of Schafer (1997), p. 156, is as follows: let $\mathbf{S} = \sum_{i=1}^{n} (\mathbf{Y}_i - \boldsymbol{\beta})(\mathbf{Y}_i - \boldsymbol{\beta})^T$ and let $\mathbf{S}^{\star}$ be a matrix with diagonal elements $\mathbf{S}^{\star}_{ii} = \mathbf{S}_{ii}$, and off diagonal elements $\mathbf{S}^{\star}_{ij} = 0$, $i \neq j$. Then replace (14.2) by

$$f(\boldsymbol{\Omega}^{-1}|\boldsymbol{\beta}, \mathbf{Y}) \sim \mathrm{W}\left[n + \nu, \left\{ \mathbf{S}_P^{-1} + \left(\frac{\lambda}{n+\lambda}\right) \mathbf{S}^{\star} + \left(\frac{n}{n+\lambda}\right) \mathbf{S} \right\}^{-1}\right].$$

We choose λ large enough so that this empirical prior stabilises the covariance matrix by down-weighting the off-diagonal terms.

In linear regression with covariates, one can show (Hoerl and Kennard, 1970) that ridge regression is equivalent to minimising the sum of squared residuals, subject to the constraint that the sum of the squared regression parameters is less than a constant. The greater the λ, the smaller the absolute values of β.

In multiple imputation, the usual guidance is to err on the side of complexity in building imputation models, in the expectation that this will recover more information from the data about the distribution of the missing values. Unlike the final model, the imputation model does not aim at a parsimonious description of the data. Consistent with this, it is appropriate to choose λ large enough to allow stable estimates of $\boldsymbol{\beta}$, without imposing marked shrinkage.

Ridge regression is attractive for imputation with a large number of variables, since we only have one shrinkage parameter. In contrast the methods below require specification of which coefficients or elements of $\boldsymbol{\beta}$, should be estimated and which set to zero.

Under the joint modelling approach, with a mix of variable types, categorical and ordinal variables impose constraints on the covariance matrix. In this setting, we might impose ridge shrinkage on the part of the covariance matrix for the continuous covariates. In practice, this is most easily done by re-ordering the data so that the q continuous variables come first and correspond to the top $q \times q$ submatrix of $\boldsymbol{\Omega}$. Then we add $\lambda \tilde{\boldsymbol{I}}$ to instead of $\lambda \boldsymbol{I}_p$ in (14.2), where $\tilde{\boldsymbol{I}}$ has the first q diagonal elements 1 and the remaining elements 0.

14.8.2 Shrinkage by constraining parameters

The alternative approach to apply shrinkage to all the parameters, $\boldsymbol{\beta}$, is to explicitly specify which should be set equal to zero. In the FCS approach, for a variable $j \in 1, \dots, p$, this corresponds to specifying which of the $(p-1)$ covariates should be excluded when imputing $\mathbf{Y}_j$, i.e. excluded from the regression model with dependent variable $\mathbf{Y}_j$.

In joint modelling terms, this corresponds to constraining terms in the inverse covariance matrix to zero. For example, suppose we have $p = 5$ continuous variables and we constrain $\mathbf{\Omega}^{-1}$ so that

$$\mathbf{\Omega}^{-1} = \begin{pmatrix} \omega_{11} & \omega_{12} & \omega_{13} & 0 & 0 \\ \omega_{21} & \omega_{22} & \omega_{23} & \omega_{24} & 0 \\ \omega_{31} & \omega_{32} & \omega_{33} & \omega_{34} & \omega_{35} \\ 0 & \omega_{42} & \omega_{43} & \omega_{44} & \omega_{45} \\ 0 & 0 & \omega_{53} & \omega_{54} & \omega_{55} \end{pmatrix},$$

where as usual, the matrix is symmetric so $\omega_{ij} = \omega_{ji}$. When the non-zero terms follow this banded pattern, the resulting covariance matrix is said to have an antedependence structure, and such matrices play a role in the modelling of non-stationary time-ordered data (Zimmerman and Núnez-Antón, 2010).

This is equivalent to the following conditional specification:

$$Y_{i,1} = \beta_{0,1} + \beta_{1,1}Y_{i,2} + \beta_{3,1}Y_{i,3} + e_{i,1}, \quad e_{i,1} \overset{i.i.d.}{\sim} N(0, \sigma_1^2),$$

$$Y_{i,2} = \beta_{0,2} + \beta_{1,2}Y_{i,1} + \beta_{2,3}Y_{i,3} + \beta_{3,3}Y_{i,4} + e_{i,2}, \quad e_{i,1} \overset{i.i.d.}{\sim} N(0, \sigma_1^2),$$

$$Y_{i,3} = \beta_{0,3} + \beta_{1,3}Y_{i,1} + \beta_{2,3}Y_{i,2} + \beta_{3,3}Y_{i,4} + \beta_{4,3}Y_{i,5} + e_{i,3}, \quad e_{i,3} \overset{i.i.d.}{\sim} N(0, \sigma_3^2),$$

$$Y_{i,4} = \beta_{0,4} + \beta_{1,4}Y_{i,2} + \beta_{2,4}Y_{i,3} + \beta_{3,4}Y_{i,5} + e_{i,4}, \quad e_{i,4} \overset{i.i.d.}{\sim} N(0, \sigma_4^2),$$

$$Y_{i,5} = \beta_{0,5} + \beta_{1,5}Y_{i,3} + \beta_{2,5}Y_{i,4} + e_{i,5}, \quad e_{i,5} \overset{i.i.d.}{\sim} N(0, \sigma_5^2).$$

In applications, with FCS, we can either specify which coefficients are set to zero in advance, or we can use variable selection in an initial stage of the algorithm. Neither approach is wholly satisfactory with large datasets. For example, for imputing a questionnaire with 100 questions, it is hard to know in advance which coefficients should be set to zero. Conversely, we should be wary of selection based on significance tests. One approach is to use non-parametric methods which impose shrinkage, see Shah *et al.* (2014), and for a promising application of the Bayesian lasso Zhao and Long (2016).

In longitudinal data, the temporal element can be used to resolve some of these issues. If we have k variables at waves $1, 2, \ldots, t$, (e.g. annual follow-up) when imputing wave t we can restrict to data from wave $t - 1, t, t + 1$. This leads to Nevalainen *et al.* (2009)'s proposal for 'twofold' MI:

1. at time $t = 1$, use FCS to impute the k variables, using as covariates (but not imputing) the k variables at time $t = 2$;

2. for times $t = 2, \ldots, t - 1$: use FCS to impute the k variables, using as covariates (but not imputing) the k variables at time $t - 1$ and the k variables at time $t + 1$; and

3. at time t, use FCS to impute the k variables, using (but not imputing) the k variables from time $t - 1$.

FCS at each time t is run for C_w 'within' time cycles, and the whole algorithm is run for C_a 'among' (or 'across') time cycles. The 'window' of time, which is $t \pm 1$ above, can clearly be made wider, and/or only a selection of the k covariates available at any specific time are included in certain imputation models.

Nevalainen *et al.* (2009) report the results of a simulation study with three time points and a mix of variable types, where the algorithm imputes with minimal bias and good coverage; they advise that C_w should be an order of magnitude greater than C_a; for example 10 within cycles and 5 across cycles.

Welch *et al.* (2014) explore the application for imputation of general practice patient record data, as illustrated in Figure 14.3. Here, over the time period of interest, patients may register with the practice, and leave the practice. While certain key health variables, such as smoking and alcohol use, blood pressure, and weight should be measured at registration, and subsequently, very often some or all of them are missing, particularly for relatively healthy patients. They apply the algorithm above, imputing individuals' clinical measurements using a measurement in a surrounding window. This avoids issues with overfitting the imputation model. Strictly following the approach of Nevalainen *et al.* (2009), the imputation window is only run forward through the dataset; however, it may be advantageous to run it forwards and backwards through the data. A comprehensive simulation study reported by Welch *et al.* (2014) shows promising performance. It suggests that longitudinal correlations beyond the 'window width' (e.g. if the window with is one year, correlations between blood pressure measurements at 2,3, … years) can be recovered with small bias, but substantially more imputations are required for convergence – a finding highlighted

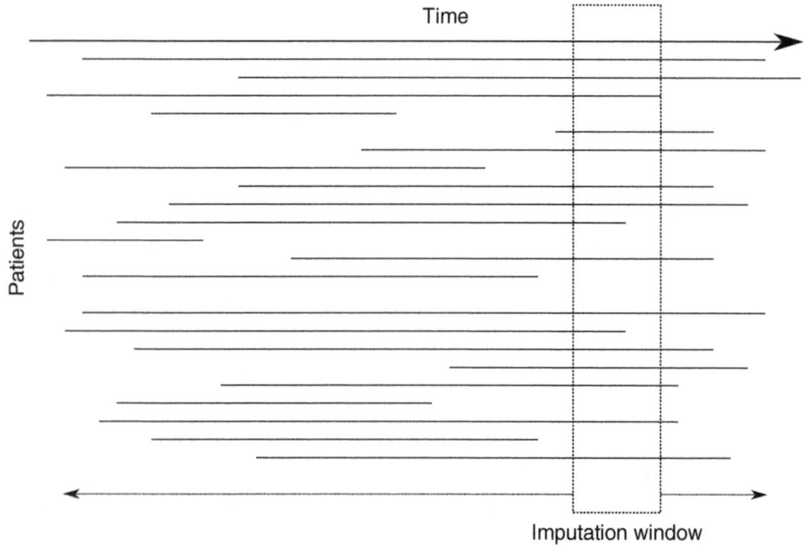

Figure 14.3 Schematic for imputation of longitudinal clinical record data using approach of Nevalainen et al. *(2009).*

by Kalaycioglu *et al.* (2015). In particular, unlike in the three-timepoint setting considered by Nevalainen *et al.* (2009), C_a should now be an order of magnitude greater than C_w : for a one-year time window: say $C_a = 30$ and $C_w = 10$.

An alternative approach, which to our knowledge has not been explored, is to 'rotate' the window in Figure 14.3. Thus, we model longitudinal measurements for each variable (or group of variables) in turn (say weight, blood pressure, smoking history) conditional on the others; we then cycle round the variables in turn, in the manner of FCS. Each imputation model now needs to be a multi-level imputation model. Such multi-level imputation models are discussed in Chapter 9.

14.8.3 Comparison of the two approaches

Shrinkage using the Ridge parameter λ in univariate linear regression can be shown to shrink with respect to the orthonormal basis formed by the principal components. Furthermore, components with the smallest variance are shrunk more. Applying such data-based shrinkage to the multivariate imputation model thus seems preferable to the alternative approach of setting some coefficients to zero, unless time-ordering, or some other natural property of the data, point to likely coefficients. In the absence of this, ridge regression does, by its construction, concentrate shrinkage where it will have the least effect on prediction.

Note that we can also use ridge regression to stabilise each of the conditional regressions in FCS; this entails working out the steps for drawing the conditional variance and regression parameters consistent with the ridge parameter. However, this does not correspond directly to the joint modelling case. An attraction of applying shrinkage through the joint model is that it allows a unified approach across response types through the latent normal structure, in a way which that does not have a direct analogue in the FCS approach.

14.9 Multiple imputation and record linkage

In many social and health applications, we wish to link individual records across different databases; for example hospital and registry data, or different surveys. Typically, the aim is to add particular variables of interest to the data, for example date and cause of death to hospital records, or information on hospital episodes to general practice research databases.

If we wish to link individuals in a primary and secondary database, we first identify a set of variables, for example surname, date of birth and gender, available in both databases. Ideally, these would give a unique match for all individuals. Unfortunately, this is rarely the case due to errors and omissions in data recording. Individuals in the primary database without a unique match in the secondary database may be discarded from the analysis, or may be assigned their 'most likely' match. Assigning a single 'most likely' match does not reflect the uncertainty in the matching process, though.

An alternative, proposed by Goldstein *et al.* (2012), is to use *prior informed imputation* (PII) . The idea is that, for each individual in the primary database who does not have a unique match, we use the matching weights to calculate a prior distribution for the missing variable. Then, when we impute, we take this as the prior for our variable in the imputation model.

Specifically, suppose we wish to link a categorical variable, with possible values $m = 1, \dots, M$, from the secondary database. For individual i in the primary database, we suppose we have a set weights w_{ij} representing the plausibility of a match to individual j in the secondary database, normalised to sum to one. In the event of a perfect match of i and j', then $w_{ij'} = 1$ and the remaining weights are zero. For an imperfect match, a number of the weights will be non-zero.

Construction, or estimation, of the w_{ij} is a specialist area of its own; see for example Clark (2004), Jaro (1995). Essentially, suppose individual i in the primary database and j in the secondary database have a particular pattern p among the matching variables. Then we use individuals where we (i) are sure of a match, to estimate $P(p|\text{match})$, and (ii) are sure that there is no match, to estimate $P(p|\text{no match})$. The traditional record linkage procedure then computes $w_{ij} \propto \log_2\{\Pr(p|\text{match})/\Pr(p|\text{no match})\}$.

Assuming we have the w_{ij}, and recalling that the variable we wish to link from the secondary database is categorical with M levels, then for individual i, we compute the prior probability that the variable takes value m as

$$p_{im} = \sum_j w_{ij}\delta_{jm} \sum_j w_{ij} , \tag{14.3}$$

where $\delta_{jm} = 1$ if individual j in the secondary database has a value of m for the categorical variable to be linked, and 0 otherwise.

For each individual i in the primary database, we therefore have a prior for imputing the value from the secondary database. For a perfect match, this uniquely identifies one value; for an imperfect match, it gives a range of probable values. During imputation, we can either:

1. impute the missing value, ignoring the prior, using the current estimate of the distribution of the missing given the observed data (i.e. as in standard MI); or

2. impute the linked value by combining (14.3) with an imputation distribution estimated from the rest of the data.

Goldstein *et al.* (2012) point out that option 1 will work reasonably well for small amounts of unmatched data under the assumption of MAR. They comment that in practice, this will often be adequate. They caution, however, against doing this if it is suspected that the probability of a correct match is associated with the values of the variables in the secondary database being linked in. They suggest that in this case, option 2 will perform better. They further report describing the extension of this approach to handle continuous data and present a simulation study which gives promising results.

The advantage of this approach is that we can use multiple imputation to unify the handling of missing data and linkage, so that the analysis both increases the number of individuals contributing to the analysis (by including those with an uncertain link) and takes proper account of uncertainty in the linkage process. There is a natural link to measurement of error problems, where we can use external data to identify a probability distribution for an individual's underlying value of a variable, given their observed value (see Chapter 11).

14.10 Setting random number seeds for multiple imputation analyses

If multiple imputation were based on genuinely random numbers, Monte Carlo error means we would obtain a different result for analysis. In practice, software uses *pseudo*-random numbers to draw imputations. This means that we can set a 'seed' to determine the initial state of the pseudo-random number generator. By doing so, we can repeat a multiple imputation procedure twice and produce identical results, which is an advantage of pseudo-random numbers in terms of reproducibility and having an audit trail. It is always advisable to set the seed for a multiple imputation analysis. Any implementation of multiple imputation that does not permit seed-setting is of dubious quality.

Note that random number seeds do not map across software, so there is no correspondence between the random numbers produced after `set seed 1` in Stata and `set.seed(1)` in R. Further, exact reproducibility can also depend on software version, operating system, method of random number generation, that the dataset is sorted in the same order and (in unusual cases) that the variables are in the same order.

14.11 Simulation studies including multiple imputation

14.11.1 Random number seeds for simulation studies including multiple imputation

In the context of simulation studies that include multiple imputation, some care needs to be taken about setting the seed to ensure not only (i) the set of simulations is reproducible but also (ii) the simulated data and the imputation analysis have the correct variability.

Consider the following pseudocode:

```
SET RandomSeed to A
FOR Repetition 1 to n_reps by 1
  SIMULATE Incomplete Dataset
  SET RandomSeed to B
  MULTIPLY_IMPUTE
  ...
END FOR
```

During repetition 1, the seed is set to `B` just after simulating the incomplete data. At the start of each subsequent repetition, the seed will be the same. Thus, the simulation study will contain $n_{\text{reps}} - 1$ identical simulated datasets and multiple imputation analysis. We have seen this issue missed when checking simulation code.

The solution is to avoid setting the random number seed anywhere within the loop, such as prior to conducting multiple imputation within a simulation study. The initial setting of the seed to `A` outside of the simulation loop ensures reproducibility in this context.

However, it is desirable to *record* the state of the random number generator before each iteration. This means that, after the simulation has run (or if it unexpectedly crashes at any point), specific incomplete datasets and corresponding imputation analyses can be re-run and examined in detail; see Morris *et al.* (2019). Note that Stata will return the state immediately prior to multiple imputation as `r(rngstate)`.

Thus, our preferred pseudocode is

```
SET RandomSeed to A
FOR Repetition 1 to n_reps by 1
  RECORD random_number_state
  GENERATE Incomplete Dataset
  MULTIPLY_IMPUTE
  ...
END FOR
```

Alternatively, it may be more practical to generate and save n_{reps} partially observed datasets separately to imputing each of them – but again, the same seed should not be used for each imputation analysis.

14.11.2 Repeated simulation of all data or only the missingness mechanism?

In simulation studies which evaluate the properties of analysis methods to handle missing data, authors typically simulate a complete dataset, then simulate the missing data indicators (a selection model approach). The latter are applied to the complete data to produce an incomplete dataset. The procedure is repeated n_{reps} times. Some authors consider that – because the aim of their simulation study is to investigate methods for handling missing data – it is sufficient to generate a *single* complete dataset before simulating the missing values n_{reps} times. Examples include Brand *et al.* (2003) and Rodwell *et al.* (2014).

This approach should not be used in general. It is only justifiable when the complete-data analysis is known to have good performance and interest is *only* in bias of methods (such as a complete records, or MI analysis) caused by missing data. In this case, the bias of various procedures to handle missing data can then be estimated and attributed to these procedures.

More generally, when the aim is to evaluate the frequentist inferential properties of a procedure (accuracy of model-based variance estimates, confidence interval coverage, etc.) it will give the wrong answers.

To see why, note that as part of our simulation study, we will usually want to look at the performance of the complete-data estimation method (i.e. before data are made missing). Suppose the complete-data estimator has good frequentist performance: it is unbiased, efficient, and confidence intervals have 95% coverage. If we fix the complete data across repetitions, then:

(a) The complete data analysis will have estimated coverage of either 100% or 0% – because the confidence interval constructed for the complete data analysis will be identical across repetitions and so either include the true parameter value in all repetitions or in none. In other words, if we were to replicate the whole simulation study, coverage would be estimated to be 100% with 95% probability or 0% with 5% probability. Because this approach cannot assess the inferential properties of the complete data analysis, it cannot assess the inferential properties of any analysis method applied to the partially observed data.

(b) We cannot compare the efficiency of methods for handling missing data with the efficiency of the complete data analysis. This is because, as the complete data analysis will have estimated variance of zero, any methods for handling missing data will by definition have greater or equal variance. This sounds superficially reasonable, but it is not. Meng (1994) and Rubin (1996) give examples in which multiple imputation procedures possess the *superefficiency* property, meaning that they are more efficient than the complete data procedure. When the variance of the complete data procedure is artificially fixed to zero, superefficiency will go undetected.

14.11.3 How many imputations for simulation studies?

Simulation studies that include multiple imputation methods frequently use a fixed, small, number of imputations (often $K = 5$ or 10) within each repetition. The primary reason is to reduce computational time. Given that multiple imputation is computationally intensive, and that simulation studies involve hundreds to millions of repetitions, this is an important consideration. However, using few imputations does not seem to follow the advice in Section 14.6. Is this a contradiction?

Using a relatively small number of imputations in simulation studies may often be appropriate. This is because multiple imputation inferences (point estimates, standard errors, p-values, and confidence intervals) are valid with a small number of imputations. So if the simulation study is investigating the inferential properties of MI in a particular setting, the results about bias and coverage will be stochastically equivalent with $K = 5$ or $K = 500$.

While the above is correct, it arguably misses an important point and may make MI appear inefficient relative to other procedures. To illustrate this, suppose a simulation study investigates two incomplete data proportions: 0.25 and 0.5. We assume that these proportions are roughly equal to the fraction of missing information γ for the parameter estimate of interest. For multiple imputation, we plan to use

$K = 5$ imputations. In Chapter 2, we discussed the relative efficiency of K versus ∞ imputations (see equation (2.28) and Figure 2.1). In this case, the relative per cent efficiency of $K = 5$ imputations is

$$100 \times \left(1 + \frac{\gamma}{5}\right)^{-1},$$

which is 95% of full efficiency for $\gamma = 0.25$ and just 91% for $\gamma = 0.5$. So using a small number of imputations in a simulation study will make MI appear inefficient relative to other procedures (the empirical standard errors would be large), but it would be a mistake to attribute this to the multiple imputation method – it is a consequence of choosing a small value of K.

This point does not mean it is wrong to use a small number of imputations, but that the choice of K should be considered and justified. If the simulation study is designed to show the performance of a multiple imputation procedure in settings where computing resource constraints are an issue, a low number of imputations may be justified. If the simulation study aims to compare multiple imputation with maximum likelihood estimation, many imputations may be required, because formal equivalence between MI and maximum likelihood estimation requires $K \to \infty$. It may be desirable to control the relative efficiency (2.28) of using MI across different values of FMI, in which case K will need to be changed across settings. In the above example, supposing we wish to have 0.99 relative efficiency, then this would require $K = 25$ for 0.25 missing and $K = 50$ for 0.5 missing.

14.11.4 Multiple imputation for data simulation

A common challenge faced by researchers planning simulation studies is how to simulate data with a 'realistic' structure which mimics some real data. The approach we outline below exploits key aspects of the monotone FCS MI algorithm for multivariate imputation. It is related to the approach of Audigier *et al.* (2018); see also Welch *et al.* (2014).

The underlying idea is to build up the full distribution through a series of conditional steps, beginning with a univariate marginal distribution. For a dataset that itself contains missing values, some initial step is needed, such as restricting to the complete cases or using a single imputation method to impute the missing values. Note that some of the variables may be fixed or resampled with replacement into the simulated dataset.

We illustrate with a simple example. Suppose we have a fixed variable and wish to simulate a $n_{\text{obs}} \times 3$ dataset with four variables, X which is a covariate to be fixed, and (Y_1, Y_2, Y_3), which will be simulated. The approach is as follows:

1. Take the real dataset and add n_{obs} empty rows.
2. Decide on the conditional sequence for simulating the data. Any fixed variable such as X will be populated first. The subsequent sequence should (i) keep the conditional models as simple as possible, and (ii) ideally use conditional

models whose appropriateness can readily be contextually confirmed (e.g. in a medical setting by checking the effects of age are correct).
Models may be used such as multinomial logistic regression for unordered categorical variables, predictive mean matching for positively bounded or skewed variables, and so on.
In our example, we will generate $Y_1|X$, then $Y_2|Y_1, X$, and then $Y_3|Y_1, Y_2, X$.

3. Fit the chosen models and estimate their parameters for the regression of Y_1 on X the regression of Y_2 on Y_1, X and the regression of Y_3 on Y_1, Y_2, X.

4. Use maximum-likelihood multiple imputation to fill in the n_{sim} blank values of Y_1, then $Y_2|Y_1$ and finally $Y_3|Y_1, Y_2$.

5. Detach the original dataset and proceed with the $n_{\text{obs}} \times 3$ simulated dataset.

Maximum likelihood multiple imputation is necessary to ensure that the 'true' values of parameters from which data are simulated are the same across repetitions. It can be implemented in the `mice` R package with `mice.impute.norm.nob` and in Stata's `ice` command using the '`nodraw`' option (it does not seem to be available in Stata's `mi impute`).

14.12 Discussion

A key point of Chapter 1 was that missing data introduces additional ambiguity into inferences. This ambiguity entails additional assumptions. The focus of this book has been showing how to use MI to obtain valid inferences – in a wide range of settings – under plausible assumptions about the distribution of the missing data. Readily available MI software means that multiple imputation analyses are now computationally easy – but it is important to remember a good MI analysis is a thought-intensive (as well as a computer-intensive) process. When applied carelessly, it is possible for multiple imputation create more bias than an inappropriate complete records analysis, even when data are missing at random; cautionary tales can be found in Tilling *et al.* (2016) and Morris *et al.* (2014b).

Therefore, this chapter has highlighted a number of general issues relating to the application of MI for data analysis and simulation studies. For the former, the discussion underlined the importance of analysts critically evaluating their assumptions and models, alongside careful consideration of the data (in particular, how it was collected) and the broader research context. Of course, this does not guarantee valid inferences, but it should dramatically reduce the risk of major errors and improve the quality, transparency, reporting, and reproducibility of multiple imputation analyses.

Exercises

The following exercises are intended to stimulate reflection and discussion about the application of MI. Therefore, there are no 'correct' answers.

1. Consider some objections to multiple imputation and write down an explanation of why they are either well founded, unfounded, or context-dependent. For example:
   - 'Multiple imputation is "making up data".'
   - 'If results from statistical analyses obtained from multiple imputation differ substantially from those of complete records analysis, the results of multiple imputation must be wrong.'
   - 'Multiple imputation can be used only when data are missing completely at random.'
   - 'Multiple imputation of baseline variables should not use information from variables measured in the future (later in time).'
2. Take a 'completed' multiple imputation analysis from one of the earlier exercises in the book (e.g. Chapter 6) and assume you are reporting it in a research article. In your answer, emphasise clarity over brevity (assuming that your report will be included in the article's supplementary material, which is not covered by a word limit).
   (a) Write out your methods in sufficient detail that you think someone with your dataset but without your code could replicate your multiple imputation analysis.
   (b) As well as explaining *what* you did, provide the rationale for each choice.
3. Search a journal from your field for the term *multiple imputation* and pick a research paper.
   (a) How much detail was given regarding the methods they used? Supposing you had their dataset and code to fit the substantive model. How confident would you be of replicating their imputation analysis?
   (b) If you would not be confident in being able to replicate their multiple imputation analyses, what further details would you require?
   (c) Did authors give the rationale for their imputation modelling choices? Did they consider sensitivity analysis? Do you think their inferences are valid?
4. Section 14.6 described two existing rules for choosing the number of imputations K. The first (linear rule) is due to Bodner (2008) and further justified by White *et al.* (2011); the second (two-step quadratic rule) is due to Von Hippel (2009). We proposed a third in Section 14.6.1, based directly on the Monte Carlo standard error of a statistic. In this exercise, we compare how these rules perform using an example dataset (for example the fictional heart attack data available from the Stata website (StataCorp, 2021a).
   The aim of the exercise is to see which approach gives the most reproducible answers, i.e. having chosen the number of decimal places to which the MI analysis for a particular statistic should be reproducible, which approach leads to a choice of K which achieves this?

The last three columns in the dataset are variables created by Stata when you set the data up for imputation. These are Stata variables that can be deleted or ignored in the imputation process if using other software.
The substantive model used in the Stata help files is a logistic regression with binary outcome `attack` and covariates `smokes`, `age`, `bmi`, `hightar`, `hsgrad`, and `female`, with continuous covariates treated as linear. For this exercise, choose a particular statistic to focus on, such as the estimated standard error for a certain parameter, or a p-value.

(a) Draw the number of imputations corresponding to the linear rule, i.e. having specified an imputation model, draw K imputations equal to the percentage of incomplete cases.

(b) Now implement the von Hippel (2020) two-step quadratic rule based on the point estimate of γ (see equation (14.1)), i.e. draw a small initial number of imputations K^{init} (say five), fit the substantive model to estimate the FMI, γ, estimate the total number of imputations needed. K^{total} and draw ($K^{\text{total}} - 5$) more.

(c) Now implement the new proposal for a two-step rule, i.e. draw the same number of imputations K^{init} as above but, instead of estimating FMI, estimate the Monte Carlo standard errors for statistics of your substantive model (in Stata, this is easily done with the `mcerror` option for `mi estimate:`). As before, estimate how many more imputations are needed and draw this number to give K^{total}.

Compare the three methods above in terms of the total number of imputations. Recall that the first method is deterministic but the latter two are subject to Monte Carlo error because they rely on an initial estimate which itself was subject to Monte Carlo error (which may be conservative or liberal). For all three methods, change the random number seed and repeat.

(a) How different are the estimated total numbers of imputations?

(b) Consider your chosen statistic: to how many decimal places do the estimates, obtained from the original and repeated analyses, agree?

(c) Is any rule too liberal, *i.e.*, suggests a value of K that turns out to be too low in the sense that the estimated Monte Carlo standard error after K imputations is bigger or smaller than the desired value?

Appendix A

Markov Chain Monte Carlo

Here we briefly describe two Markov Chain Monte Carlo (MCMC) methods for drawing samples from a Bayesian posterior. For a detailed discussion of MCMC methods and their application, we refer the reader to Gilks *et al.* (1996) and Gelman *et al.* (1995).

Suppose we have observed data $\mathbf{Y}$ (typically n observations on q variables), and we have a statistical model which gives a likelihood for the data given parameter $\boldsymbol{\theta}$. In frequentist inference, we typically write this $f(\mathbf{Y};\boldsymbol{\theta})$, denoting the probability distribution of the data $\mathbf{Y}$ at the particular parameter value $\boldsymbol{\theta}$. However, in Bayesian inference, the parameters themselves are random variables, so it is more convenient to write $f(\mathbf{Y}|\boldsymbol{\theta})$ when we are thinking about the distribution of $\mathbf{Y}$ given $\boldsymbol{\theta}$, and $f(\boldsymbol{\theta}|\mathbf{Y})$ when we are thinking about the distribution of $\boldsymbol{\theta}$ given $\mathbf{Y}$.

For example, if we have $Y_i \overset{i.i.d.}{\sim} N(\theta, 1)$, $i \in (1, \dots, n)$, then $f(\mathbf{Y}|\theta) \sim N(\theta \boldsymbol{1}_n, \boldsymbol{I}_n)$ and $f(\theta|\mathbf{Y}) \sim N(\overline{Y}, n^{-1})$. More generally, f is the multivariate normal model for $\mathbf{Y}$, with unstructured mean and covariance, as in (3.4).

Suppose we have a prior distribution for $\boldsymbol{\theta}$, denoted $f(\boldsymbol{\theta}|\boldsymbol{\gamma})$, where $\boldsymbol{\gamma}$ are the parameters of the prior distribution, chosen by the analyst. For simplicity, we suppress these in the following, writing $f(\boldsymbol{\theta})$ for the prior.

Then, under Bayes theorem, the posterior distribution of the parameters given the data, $f(\boldsymbol{\theta}|\mathbf{Y})$, is given by

$$f(\boldsymbol{\theta}|\mathbf{Y}) = \frac{f(\mathbf{Y}|\boldsymbol{\theta})f(\boldsymbol{\theta})}{\int f(\mathbf{Y}|\boldsymbol{\theta})f(\boldsymbol{\theta})\, d\boldsymbol{\theta}} \propto f(\mathbf{Y}|\boldsymbol{\theta})f(\boldsymbol{\theta}). \tag{A.1}$$

For certain choices of likelihood and prior, when $\mathbf{Y}$ is fully observed, the posterior distribution can be calculated exactly. More commonly, we will be unable to derive the posterior analytically. However, using a technique known as MCMC, we can set up an iterative sampling algorithm to draw a sequence – known as a chain – of

Multiple Imputation and its Application, Second Edition.
James R. Carpenter, Jonathan W. Bartlett, Tim P. Morris, Angela M. Wood, Matteo Quartagno and Michael G. Kenward.

parameter values $\boldsymbol{\theta}^0, \boldsymbol{\theta}^1, \dots, \boldsymbol{\theta}^r, \dots$ whose stationary distribution is the posterior distribution (A.1). Thus, running this algorithm from initial values, after discarding the early values of the chain – known as the 'burn in' – we end up with a (correlated) sample from the posterior. We can use this sample to estimate aspects of the posterior distribution of interest (e.g. mean, mode, variance).

We now describe two algorithms for setting up the chain $\boldsymbol{\theta}^0, \boldsymbol{\theta}^1, \dots, \boldsymbol{\theta}^r, \dots$; a general algorithm, known as the Metropolis Hastings sampler, and a special case called the Gibbs sampler.

A.1 Metropolis Hastings sampler

Recall that the parameter vector is $\boldsymbol{\theta} = (\theta_1, \theta_2, \dots, \theta_p)^T$. Let $\boldsymbol{\theta}_{-j} = (\theta_1, \dots, \theta_{j-1}, \theta_{j+1}, \dots, \theta_p)^T$, i.e. the parameter vector with parameter θ_j removed.

The algorithm proceeds as follows:

1. Choose initial values for each element of $\boldsymbol{\theta}$ and denote these $\boldsymbol{\theta}^0$.
2. At update step $r = 1, 2, \dots,$ initially set $\boldsymbol{\theta}^r = \boldsymbol{\theta}^{r-1}$. Then, for $j = 1, \dots, p$ in turn:
   (a) Sample a proposed new value for θ_j^r from an appropriate proposal distribution, $\theta_j^{r*} \sim f(\theta | \theta_j^r, \boldsymbol{\theta}_{-j}^r)$.
   (b) calculate the acceptance probability
   $$p = \min\left(1, \frac{\{f(\mathbf{Y}|\theta_j^{r*}, \boldsymbol{\theta}_{-j}^r)f(\theta_j^{r*}, \boldsymbol{\theta}_{-j}^r)\}f(\theta_j^r|\theta_j^{r*}, \boldsymbol{\theta}_{-j}^r)}{\{f(\mathbf{Y}|\theta_j^r, \boldsymbol{\theta}_{-j}^r)f(\theta_j^r, \boldsymbol{\theta}_{-j}^r)\}f(\theta_j^{r*}|\theta_j^r, \boldsymbol{\theta}_{-j}^r)}\right) \quad \text{(A.2)}$$
   then draw $u \sim$ uniform $[0, 1]$ and accept θ^* if $u < p$, in other words, accept the proposal with probability p.
   (c) If the proposal is accepted, replace the current value of θ_j^r of $\boldsymbol{\theta}^r$ with the proposal, θ_j^{r*}; otherwise, retain the current value.
   (d) Return to step 2(a) to update the next element of the parameter vector.

The term
$$\frac{f(\theta_j^r|\theta_j^{r*}, \boldsymbol{\theta}_{-j}^r)}{f(\theta_j^{r*}|\theta_j^r, \boldsymbol{\theta}_{-j}^r)}$$
in (A.2) is known as the Hastings ratio.

Two kinds of proposal distribution are common in practice: (i) where the proposal distribution is a marginal distribution for θ_j, so that no conditioning is involved, and (ii) where the proposal distribution is symmetric, so that $f(\theta_j^r|\theta_j^{r*}) = f(\theta_j^{r*}|\theta_j^r)$. In the latter case, the Hastings ratio is 1. In almost every setting in this book, we create proposals by drawing $\Delta^* \sim N(0, \sigma^2)$ and then setting $\theta_j^{r*} = \theta_j^r + \Delta^*$. This means that $f(\theta_j^{r*}|\theta_j^r) = f(\Delta^*) = f(-\Delta^*) = f(\theta_j^r|\theta_j^{r*})$, so that the Hastings ratio is 1.

In applications, it is good practice to plot θ_j^r against r for each parameter $j = 1, \dots, p$ to check the sampler has passed the 'burn in' phase and that it is 'mixing' (i.e. exploring the posterior distribution) well. If the sampler is still in the burn-in phase, i.e. moving towards the stationary posterior distribution, then one or more of these will show a trend in the mean of θ_j^r with r. Once the stationary distribution has been reached, the graphs should show random variation but no trend.

If we have a good proposal distribution for a parameter, then it should update roughly 50% of the time, resulting in a chain with relatively low auto-correlation. If the proposal distribution has too great a variance, then the majority of the proposals will be rejected, and the chain will 'stick' and occasionally make larger jumps. Conversely, if the proposal distribution has too small a variance, the posterior distribution will only be explored slowly.

It is important to realise that the algorithm above will update even if the underlying model, $f(\mathbf{Y}|\boldsymbol{\theta})f(\boldsymbol{\theta})$ is wrongly specified (for example, by having the same covariate included twice, or in a multivariate response model including the same response variable twice). This is another reason for monitoring the chains, which typically quickly reveal that something is wrong.

Most software packages, including `REALCOM-impute`, have options for displaying the chains, and a number allow more formal diagnostic checks of the convergence of the sampler.

To improve the mixing of the sampler, it is useful to standardise continuous variables to have mean 0 and variance 1 before fitting the model. If this is done, we have found that a burn in of 1000 is typically sufficient, with updates of 500–1000 between drawing imputed datasets. Schafer (1997), p. 87 points out that slow convergence of the chains for one or more parameters when using the MCMC algorithm with missing data will likely indicate there is little information remaining in the observed data about that parameter. This in turn means that inference and imputed data are may be more dependent on the imputation model chosen. In practice, it may be helpful to use an expectation–maximisation (EM) algorithm to find starting values for the MCMC sampler for the imputation model, or where possible a direct (restricted) maximum likelihood fit of the imputation model, to highlight any such problems. Schafer (1997) gives appropriate EM algorithms for the multivariate normal model, the log-linear model for categorical data, and the general location model for a mix of categorical and multivariate normal data.

A.2 Gibbs sampler

If, in the update step, we are able to choose the proposal distribution for θ_j to be the $f(\theta_j|\boldsymbol{\theta}_{-j}, \mathbf{Y})$, then the acceptance probability (A.2) is always 1. This special case of proposal distribution is known as the Gibbs sampler. Using the Gibbs sampler, we do not have to be concerned about poor mixing due to the chain not updating, or about the choice of variance for the proposal distribution. We therefore use this whenever possible.

Note that, while above we have updated each component, θ_j of the parameter vector $\boldsymbol{\theta}$ in turn, in practice we can update blocks of parameters together. For example, when fitting the multivariate normal model, we will see that we can update all elements of the covariance matrix together, and all elements of the mean vector together.

A.3 Missing data

Now suppose that we have missing data and partition $\mathbf{Y} = (\mathbf{Y}_O, \mathbf{Y}_M)$. Assuming MAR, then modelling $f(\mathbf{Y}_O|\boldsymbol{\theta})$ gives valid inference for $\boldsymbol{\theta}$. However, this is typically awkward in practice, because we have to derive $f(\mathbf{Y}_O|\boldsymbol{\theta})$ from $f(\mathbf{Y}|\boldsymbol{\theta})$ by integrating out the missing data.

Fortunately, it turns out that using MCMC methods this is not necessary. We may simply regard the missing data as another set of parameters and update these in their turn. Thus, under a Gibbs sampling approach we would first construct the conditional distributions $f(\mathbf{Y}_M|\mathbf{Y}_O, \boldsymbol{\theta}), f(\theta_j|\boldsymbol{\theta}_{-j}, \mathbf{Y}), j = 1, \dots, p$ and then, having chosen starting values $\mathbf{Y}_M^0, \boldsymbol{\theta}^0$, at update r

1. draw $\boldsymbol{\theta}^r$ from $f(\boldsymbol{\theta}|\mathbf{Y}_O, \mathbf{Y}_M^{r-1})$, then
2. draw $\mathbf{Y}_M^r$ from $f(\mathbf{Y}_M|\mathbf{Y}_O, \boldsymbol{\theta}^r)$.

In practice, as discussed above, in step 1, it will often be convenient to subdivide step 1, updating subsets of the parameters conditional on the current draws of the remaining parameters and the missing data.

As an illustration of step 2, If the data follow a multivariate normal distribution, then for each unit with missing data, we calculate the conditional normal distribution of their missing data given their observed data and current draws of the parameters, $\boldsymbol{\theta}$. We then update their missing values with a draw from this distribution.

An advantage of using a MCMC approach for fitting imputation models is that we can use the same procedure for updating the parameters, in step 1, regardless of the pattern of missing data. In the context of MI, an MCMC approach also naturally incorporates the uncertainty in the parameter estimates so that the between imputation variance is correctly incorporated.

The data augmentation algorithm (Tanner and Wong (1987), Schafer (1997), p. 71) is is closely related to the Gibbs sampler. Essentially, instead of updating a single pair, $(\mathbf{Y}_M^r, \boldsymbol{\theta}^r)$, we update m pairs $(\mathbf{Y}_M^{r,1}, \boldsymbol{\theta}^{r,1}), \dots, (\mathbf{Y}_M^{r,m}, \boldsymbol{\theta}^{r,m})$. This requires a minor modification to the update process. However, choosing $m = 1$ gives a valid data augmentation algorithm, which is then equivalent to a particular Gibbs sampler.

Appendix B

Probability distributions

Here we give the commonly used probability density functions (pdfs) in this book and summarise some results for the multivariate normal distribution.

Univariate normal distribution

The univariate normal probability density function (pdf) of a random variable Y is

$$f(Y|\mu, \sigma^2) = \frac{1}{\sqrt{2\pi\sigma^2}} \exp\left\{-\frac{1}{2\sigma^2}(Y-\mu)^2\right\},$$

where Y, μ can take any real value and $\sigma^2 > 0$.

$\mathrm{E}(Y) = \mu$ and $\mathrm{Var}(Y) = \sigma^2$.

Multivariate normal distribution

The multivariate normal pdf of a $p \times 1$ vector of random variables $\mathbf{Y} = (Y_1, \dots, Y_p)^T$ is

$$f(\mathbf{Y}|\mu, \mathbf{\Omega}) = |2\pi\mathbf{\Omega}|^{-1/2} \exp\left\{-\frac{1}{2}(\mathbf{Y}-\mu)^T \mathbf{\Omega}^{-1}(\mathbf{Y}-\mu)\right\},$$

where elements of $\mathbf{Y}$ can take any real value, $\mu = (\mu_1, \dots, \mu_p)^T$ is a $p \times 1$ vector of real numbers with $\mathrm{E}(Y_j) = \mu_j, j = 1, \dots, p$, and $\mathbf{\Omega}$ a $p \times p$ positive definite matrix with $\mathrm{Var}(\mathbf{Y}) = \mathbf{\Omega}$.

We may also write this density in terms of the precision matrix $\mathbf{\Lambda} = \mathbf{\Omega}^{-1}$ giving

$$f(\mathbf{Y}|\mu, \mathbf{\Lambda}) = (2\pi)^{-p/2}|\mathbf{\Lambda}|^{1/2} \exp\left\{-\frac{1}{2}(\mathbf{Y}-\mu)^T \mathbf{\Lambda}(\mathbf{Y}-\mu)\right\}.$$

Multiple Imputation and its Application, Second Edition.
James R. Carpenter, Jonathan W. Bartlett, Tim P. Morris, Angela M. Wood, Matteo Quartagno and Michael G. Kenward.

Conditional normal distribution

Suppose $\mathbf{Y}$, of dimension $p \times 1$, follows a multivariate normal distribution with mean μ and variance–covariance matrix $\boldsymbol{\Omega}$. Suppose we partition $\mathbf{Y} = (Y_1, \dots, Y_p)^T$ into $\mathbf{Y}_q, \mathbf{Y}_r$, where $p = q + r$, $\mathbf{Y}_q = (Y_1, \dots, Y_q)^T$ and $\mathbf{Y}_r = (Y_{q+1}, \dots, Y_p)^T$. Thus, $\mathbf{Y}^T = (\mathbf{Y}_q^T, \mathbf{Y}_r^T)$.

Partition the mean μ in the same way into μ_p, μ_r, and partition the $p \times p$ variance–covariance matrix as

$$\boldsymbol{\Omega} = \begin{pmatrix} \boldsymbol{\Omega}_q & \boldsymbol{\Omega}_{qr} \\ \boldsymbol{\Omega}_{rq} & \boldsymbol{\Omega}_r \end{pmatrix},$$

where $\boldsymbol{\Omega}_q$ has dimension $q \times q$, $\boldsymbol{\Omega}_r$ dimension $r \times r$, $\boldsymbol{\Omega}_{qr}$ dimension $q \times r$, $\boldsymbol{\Omega}_{rq}$ dimension $r \times q$ and $\boldsymbol{\Omega}_{rq}^T = \boldsymbol{\Omega}_{qr}$.

Then $\mathbf{Y}_q$ has a multivariate normal distribution with mean μ_q and variance $\boldsymbol{\Omega}_q$, and the conditional distribution $f(\mathbf{Y}_r|\mathbf{Y}_q)$ is multivariate normal with mean

$$\mu_r + (\mathbf{Y}_q - \mu_q)\,\boldsymbol{\Omega}_{qq}^{-1}\boldsymbol{\Omega}_{qr}$$

and variance

$$\boldsymbol{\Omega}_r - \boldsymbol{\Omega}_{rq}\boldsymbol{\Omega}_{qq}^{-1}\boldsymbol{\Omega}_{qr}.$$

Gamma distribution

The gamma pdf of a random variable $Y > 0$ is

$$f(Y|\alpha, r) = \frac{\alpha}{\Gamma(r)}(\alpha Y)^{r-1}e^{-\alpha Y},$$

where $r > 0$, $\alpha > 0$ and $Y > 0$.

Here, the gamma function, $\Gamma(r)$ is defined for $r > 0$, as

$$\Gamma(r) = \int_0^\infty x^{r-1}e^{-x}\,dx.$$

For integer r, $\Gamma(r) = (r-1)(r-2), \dots, 1 = (r-1)!$

Then $\mathrm{E}(Y) = r/\alpha$ and $\mathrm{Var}(Y) = r/\alpha^2$.

In the special case that $r = 1$, Y follows an exponential distribution.

χ^2 distribution

In the definition of the gamma distribution, if $\alpha = 1/2$ and $r = n/2$, then we say Y follows a χ^2_n distribution, with mean n and variance $2n$.

t-distribution

If $X \sim N(0,1)$ and independently $Y \sim \chi^2_n$, then

$$\frac{X}{\sqrt{Y/n}}$$

follows a t distribution with n degrees of freedom, denoted as t_n.

The probability density function is

$$f(Y) = \frac{\Gamma\left(\frac{n+1}{2}\right)}{\sqrt{n\pi}\Gamma\left(\frac{n}{2}\right)}\left(1 + \frac{Y^2}{n}\right)^{-\frac{n+1}{2}}.$$

The t_n distribution has mean 0 and variance $n/(n-2)$ for $n > 2$. For $n = 1,2$ the variance is undefined.

F-distribution

If $X \sim \chi^2_p$ and independently $Y \sim \chi^2_q$, then

$$\frac{X/p}{Y/q}$$

follows and F distribution on p and q degrees of freedom.

This has mean $q/(q-2)$ for $q > 2$ and variance

$$\frac{2q^2(p+q-2)}{p(q-2)^2(q-4)}$$

for $q > 4$.

Wishart distribution

The Wishart distribution of a positive definite matrix $\mathbf{W}$ has probability density function

$$\mathrm{W}(n, \mathbf{\Lambda}) = f(\mathbf{W}|n, \mathbf{\Lambda}) = \frac{|\mathbf{W}|^{(n-p-1)/2}}{2^{(np)/2}|\mathbf{\Lambda}|^{n/2}\Gamma_p(\frac{n}{2})} \exp\left\{-\frac{1}{2}\mathrm{tr}(\mathbf{\Lambda}^{-1}\mathbf{W})\right\},$$

where p is the dimension of $\mathbf{W}$, $n > (p-1)$ is the degrees of freedom (which is not restricted to being integer), and $\mathbf{\Lambda}$ is a positive definite matrix.

Here tr means the trace of the matrix, defined as the sum of its diagonal elements. $\Gamma_p(n/2)$ is the multivariate gamma function, defined as

$$\Gamma_p\left(\frac{n}{2}\right) = \pi^{\frac{p(p-1)}{4}} \prod_{j=1}^{p} \Gamma\left(\frac{n+(1-j)}{2}\right).$$

The Wishart distribution has mean $n\mathbf{\Lambda}$ and variance $\mathrm{Var}(\mathbf{W}_{ij}) = n(\mathbf{\Lambda}_{ij}^2 + \mathbf{\Lambda}_{ii}\mathbf{\Lambda}_{jj})$.

The χ_n^2 distribution is the special case of the Wishart distribution with $p = 1$, $\Lambda = 1$.

Inverse gamma distribution

The inverse gamma pdf of a random variable $Y > 0$ is

$$f(Y|\alpha, r) = \frac{\alpha}{\Gamma(r)}\alpha^{r-1}Y^{-(r+1)}e^{-\alpha/Y},$$

where $r > 0$, $\alpha > 0$ and $Y > 0$.

Then $\mathrm{E}(Y) = \alpha/(r-1)$ and $\mathrm{Var}(Y) = \alpha^2/(r-1)^2(r-2)$ for $r > 2$.

Inverse Wishart distribution

If the matrix $\mathbf{W}$ has a $\mathrm{W}(n, \mathbf{\Lambda})$ distribution, then its inverse $\mathbf{V} = \mathbf{W}^{-1}$ has an inverse Wishart $W^{-1}(n, \mathbf{\Lambda}^{-1})$ with probability density function

$$f(\mathbf{V}|n, \mathbf{\Lambda}) = \frac{|\mathbf{V}|^{-(n+p+1)/2}}{2^{(np)/2}|\mathbf{\Lambda}|^{n/2}\Gamma_p(\frac{n}{2})} \exp\left\{-\frac{1}{2}\mathrm{tr}(\mathbf{\Lambda}^{-1}\mathbf{V}^{-1})\right\}.$$

Under the inverse Wishart distribution,

$$E(\mathbf{V}) = \frac{1}{n-p-1}\mathbf{\Lambda}^{-1}.$$

B.1 Posterior for the multivariate normal distribution

Suppose we have a sample of size n from the p-dimensional multivariate normal distribution, denoted as $\mathbf{Y}_i = (Y_{i1}, \ldots, Y_{ip})^T$, $i \in (1, \ldots, n)$. If we parameterise this in terms of the mean, μ and precision matrix $\mathbf{\Lambda}$, the likelihood of the parameters is

$$\begin{aligned} L(\mu, \mathbf{\Lambda}|\mathbf{Y}) &= \prod_{i=1}^{n} \frac{|\mathbf{\Lambda}|^{1/2}}{(2\pi)^{p/2}} \exp\left\{-\frac{1}{2}(\mathbf{Y}_i - \mu)^T\mathbf{\Lambda}(\mathbf{Y}_i - \mu)\right\} \\ &\propto |\mathbf{\Lambda}|^{n/2} \exp\left\{-\frac{1}{2}\sum_{i=1}^{n}(\mathbf{Y}_i - \mu)^T\mathbf{\Lambda}(\mathbf{Y}_i - \mu)\right\} \\ &= |\mathbf{\Lambda}|^{n/2} \exp\left\{-\frac{1}{2}\mathrm{tr}(\mathbf{S}\mathbf{\Lambda}) - \frac{n}{2}(\overline{\mathbf{Y}} - \mu)^T\mathbf{\Lambda}(\overline{\mathbf{Y}} - \mu)\right\}. \qquad \text{(B.1)} \end{aligned}$$

Here $\overline{\mathbf{Y}} = \sum_{i=1}^{n} \mathbf{Y}_i/n$,

$$\mathbf{S} = \sum_{i=1}^{n}(\mathbf{Y}_i - \overline{\mathbf{Y}})(\mathbf{Y}_i - \overline{\mathbf{Y}})^T,$$

and the last equality can be derived by noting that, for example,

$$\begin{aligned}\mathbf{Y}_i^T\boldsymbol{\Lambda}\mathbf{Y}_i &= \mathrm{tr}\{\boldsymbol{\Lambda}(\mathbf{Y}_i\mathbf{Y}_i^T)\}\\ &= \mathrm{tr}\{(\mathbf{Y}_i\mathbf{Y}_i^T)\boldsymbol{\Lambda}\} \text{ for symmetric matrices } \boldsymbol{\Lambda}, (\mathbf{Y}\mathbf{Y}^T).\end{aligned}$$

Suppose we choose priors for $\mu, \boldsymbol{\Lambda}$ as $\mu \sim \mathrm{N}_p\{\mathbf{0}, (\lambda\boldsymbol{\Lambda})^{-1}\}$, and $\boldsymbol{\Lambda} \sim \mathrm{W}(\nu, \mathbf{S}_p)$. Then the prior for $(\mu, \boldsymbol{\Lambda})$ is proportional to

$$|\lambda\boldsymbol{\Lambda}|^{1/2}|\boldsymbol{\Lambda}|^{(\nu-p-1)/2}\exp\left\{-\frac{1}{2}\mathrm{tr}(\mathbf{S}_p^{-1}\boldsymbol{\Lambda}) - \frac{1}{2}\mu^T(\lambda\boldsymbol{\Lambda})\mu\right\}.$$

It follows that the posterior is

$$\begin{aligned}f(\mu, \boldsymbol{\Lambda}|\mathbf{Y}) &\propto |\lambda\boldsymbol{\Lambda}|^{1/2}\exp\left\{-\frac{n}{2}(\overline{\mathbf{Y}} - \mu)^T\boldsymbol{\Lambda}(\overline{\mathbf{Y}} - \mu) - \frac{\lambda}{2}\mu^T\boldsymbol{\Lambda}\mu\right\}\\ &\quad \times |\boldsymbol{\Lambda}|^{(n+\nu-p-1)/2}\exp\left\{-\frac{1}{2}\mathrm{tr}[(\mathbf{S}_p^{-1} + \mathbf{S})\boldsymbol{\Lambda}]\right\}\\ &\propto f(\mu|\boldsymbol{\Lambda}, \mathbf{Y})f(\boldsymbol{\Lambda}|\mathbf{Y}),\end{aligned}$$

where

(a) $f(\mu|\boldsymbol{\Lambda}, \mathbf{Y})$ is $N_p\{\mu^\star, (\boldsymbol{\Lambda}^\star)^{-1}\}$ with

$$\mu^\star = \overline{\mathbf{Y}}\left(\frac{n}{n+\lambda}\right), \quad \text{and} \quad \boldsymbol{\Lambda}^\star = (n+\lambda)\boldsymbol{\Lambda};$$

(b) $f(\boldsymbol{\Lambda}|\mathbf{Y})$ is $\mathrm{W}\{n+\nu, [\mathbf{S}_p^{-1} + \mathbf{S} + \overline{\mathbf{Y}}\overline{\mathbf{Y}}^T(n\lambda)/(\lambda+n)]^{-1}\}$.

If we make the prior for the mean, μ less and less informative by letting $\lambda \to 0$, then the $f(\mu|\boldsymbol{\Lambda}, \mathbf{Y}) \to N_p\{\overline{\mathbf{Y}}, (n\boldsymbol{\Lambda})^{-1}\}$.

We note that in the case $p = 1$, this corresponds to $\mu \sim N(\overline{Y}, \sigma^2/n)$ and $\sigma^2 \sim \{S_p^{-1} + \sum(Y_i - \overline{Y})^2\}/\chi^2_{n+\nu}$.

It remains to choose the parameters of the Wishart prior, $\nu, \mathbf{S}_p$. One option is to choose $\mathbf{S}_p = \mathbf{S}^{-1}$, with $\mathbf{S}$ estimated from the observed data, and ν_p just greater than its minimum permissible value of $(p-1)$. In other words, the smallest possible degrees of freedom (representing the greatest uncertainty) about an estimate of S based on the observed data.

An alternative arises if we note that when looking at the posterior for $\mu, \boldsymbol{\Sigma}$, we may relax the constraints on the parameters required for the prior to be a proper probability distribution, provided the posterior remains a proper probability distribution. Thus, we may allow $\mathbf{S}_p^{-1} \to 0$. In the univariate case, this now gives

$$\sigma^2 \sim \sum(Y_i - \overline{Y})^2/\chi^2_{n+\nu}.$$

Applying the same argument to ν, we let $\nu \to -1$, so that the posterior for σ^2 tends to the sampling distribution for σ^2,

$$\sigma^2 \sim \sum (Y_i - \overline{Y})^2 / \chi^2_{n-1}.$$

Bringing all this together, letting $\lambda \to 0$, $\mathbf{S}_p^{-1} \to 0$ and $\nu \to -1$ gives

$$\begin{aligned} \mu &\sim N\{\mathbf{Y}, (n\Lambda)^{-1}\}, \\ \mathbf{\Lambda} &\sim \mathrm{W}(n-1, S^{-1}). \end{aligned} \tag{B.2}$$

Schafer (1997), p. 154–155 discuss this in more detail, noting that posterior (B.2) can be derived from the Jeffrey's invariance principle.

In multiple imputation (MI) especially if the means (or more generally regression parameters) are the focus of inferential interest, provided the degrees of freedom of the Wishart prior are kept low, precise choices are unlikely to have a substantive impact on the results.

Appendix C

Overview of multiple imputation in R, Stata

C.1 Basic multiple imputation using R

Here we outline how a basic fully conditional specification multiple imputation analysis can be performed in R using the `mice` package. For further details, please consult the package documentation, and for a comprehensive guide see van Buuren (2018).

The first step is to load the `mice` package:

```
library(mice)
```

To create multiple imputations of missing values for partially observed variables in a dataframe `dataf`, we use the `mice` function:

```
imps <- mice(dataf, m=10, seed=7244)
```

Here we have specified 10 imputations and set the seed of the random number generator so that our results are reproducible. By default, `mice` will impute all missing values in the data frame and will impute each variable using an imputation method chosen to match its assessment of the variable's type. For continuous (numeric) variables, the default method is predictive mean matching (see Section 6.3.4). If we instead wanted to impute numeric variables using normal linear regression, we can modify the `defaultMethod` argument:

```
imps <- mice(dataf, m=10, seed=7244,
          defaultMethod=c("norm", "logreg", "polyreg", "polr")
```

This specifies that normal linear regression can be used for numeric variables, logistic regression for binary variables, polytomous logistic regression (multinomial

Multiple Imputation and its Application, Second Edition.
James R. Carpenter, Jonathan W. Bartlett, Tim P. Morris, Angela M. Wood, Matteo Quartagno and Michael G. Kenward.

logistic regression) for unordered factor (categorical) variables, and the proportional odds model for ordered factor variables.

Having created the multiple imputations, we can then apply our chosen analysis method (fit our substantive model) to each. This is achieved using `with`, for example:

```
fit <- with(imps, lm(y1~1))
```

This fits a linear regression model to each imputed dataset with the variable `y1` as dependent variable and no covariates (just an intercept), saving the estimates and within-imputation variances. The intercept in such a model thus corresponds to the mean of the dependent variable, and so this is a convenient approach when we are interested in estimating the mean of one of the variables.

To apply Rubin's rules to the estimates and within-imputation variances, we use the `pool` function:

```
summary(pool(fit), conf.int=TRUE)
```

The output is of the following form:

```
  term  estimate std.error statistic df     p. val  2.5%   97.5%
1 (Int) 0.291    0.456     0.638     27.26 0.529 -0.644 1.227
```

The `estimate` and `std.error` show the Rubin's rules estimate and standard error of the parameter of interest (in this case the mean of `y1`). The subsequent columns show the test statistic for testing the null hypothesis that the parameter equals zero, the degrees of freedom, the p-value corresponding to testing this null, and limits of the 95% confidence interval.

C.2 Basic MI using Stata

Multiple imputation in Stata uses the `mi` suite of commands. Full details are given in the manuals (StataCorp, 2021b). For descriptions of missing data, the `misstable` commands are useful. There are four key commands for multiple imputation:

`mi set`	Tell Stata how to store imputed datasets
`mi register`	Tell Stata which variables will be imputed
`mi impute`	Perform multiple imputation
`mi estimate`	Analyse imputed data and combine results using Rubin's rules

The first step is to declare to Stata that you are going to use multiple imputation. This is achieved with

`mi set` *`style`*

The *style* refers to how Stata will store imputed datasets. We will describe the styles using an example, Table C.1 after describing two more commands.

Having set a style, the second step is to 'register' the variables that will be used. Suppose we wish to impute a single incomplete variable `y1`. This must be registered in advance using

Table C.1 Depiction of Stata's `mi styles`.

<table>
<tr><th>Style</th><th>Example of storage format</th></tr>
<tr><td>Incomplete data</td><td>
<table>
<tr><td>y0</td><td>y1</td></tr>
<tr><td>1</td><td>0</td></tr>
<tr><td>0</td><td>.</td></tr>
</table>
</td></tr>
<tr><td><code>wide</code></td><td>
<table>
<tr><td>y0</td><td>y1</td><td>_1_y1</td><td>_2_y1</td><td>_mi_miss</td></tr>
<tr><td>1</td><td>0</td><td>0</td><td>0</td><td>0</td></tr>
<tr><td>0</td><td>.</td><td>2</td><td>5</td><td>1</td></tr>
</table>
</td></tr>
<tr><td><code>mlong</code></td><td>
<table>
<tr><td>y0</td><td>y1</td><td>_mi_miss</td><td>_mi_m</td><td>_mi_id</td></tr>
<tr><td>1</td><td>0</td><td>0</td><td>0</td><td>1</td></tr>
<tr><td>0</td><td>.</td><td>1</td><td>0</td><td>2</td></tr>
<tr><td>0</td><td>2</td><td>.</td><td>1</td><td>2</td></tr>
<tr><td>0</td><td>5</td><td>.</td><td>2</td><td>2</td></tr>
</table>
</td></tr>
<tr><td><code>flong</code></td><td>
<table>
<tr><td>y0</td><td>y1</td><td>_mi_miss</td><td>_mi_m</td><td>_mi_id</td></tr>
<tr><td>1</td><td>0</td><td>0</td><td>0</td><td>1</td></tr>
<tr><td>0</td><td>.</td><td>1</td><td>0</td><td>2</td></tr>
<tr><td>1</td><td>0</td><td>0</td><td>1</td><td>1</td></tr>
<tr><td>0</td><td>2</td><td>.</td><td>1</td><td>2</td></tr>
<tr><td>1</td><td>0</td><td>0</td><td>2</td><td>1</td></tr>
<tr><td>0</td><td>5</td><td>.</td><td>2</td><td>2</td></tr>
</table>
</td></tr>
</table>

```
mi register imputed y1
```

To multiply impute `y1` using (for example) linear regression imputation with `y0` as a covariate, we use the command:

```
mi impute regress y1 y0
```

Various options are available instead of regress (pmm for predictive mean matching, logit for logistic regression imputation and so on). The multiply imputed data can now be analysed. To estimate the mean of `y1`, for example, we use

```
mi estimate: regress y1
```

Here, we simply prefixed '`mi estimate:`' to the command that fits our substantive model (`regress y1`). Stata fits this model in each imputed dataset and combines the multiple results using Rubin's rules. To see the estimated Monte Carlo error for the table of results, the option mcerror is added before the colon as follows:

```
mi estimate, mcerror: regress y1
```

More details about the imputation process can be found using the `vartable` option, which gives information such as the within- and between-imputation variance and the fraction of missing information:

```
mi estimate: regress y1, vartable
```

For a similar table to return to the original data (and clear the imputations), we can type:

```
mi extract 0, clear
```

We now describe the *`styles`* for storing multiply imputed data, which are depicted in Table C.1. The top row depicts a simple incomplete dataset with two variables, `y0` and `y1`, and two rows of data. The only missing value, denoted by a dot `.` is in the second row of variable `y1`. This value is imputed twice: first as 2 and then as 5.

The `wide` storage style creates two variables, `_1_y1` and `_2_y1`, containing these imputed values, but also containing the observed value for the complete case (row 1). Note that this is done only for the variable that was imputed, not for the fully observed variable y0. The `wide` style also creates a variable `_mi_miss` that is an indicator of whether a row contained a missing value.

The `mlong` format stores imputations in rows below the incomplete data. Rather than creating a new variable for each imputation, it creates a categorical variable `_mi_m` denoting the imputation number, where the value 0 is given to the original partially observed dataset. The imputations are then stored for rows that had data imputed. A third variable, `_mi_id`, is a row-identifier that is common across imputed datasets so that we can see, for example the values imputed for a given individual.

The `flong` style is similar to `mlong` in structure except that complete rows are also duplicated for imputed datasets (i.e. `_mi_mi` > 0).

Once a style has been chosen, it is straightforward to convert between styles. For example, if the initially chosen style was `mlong`, it can be changed to `wide` using

```
mi convert wide, clear
```

Different storage styles have different advantages. Some are better suited to inspecting or plotting imputed data, some make estimation (slightly) faster. If you do not know which style you need, you do not need to worry about it: pick one and Stata will work with it.

A final style is called `flongsep` and similar flong except each imputed dataset is saved as a separate dataset; this is for very large datasets or especially large numbers of imputations, such that holding them in memory simultaneously is too much of a burden.

Stata knows how to work with all these storage types. By telling Stata, the `mi style`, commands like `mi impute` and `mi estimate` know how the imputed datasets are stored and will work automatically.

To better understand the storage styles, there is a useful toy dataset available online called '`miproto.dta`'. It can be loaded into Stata from https://www.stata-press.com/data/r17/miproto.dta (Stata version 17). Look at the dataset and try converting between styles to check your understanding of the styles.

References

Abadie, A. and Imbens, G. W. (2016) Matching on the estimated propensity score. *Econometrica*, 84(2), 781–807.

Afifi, A. and Elashoff, R. (1966) Missing observations in multivariate statistics I: Review of the literature. *Journal of the American Statistical Association*, 61, 595–604.

Aitchison, J. and Bennett, J. A. (1970) Polychotomous quantal response by maximum indicant. *Biometrika*, 57, 253–262.

Albert, J. H. and Chib, S. (1993) Bayesian analysis of binary and polychotomous response data. *Journal of the American Statistical Association*, 88, 669–679.

Albert, P. S. and Follman, D. A. (2009) Shared parameter models. In *Longitudinal Data Analysis: A Handbook of Modern Statistical Methods* (Eds M. Davidian, G. Fitzmaurice, G. Molenberghs and G. Verbeke), pp. 433–452. Chapman & Hall/CRC.

Allison, P. D. (2002) *Missing Data*. Thousand Oaks, CA: Sage.

Andridge, R. R. and Little, R. J. A. (2010) A review of hot deck imputation for survey non-response. *International Statistical Review*, 78, 40–64.

Atkinson, A., Kenward, M. G., Clayton, T. and Carpenter, J. (2019) Reference-based sensitivity analysis for time-to-event data. *Pharmaceutical Statistics*, 18(6), 645–658.

Atkinson, A., Cro, S., Carpenter, J. and Kenward, M. (2021) Information anchored reference based sensitivity analysis for truncated normal data with application to survival analysis. *Statistica Neerlandica*, 75(4), 500–523.

Audigier, V. and Resche-Rigon, M. (2019) *micemd: Multiple Imputation by Chained Equations with Multilevel Data*. R package version 1.6.0.

Audigier, V., White, I. R., Jolani, S., Debray, T. P. A., Quartagno, M., Carpenter, J., van Buuren, S. and Resche-Rigon, M. (2018) Multiple imputation for multilevel data with continuous and binary variables. *Statistical Science*, 33(2), 160–183.

Ayieko, P., Ntoburi, S., Wagai, J., Opondo, C., Opiyo, N., Migiro, S., Wamae, A., Mogoa, W., Were, F., Wasunna, A., Fegan, G., Irimu, G. and English, M. (2011) A multifaceted intervention to implement guidelines and improve admission paediatric care in Kenyan district hospitals: a cluster randomised trial. *PLOS Medicine*, 8, e1001018.

Bahadur, R. R. (1961) A representation of the joint distribution of responses to n dichotomous items. In *Studies in Item Analysis and Prediction* (Ed. H. Solomon). Stanford, CA: Stanford University Press.

Multiple Imputation and its Application, Second Edition.
James R. Carpenter, Jonathan W. Bartlett, Tim P. Morris, Angela M. Wood, Matteo Quartagno and Michael G. Kenward.

Barnard, J. and Rubin, D. (1999) Small-sample degrees of freedom with multiple imputation. *Biometrika*, 86, 948–955.

Bartlett, J. W. (2019) smcfcs for covariate measurement error correction. https://cran.r-project.org/web/packages/smcfcs/vignettes/smcfcs_coverror-vignette.html.

Bartlett, J. W. (2021) Reference-based multiple imputation—what is the right variance and how to estimate it. *Statistics in Biopharmaceutical Research*, 15(1), 178–186.

Bartlett, J. W. and Hughes, R. A. (2020) Bootstrap inference for multiple imputation under uncongeniality and misspecification. *Statistical Methods in Medical Research*, 29(12), 3533–3546.

Bartlett, J. W. and Keogh, R. H. (2018) Bayesian correction for covariate measurement error: a frequentist evaluation and comparison with regression calibration. *Statistical Methods in Medical Research*, 27(6), 1695–1708.

Bartlett, J. W. and Morris, T. P. (2015) Multiple imputation of covariates by substantive-model compatible fully conditional specification. *The Stata Journal*, 15(2), 437–456.

Bartlett, J. A. and Shao, J. F. (2009) Successes, challenges, and limitations of current antiretroviral therapy in low-income and middle-income countries. *Lanced Infections Diseases*, 9, 637–649.

Bartlett, J. W. and Taylor, J. M. G. (2016) Missing covariates in competing risks analysis. *Biostatistics*, 17(4), 751–763.

Bartlett, J. W., De Stavola, B. L. and Frost, C. (2009) Linear mixed models for replication data to efficiently allow for covariate measurement error. *Statistics in Medicine*, 28(25), 3158–3178.

Bartlett, J. W., Carpenter, J. R., Tilling, K. and Vansteelandt, S. (2014) Improving upon the efficiency of complete case analysis when covariates are MNAR. *Biostatistics*, 15(4), 719–730.

Bartlett, J. W., Harel, O. and Carpenter, J. R. (2015a) Asymptotically unbiased estimation of exposure odds ratios in complete records logistic regression. *American Journal of Epidemiology*, 182(8), 730–736.

Bartlett, J. W., Seaman, S., White, I. R. and Carpenter, J. R. (2015b) Multiple imputation of covariates by fully conditional specification: accommodating the substantive model. *Statistical Methods in Medical Research*, 24, 462–487.

Beesley, L. J. and Taylor, J. M. (2021) A stacked approach for chained equations multiple imputation incorporating the substantive model. *Biometrics*, 77(4), 1342–1354.

Bernaards, C. A., Belin, T. R. and Schafer, J. L. (2007) Robustness of a multivariate normal approximation for imputation of incomplete binary data. *Statistics in Medicine*, 26(6), 1368–1382.

Blatchford, P., Goldstein, H., Martin, C. and Browne, W. (2002) A study of class size effects in English school reception year classes. *British Educational Research Journal*, 28, 169–185.

Bodner, T. E. (2008) What improves with increased missing data imputations? *Structural Equation Modeling: A Multidisciplinary Journal*, 15(4), 651–675.

Bonora, B. M., Avogaro, A. and Fadini, G. P. (2020) Extraglycemic effects of SGLT2 inhibitors: a review of the evidence. *Diabetes, Metabolic Syndrome and Obesity: Targets and Therapy*, 13, 161–174.

Borgan, O. and Samuelsen, S. O. (2013) Nested case-control and case-cohort studies. In *Handbook of Survival Analysis* (Eds. J. P. Klein, H. C. van Houwelingen, J. G. Ibrahim, T. H. Scheike), pp. 343–367. CRC Press.

Bornkamp, B., Rufibach, K., Lin, J., Liu, Y., Mehrotra, D. V., Roychoudhury, S., Schmidli, H., Shentu, Y. and Wolbers, M. (2021) Principal stratum strategy: potential role in drug development. *Pharmaceutical Statistics*, 20(4), 737–751.

Boulle, A., Bock, P., Osler, M., Cohen, K., Channing, L., Hilderbrand, K., Mothibi, E., Zweigenthal, V., Slingers, N., Cloete, K. and Abdullah, F. (2008) Antiretroviral therapy and early mortality in South Africa. *Bulletin of the World Health Organization*, 86, 657–736.

Bowman, D. and George, E. O. (1995) A saturated model for analyzing exchangeable binary data: applications to clinical and developmental toxicity studies. *Journal of the American Statistical Association*, 90, 871–879.

Brand, J. P., Buuren, S., Groothuis-Oudshoorn, K. and Gelsema, E. S. (2003) A toolkit in SAS for the evaluation of multiple imputation methods. *Statistica Neerlandica*, 57(1), 36–45.

Brand, J., van Buuren, S., le Cessie, S. and van den Hout, W. (2019) Combining multiple imputation and bootstrap in the analysis of cost-effectiveness trial data. *Statistics in Medicine*, 38(2), 210–220.

Brinkhof, M. W. G., Dabis, F., Myer, L., Bangsberg, D. R., Boulle, A., Nash, D., Schechter, M., Laurent, C., Keiser, O., May, M., Sprinz, E., Egger, M., Anglaret, X. and for the ART-LINC of IeDEA collaboration (2008) Early loss of HIV-infected patients on potent antiretroviral therapy programmes in lower-income countries. *Bulletin of the World Health Organization*, 86, 497–576.

Brinkhof, M. W. G., Pujades-Rodreguez, M. and Egger, M. (2009) Lost to follow-up in antiretroviral treatment programmes in resource-limited settings: systematic review and meta-analysis. *PLoS ONE*, 4, e5790.

Brinkhof, M. W. G., Spycher, B. D., Yiannoutsos, C., Weigel, R., Wood, R., Messou, E., Boulle, A., Egger, M. and Sterne, J. A. C. (2010) Adjusting mortality for loss to follow-up: analysis of five art programmes in sub-Saharan Africa. *PLoS ONE*, 5, e14149.

Browne, W. J. (2006) MCMC algorithms for constrained variance matrices. *Computational Statistics and Data Analysis*, 50, 1655–1677.

Burgess, S., White, I. R., Resche-Rigon, M. and Wood, A. M. (2013) Combining multiple imputation and meta-analysis with individual participant data. *Statistics in Medicine*, 32(26), 4499–4514.

Busse, W. W., Chervinsky, P., Condemi, J., Lumry, W. R., Petty, T. L., Rennard, S. and Townley, R. G. (1998) Budesonide delivered by Turbuhaler is effective in a dose-dependent fashion when used in the treatment of adult patients with chronic asthma. *Journal of Allergy and Clinical Immunology*, 101, 457–463.

van Buuren, S. (2007) Multiple imputation of discrete and contiuous data by fully conditional specification. *Statistical Methods in Medical Research*, 16, 219–242.

van Buuren, S. (2011) Multiple imputation of multilevel data. In *The Handbook of Advanced Multilevel Analysis* (Ed. J. K. R. Joop Hox), pp. 173–196. New York: Routledge.

van Buuren, S. (2018) *Flexible Imputation of Missing Data*. CRC Press.

van Buuren, S. and Groothuis-Oudshoorn, K. (2011) MICE: Multivariate imputation by chained equations in R. *Journal of Statistical Software*, 45(3), 1–67.

van Buuren, S., Boshuizen, H. C. and Knook, D. L. (1999) Multiple imputation of missing blood pressure covariates in survival analysis. *Statistics in Medicine*, 18, 681–694.

van Calster, B., McLernon, D. J., van Smeden, M., Wynants, L. and Steyerberg, E. W. (2019) Calibration: the Achilles heel of predictive analytics. *BMC Medicine*, 17(1), 230.

Carpenter, J. R. and Kenward, M. G. (2008) *Missing Data in Clinical Trials — A Practical Guide*. Birmingham: National Health Service Co-ordinating Centre for Research Methodology.

Carpenter, J. and Kenward, M. (2009) Multiple imputation. In *Longitudinal Data Analysis: A Handbook of Modern Statistical Methods* (Eds M. Davidian, G. Fitzmaurice, G. Molenberghs and G. Verbeke), pp. 477–500. Chapman & Hall/CRC.

Carpenter, J. and Plewis, I. (2011) Analysing longitudinal studies with non-response: issues and statistical methods. In *The SAGE Handbook of Innovation in Social Research Methods* (Eds M. Williams and P. Vogt), pp. 498–523. London: Sage.

Carpenter, J. R. and Smuk, M. (2021) Missing data: a statistical framework for practice. *Biometrical Journal*, 63(5), 915–947.

Carpenter, J., Pocock, S. and Lamm, C. J. (2002) Coping with missing data in clinical trials: a model based approach applied to asthma trials. *Statistics in Medicine*, 21, 1043–1066.

Carpenter, J. R., Kenward, M. G. and Vansteelandt, S. (2006) A comparison of multiple imputation and inverse probability weighting for analyses with missing data. *Journal of the Royal Statistical Society, Series A (Statistics in Society)*, 169, 571–584.

Carpenter, J. R., Kenward, M. G. and White, I. R. (2007) Sensitivity analysis after multiple imputation under missing at random — a weighting approach. *Statistical Methods in Medical Research*, 16, 259–275.

Carpenter, J. R., Goldstein, H. and Kenward, M. G. (2011a) REALCOM-IMPUTE software for multilevel multiple imputation with mixed response types. *Journal of Statistical Software*, 45, e1–e14.

Carpenter, J. R., Rücker, G. and Schwarzer, G. (2011b) Assessing the sensitivity of meta-analysis to selection bias: a multiple imputation approach. *Biometrics*, 67, 1066–1072.

Carpenter, J. R., Kenward, M. G. and Goldstein, H. (2012) Statistical modelling of partially observed data using multiple imputation: principles and practice. In *Modern Methods for Epidemiology* (Eds Y. Tu and D. Greenwood), pp. 15–31. New York: Springer.

Carpenter, J. R., Roger, J. H. and Kenward, M. G. (2013) Analysis of longitudinal trials with protocol deviation: a framework for relevant, accessible assumptions, and inference via multiple imputation. *Journal of Biopharmaceutical Statistics*, 23, 1352–1371.

Carroll, O. (2022) *Strategies for imputing missing covariate values in observational data*. Ph.D. thesis, London School of Hygiene & Tropical Medicine, London, UK.

Carroll, O. U., Morris, T. P. and Keogh, R. H. (2020) How are missing data in covariates handled in observational time-to-event studies in oncology? A systematic review. *BMC Medical Research Methodology*, 20(1), 134.

Carroll, R. J., Ruppert, D., Stefanski, L. A. and Crainiceanu, C. M. (2006) *Measurement Error in Nonlinear Models: A Modern Perspective*. Chapman and Hall/CRC.

Çay, F., Firat, M. Z. and Kaçar, C. (2021) Comparison of methods dealing with missing data in a longitudinal rheumatologic study. *Akdeniz Medical Journal*, 7(2), 268–276.

Chib, S. and Greenburg, E. (1998) Analysis of multivariate probit models. *Biometrika*, 85, 347–361.

Clark, D. (2004) Practical introduction to record linkage for injury research. *Injury Prevention*, 10, 186–191.

Clark, T. P., Kahan, B. C., Phillips, A., White, I. and Carpenter, J. R. (2022) Estimands: bringing clarity and focus to research questions in clinical trials. *BMJ Open*, 12(1), 1–7.

Clayton, D. G. (1991) A Monte Carlo method for Bayesian inference in frailty models. *Biometrics*, 47, 467–485.

Clayton, D., Spiegelhalter, D., Dunn, G. and Pickles, A. (1998) Analysis of longitudinal binary data from multi-phase sampling (with discussion). *Journal of the Royal Statistical Society, Series B (Statistical Methodology)*, 60(1), 71–87.

Cole, S. R., Chu, H. and Greenland, S. (2006) Multiple-imputation for measurement-error correction. *International Journal of Epidemiology*, 35, 1074–1081.

Collins, L. M., Schafer, J. L. and Kam, C. M. (2001) A comparison of inclusive and restrictive strategies in modern missing-data procedures. *Psychological Methods*, 6, 330–351.

Committee for Medicinal Products for Human Use (2010) *Guideline on Missing Data in Confirmatory Clinical Trials*. London: European Medicines Agency.

Copas, J. B. and Shi, J. Q. (2000) Meta-analysis, funnel plots and sensitivity analysis. *Biostatistics*, 1(3), 247–262.

Cowles, M. K. (1996) Accelerating Monte Carlo Markov chain convergence for cumulative-link generalized linear models. *Statistics and Computing*, 6, 101–110.

Cro, S., Morris, T. P., Kenward, M. G. and Carpenter, J. R. (2016) Reference-based sensitivity analysis via multiple imputation for longitudinal trials with protocol deviation. *The Stata Journal*, 16, 443–463.

Cro, S., Carpenter, J. R. and Kenward, M. G. (2019) Information anchored sensitivity analysis. *Journal of the Royal Statistical Society, Series A (Statistics in Society)*, 182(2), 623–645.

Cro, S., Morris, T. P., Kenward, M. G. and Carpenter, J. R. (2020) Sensitivity analysis for clinical trials with missing continuous outcome data using controlled multiple imputation: a practical guide. *Statistics in Medicine*, 39(21), 2815–2842.

Cro, S., Kahan, B. C., Rehal, S., Ster, A. C., Carpenter, J. R., White, I. R. and Cornelius, V. R. (2022) Evaluating the clarity of the questions being addressed in randomised trials: a systematic review of estimands. *BMJ: British Medical Journal*, 378, e070146.

Croxford, L., Ianelli, C. and Shapira, M. (2007) Documentation of the Youth Cohort Time-Series Datasets, UK Data Archive Study Number 5765, Economic and Social Data Service.

Daniel, R. M., Kenward, M. G., Cousens, S. N. and Stavola, B. L. D. (2011) Using causal diagrams to guide analysis in missing data problems. *Statistical Methods in Medical Research*, 21, 243–256.

Daniel, R., Zhang, J. and Farewell, D. (2021) Making apples from oranges: comparing noncollapsible effect estimators and their standard errors after adjustment for different covariate sets. *Biometrical Journal*, 63(3), 528–557.

Daniels, M. J. and Hogan, J. W. (2000) Reparameterizing the pattern mixture model for sensitivity analysis under informative dropout. *Biometrics*, 56, 1241–1248.

Daniels, M. J. and Hogan, J. W. (2008) *Missing Data in Longitudinal Studies*. London: Chapman & Hall.

Demirtas, H. and Schafer, J. L. (2003) On the performance of random-coefficient pattern-mixture models for non-ignorable drop-out. *Statistics in Medicine*, 22, 2553–2575.

Demirtas, H., Freels, S. A. and Yucel, R. M. (2008) Plausibility of multivariate normality assumption when multiply imputing non-Gaussain continous outcomes: a simulation assessment. *Journal of Statistical Computation and Simulation*, 78, 69–84.

Dempster, A. P., Laird, N. M. and Rubin, D. B. (1977) Maximum likelihood from incomplete data via the *EM* algorithm (with discussion). *Journal of the Royal Statistical Society, Series B (Statistical Methodology)*, 39, 1–38.

DiazOrdaz, K. and Carpenter, J. (2019) Local average treatment effects estimation via substantive model compatible multiple imputation. *Biometrical Journal*, 61(6), 1526–1540.

Diggle, P. J. and Kenward, M. G. (1994) Informative dropout in longitudinal data analysis (with discussion). *Journal of the Royal Statistical Society, Series C (Applied Statistics)*, 43, 49–94.

Ding, P. and Li, F. (2018) Causal inference: a missing data perspective. *Statistical Science*, 33(2), 214–237.

Drechsler, J. (2011) Multiple imputation in practice—a case study using a complex german establishment survey. *Advances in Statistical Analysis*, 95, 1–26.

Efron, B. (1992) Jackknife-after-bootstrap standard errors and influence functions. *Journal of the Royal Statistical Society, Series B (Methodological)*, 54(1), 83–127.

Efron, B. (1994) Missing data, imputation, and the bootstrap. *Journal of the American Statistical Association*, 89, 463–475.

Eiset, A. H. and Frydenberg, M. (2022) Considerations for using multiple imputation in propensity score-weighted analysis–a tutorial with applied example. *Clinical Epidemiology*, 14, 835.

Enders, C. K., Keller, B. T. and Levy, R. (2018) A fully conditional specification approach to multilevel imputation of categorical and continuous variables. *Psychol Methods*, 23(2), 298–317.

Erler, N. S., Rizopoulos, D., van Rosmalen, J., Jaddoe, V. W. V., Franco, O. H. and Lesaffre, E. M. E. H. (2016) Dealing with missing covariates in epidemiologic studies: a comparison between multiple imputation and a full Bayesian approach. *Statistics in Medicine*, 35(17), 2955–2974.

Erler, N. S., Rizopoulos, D. and Lesaffre, E. M. E. H. (2021) JointAI: Joint analysis and imputation of incomplete data in R. *Journal of Statistical Software*, 100(20), 1–56.

Fay, R. E. (1992) When are inferences from muliple imputation valid? *Proceedings of the Survey Research Methodology Section of the American Statistical Association*, pp. 227–232.

Fay, R. (1993) Valid inferences from imputed survey data. *Proceedings of the Survey Research Methodology Section of the American Statistical Association*, pp. 41–48.

Firth, D. (1993) Bias reduction of maximum likelihood estimates. *Biometrika*, 80, 27–38.

Fletcher Mercaldo, S. and Blume, J. D. (2018) Missing data and prediction: the pattern submodel. *Biostatistics*, 21(2), 236–252.

Frangakis, C. E. and Rubin, D. B. (2002) Principal stratification in causal inference. *Biometrics*, 58(1), 21–29.

Freedman, L. S., Fainberg, V., Kipnis, V., Midthune, D. and Carroll, R. J. (2004) A new method for dealing with measurement error in explanatory variables of regression models. *Biometrics*, 60(1), 172–181.

Freedman, L. S., Midthune, D., Carroll, R. J. and Kipnis, V. (2008) A comparison of regression calibration, moment reconstruction and imputation for adjusting for covariate measurement error in regression. *Statistics in Medicine*, 27(25), 5195–5216.

Gachau, S., Quartagno, M., Njeru Njaga, E., Owuor, N., English, M. and Ayieko, P. (2020) Handling missing data in modelling quality of clinician-prescribed routine care: Sensitivity analysis of departure from missing at random assumption. *Statistical Methods in Medical Research*, 29, 3076–3092. doi:10.1177/0962280220918279.

Gasparini, A. (2022) `mice.mcerror`. https://github.com/ellessenne/mice.mcerror. Online; accessed 2022-09-02.

Gelman, A., Carlin, J. B., Stern, H. S. and Rubin, D. B. (1995) *Bayesian Data Analysis*. Boca Raton: CRC Press.

Gelman, A. G., Roberts, G. O. and Gilks, W. R. (1996) Efficient Metropolis jumping rules. In *Bayesian Statistics V* (Eds J. M. Bernardo, J. O. Berger, A. F. Dawid and A. F. M. Smith), pp. 599–608. Oxford: Oxford University Press.

Gilks, W. R., Richardson, S. and Spiegelhalter, D. J. (1996) *Markov Chain Monte-Carlo in Practice*. London: Chapman and Hall.

Goldstein, H. (2010) *Multilevel Statistical Models. Fourth Edition*. Chichester: Wiley.

Goldstein, H., Carpenter, J., Kenward, M. and Levin, K. (2009) Multilevel models with multivariate mixed response types. *Statistical Modelling*, 9, 173–197.

Goldstein, H., Harron, K. and Wade, A. (2012) The analysis of record-linked data using multiple imputation with data value priors. *Statistics in Medicine*, 31(28), 3481–3493.

Goldstein, H., Carpenter, J. R. and Browne, W. (2014) Fitting multilevel multivariate models with missing data in responses and covariates, which may include interactions and non-linear terms. *Journal of the Royal Statistical Society, Series A*, 177, 553–564.

Gower-Page, C., Noci, A. and Wolbers, M. (2022) rbmi: AR package for standard and reference-based multiple imputation methods. *Journal of Open Source Software*, 7(74), 4251.

Grace, Y. Y., Delaigle, A. and Gustafson, P. (2021) *Handbook of Measurement Error Models*. CRC Press.

Gray, C. M. (2018) *Use of the Bayesian family of methods to correct for effects of exposure measurement error in polynomial regression models*. Ph.D. thesis, London School of Hygiene & Tropical Medicine.

Grund, S., Lüdtke, O. and Robitzsch, A. (2018) Multiple imputation of missing data for multilevel models: simulations and recommendations. *Organizational Research Methods*, 21(1), 111–149.

Grund, S., Robitzsch, A. and Luedtke, O. (2019) *mitml: Tools for Multiple Imputation in Multilevel Modeling*. R package version 0.3-7.

Grund, S., Lüdtke, O. and Robitzsch, A. (2021) Multiple imputation of missing data in multilevel models with the R package mdmb: a flexible sequential modeling approach. *Behavior Research Methods*, 53(6), 2631–2649.

Gustafson, P. (2003) *Measurement Error and Misclassification in Statistics and Epidemiology: Impacts and Bayesian Adjustments*. CRC Press.

Hansen, P. C. (1998) *Rank-Deficient and Discrete Ill-posed Problems*. SIAM.

Hardt, J., Herke, M. and Leonhart, R. (2012) Auxiliary variables in multiple imputation in regression with missing X: a warning against including too many in small sample research. *BMC Medical Research Methodology*, 12(1), 1–13.

Harel, O. and Carpenter, J. R. (2012) Complete records regression with missing data: relating bias in coefficient estimates to the missingness mechanism, *submitted*.

Harel, O. and Schafer, J. L. (2003) Multiple imputation in two stages. In *Proceedings of Federal Committee on Statistical Methodology Conference*. Available from http://www.fcsm.gov/03papers/Harel.pdf, accessed April 2012.

Harel, O. and Schafer, J. L. (2009) Partial and latent ignorability in missing data problems. *Biometrika*, 96, 37–50.

Harrell, F. E. (2015) *Regression Modeling strategies: With Applications to Linear Models, Logistic and Ordinal Regression, and Survival Analysis*, section edition. Springer Cham.

Hastie, T., Tibshirani, R., Friedman, J. H. and Friedman, J. H. (2009) *The Elements of Statistical Learning: Data Mining, Inference, and Prediction*, volume 2. Springer.

Hayati Rezvan, P., White, I. R., Lee, K. J., Carlin, J. B. and Simpson, J. A. (2015) Evaluation of a weighting approach for performing sensitivity analysis after multiple imputation. *BMC Medical Research Methodology*, 15(83), 1–16.

Hayden, D., Pauler, D. K. and Schoenfeld, D. (2005) An estimator for treatment comparisons among survivors in randomized trials. *Biometrics*, 61(1), 305–310.

Hayes, T. (2019) Flexible, free software for multilevel multiple imputation: a review of blimp and jomo. *Journal of Educational and Behavioral Statistics*, 44(5), 625–641.

He, Y., Zaslavsky, A. M., Harrington, D. P., Catalano, P. and Landrum, M. B. (2010) Multiple imputation in a large-scale compelex survey: a practical guide. *Statistical Methods in Medical Research*, 19, 653–670.

Healy, M. J. R. and Westmacott, M. (1956) Missing values in experiments analyzed on automatic computers. *Applied Statistics*, 5, 203–206.

Heitjan, D. F. and Rubin, D. B. (1991) Ignorability and coarse data. *The Annals of Statistics*, 19(4), 2244–2253.

Héraud-Bousquet, V., Larsen, C., Carpenter, J., Desenclos, J.-C. and Strat, Y. L. (2012) Practical considerations for sensitivity analysis after multiple imputation applied to epidemiological studies with incomplete data. *BMC Medical Research Methodology*, 12, 73.

Hernán, M. A. and Robins, J. M. (2020) Causal inference: what if.

Higgins, J. P. T., White, I. R. and Wood, A. M. (2006) Missing outcome data in meta-analysis of clinical trials: development and comparison of methods, with recommendations for practice *Technical report, MRC Biostatistics Unit, Cambridge UK.*

von Hippel, P. T. (2007) Regression with missing Ys: an improved strategy for analyzing multiply imputed data. *Sociological Methodology*, 37(1), 83–117.

Von Hippel, P. T. (2009) How to impute interactions, squares and other transformed variables. *Sociological Methodology*, 39, 265–291.

von Hippel, P. T. (2020) How many imputations do you need? A two-stage calculation using a quadratic rule. *Sociological Methods & Research*, 49(3), 699–718.

von Hippel, P. T. and Bartlett, J. W. (2021) Maximum likelihood multiple imputation: faster imputations and consistent standard errors without posterior draws. *Statistical Science*, 36(3), 400–420.

Hippisley-Cox, J., Coupland, C., Vinogradova, Y., Robson, J., May, M. and Brindle, P. (2007) Derivation and validation of qrisk, a new cardiovascular disease risk score for the united kingdom: prospective open cohort study. *British Medical Journal*, 335, 7611–7623.

Hippisley-Cox, J., Coupland, C. and Brindle, P. (2017) Development and validation of QRISK3 risk prediction algorithms to estimate future risk of cardiovascular disease: prospective cohort study. *BMJ*, 357, j2099.

Hobert, J. P. and Casella, G. (1996) The effect of improper priors on Gibbs sampling in hierarchical linear mixed models. *Journal of the American Statistical Association*, 91(436), 1461–1473.

Hoerl, A. E. and Kennard, R. W. (1970) Ridge regression: biased estimation for nonorthogonal problems. *Technometrics*, 42, 80–86.

Hollis, S. and Campbell, F. (1999) What is meant by intention to treat analysis? Survey of published randomised controlled trials. *British Medical Journal*, 319, 670–674.

Hoogland, J., van Barreveld, M., Debray, T. P., Reitsma, J. B., Verstraelen, T. E., Dijkgraaf, M. G. and Zwinderman, A. H. (2020) Handling missing predictor values when validating and applying a prediction model to new patients. *Statistics in Medicine*, 39(25), 3591–3607.

Horton, N. J., Lipsitz, S. R. and Parzen, M. (2003) A potential for bias when rounding in multiple imputation. *The American Statistician*, 57, 229–232.

Horvitz, D. G. and Thompson, D. J. (1952) A generalisation of sampling without replacement from a finite universe. *Journal of the American Statistical Association*, 47, 663–685.

Hsu, C. and Taylor, J. M. G. (2009) Nonparametric comparison of two survival functions with dependent censoring via nonparametric multiple imputation. *Statistics in Medicine*, 28, 462–475.

Hsu, C.-H., Taylor, J. M. G., Murray, S. and Commenges, D. (2006) Survival analysis using auxiliary variables via nonparametric multiple imputation. *Statistics in Medicine*, 25, 3503–3517.

Hsu, C., Taylor, J. M. G., Murray, S. and Commenges, D. (2007) Multiple imputation for interval censored data with auxiliary variables. *Statistics in Medicine*, 26, 769–781.

Hughes, R. A., Sterne, J. A. C. and Tilling, K. (2012) Comparison of imputation variance estimators. *Technical report*, University of Bristol, Department of Social Medicine.

Hughes, R., White, I. R., Carpenter, J. R., Tilling, K. and Sterne, J. A. C. (2014) Joint modelling rationale for chained equations imputation. *BMC Medical Research Methodology*, 14, 28.

Hughes, R. A., Sterne, J. A. C. and Tilling, K. (2016) Comparison of imputation variance estimators. *Statistical Methods in Medical Research*, 25(6), 2541–2557.

Hughes, R. A., Heron, J., Sterne, J. A. C. and Tilling, K. (2019) Accounting for missing data in statistical analyses: multiple imputation is not always the answer. *International Journal of Epidemiology*, 48(4), 1294–1304.

Hui, S. L. and Walter, S. D. (1980) Estimating the error rates of diagnostic tests. *Biometrics*, 36(1), 167–171.

Huque, M. H., Moreno-Betancur, M., Quartagno, M., Simpson, J. A., Carlin, J. B. and Lee, K. J. (2020) Multiple imputation methods for handling incomplete longitudinal and clustered data where the target analysis is a linear mixed effects model. *Biometrical Journal*, 62(2), 444–466.

Hussain, J. A., White, I. R., Johnson, M. J., Byrne, A., Preston, N. J., Haines, A., Seddon, K. and Peters, T. J. (2022) Development of guidelines to reduce, handle and report missing data in palliative care trials: a multi-stakeholder modified nominal group technique. *Palliative Medicine*, 36(1), 59–70.

Husson, F., Josse, J., Narasimhan, B. and Robin, G. (2019) Imputation of mixed data with multilevel singular value decomposition. *Journal of Computational and Graphical Statistics*, 28(3), 552–566.

Ibrahim, J. G., Chen, M. and RLipsitz, S. (2002) Bayesian methods for generalized linear models with covariates missing at random. *Canadian Journal of Statistics*, 30(1), 55–78.

ICH (2019) Addendum on estimands and sensitivity analyses in clinical trials to the guideline on statistical principles for clinical trials, ICH E9(R1). https://database.ich.org/sites/default/files/E9-R1_Step4_Guideline_2019_1203.pdf.

Imbens, G. W. and Rubin, D. B. (1997) Estimating outcome distributions for compliers in instrumental variables models. *The Review of Economic Studies*, 64(4), 555–574.

Jack Jr., C. R., Wiste, H. J., Vemuri, P., Weigand, S. D., Senjem, M. L., Zeng, G., Bernstein, M. A., Gunter, J. L., Pankratz, V. S., Aisen, P. S. *et al.* (2010) Brain beta-amyloid measures and magnetic resonance imaging atrophy both predict time-to-progression from mild cognitive impairment to Alzheimer's disease. *Brain*, 133(11), 3336–3348.

Jackson, D., White, I. R., Seaman, S., Evans, H., Baisley, K. and Carpenter, J. (2014) Relaxing the independent censoring assumption in the cox proportional hazards model using multiple imputation. *Statistics in Medicine*, 33(27), 4681–4694.

Janssen, K. J., Vergouwe, Y., Donders, A. R. T., Harrell Jr., F. E., Chen, Q., Grobbee, D. E. and Moons, K. G. (2009) Dealing with missing predictor values when applying clinical prediction models. *Clinical Chemistry*, 55(5), 994–1001.

Jaro, M. (1995) Probabilistic linkage of large public health data files. *Statistics in Medicine*, 14, 491–498.

Jolani, S. (2018) Hierarchical imputation of systematically and sporadically missing data: an approximate Bayesian approach using chained equations. *Biometrical Journal*, 60(2), 333–351.

Jolani, S., Debray, T. P. A., Koffijberg, H., van Buuren, S. and Moons, K. G. M. (2015) Imputation of systematically missing predictors in an individual participant data meta-analysis: a generalized approach using mice. *Statistics in Medicine*, 34(11), 1841–1863.

Kalaycioglu, O., Copas, A., King, M. and Omar, R. Z. (2015) A comparison of multiple-imputation methods for handling missing data in repeated measurements observational studies. *Journal of the Royal Statistical Society, Series A (Statistics in Society)*, 179(3), 683–706.

Kang, J. D. Y. and Schafer, J. L. (2007) Demystifying double robustness: a comparison of alternative strategies for estimating a population mean from incomplete data (with discussion). *Statistical Science*, 22(4), 523–539. Argues double robustness was already known in the survey sampling world, and that MI is more reliable.

Keller, B. T. (2022) An introduction to factored regression models with Blimp. *Psych*, 4(1), 10–37.

Keller, B. T. and Enders, C. K. (2017) *Blimp User's Guide. Version 1.0.* Los Angeles, CA.

Kenward, M. G. (1998) Selection models for repeated measurements with non-random dropout: an illustration of sensitivity. *Statistics in Medicine*, 17, 2723–2732.

Kenward, M. G. and Carpenter, J. R. (2007) Multiple imputation: current perspectives. *Statistical Methods in Medical Research*, 16, 199–218.

Kenward, M. G. and Molenberghs, G. (1998) Likelihood based frequentist inference when data are missing at random. *Statistical Science*, 13(3), 236–247.

Kenward, M. G. and Rosenkranz, G. (2011) Joint modelling of outcome, observation time and missingness. *Journal of Biopharmaceutical Statistics*, 21, 252–262.

Kenward, M. G., Molenberghs, G. and Thijs, H. (2003) Pattern-mixture models with proper time dependence. *Biometrika*, 90, 53–71.

Keogh, R. H. and Bartlett, J. W. (2021) Measurement error as a missing data problem. In *Handbook of Measurement Error Models* (Eds P. Gustafson, A. Delaigle, G.Y. Yi), pp. 429–452. Chapman and Hall/CRC.

Keogh, R. H. and Morris, T. P. (2018) Multiple imputation in Cox regression when there are time-varying effects of covariates. *Statistics in Medicine*, 37(25), 3661–3678.

Keogh, R. H. and White, I. R. (2013) Using full-cohort data in nested case-control and case-cohort studies by multiple imputation. *Statistics in Medicine*, 32(23), 4021–4043.

Keogh, R. H., Strawbridge, A. D. and White, I. R. (2012) Effects of classical exposure measurement error on the shape of exposure-disease associations. *Epidemiologic Methods*, 1(1), 13–32.

Keogh, R. H., Seaman, S. R., Bartlett, J. W. and Wood, A. M. (2018) Multiple imputation of missing data in nested case–control and case–cohort studies. *Biometrics*, 74(4), 1438–1449.

Keogh, R. H., Shaw, P. A., Gustafson, P., Carroll, R. J., Deffner, V., Dodd, K. W., Küchenhoff, H., Tooze, J. A., Wallace, M. P., Kipnis, V. *et al.* (2020) Stratos guidance document on measurement error and misclassification of variables in observational epidemiology: Part 1–basic theory and simple methods of adjustment. *Statistics in Medicine*, 39(16), 2197–2231.

Kim, J. K. (2002) A note on approximate Bayesian boostrap imputation. *Biometrika*, 89, 470–477.

Kim, J. K., Brick, J. M., Fuller, W. A. and Kalton, G. (2006) On the bias of the multiple-imputation variance estimator in a survey setting. *Journal of the Royal Statistical Society, Series B (Methodological)*, 68, 509–522.

Klebanoff, M. A. and Cole, S. R. (2008) Use of multiple imputation in the epidemiologic literature. *American Journal of Epidemiology*, 168, 355–357.

Koehler, E., Brown, E. and Haneuse, S. J.-P. A. (2009) On the assessment of Monte Carlo error in simulation-based statistical analyses. *The American Statistician*, 63(2), 155–162.

Kott, P. S. (1995) A paradox of multiple imputation. *Proceedings of the Survey Research Methodology Section of the American Statistical Association*, pp. 380–383.

Lavori, P. W., Dawson, R. and Shera, D. (1995) A multiple imputation strategy for clinical trials with trunction of patient data. *Statistics in Medicine*, 14, 1913–1925.

Leacy, F. P., Floyd, S., Yates, T. A. and White, I. R. (2017) Analyses of sensitivity to the missing-at-random assumption using multiple imputation with delta adjustment: application to a tuberculosis/HIV prevalence survey with incomplete HIV-status data. *American Journal of Epidemiology*, 185(4), 304–315.

Lee, K. J. and Carlin, J. B. (2010) Multiple imputation for missing data: fully conditional specification versus multivariate normal imputation. *American Journal of Epidemiology*, 171, 624–632.

Lee, K. J. and Carlin, J. B. (2017) Multiple imputation in the presence of non-normal data. *Statistics in Medicine*, 36(4), 606–617.

Lee, K. J., Carlin, J. B., Simpson, J. A. and Moreno-Betancur, M. (2023) Assumptions and analysis planning in studies with missing data in multiple variables: moving beyond the MCAR/MAR/MNAR classification. *International Journal of Epidemiology*, https://doi.org/10.1093/ije/dyad008.

Lee, K. J., Tilling, K. M., Cornish, R. P., Little, R. J., Bell, M. L., Goetghebeur, E., Hogan, J. W. and Carpenter, J. R. (2021) Framework for the treatment and reporting of missing data in observational studies: the treatment and reporting of missing data in observational studies framework. *Journal of Clinical Epidemiology*, 134, 79–88.

Leurent, B. and Cro, S. (2022) CEMIMIX: Stata module to perform reference-based multiple imputation of cost-effectiveness data in clinical trials, *Statistical Software Components s459096*, Boston College Department of Economics. https://ideas.repec.org/c/boc/bocode/s459096.html.

Leurent, B., Gomes, M., Faria, R., Morris, S., Grieve, R. and Carpenter, J. R. (2018) Sensitivity analysis for not-at-random missing data in trial-based cost-effectiveness analysis: a tutorial. *Pharmacoeconomics*, 36(8), 889–901.

Leyrat, C., Seaman, S. R., White, I. R., Douglas, I., Smeeth, L., Kim, J., Resche-Rigon, M., Carpenter, J. R. and Williamson, E. J. (2019) Propensity score analysis with partially observed covariates: how should multiple imputation be used? *Statistical Methods in Medical Research*, 28(1), 3–19.

Li, K. H., Raghunathan, T. E. and Rubin, D. B. (1991) Large-sample significance levels from multiply-imputed data using moment-based statistics and an *F* references distribution. *Journal of the American Statistical Association*, 86, 1065–1073.

Li, X., Ge, P., Zhu, J., Li, H., Graham, J., Singer, A., Richman, P. S. and Duong, T. Q. (2020) Deep learning prediction of likelihood of ICU admission and mortality in COVID-19 patients using clinical variables. *PeerJ*, 8, e10337.

Lipkovich, I., Ratitch, B., Qu, Y., Zhang, X., Shan, M. and Mallinckrodt, C. (2022) Using principal stratification in analysis of clinical trials. *Statistics in Medicine*, 41(19), 3837–3877.

Little, R. J. and Yau, L. H. (1998) Statistical techniques for analyzing data from prevention trials: treatment of no-shows using Rubin's causal model. *Psychological Methods*, 3(2), 147.

Little, R. J. and Zhang, N. (2011) Subsample ignorable likelihood for regression analysis with missing data. *Journal of the Royal Statistical Society, Series C (Applied Statistics)*, 60, 591–605.

Little, R. J., Carpenter, J. R. and Lee, K. J. (2022) A comparison of three popular methods for handling missing data: complete-case analysis, inverse probability weighting, and multiple imputation. *Sociological Methods & Research*, https://doi.org/10.1177/00491241221113873.

Little, R. J. A. (1994) A class of pattern-mixture models for multivariate incomplete data. *Biometrika*, 81, 471–483.

Little, R. J. A. and Rubin, D. B. (1987) *Statistical Analysis with Missing Data*. Chichester: Wiley.

Little, R. J. A. and Rubin, D. B. (2019) *Statistical Analysis with Missing Data. Third Edition*. John Wiley & Sons.

Little, R. J. A. and Yau, L. (1996) Intent-to-treat analysis for longitudinal studies with drop-outs. *Biometrics*, 52, 471–483.

Liu, J., Gelman, A., Hill, J., Su, Y.-S. and Kropko, J. (2013) On the stationary distribution of iterative imputations. *Biometrika*, 101, 155–173.

Lo, A. Y. (1986) Bayesian statistical inference for sampling from a finite population. *Annals of Statistics*, 14, 1226–1233.

Louis, T. (1982) Finding the observed information matrix when using the EM algorithm. *Journal of the Royal Statistical Society, Series B (Methodological)*, 44, 226–233.

Lunceford, J. K. and Davidian, M. (2004) Stratification and weighting via the propensity score in estimation of causal treatment effects: a comparative study. *Statistics in Medicine*, 23(19), 2937–2960.

Magder, L. S. (2003) Simple approaches to assess the possible impact of missing outcome information on estimates of risk ratios, odds ratios, and risk differences. *Controlled Clinical Trials*, 24(4), 411–421.

Mallinckrodt, C., Molenberghs, G., Lipkovich, I. and Ratitch, B. (2019) *Estimands, Estimators and Sensitivity Analysis in Clinical Trials*. Chapman and Hall/CRC.

Mallinckrodt, C., Bell, J., Liu, G., Ratitch, B., O'Kelly, M., Lipkovich, I., Singh, P., Xu, L. and Molenberghs, G. (2020) Aligning estimators with estimands in clinical trials: putting the ICH E9 (R1) guidelines into practice. *Therapeutic Innovation & Regulatory Science*, 54(2), 353–364.

Mardia, K. V., Kent, J. T. and Bibby, J. M. (1979) *Multivariate Analysis*. Academic Press.

Marshall, G., Warner, B., MaWhinney, S. and Hammermeister, K. (2002) Prospective prediction in the presence of missing data. *Statistics in Medicine*, 21(4), 561–570.

Marshall, A., Altman, D. G., Holder, R. L. and Royston, P. (2009) Combining estimates of interest in prognostic modelling studies after multiple imputation: current practice and guidelines. *BMC Medical Research Methodology*, 9(1), 57.

Mason, A. J., Gomes, M., Grieve, R., Ulug, P., Powell, J. T. and Carpenter, J. R. (2017) Development of a practical approach to expert elicitation for randomised controlled trials with missing health outcomes: application to the improve trial. *Clinical Trials*, 14, 357–367.

McCullagh, P. (1980) Regression models for ordinal data (with discussion). *Journal of the Royal Statistical Society, Series B (Methodological)*, 42, 109–142.

Meng, X. L. (1994) Multiple-imputation inferences with uncongenial sources of input (with discussion). *Statistical Science*, 10, 538–573.

Meng, X.-L. and Romero, M. (2003) Discussion: efficiency and self-efficiency with multiple imputation inference. *International Statistical Review*, 71, 607–618.

Meng, X. and Rubin, D. (1992) Performing likelihood ratio tests with multiply-imputed data sets. *Biometrika*, 89, 267–278.

Mistler, S. A. and Enders, C. K. (2017) A comparison of joint model and fully conditional specification imputation for multilevel missing data. *Journal of Educational and Behavioral Statistics*, 42(4), 432–466.

Mitra, R. and Reiter, J. P. (2016) A comparison of two methods of estimating propensity scores after multiple imputation. *Statistical Methods in Medical Research*, 25(1), 188–204.

Mohan, K. and Pearl, J. (2020) Graphical models for processing missing data. *Journal of the American Statistical Association*, 116(534), 1023–1037.

Molenberghs, G. and Kenward, M. G. (2007) *Missing Data in Clinical Studies*. Chichester: Wiley.

Molenberghs, G., Michiels, B., Kenward, M. G. and Diggle, P. J. (1998) Missing data mechanisms and pattern-mixture models. *Statistica Neerlandica*, 52, 153–161.

Moreno-Betancur, M., Lee, K. J., Leacy, F. P., White, I. R., Simpson, J. A. and Carlin, J. B. (2018) Canonical causal diagrams to guide the treatment of missing data in epidemiologic studies. *American Journal of Epidemiology*, 187(12), 2705–2715.

Morris, T. P., White, I. R. and Royston, P. (2014a) Tuning multiple imputation by predictive mean matching and local residual draws. *BMC Medical Research Methodology*, 14(1), 75.

Morris, T. P., White, I. R., Royston, P., Seaman, S. R. and Wood, A. M. (2014b) Multiple imputation for an incomplete covariate that is a ratio. *Statistics in Medicine*, 33, 88–104.

Morris, T. P., White, I. R., Carpenter, J. R., Stanworth, S. J. and Royston, P. (2015) Combining fractional polynomial model building with multiple imputation. *Statistics in Medicine*, 34(25), 3298–3317.

Morris, T. P., White, I. R. and Crowther, M. J. (2019) Using simulation studies to evaluate statistical methods. *Statistics in Medicine*, 38(11), 2074–2102.

Morris, T. P., Walker, A. S., Williamson, E. J. and White, I. R. (2022) Planning a method for covariate adjustment in individually randomised trials: a practical guide. *Trials*, 23(1), 1–17.

Musoro, J. Z., Zwinderman, A. H., Puhan, M. A., ter Riet, G. and Geskus, R. B. (2014) Validation of prediction models based on lasso regression with multiply imputed data. *BMC Medical Research Methodology*, 14(1), 1–13.

Muthén, L. K. and Muthén, B. O. (2011) *Mplus User's Guide. Sixth Edition*. Los Angeles, CA.

Nevalainen, J., Kenward, M. G. and Virtanen, S. M. (2009) Missing values in longitudinal dietary data: a multiple imputation approach based on a fully conditional specification. *Statistics in Medicine*, 28, 3657–3669.

Nielsen, S. F. (2003) Proper and improper multiple imputation. *International Statistical Review*, 71, 593–627.

Nur, U., Shack, L. G., Rachet, B., Carpenter, J. R. and Coleman, M. P. (2010) Modelling relative survival in the presence of incomplete data: a tutorial. *International Journal of Epidemiology*, 39, 118–128.

Olarte Parra, C., Daniel, R. M. and Bartlett, J. W. (2022) Hypothetical estimands in clinical trials: a unification of causal inference and missing data methods. *Statistics in Biopharmaceutical Research*, (just-accepted), 1–26.

Olkin, I. and Tate, R. F. (1961) Multivariate correlation models with mixed discrete and continuous variables. *Annals of Mathematical Statistics*, 32, 448–465.

Orchard, T. and Woodbury, M. (1972) A missing information principle: theory and applications. In *Proceedings of the Sixth Berkely Symposium on Mathematics, Statistics and Probability*, Volume 1 (Eds L. M. L. Cam, J. Neyman and E. L. Scott), pp. 697–715. Berkeley: University of California Press.

Panel on Handling Missing Data in Clinical Trials. Committee on National Statistics, Division of Behavioral and Social Sciences and Education (2010) *The Prevention and Treatment of Missing Data in Clinical Trials*. Washington, DC: The National Academies Press, National Research Council.

Pencina, M. J., D'Agostino, Sr, R. B. and Demler, O. V. (2012) Novel metrics for evaluating improvement in discrimination: net reclassification and integrated discrimination improvement for normal variables and nested models. *Statistics in Medicine*, 31(2), 101–113.

Peto, R. (1973) Experimental survival curves for interval-censored data. *Journal of the Royal Statistical Society, Series C (Applied Statistics)*, 22, 86–91.

Pham, T. M., Carpenter, J. R., Morris, T. P., Wood, A. M. and Petersen, I. (2018) Population-calibrated multiple imputation for a binary/categorical covariate in categorical regression models. *Statistics in Medicine*, 38(5), 792–808.

Pham, T. M., White, I. R., Kahan, B. C., Morris, T. P., Stanworth, S. J. and Forbes, G. (2021) A comparison of methods for analyzing a binary composite endpoint with partially observed components in randomized controlled trials. *Statistics in Medicine*, 40(29), 6634–6650.

Plewis, I. (2007) Non-response in a birth cohort study: the case of the millennium cohort study. *International Journal of Social Research Methodology*, 10(5), 325–334.

Plumpton, C. O., Morris, T. P., Hughes, D. A. and White, I. R. (2016) Multiple imputation of multiple multi-item scales when a full imputation model is infeasible. *BMC Research Notes*, 9(1), 1–15.

Qu, Y. and Lipkovich, I. (2009) Propensity score estimation with missing values using a multiple imputation missingness pattern (MIMP) approach. *Statistics in Medicine*, 28(9), 1402–1414.

Quartagno, M. and Carpenter, J. R. (2016) Multiple imputation for IPD meta-analysis: allowing for heterogeneity and studies with missing covariates. *Statistics in Medicine*, 35(17), 2938–2954.

Quartagno, M. and Carpenter, J. (2023) *jomo: A package for Multilevel Joint Modelling Multiple Imputation*, https://CRAN.R-project.org/package=jomo.

Quartagno, M., Grund, S. and Carpenter, J. (2019) Jomo: a flexible package for two-level joint modelling multiple imputation. *The R Journal*, 11(2), 205–228.

Quartagno, M., Carpenter, J. R. and Goldstein, H. (2020) Multiple imputation with survey weights: a multilevel approach. *Journal of Survey Statistics and Methodology*, 8, 965–989.

Raghunathan, T. E., Lepkowski, J. M., Van Hoewyk, J. and Solenberger, P. (2001) A multivariate technique for multiply imputing missing values using a sequence of regression models. *Survey Methodology*, 27, 85–95.

Rao, J. N. K. and Wu, C. F. J. (1988) Resampling inference with complex survey data. *Journal of the American Statistical Association*, 83, 231–241.

Reiter, J. P. (2007) Small-sample degrees of freedom for multi-component significance tests with multiple imputation for missing data. *Biometrika*, 92, 502–508.

Reiter, J. P. (2008) Multiple imputation when records used for imputation are not used or disseminated for analysis. *Biometrika*, 95(4), 933–946.

Reiter, J. (2017) Discussion: dissecting multiple imputation from a multi-phase inference perspective: What happens when god's imputer's and analyst's models are uncongenial? *Statistica Sinica*, 27(4), 1578–1583.

Resche-Rigon, M. and White, I. R. (2018) Multiple imputation by chained equations for systematically and sporadically missing multilevel data. *Statistical Methods in Medical Research*, 27(6), 1634–1649.

Rizopoulos, D. (2012) *Joint Models for Longitudinal and Time-to-Event Data: With Applications in R*. CRC Press.

Robins, J. M. and Gill, R. (1997) Non-response models for the analysis of non-monotone ignorable missing data. *Statistics in Medicine*, 16, 39–56.

Robins, J. M. and Rotnitzky, A. (1995) Semiparametric efficiency in multivariate regression models with missing data. *Journal of the American Statistical Association*, 90, 122–129.

Robins, J. M. and Wang, N. (2000) Inference for imputation estimators. *Biometrika*, 85, 113–124.

Robins, J. M., Rotnitzky, A. and Zhao, L. P. (1994) Estimation of regression coefficients when some regressors are not always observed. *Journal of the American Statistical Association*, 89, 846–866.

Robitzsch, A. and Luedtke, O. (2020) *mdmb: Model Based Treatment of Missing Data*. R package version 1.4-12.

Rodwell, L., Lee, K. J., Romaniuk, H. and Carlin, J. B. (2014) Comparison of methods for imputing limited-range variables: a simulation study. *BMC Medical Research Methodology*, 14(1), 57.

Rosenbaum, P. R. and Rubin, D. B. (1983) The central role of the propensity score in observational studies for causal effects. *Biometrika*, 70, 41–55.

Royall, R. M. (1992) The model based (prediction) approach to finite population sampling theory. In *Current Isuues in Statistial Inference: Essays in Honor of D Basu* (Eds M. Ghosh and P. K. Patahak), pp. 225–240. Instituite of Mathematical Statistics.

Royston, P. and Sauerbrei, W. (2008) *Multivariable Model-Building*. Chichester: Wiley.

Rubin, D. B. (1976) Inference and missing data. *Biometrika*, 63, 581–592.

Rubin, D. B. (1981) The Bayesian bootstrap. *Annals of Statistics*, 9, 130–134.

Rubin, D. B. (1987) *Multiple Imputation for Nonresponse in Surveys*. New York: Wiley.

Rubin, D. (1996) Multiple imputation after 18+ years. *Journal of the American Statistical Association*, 91(434), 473–490.

Rubin, D. B. (1998) More powerful randomization-based p-values in double-blind trials with non-compliance. *Statistics in Medicine*, 17(3), 371–385.

Rubin, D. B. (2003) Discussion on multiple imputation. *International Statistical Review*, 71, 619–625.

Rubin, D. B. and Schenker, N. (1986) Multiple imputation for interval estimation from simple random samples with ignorable nonresponse. *Journal of the American Statistical Association*, 81, 366–374.

Ryan, L., Lam, C., Mataraso, S., Allen, A., Green-Saxena, A., Pellegrini, E., Hoffman, J., Barton, C., McCoy, A. and Das, R. (2020) Mortality prediction model for the triage of COVID-19, pneumonia, and mechanically ventilated ICU patients: a retrospective study. *Annals of Medicine and Surgery*, 59, 207–216.

Sanders, A. E., Divaris, K., Naorungroj, S., Heiss, G. and Risques, R. A. (2014) Telomere length attrition and chronic periodontitis: an ARIC study nested case-control study. *Journal of Clinical Periodontology*, 42(1), 12–20.

Särndal, C.-E., Swensson, B. and Wretman, J. (1992) *Model Assisted Survey Sampling*. Springer.

Särndal, C. E., Swensson, B. and Wretman, J. (2003) *Model Assisted Survey Sampling. Second edition*. New York: Springer.

Schafer, J. L. (1997) *Analysis of Incomplete Multivariate Data*. London: Chapman and Hall.

Schafer, J. (1999a) `MIX` software for multiple imputation of a mix of categorical and continuous data in s+.

Schafer, J. L. (1999b) Multiple imputation: a primer. *Statistical Methods in Medical Research*, 8, 3–15.

Scharfstein, D. O., Rotnitzky, A. and Robins, J. M. (1999) Adjusting for nonignorable drop-out using semi-parametric nonresponse models (with comments). *Journal of the American Statistical Association*, 94, 1096–1146.

Schomaker, M. and Heumann, C. (2018) Bootstrap inference when using multiple imputation. *Statistics in Medicine*, 37(14), 2252–2266.

Schroter, S., Black, N., Evans, S., Carpenter, J., Godlee, F. and Smith, R. (2004) Effects of training on quality of peer review: randomised controlled trial. *British Medical Journal*, 328, 673–675.

Seaman, S. and White, I. (2014) Inverse probability weighting with missing predictors of treatment assignment or missingness. *Communications in Statistics – Theory and Methods*, 43(16), 3499–3515.

Seaman, S., White, I. R., Copas, A. J. and Li, L. (2012a) Combining multiple imputation and inverse-probability weighting. *Biometrics*, 68, 129–137.

Seaman, S. R., Bartlett, J. W. and White, I. R. (2012b) Multiple imputation of missing covariates with non-linear effects and interactions: evaluation of statistical methods. *BMC Medical Research Methodology*, 12, 46.

Seaman, S. R., White, I. R. and Leacy, F. P. (2014) Comment on "analysis of longitudinal trials with protocol deviations: a framework for relevant, accessible assumptions, and inference via multiple imputation," by Carpenter, Roger, and Kenward. *Journal of Biopharmaceutical Statistics*, 24(6), 1358–1362.

Ségalas, C., Leyrat, C., Carpenter, J. and Williamson, E. (2023) Propensity score matching after multiple imputation when a confounder has missing data. *Statistics in Medicine, https://doi.org/10.1002/sim.9658.*

Shah, A. D., Bartlett, J. W., Carpenter, J. R., Nicholas, O. and Hemingway, H. (2014) Comparison of random forest and parametric imputation models for imputing missing data using MICE: a CALIBER study. *American Journal of Epidemiology*, 179, 764–774.

Sharp, S. J., Poulaliou, M., Thompson, S. G., White, I. R. and Wood, A. M. (2014) A review of published analyses of case-cohort studies and recommendations for future reporting. *PLoS ONE*, 9(6), e101176.

Shaw, P. A., Gustafson, P., Carroll, R. J., Deffner, V., Dodd, K. W., Keogh, R. H., Kipnis, V., Tooze, J. A., Wallace, M. P., Küchenhoff, H. *et al.* (2020) Stratos guidance document on measurement error and misclassification of variables in observational epidemiology: part 2–more complex methods of adjustment and advanced topics. *Statistics in Medicine*, 39(16), 2232–2263.

Siddique, J. and Belin, T. R. (2008) Multiple imputation using an iterative hot-deck with distance-based donor selection. *Statistics in Medicine*, 27(1), 83–102.

van Smeden, M., Groenwold, R. H. H. and Moons, K. G. M. (2020) A cautionary note on the use of the missing indicator method for handling missing data in prediction research. *Journal of Clinical Epidemiology*, 125, 188–190.

Smuk, M. J. (2015) *Missing data methodology: sensivitiy analysis after multiple imputation.* Ph.D. thesis, London School of Hygiene & Tropical Medicine, Keppel Street, London, WC1E7HT.

Sperrin, M., Martin, G. P., Sisk, R. and Peek, N. (2020) Missing data should be handled differently for prediction than for description or causal explanation. *Journal of Clinical Epidemiology*, 125, 183–187.

Spiegelhalter, D., Best, N., Carlin, B. P. and Van der Linde, A. (2002) Bayesian measures of model complexity and fit (with discussion). *Journal of the Royal Statistical Society, Series B*, 64, 583–640.

Spiegelman, D., Rosner, B. and Logan, R. (2000) Estimation and inference for logistic regression with covariate misclassification and measurement error, in main study/validation study designs. *Journal of the American Statistical Association*, 95, 51–61.

Spratt, M., Carpenter, J. R., Sterne, J. A. C., Carlin, B., Heron, J., Henderson, J. and Tilling, K. (2010) Strategies for multiple imputation in longitudinal studies. *American Journal of Epidemiology*, 172, 478–487.

StataCorp (2021a) (Fict. heart attack data; BMI, age, hightar, & smokes missing; arbitrary pattern). https://www.stata-press.com/data/r17/mheart10s0.dta. Online; accessed 2022-07-22.

StataCorp (2021b) *Stata 17 Multiple Imputation Reference Manual.* College Station, TW: Stata Press.

Steele, F., Goldstein, H. and Browne, W. (2004) A general multilevel multistate competing risks model for event history data, with an application to a study of contraceptive use dynamics. *Statistical Modelling*, 4, 145–159.

Sterne, J. A. C., White, I. R., Carlin, J. B., Spratt, M., Royston, P., Kenward, M. G., Wood, A. M. and Carpenter, J. R. (2009) Multiple imputation for missing data in epidemiological and clinical research: potential and pitfalls. *British Medical Journal*, 339, 157–160.

Steyerberg, E. W. (2019) *Clinical Prediction Models.* Second Edition. Statistics for Biology and Health. Cham, Switzerland: Springer Nature.

Sullivan, T. R., Salter, A. B., Ryan, P. and Lee, K. J. (2015) Bias and precision of the "multiple imputation, then deletion" method for dealing with missing outcome data. *American Journal of Epidemiology*, 182(6), 528–534.

Tanboğa, I. H., Canpolat, U., Özcan Çetin, E. H., Kundi, H., Çelik, O., Çağlayan, M., Ata, N., Özeke Ö., Çay, S., Kaymaz, C. and Topaloğlu, S. (2021) Development and validation of clinical prediction model to estimate the probability of death in hospitalized patients with COVID-19: insights from a nationwide database. *Journal of Medical Virology*, 93(5), 3015–3022.

Tanner, M. A. (1996) *Tools for Statistical Inference. Third Edition*. New York: Springer.

Tanner, M. and Wong, W. (1987) The calculation of posterior distributions by data augmentation (with discussion). *Journal of the American Statistical Association*, 82, 528–550.

Taylor, J. M. G., Murray, S. and Hsu, C. (2002) Survival estimation and testing via multiple imputation. *Statistics and Probability Letters*, 58, 221–232.

Thijs, H., Molenberghs, G., Michiels, B., Verbeke, G. and Curran, D. (2002) Strategies to fit pattern-mixture models. *Biostatistics*, 3, 245–265.

Thoemmes, F. and Rose, N. (2014) A cautious note on auxiliary variables that can increase bias in missing data problems. *Multivariate Behavioral Research*, 49(5), 443–459.

Tierney, N. J. and Cook, D. H. (2018) Expanding tidy data principles to facilitate missing data exploration, visualization and assessment of imputations.

Tierney, N., Cook, D., McBain, M., Fay, C., O'Hara-Wild, M., Hester, J., Smith, L. and Heiss, A. (2021) *naniar: Data Structures, Summaries, and Visualisations for Missing Data*. R package version 0.6.1.

Tilling, K., Williamson, E. J., Spratt, M., Sterne, J. A. and Carpenter, J. R. (2016) Appropriate inclusion of interactions was needed to avoid bias in multiple imputation. *Journal of Clinical Epidemiology*, 80, 107–115.

Tompsett, D. M., Leacy, F., Moreno-Betancur, M., Heron, J. and White, I. R. (2018) On the use of the not-at-random fully conditional specification (NARFCS) procedure in practice. *Statistics in Medicine*, 37(15), 2338–2353.

Tsiatis, A. A. (2006) *Semiparametric Theory and Missing Data*. New York: Springer.

Tsvetanova, A., Sperrin, M., Peek, N., Buchan, I., Hyland, S. and Martin, G. P. (2021) Missing data was handled inconsistently in UK prediction models: a review of method used. *Journal of Clinical Epidemiology*, 140, 149–158.

Tuti, T., Bitok, M., Malla, L., Paton, C., Muinga, N., Gathara, D., Gachau, S., Mbevi, G., Nyachiro, W., Ogero, M., Julius, T., Irimu, G. and English, M. (2016) Improving documentation of clinical care within a clinical information network: an essential initial step in efforts to understand and improve care in Kenyan hospitals. *BMJ Global Health*, 1, e000028. doi: 10.1136/bmjgh-2016-000028.

UK Data Archive (2007) Youth Cohort Time Series for England, Wales and Scotland, 1984–2002 [computer file]. First Edition, Colchester, Essex: UK Data Archive [distributor], November 2007. SN 5765.

Vansteelandt, S. and Daniel, R. M. (2014) On regression adjustment for the propensity score. *Statistics in Medicine*, 33(23), 4053–4072.

Vansteelandt, S., Carpenter, J. R. and Kenward, M. G. (2009) Analysis of incomplete data using inverse probability weighting and doubly robust estimators. *Methodology: European Journal of Research Methods for the Behavioral and Social Sciences*, 6(1), 37–48.

Verbyla, A. P., Cullis, B. R., Kenward, M. G. and Welham, S. J. (1999) The analysis of designed experiments and longitudinal data by using smoothing splines. *Journal of the Royal Statistical Society, Series C (Applied Statistics)*, 48, 269–311.

Vergouwe, Y., Royston, P., Moons, K. G. M. and Altman, D. G. (2010) Development and validation of a prediction model with missing predictor data: a practical approach. *Journal of Clinical Epidemiology*, 63(2), 205–214.

Verzilli, C. and Carpenter, J. R. (2002) A Monte Carlo EM algorithm for random-coefficient-based dropout models. *Journal of Applied Statistics*, 29, 1011–1021.

Vidotto, D., Vermunt, J. K. and van Deun, K. (2018) Bayesian multilevel latent class models for the multiple imputation of nested categorical data. *Journal of Educational and Behavioral Statistics*, 43(5), 511–539.

Wahl, S., Boulesteix, A.-L., Zierer, A., Thorand, B. and van de Wiel, M. A. (2016) Assessment of predictive performance in incomplete data by combining internal validation and multiple imputation. *BMC Medical Research Methodology*, 16(1).

Wang, N. and Robins, J. M. (1998) Large-sample theory for parametric multiple imputation procedures. *Biometrika*, 85, 935–948.

Wang, C., Zhang, Y., Mealli, F. and Bornkamp, B. (2022) Sensitivity analyses for the principal ignorability assumption using multiple imputation. *Pharmaceutical Statistics*.

Welch, C., Petersen, I., Bartlett, J. W., White, I. R., Marston, L., Morris, R. W., Nazareth, I., Walters, K. and Carpenter, J. R. (2014) Evaluation of two-fold fully conditional specification multiple imputation for longitudinal electronic health record data. *Statistics in Medicine*, 33, 3725–3737.

Welham, S. (2010) Smoothing spline models for lonigitudinal data. In *Longitudinal Data Analysis: A Handbook of Modern Statistical Methods* (Eds M. Davidian, G. Fitzmaurice, G. Molenberghs and G. Verbeke), pp. 253–290. Chichester: Wiley.

Westreich, D., Edwards, J. K., Cole, S. R., Platt, R. W., Mumford, S. L. and Schisterman, E. F. (2015) Imputation approaches for potential outcomes in causal inference. *International Journal of Epidemiology*, 44(5), 1731–1737.

White, I. R. (2006) Commentary: dealing with measurement error: multiple imputation or regression calibration. *International Journal of Edpidemiology*, 35, 1081–1082.

White, I. R. and Royston, P. (2009) Imputing missing covariate values for the cox model. *Statistics in Medicine*, 28, 1982–1998.

White, I., Carpenter, J., Evans, S. and Schroter, S. (2007) Eliciting and using expert opinions about non-response bias in randomised controlled trials. *Clinical Trials*, 4, 125–139.

White, I. R., Daniel, R. and Royston, P. (2010) Avoiding bias due to perfect prediction in multiple imputation of incompete categorical variables. *Computational Statistics and Data Analysis*, 54, 2267–2275.

White, I. R., Royston, P. and Wood, A. M. (2011) Multiple imputation using chained equations: issues and guidance for practice. *Statistics in Medicine*, 30(4), 377–399.

White, I. R., Carpenter, J. and Horton, N. J. (2012) Including all individuals is not enough: lessons for intention-to-treat analysis. *Clinical Trials*, 9(4), 396–407.

White, I., Joseph, R. and Best, N. (2019) A causal modelling framework for reference-based imputation and tipping point analysis in clinical trials with quantitative outcome. *Journal of Biopharmaceutical Statistics*, 30(2), 334–350.

Wood, A. M., White, I. R. and Royston, P. (2008) How should variable selection be performed with multiply imputed data? *Statistics in Medicine*, 27(17), 3227–3246.

Wood, A. M., Royston, P. and White, I. R. (2015) The estimation and use of predictions for the assessment of model performance using large samples with multiply imputed data. *Biometrical Journal*, 4, 614–632.

Wynants, L., Calster, B. V., Collins, G. S., Riley, R. D., Heinze, G., Schuit, E., Albu, E., Arshi, B., Bellou, V., Bonten, M. M. J., Dahly, D. L., Damen, J. A., Debray, T. P. A., de Jong, V. M. T., Vos, M. D., Dhiman, P., Ensor, J., Gao, S., Haller, M. C., Harhay, M. O., Henckaerts, L., Heus, P., Hoogland, J., Hudda, M., Jenniskens, K., Kammer, M., Kreuzberger, N., Lohmann, A., Levis, B., Luijken, K., Ma, J., Martin, G. P., McLernon, D. J., Navarro, C. L. A., Reitsma, J. B., Sergeant, J. C., Shi, C., Skoetz, N., Smits, L. J. M., Snell, K. I. E., Sperrin, M., Spijker, R., Steyerberg, E. W., Takada, T., Tzoulaki, I., van Kuijk, S. M. J., van Bussel, B. C. T., van der Horst, I. C. C., Reeve, K., van Royen, F. S., Verbakel, J. Y., Wallisch, C., Wilkinson, J., Wolff, R., Hooft, L., Moons, K. G. M. and van Smeden, M. (2020) Prediction models for diagnosis and prognosis of COVID-19: systematic review and critical appraisal. *BMJ*, 369, m1328.

Xie, X. and Meng, X.-L. (2017) Dissecting multiple imputation from a multi-phase inference perspective: what happens when God's, imputer's and analyst's models are uncongenial? *Statistica Sinica*, 27(4), 1485–1545.

Yu, L. M., Burton, A. and Revero-Arias, O. (2007) Evaluation of software for multiple imputation of semi-continuous data. *Statistical Methods in Medical Research*, 16, 243–258.

Yucel, R. M. (2011) Random covariances and mixed-effects models for imputing multivariate multilevel continuous data. *Statistical Modelling*, 11, 351–370.

Zaslavsky, A. (1994) Comment on Meng, X.L., 'Multiple-imputation inferences with uncongenial sources of input.'. *Statistical Science*, 9, 563–566.

Zhao, J. H. and Schafer, J. L. (2018) *pan: Multiple imputation for multivariate panel or clustered data*. R package version 1.6.

Zhao, Y. and Long, Q. (2016) Multiple imputation in the presence of high-dimensional data. *Statistical Methods in Medical Research*, 25(5), 2021–2035. PMID: 24275026.

Zimmerman, D. L. and Núnez-Antón, V. A. (2010) *Antedependence Models for Longitudinal Data*. Chapman & Hall/CRC.

Author Index

Multiple Imputation and its Application, Second Edition.
James R. Carpenter, Jonathan W. Bartlett, Tim P. Morris, Angela M. Wood, Matteo Quartagno and Michael G. Kenward.

Index of Examples

Multiple Imputation and its Application, Second Edition.
James R. Carpenter, Jonathan W. Bartlett, Tim P. Morris, Angela M. Wood, Matteo Quartagno and Michael G. Kenward.

Subject Index

Multiple Imputation and its Application, Second Edition.
James R. Carpenter, Jonathan W. Bartlett, Tim P. Morris, Angela M. Wood, Matteo Quartagno and Michael G. Kenward.